This much-needed new book provides a fresh and innovative approach to understanding medicine and the fundamental mechanisms of disease. Instead of bewildering the reader with a plethora of unnecessary detail, the text focuses on a carefully selected number of pathological processes and key diseases. These exemplars provide the student with a much deeper understanding of the molecular and cellular mechanisms and pathophysiology of the disease process; they also provide a scientific basis for understanding the medical management and treatment of broad groups of disorders. The text is supported throughout with explanatory illustrations, tables, key points and references for directed self-learning.

This novel book is designed to reflect the changing face of undergraduate medical education, with its increasing emphasis on directed self-learning and the integration of basic and clinical parts of the course. This approach, based on understanding principles rather than learning facts, will be an invaluable source of illumination and comprehension for all students of medicine.

Mechanisms of disease
An introduction to clinical science

Mechanisms of disease

An introduction to clinical science

EDITED BY

S. TOMLINSON
Professor of Medicine, University of Manchester

A. M. HEAGERTY
Professor of Medicine, University of Manchester

A. P. WEETMAN
Sir Arthur Hall Professor of Medicine, University of Sheffield

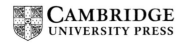
CAMBRIDGE
UNIVERSITY PRESS

PUBLISHED BY THE PRESS SYNDICATE OF THE UNIVERSITY OF CAMBRIDGE
The Pitt Building, Trumpington Street, Cambridge CB2 1RP, United Kingdom

CAMBRIDGE UNIVERSITY PRESS
The Edinburgh Building, Cambridge CB2 2RU, United Kingdom
40 West 20th Street, New York, NY 10011-4211, USA
10 Stamford Road, Oakleigh, Melbourne 3166, Australia

First published 1997

Printed in the United Kingdom at the University Press, Cambridge

Typeset in 10/13 Adobe Palatino

A catalogue record for this book is available from the British Library

Library of Congress Cataloguing in Publication data

Mechanisms of disease : an introduction to clinical science / edited
by S. Tomlinson, A. M. Heagerty, A. P. Weetman.
    p.   cm.
Includes index.
ISBN 0 521 46180 4 (hardback). – ISBN 0 521 46738 1 (paperback)
1. Physiology, Pathological.   2. Pathology, Molecular.
3. Pathology, Cellular.   I. Tomlinson, S. (Stephen), 1944–   .
II. Heagerty, A. M. (Anthony Michael)   III. Weetman, A. P. (Anthony P).
   [DNLM: 1. Disease.   2. Pathology – methods.   3. Clinical Medicine –
methods.   QZ 140 M486 1997]
RB113.M38   1997
616.07–dc21   96–39361 CIP
DNLM/DLC
for Library of Congress

ISBN 0 521 46180 4 hardback
ISBN 0 521 46738 1 paperback

CONTENTS

CONTRIBUTORS

G. Anderson *The Molecular Medicine Unit, University of Leeds, St James University Hospital, Leeds LS9 7TF, UK*

P. Bradding *University Medicine (Centre Block), Southampton General Hospital, Southampton SO9 4XY, UK*

A. M. Breckenridge *Clinical Pharmacology New Medical Building, Ashton Street, PO Box 147, Liverpool L69 3RX, UK*

D. J. Burn *Royal Victoria Infirmary, Newcastle upon Tyne, NE2 4HH, UK*

J. R. E. Davis *Department of Endocrinology, Manchester Royal Infirmary, Manchester M13 9WL, UK*

A. J. Frew *University Medicine (Centre Block), Southampton General Hospital, Southampton SO9 4XY, UK*

A. Gaw *Department of Pathological Biochemistry, Royal Infirmary, Glasgow G4 0SF, UK*

A. M. Heagerty *Department of Medicine, Manchester Royal Infirmary, Manchester M13 9WL, UK*

S. T. Holgate *University Medicine (Centre Block), Southampton General Hospital, Southampton SO9 4XY, UK*

P. G. Ince *MRC Neurochemical Pathology Unit, Newcastle General Hospital, Westgate Road, Newcastle upon Tyne NE4 6BE, UK*

D. G. Johnston *Unit of Metabolic Medicine, Imperial College School of Medicine at Norfolk Place, St Mary's Hospital, London W2 1PG, UK*

S. L. Johnston *University Medicine (Centre Block), Southampton General Hospital, Southampton SO9 4XY, UK*

P. Lackie *University Medicine (Centre Block), Southampton General Hospital, Southampton SO9 4XY, UK*

G. M. Lindsay *Department of Pathological Biochemistry, Royal Infirmary, Glasgow G4 0SF, UK*

R. A. Little *North Western Injury Research Centre, Stopford Building, Oxford Road, Manchester M13 9PT, UK*

D. R. London *Royal College of Physicians, 11 St Andrews Place, Regents Park, London NW1 4LE, UK*

A. F. Markham *The Molecular Medicine Unit, University of Leeds, St James' University Hospital, Leeds LS9 7TF, UK*

J. F. J. Morrison *The Molecular Medicine Unit, University of Leeds, St James' University Hospital, Leeds LS9 7TF, UK*

G. Neale *3 Worts Causeway, Cambridge CB1 4RJ, UK*

J. Neuberger *Liver and Hepatobiliary Unit, Queen Elizabeth Hospital, Edgbaston, Birmingham B15 2TH, UK*

H. S. Pandha *ICRF Oncology, Royal Postgraduate Medical School, Hammersmith Hospital, London W12 0NW, UK*

B. K. Park *Clinical Pharmacology, New Medical Building, Ashton Street, PO Box 147, Liverpool L69 3RX, UK*

M. Pirmohamed *Clinical Pharmacology, New Medical Building, Ashton Street, PO Box 147, Liverpool L69 3RX, UK*

S. Robinson *Unit of Metabolic Medicine, Imperial College School of Medicine at Norfolk Place, St Mary's Hospital, London W2 1PG, UK*

A. Semper *University Medicine (Centre Block), Southampton General Hospital, Southampton SO9 4XY, UK*

J. Shepherd *Department of Pathological Biochemistry, Royal Infirmary, Glasgow G4 0SF, UK*

J. Shute *University Medicine (Centre Block), Southampton General Hospital, Southampton SO9 4XY, UK*

K. Sikora *Department of Clinical Oncology, Royal Postgraduate Medical School, Hammersmith Hospital, London W12 0NW, UK*

J. G. P. Sissons *Department of Medicine, Addenbrookes Hospital, Cambridge CB2 2QQ, UK*

A. F. Walls *University Medicine (Centre Block), Southampton General Hospital, Southampton SO9 4XY, UK*

A. P. Weetman *Department of Medicine, North General Hospital, Sheffield S5 7AU, UK*

D. Wilks *Regional Infectious Disease Unit, City Hospital, Edinburgh EH10 5SB, UK*

PREFACE

This book reflects innovative approaches to the learning of core subjects and provides opportunities for in-depth study in undergraduate medicine, emphasising the understanding of principles rather than simply memorising facts. Our approach follows the direction of curricular development throughout the UK and is the expressed educational aim of the General Medical Council. In addition, higher medical training at postgraduate level will be increasingly based on the principles of clinical science; given the accelerating pace of advances in biomedical knowledge, requirements of continuing education are likely to have a strong scientific component.

The introductory section to the book sets out the essentials of molecular and cellular biology as they relate to mechanisms of disease. There is also a brief description of some established and more recently developed methodologies used in molecular and cell biology.

The book then outlines leading-edge scientific knowledge and demonstrates how this is fundamental to the practice of up-to-date clinical medicine. Each chapter focuses on one or more clinically important exemplar topics where science has helped to develop clinical practice or improved understanding of the basis of disease.

Each chapter falls broadly into two parts: the first is devoted to basic mechanisms and the second to the application of knowledge of these basic mechanisms to the understanding of pathogenesis and diagnosis of an exemplar condition. Although the emphasis is on mechanisms of disease, aspects of treatment are also included where they have explanatory value in understanding disease processes. Authors have focused usually on one specific exemplar condition, but where relevant there is comment on other diseases relevant to the section 'mechanism'.

The overriding aim of the book is to meet the need for new approaches to learning medicine; it also provides information for students undertaking special study modules, encouraging self-directed learning by study in depth of specific subjects chosen by the students themselves.

We are especially grateful to Professor David R. London, Registrar of the Royal College of Physicians of London, for the chapter on the historical development of concepts of disease, which we believe sets the scene for succeeding chapters.

S. TOMLINSON
A. M. HEAGERTY
A. P. WEETMAN

A growing mountain of factual information faces medical students and young gradu-ates, yet, much of what they are taught rapidly becomes outdated. The pace at which biomedical science advances is causing an exponential rise in new knowledge, making it increasingly difficult, if not impossible, for it all to be assimilated. The inevitable con-clusion is that there should be essential core knowledge which every student should gain, leaving them free to acquire new information as it becomes available during a full lifetime of continuing education. The recognition that doctors have to continue their education throughout their careers has made it easier to accept the idea that newly grad-uated medical students do not have to know everything there is to know about every aspect of medicine.

Defining the core principles for every student is not easy although many medical schools have attempted to do so. It is the stimulus to define a core of clinical science underlying some basic mechanisms of disease that lies behind the writing of this excel-lent book. It fills an important gap in a novel and particularly effective way. It should be seen as a supplement to, rather than as a replacement for, traditional textbooks of med-icine, which grow ever larger and encyclopaedic.

This book combines two interesting approaches. First, it outlines the scientific basis that is essential for an understanding of modern medical practice and then it uses the concept of 'exemplar diseases' to illustrate this theme in an imaginative way. The Editors are to be congratulated on achieving their highly desirable aims so successfully. They have gathered a group of excellent contributors, all recognised authorities in their fields, who have provided accessible and stimulating accounts of their areas of expertise. This book is ahead of the field and will undoubtedly appeal to medical students and junior trainees.

SIR LESLIE A. TURNBERG MD, PRCP

ABBREVIATIONS

AAV	adeno-associated virus
ABC resuscitation	airways, breathing, circulation resuscitation
ACE	angiotensin converting enzyme
ACTH	adrenocorticotrophic hormone
ADCC	antibody-dependent cell-mediated cytotoxicity
AGE	advanced glycosylation end-products
AP-1	activator protein 1
APC	antigen-presenting cell
ApoE	apolipoprotein E
APP	amyloid precursor protein
ARDS	adult respiratory distress syndrome
ARMs	amplification refractory mutation system
ATF	activating transcriptional factor
BAL	bronchoalveolar lavage
BMR	basal metabolic rate
BPI	bactericidal/permeability-increasing protein
CCK	cholecystokinin
CD4O-L	CD40 ligand
cDNA	complementary DNA
CDRs	complementarity determining regions
CEA	carcinoembryonic antigen
CF	cystic fibrosis
CFTR	cystic fibrosis transmembrane conductance regulator
CGRP	calcitonin gene-related peptide
CHD	coronary heart disease
CRC	colorectal cancer
CRE	cyclic AMP response element
CREB	cyclic AMP response element binding protein
CREM	cyclic AMP response element modulator
CRF	corticotrophin releasing factor
CSF	colony-stimulating factor
cyclicADPR	cyclic adenosine diphosphate-ribose
DAG	diacylglycerol
DMD	Duchenne muscular dystrophy

EAR	early asthmatic response
EAT	experimental autoimmune thyroiditis
ECP	eosinophil cationic protein
EDN	eosinophil-derived neurotoxin
EFA	essential fatty acid
EGF	epidermal growth factor
ELAM-1	endothelial leucocyte adhesion molecule 1
EPO	eosinophil peroxidase
ES cells	embryonic stem cells
EST	expressed sequence tag
FACS	fluorescent-activated cell sorting
FAP	familial adenomatous polyposis
FcεR	Fc ε-receptor
FISH	fluorescence *in situ* hybridisation
G-CSF	granulocyte colony stimulating factor
GABA	gamma-aminobutyric acid
GAD	glutamic acid decarboxylase
GDP	guanosine diphosphate
GM-CSF	granulocyte-macrophage colony stimulating factor
GTP	guanosine triphosphate
HA	haemagglutinin
HBV	hepatitis B virus
HDL	high density lipoprotein
HIV	human immunodeficiency virus
HLA	human leucocyte antigen
hnRNA	heterogeneous nuclear RNA
hsp	heat shock protein
ICAM	intercellular adhesion molecule
IDDM	insulin-dependent diabetes mellitus
IFN	interferon
Ig	immunoglobulin
IGF-I -II	insulin-like growth factor I and II
IL	interleukin
IL-1RA	IL-1 receptor antagonist
IP_3	inositol 1,4,5-triphosphate
KGF	keratinocyte growth factor
LAR	late-phase asthmatic response
LDL	low density lipoprotein
LFA	lymphocyte function associated antigen
LH	luteinising hormone
LOH	loss of heterozygosity
LPS	lipopolysaccharide
LTC_4	leukotriene C_4
mRNA	messenger RNA

MAP	microtubule-associated protein
MBP	major basic protein
MCP-1	monocyte chemoattractant protein-1
M-CSF	macrophage colony stimulating factor
MHC	major histocompatibility complex
MMP	metalloproteinase
MODY	maturity-onset diabetes of the young
NEFA	non-esterified fatty acids
NIDDM	non-insulin-dependent diabetes mellitus
NK	natural killer
NOD	non-obese diabetic (mice)
NPY	neuropeptide Y
NSAID	non-steroidal anti-inflammatory (drugs)
NSBR	non-specific bronchial responsiveness
NTS	nerve terminal spike
OMPs	outer membrane proteins
oxLDL	oxidised low density lipoprotein
PAF	platelet activating factor
PCR	polymerase chain reaction
PDGF	platelet-derived growth factor
PGD_2	prostaglandin D_2
PGF	peptide growth factor
PHF	paired helical filaments
PI	phosphatidylinositol
PIC	polymorphism information content
PIP2	phosphatidylinositol 4,5-bisphosphate
PUFA	polyunsaturated fatty acids
RFLPs	restriction fragment length polymorphisms
RNA	ribonucleic acid
ROC	receptor-operated calcium channels
rt-PCR	reverse transcription PCR
SFT	skin fold thickness
SIRS	systemic inflammatory response syndrome
SLE	systemic lupus erythematosus
SMOC	second messenger-operated calcium channels
SSCP	single-stranded conformational polymorphism
TCR	T cell receptor
TG	thyroglobulin
TGF	transforming growth factor
T_H cells	T helper cells
TIAs	transient ischaemic attacks
TIMP	tissue inhibitor of MMP
TNF	tumour necrosis factor
TNFR-1	TNF receptor 1

TPA	12-*O*-tetradecanoylphorbol 13-acetate (mimics DAG)
TRE	TPA response element
tRNA	transfer RNA
TSH	thyroid-stimulating hormone
TSH-R	TSH receptor
TSS	toxic shock syndrome
TSST-1	toxic shock syndrome toxin 1
VCAM-1	vascular cell adhesion molecule 1
VEGF	vascular endothelial growth factor
VIP	vasoactive intestinal peptide
VLDL	very low density lipoprotein
VNTRs	variable number of tandem repeats
VOC	voltage-operated calcium channels
VSG	variable surface glycoprotein
YAC	yeast artificial chromosome

1

Historical development

D. R. LONDON

- The development of concepts regarding disease is outlined in the context of the philosophy and observational technology of the time.

- At first the causes of disease were linked to punishment and retribution. Then the Rationalist movement and advances in scientific instrumentation stimulated a fresh approach.

- As instrumentation improved, allowing the application of empiricism, the new methodology was brought to bear on describing normal functions, then disease states. Infectious agents, their presence suspected since earliest times, were identified following advances in microscopy.

- The development of biochemistry and then immunology provided new insights into disease, with a coming together of an understanding of molecular processes and recognition of the importance of genetically determined susceptibilities.

- The recent explosion in knowledge about disease mechanisms stems from the invention of new scientific instruments and computer technology, which has made acquiring and communicating information much easier.

In medicine, as in other areas where hypotheses are constructed to explain natural phenomena, theories of causation are greatly influenced by the prevailing philosophies of the time and by the methodology available to test them. In this way, our current ideas on the causes of disease have evolved over the centuries. What we consider now to be the last word will, if history is to remain true to itself, be thought simple and naive by generations to come, even possibly by the current one given the rate at which technology and information science are progressing. Nevertheless, it is sobering to reflect that our current ideas have come from ideas that were first elaborated in the golden age of Greek learning nearly 25 centuries ago.

In this chapter, the development of these ideas in the West is traced as a background to the main substance of this book, setting the developments in the context of the contemporary intellectual currents and of the instrumentation available to produce observations on which they were based and that were used to test them. In a brief review of this sort, movements have been linked to names, and the names are few. This puts a simplistic gloss on events. There are indeed giants who 'bestride the narrow world like a Colossus' and with the power of their minds have alone translated the sum of knowledge to a new order of magnitude. Some of these are so great that they would find their way into any history however superficial. Others, important though they are, have not been mentioned, as arbitrary choices have had to be made for a chapter that is but an introduction to other topics. There are two further groups who would remain anonymous in any current account, one because their contributions, though adding bricks to the edifice of knowledge, are judged small and they are too numerous to quote, and the other because the chronicles of the time never recorded who they were nor indeed what they were thinking and doing.

Medicine has its roots in superstition and the occult: voodoo and the medicine man, magic and sorcery. Primitive societies still regard illness in this way. The body is possessed by some evil spirit either because one has sinned or broken a taboo or because one's enemies have willed it. Illness is seen as a punishment. Just as harm may come through the invasion of the body by a spear or an arrow, so something unseen can have an equal effect and result in disease and death. Stigma was attached to illness. To some extent it still is. The *hubris*, offending the gods, of the Greek philosophers meets its comeuppance in *nemesis*, the punishment. The suggestion that there may be hidden forces behind illness and disease is a strong one; as recently as the seventeenth century, a distinguished physician of the day, Thomas Browne (1605–82), was called upon to give his professional opinion in a witchcraft trial. And even now there are a few moralists who believe that AIDS is retribution for what they regard as abnormal practices or that smoking-related diseases are deserved by those suffering from them.

What has changed these ideas? There are three factors: the coming of rationalist thought, starting in the West with the Greeks; the development of scientific instrumentation; and, most recent of all, the new technology to facilitate the acquisition, storage, transfer and retrieval of information. The threads of the first two of these are woven into the account in the remainder of this chapter. The third is dealt with here.

In the beginning, information was passed by word of mouth. Then came writing and then printing. It was not until the printing press appeared that ideas and knowledge were available to more than the few, and with it began the decline of the influence of the Church; reason was given the wherewithal to challenge faith. Printing was initially for books. Scientific journals came later, first as records of transactions of learned societies, then as vehicles for the publication of experimental observations. Journals have their origin in the Age of Enlightenment in the seventeenth and eighteenth centuries and were partially responsible for it. They multiplied in the following century as scientific experimentation expanded, with a consequent requirement for the dissemination of its results. The twentieth century has seen scientific endeavour grow almost at a geometric rate. This can be attributed to a number of causes, many of which feed on each other. The apparatus of science has improved to the extent that experiments can be done faster and more easily, so there is more to publish. Fundamental to this is the use of electronics in equipment design, automation and the use of computers in instrument control and data processing. The computer has also made easier the preparation of material for publication, through the invention of the word processor and the introduction of electronic publishing. This in turn improves storage and speeds the availability of information. All this is of direct relevance to medical research, one of the highest of human activities; humans wish to know about themselves as a manifestation of the spirit of inquiry. And rather than accepting disease as something driven by unseen forces, they wish to understand how it has come about in order that it may be overcome. The remainder of this chapter outlines that history.

The earliest theories

Although the ancient civilisations of China, Egypt and India had well developed systems of medicine, the Western tradition owes its origins to Greece, in particular to Hippocrates (*c*. 460–377 BC) and his school. His contribution has laid the foundation for all that has followed. In addition to the setting out of a code of practice, followed to this day, he was the first to construct theories of the causes of disease based on what he had observed in his patients. Although his statements have been elaborated and modified over time, the fundamental truth that he enunciated has remained unchanged. It is that there are two factors acting alone or in combination which cause illness: the intrinsic or constitutional make-up of the person, and an extrinsic or environmental agent.

Hippocrates recognised four humours: blood, bile, black bile and phlegm. The role of blood was equivocal, but black bile was certainly bad. The balance of the humours was an important determinant of disease, although it is not absolutely clear whether these humours are intrinsic to the body or come from the outside. These ideas derived ultimately from the philosophies of the day. Among the most influential were those of Heraclitus (*c*. 500 BC), who proposed that matter was in a state of constant flux, with fire and water fighting it out like the lion and the unicorn, and Empedocles (*c*. 430 BC) who added a further two elements, earth and air, but who proposed, in contrast to Heraclitus, that a steady state could be achieved. The Hippocratic writings also introduced the important concept of external causes of disease with the use of the word 'miasma', meaning a polluting agent, usually bad air, and attributed many disorders to environmental factors and to way of life, remarkable in the way they anticipated modern thought.

As we shall see, these two themes have pervaded thinking about pathology to the present day.

The Hippocratic aftermath

The synthesis of these ideas is ascribed to Galen (129–200 AD), a Greek physician of the second century who moved to Rome where he held a fashionable position and was of great influence. He took up the humoral hypothesis and popularised it into a scheme whereby the constitution of the individual was determined by the proportion in which these elements were mixed, giving four temperaments: sanguine, choleric, melancholic and phlegmatic. Each temperament predisposed to a particular group of diseases. Besides his dissemination of the Hippocratic tradition, Galen was important for his role in developing anatomical considerations. Although his work was done on animals and many of his conclusions were wrong, his introduction of the structural dimension marked a significant step forward in leading to an understanding of the processes of disease.

The Renaissance

The flowering of the arts that took place in Europe after the Dark Ages had its parallel in science and medicine. As in other areas of intellectual endeavour, there was little progress after the crumbling of the Roman empire; the school of Galen held sway for many centuries.

Advances in thinking came in several ways. First there was introduced the dissection of the human body in Bologna and Padua, culminating in the work of Vesalius (1514–64) in the sixteenth century, defining an anatomical platform on which the great pathological tradition was founded. Then there were the ideas of Frascatorius (1478–1553), who raised the possibility of contagions with his 'seeds of disease' and of the French physician Jean Fernel (1497–1558) who compiled reports on autopsies carried out on some of the notables of the time – it was apparently considered rather smart to have one's body treated in this way. Not that one was in a position to know much about it! Fernel produced a classification of disease according to its location and localisation within the body. Fernel's other contribution is his conclusion about the nature of disease, a question that had teased physicians ever since they started recording their thoughts, namely 'whether in disease there is not something supernatural'. His conclusion, an important one because it confirmed rationalism as the basis of medical thought, was that disease existed as a material phenomenon. This may appear surprising, but even though the Greek philosophers many centuries previously had set out the rationalist's stall, superstition remained a powerful force in science and medicine, gaining strength particularly in the Middle Ages.

Contemporary with Fernel was the Swiss physician Paracelsus (1493–1541). Although he was equivocal about the origins of disease, stressing the spiritual and the occult, he was another key figure in the development of medical thought for a number of reasons. First, through his travels and teachings he was a powerful voice in reducing the influence of humoralistic theories as popularised by Galen. Second, he encouraged research and experiment; third, he contributed to the thinking on pathological mechanisms by postulating that factors which caused disease came from without and had local rather than systemic effects.

The scientific revolution

The quest for knowledge, reawakened in the Renaissance after the Dark Ages, grew ever stronger in the second half of the sixteenth and in the seventeenth centuries. The foundation of modern science had its roots in the latter part of the Renaissance with the growth of observational astronomy. Initially, Copernicus (1473–1543) reported what he saw and drew conclusions even though they conflicted with the established teachings of the all-powerful Church. Then Galileo (1564–1642) used the refracting telescope that he had perfected to confirm the Copernican theory of the heliocentricity of the universe – and incidentally getting himself into trouble with the Church for doing so. In the same period, Kepler (1571–1630) with his astronomical calculations laid the foundations of Newtonian physics. Finally, Newton (1642–1727) himself made his epoch-making advances in science and, simultaneously with Leibniz, in mathematics, with the invention of the differential and integral calculus.

This scientific ferment had its philosophical counterpart. Two schools of thought grew up, one in England the other in France. Both were to have a profound effect on science and medicine. The Englishman was Francis Bacon (1561–1626). He pioneered the modern scientific method, that is that knowledge comes from experimentation as well as observation, with the former distinguished from the latter by being a contrived event, not just one encountered by chance. This contrasts with the philosophy of the Frenchman Rene Decartes (1596–1650), who enunciated the tenet 'I think, therefore I am (*cogito ergo sum*)'. These two schools, the one empirical the other centred on the observer, have in their complementary ways formed the basis of the experimental approach to solving problems and providing answers in all branches of science, including medicine. In addition to his monumental contribution to philosophical thought, Decartes postulated that living organisms obeyed the laws of physics, although he did allow himself a let out in the case of 'Man', who had a mind separate from the body.

The greatest medical scientist of the time was William Harvey (1578–1657), who, working as a physician, applied the new philosophy using the experimental method to ascertain the 'action, function and purpose' of the parts, out of which he described the circulation of the blood. Although his starting point was anatomical, his work was the foundation of modern physiology. Others taking a lead from Harvey, in the spirit of the age and with the newly developed scientific instruments, carried out experiments that were to expand the new subject by experimental observation. Once normal function had been described, it was but a step to investigate states of disease, delineate abnormalities of function and relate them to the symptomatology of the patient and to the underlying disease process.

The other development that came form this period, but which had to wait for nearly 200 years before it was systematically applied to medicine, was the invention of the microscope.

By the end of the seventeenth century, all the basic disciplines, bar one, necessary for the study of the mechanisms of disease were in place. The only one lacking was biochemistry. Although one might consider that the concept of the humours represented a primitive approach to a chemical model for disease, the subject itself progressed slowly and became much bound up with alchemy. It was not until later that it became sufficiently advanced to be applicable to the study of disease.

There remained, however, a further matter without which disease mechanisms could not be assigned, namely the systematic description and classification of disease itself. The first proper attempt at a classification together with a recognition that, if the study of medicine was to progress, classification was necessary came from Thomas Sydenham (1624–89), who was known as the 'English Hippocrates'. Not only did he assert that diseases could be categorised despite their presentation varying from individual to individual, but he also indicated that each disease had its own specific cause with, incidentally, its own specific cure.

The synthesis of ideas

The thirst for knowledge, reborn in the Renaissance, resulted in an explosion in activities designed for its acquisition, the development of instrumentation to allow this to happen and of philosophies to explain what had been revealed. Laws, set out as general explanations of natural phenomena, were testable by further experimentation. But as the influence of the Church declined, with matters spiritual being replaced by the materialism of the modern age, so the philosophy-driven quest towards explaining disease was replaced by a methodology-led process.

The remainder of this chapter will trace the rise of the various disciplines that have contributed to this knowledge about the origins of disease.

The classification of disease

As has been stated above, in order to understand the mechanisms of disease there must be a satisfactory classification and description of the diseases themselves. This could be said to have begun with Sydenham and was brought on by Linnaeus (1707–78), better known for his taxonomy of the plant and animal kingdoms, and Francois Boissier de Sauvages (1706–67), both of whom employed symptom-based classifications. Their work was simplified by William Cullen (1710–90), who reduced their classifications to three classes of generalised illness – pyrexia, neuroses and cachexia – based on the physiological systems of the day: vital, animal and natural functions. A fourth class, which did not fit into this scheme, was local disease. This was a significant advance as it reconciled generalised and localised diseases into a single scheme. Thereafter, the elaboration and refining of the classification of disease has been based on a synergy between clinical and non-clinical studies, with the latter depending increasingly on advances in the basic sciences of biology, physics and chemistry, with general pathology emerging fully fledged halfway through the nineteenth century and molecular biology arriving 100 years later.

The morphological basis of disease

The seeds of general pathology were sown in the fifteenth century primarily for forensic reasons, although it was also considered fashionable and chic to be the subject of an autopsy. Serious morbid anatomy grew up in the eighteenth century in Italy and France, with the desire to correlate post-mortem appearances with the clinical diagnosis. The pioneers in this respect were Morgagni (1682–1771), who described a number of pathological conditions as well as linking case histories with autopsy findings, and Bichat (1771–1802), who with the help only of a hand lens conceived the idea that organs were made up of tissues, thereby introducing histology as a subject. The microscope at that time was thought too primitive to be a tool usable in pathology.

Although there was some work with the microscope in the early nineteenth century, on such topics as inflammation and healing, it was not until later that the studies of Virchow (1821–1902) laid the foundations of modern morbid anatomy with the concept that the pathological process was centred on the cell, with the pathological cell derived from the normal cell: 'Omnis cellula e cellula'. This line of thinking has formed the basis of the modern use of pathology for the diagnosis of disease in life, through the introduction first of biopsy using the whole tissue and latterly with less traumatic techniques such as aspiration for tissue cytology and the non-invasive examination of body fluids. The introduction of special stains, based first on the aniline dyes and later on more derivative techniques such as immunocytochemistry, the invention of new ways of using the light microscope, for example phase contrast, and the advent of electron microscopy have ensured that the Virchow approach continues to be of fundamental importance in diagnostic pathology. This approach has also led to an understanding of the causes of disease through studies of cellular mechanisms but, as we shall see, through its rejection of humoralism is restrictive in its view by failing to take into account the interaction of cells and tissues and the systemic effects of external agents.

Advances in imaging techniques, beginning with radiography and moving on to the use of radioisotopes and the introduction of computed tomography, magnetic resonance imaging and, most recently, positron emission imaging tomography (PET), have added not only to the diagnostic power of clinical morphology but also to furthering an understanding of the causes of disease, for example, the use of PET in the investigation of brain mechanisms in mental illness.

Infection

Cellular pathology as a subject worthy of study would not have progressed without the microscope. A similar statement can be made about microbiology. However, the concept of infection, from which microbiology grew, goes back to the very beginnings of thoughts on the origin of disease with the Hippocratic writings on 'Airs, Waters and Places' and the idea of miasmata, leading via Frascatorius to the concept of contagions, with the disease passing from person to person or being acquired from inanimate objects. But not only were diseases thought to be transmitted in this way; sin was too. While Frascatorius might be given a place as the founding father of the science of infection, and even of epidemiology, his credentials are compromised by his having postulated that certain caballistic manifestations could thereby be transmitted. Even though the ideas of the time still flirted with the supernatural in addition to the physical, they did give substance to the likelihood that something in the environment might be involved in the causation of disease to the point where there was speculation about the possible existence of live disease-causing agents.

It was recognised in the seventeenth and eighteenth centuries that fevers might be contagious, but these were deemed to be disease processes in themselves rather than manifestations of disease, associated by the thinkers of the time with the Hippocratic 'Air, Waters and [particularly] Places'. The twentieth century reader is amazed to learn that the introduction of vaccination at the end of the eighteenth century to immunise against smallpox and the nineteenth century removal of the Broad St pump to end a cholera epidemic in London were both carried out before it was known for sure that disease could be transmitted by live agents. The former owes its origin in the West to a traveller's tale and the latter was based on some clever detective work and the application of the Utilitarian principle of 'greatest happiness' with security having primacy over liberty.

As for cellular pathology, it took the microscope to transform speculation into observable reality. Clinical microbiology owes its origins to Jacob Henle (1809–85), the teacher of Robert Koch (1843–1910), who took the hypothesis of Agostino Bassi (1773–1856) concerning the possible role of a living agent of microscopic size in causing a disease of silkworms and translated it to disorders in the human. Henle without any experimental support enumerated what were later, on the basis of hard data, to become known as 'Koch's postulates'. Koch himself derived his ideas from the work of Louis Pasteur (1822–95) who showed that living organisms coming from the atmosphere were responsible for fermentation and putrefaction. Koch, on the basis of the Germ Theory proved by Pasteur, showed that organisms visible under the microscope were the cause of anthrax. Soon other conditions, such as tuberculosis and diphtheria, were also found to be caused by specific bacteria. As a further advance, an identical organism was identified in two dissimilar conditions: boils and acute osteomyelitis. The other significant contribution that Koch made to his subject was the introduction of methods of staining and culture, thereby enabling a vast increase in the number of identifiable features differentiating one organism from another; a further example of how expansion of knowledge may follow technical progress.

The same process occurred for viruses. Their initial recognition and the identification of their role as infective agents depended first on improvements in the optical microscope, which allowed the larger viruses to be visualised, and then on the development of the electron microscope for the detection of the smaller ones. Latterly, DNA and RNA analyses for the smallest particles demonstrated once again the part that improvements in technology and instrumentation have played in the advance of knowledge. As resolution improves still further, the prion has been found, an infective agent that, despite a capacity to reproduce, contains no nucleic acids.

Immune mechanisms

Immunology was born out of microbiology, with which it spent its early years. Only in its maturity has its full parenthood been revealed. The initial studies concentrated on the microbial agent as a stimulus for an immune response that could be harnessed for therapeutic purposes. The theory behind this approach, as reasoned by Pasteur and Koch from the writings of Sydenham, was that specific causes had specific cures; so once it had been shown that bacteria could produce toxins, efforts were made to generate antitoxins. This was accomplished through the work of Emile Roux (1853–1933) and Emile Behring (1854–1919). An alternative avenue was explored by Elie Metchnikoff (1845–1916), ultimately to lead to the epoch-making achievements in the second half of the twentieth century. Metchnikoff concentrated on the response of the infected individual, with the proposal that inflammation was protective and that immunity had survival value in the Darwinian sense. While he thought the cell all-important, experiments a few years later showing the synergistic effect of immune serum on the activity of the white cells linked his ideas with those of the 'humoralists' who favoured a primary role for the non-cellular constituents of the blood. This scheme has formed the basis of all that has subsequently been achieved in elucidating cellular and immune responses to noxious agents.

Following the early studies that concentrated on the relationships between immunity and infection, with immunity being considered to be beneficial, hypersensitivity and other adverse reactions involving the formation of antibodies, as they had come to be called, were observed as examples of immune mechanisms causing disease. The initial demonstrations resulted from provocation by external agents, but subsequently they were noted to occur without any apparent exogenous cause, giving rise to the concept of autoimmunity as an immunopathological mechanism, with the recent recognition of immunodeficiency as a further way in which abnormalities of the immune system can lead to disease.

The idea of autoimmunity implies that under normal circumstances the body is able to recognise its own components, which in turn carries the assumption that there is an individuality of the immune system just as there is for height, shape of the nose, voice and all other characteristics that confer uniqueness. That this is indeed so was first shown by Karl Landsteiner (1868–1943) through his demonstration of the main blood groups, with others later identifying minor blood groups and finally histocompatibility antigens on leucocytes. The linking of certain of these antigens to susceptibility to disease has been one of the major advances of recent years. In some instances, there is a direct immunological reason, but in other cases it is through studies of linkage with these antigens that light has been shed on mechanisms of disease.

The genetic connection

In the previous paragraph, reference was made to a genetic basis for disease. It has been long known that certain disorders run in families. It is, therefore, germane briefly to examine the recent history of this area, particularly as it is only comparatively recently that the definition by Gregor Mendel (1822–84) of the laws of genetics (based on his studies with peas) has made it possible accurately to relate heredity to disease. In medicine, two names stand out: William Bateson (1861–1926) and Archibald Garrod (1857–1935). Although others had observed that certain disorders were transmitted from generation to generation in families on a Mendelian basis, it was Bateson, a geneticist, advising Garrod, a physician, who brought the subject into prominence in medicine. Garrod made two major contributions. First through his documentation of families with metabolic disease he was able to establish a genetic basis for certain biochemical abnormalities; and, second, he was able to show that there were certain susceptibilities to non-metabolic disorders that were carried on the genes. The identification of chromosomes and the characterisation of the human karyotype led to a further understanding of the inherited transmissibility of disease. But the most significant development, possibly one of the most important advances in the history of humans, and most certainly the most important recent advance in the history of medicine, has been the localisation of genetic information to DNA and the breaking of the genetic code. This gigantic discovery, not yet 50 years old, has transformed medicine, allowing mechanisms of inherited disease to be defined at the molecular level. Through the application of immunogenetics and the identification through molecular biology (see below) of susceptibility genes, it has cast light on disorders that until now seemed to be without a genetic basis. Gene mapping has led to the definition of specific biochemical lesions through the identification of gene products.

Metabolic disorders and chemical pathology

What above all distinguishes the modern era from previous studies is the introduction of chemistry into medicine. It could be said that the naming of diabetes mellitus by Aretaeus (*c.* 100 AD) through his detection of sweetness in the urine of sufferers was the first recorded instance of diagnostic chemical pathology. But chemistry as a discipline did not emerge from alchemy until the early seventeenth century and the coming of the scientific revolution that introduced system into scientific observation. Paracelsus and his contemporaries attempted to put disease on a chemical basis but were unable to distinguish between the material and the occult. Thomas Willis (1621–75) is said to have been the first to identify sugar as such in the urine of diabetic subjects, but it was not until two centuries later that there was a sustained effort to demonstrate in disease abnormal chemical constituents or normal constituents in abnormal amounts and to explain how this had come about.

With the appearance of modern biochemistry, 100 years ago, followed by its flowering in the twentieth century, with studies in the whole organism and then in tissues, the concept of the 'biochemical lesion' at the cellular and then the subcellular level was developed. This culminated most recently in the arrival of molecular biology as a subject linking genetics and biochemistry to explain how some diseases come about. As the methodology has become refined, drawing on techniques borrowed from 'big science', such as the use of radioisotopes, X-ray diffraction crystallography, magnetic resonance imaging and computer modelling, it is proving possible not only to shed light on mechanisms of disease but also to describe new disorders. This again is an example of how knowledge of the natural world depends on the techniques available for its acquisition; for example, radioastronomy and the Hubble telescope are providing new information about our universe. In order to dispel the impression that this traffic is only one way, the reader will also know that methodologies can themselves only be developed on the basis of prior knowledge.

The physiological approach

It could reasonably be said that Harvey was the father of human physiology. The ancients speculated; Harvey observed and experimented and, on that basis, constructed hypotheses that could be tested by further experimentation. Indeed, shortly after Harvey had predicted their existence, Marcello Malpighi (1628–94), using the newly invented microscope, discovered the capillaries. There followed a steady accretion of knowledge about the function of the human body based on the inter-related intellectual processes of observation, experimentation and hypothesis.

The next leap in ideas came from Claud Bernard (1813–78), who coined the phrase *milieu interieur* to encapsulate two concepts, both of which have remained central to medical thinking. The first is that the body functions as an integrated whole and the second is that this integration works to maintain stability of the internal environment, a regression to a physiological mean. This idea spawned models of disease based on notions of over- or underactivity. His importance, however, is not limited to his overarching view of the integration of bodily function. He also extended the range of physiological experimentation by introducing a biochemical dimension and took explanations of disease from a static morbid anatomical base into the realms of dynamic disorders of physiology and biochemistry, concepts that have survived to underpin current investigative medicine and its search for causes.

Defining disease

The preceding sections of this chapter have traced the development of ideas concerning the causes of disease without attempting a definition of what is understood by the term itself. This omission requires redressing.

Disease produces morbidity or the potential for morbidity. 'Disease must be distinguished from 'illness'. Illness is the clear manifestation of disease, as judged either by the sufferer or by the clinical observer, both of whom have been conditioned by subjective values inculcated into them by society. 'Disease' and 'illness' can also be defined epidemiologically as having measurable characteristics that lie outside a normal range. Disease is dysfunction. Such a definition is of general service but it runs into trouble in regard to the comparator. The elderly have dysfunctions associated with age. Does this then make them diseased? Within a definition generalised to the whole population, it does, if disease carries with it a threat to survival, which the elderly have because of their age, or to reproduce, which the elderly also have, or an impaired capacity to carry out the normal functions of day-to-day living, which the elderly also have. The logical conclusion of this argument must be that old age is a disease. This clearly is an absurdity. One can, therefore, qualify the definition of disease as a dysfunction by requiring that the comparator is relevant to the individual or group being tested. Thus, the 'normal' elderly are no more abnormal among the elderly than pygmies are among pygmies, particularly if it is shown there is no special morbidity within the group.

Summary

Prior to a rational view of the universe developed by the Greek philosophers approximately five centuries BC, the Western tradition of medicine was founded on the idea that supernatural forces caused disease. It was Hippocrates and his disciples, followed by Galen, who led the way into a physical approach, with their description of illnesses and speculations as to cause. The Galenic system held sway until the Renaissance when a fresh spirit of enquiry, accompanying a resurgence of art and learning, stimulated a new interest in the human body, both healthy and diseased, and led to the birth of morphological pathology as a discipline. As science grew, with the introduction of the scientific method and the philosophy underpinning it and with advances in instrumentation, so an understanding of the mechanics of disease moved forward; first, pathology was put on an observational footing with the introduction of gross morbid anatomy and then microscopic histopathology developed. With advancing technology, with refinements in optics and then in electronic imaging, culminating in the introduction of computed tomography, magnetic resonance imaging and positron emission tomography (PET), the morphological approach to investigational pathology received new tools and hence the acquisition of new knowledge occurred. Imaging, initially through the optical microscope and latterly through the electron microscope, has also given material substance to theories of infection dating back to Hippocrates.

Most recently, biochemistry, which arose out of alchemy and chemistry, has contributed to a further understanding of infection as it has to mechanisms of disease more generally, including those with an immune and/or genetic basis.

The physiological approach is relatively recent, dating from the work of Harvey in the seventeenth century. This has now come together with biochemistry to enable disease processes to be studied ever more closely. And biochemical pathology in its turn, through PET, can now be viewed in the context of structure. The introduction and use of computing have not only made many of these developments possible but have also provided the wherewithal to facilitate the diffusion of the knowledge thereby acquired. Thus, progress in understanding disease mechanisms has come about through the application of new technology in an ever evolving cultural environment.

FURTHER READING

Bynum, W.F. & Porter, R. (eds.) (1993). *Companion Encyclopaedia of the History of Medicine*. London: Routledge.

Conrad, L.I., Neve, M., Nutton, V., Porter, R. & Wear, A. (1995) *The Western Medical Tradition*. Cambridge: Cambridge University Press.

Foucault, M. (1973). *The Birth of the Clinic*. London: Tavistock.

Medawar, P.B. (1967). *The Art of the Soluble*. London: Methuen.

Russell, B. (1984). *A History of Western Philosophy*. London: Unwin Paperbacks.

Singer C. & Underwood, E.A. (1962). *A Short History of Medicine*. Oxford: Oxford University Press.

2

Molecular and cell biology

J. R. E. DAVIS

- The human genome functions through transcription of coding regions (exons) of DNA to messenger RNA (mRNA) and translation of mRNA into protein.

- Normal cell function and growth are controlled by intracellular signalling systems that couple external stimuli to cellular responses.

- Gene expression can be studied *in vitro* by cloning of DNA, sequence analysis, analysis of DNA–protein interactions *in vivo* and by gene transfer, including the use of transgenic animals.

- Such studies have led to identification of genetic defects in diseases such as cystic fibrosis and the genetic events underlying cancer formation, and they have directed the first applications of gene therapy.

- Molecular and cell biology, as techniques used to understand normal cellular mechanisms, are themes that run through each chapter of this book in exploring mechanisms of disease.

Molecular biology

The human genome and gene structure

The genome comprises the total of the inherited material passed on from one generation to the next. In humans, it consists of the 23 pairs of chromosomes in the nucleus, together with a small amount of mitochondrial DNA. Chromosomal DNA is a tightly packaged array of genes (the units of inheritance) together with long tracts of intergenic DNA whose function is still largely unknown. The overall organisation and structure of the human genome is under intense study at present, and this chapter will focus only on small parts of this overall structure in order to describe some of the essential elements of molecular biology involved in mechanisms of disease. In Chapter 3, changes in chromosomes and genes relating to hereditary diseases will be described. Later sections of this chapter will outline intracellular signalling systems, especially as they relate to the control of gene expression and growth regulation. Finally, some of the methods of analysis currently used in molecular and cell biology will be reviewed.

The basic chemical composition of chromosomes – DNA and protein – was generally understood long before it was clear which functioned as genes. Work by Griffith and

Avery showed that DNA was the most likely candidate and experiments by Hershey and Chase in 1952 showed that only DNA from bacteriophages entered the host cell and initiated the production of viral particles. The double helix structure of DNA, defined by Watson and Crick, comprising two antiparallel strands with the sugar phosphate backbones on the outside and the purine–pyrimidine base pairs on the inside, forms the basis of our concepts of replication and utilisation of genes. A consequence of this hydrogen bonded pairing of the two DNA strands is that the strands can be separated by conditions that break hydrogen bonds (heat or extremes of pH) and then allowed to rejoin or anneal under less stringent conditions. Because of the obligatory complementary binding, strands that are complementary in sequence will bond to form a double helix. This is the basis of many of the experimental studies that allow related genes to be identified and probes of known sequence to be 'annealed' or bound to sections of DNA (see below).

The linear sequence of nucleotides forms a genetic code in which triplets of nucleotides code for each amino acid. The possible permutations of nucleotides allows some degeneracy (more than one code for an amino acid) and for start and stop codons.

Chromosomes are generally organised in pairs, one inherited from each parent, and in each pair genetic material undergoes rearrangement by crossing over of paired segments during meiosis in paternal or maternal gametes. Thus, each chromosome contains newly arranged genetic material, but with conserved overall structure in homologous pairs of chromosomes. Most genes will be represented by a maternal and a paternal 'allele', (alternative forms of the same gene), which in turn can undergo pairing in meiosis to form the next generation of gametes.

Genes contain structural information that ultimately dictates the sequence of a protein, for example a peptide hormone, an enzyme or a structural protein. The linear sequence of deoxynucleotides determines the properties of the gene and its protein product. However, this protein-coding information is not an unbroken stretch of DNA but instead consists (in most mammalian genes) of separate coding regions, exons, interspersed with non-coding introns. Each gene also contains characteristic flanking sequences, both upstream and downstream of the coding region (Fig 2.1).

The function of much of the intergenic DNA is unknown: it occupies a large percentage of the genome, proportionately more in humans than in simpler organisms. Some of this material has obvious structural functions, for example several megabases of DNA in the centromere of most chromosomes are involved in the formation of the mitotic spindle in cell division. Other parts of chromosomes contain long stretches of repetitive non-coding sequences, such as tandem repeats, whose function is still unknown.

Repetitive sequences have, in some cases, been found to have major significance, as illustrated by the discovery of genetic alterations in repetitive DNA in a number of disorders, exemplified by Huntington's disease. The Huntington's disease gene on chromosome 4 contains an expanded unstable region of DNA comprising a series of CAG repeats whose overall length changes during gamete formation: this repetitive DNA stretch is longer in patients with Huntington's disease than in non-affected people, and the more CAG repeats that occur the earlier the disease develops. Such alterations in the

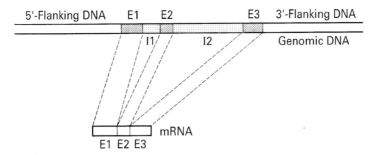

Fig. 2.1. Gene structure. Exons (E1, E2 and E3) contain the sequences that code for proteins. Exons are separated by regions of non-coding DNA, introns (I1 and I2).

length of this DNA region may favour the assembly of *nucleosomes*. These are complexes of chromosomal DNA with histone proteins that hinder the access of regulatory proteins to control elements of genes and hence they will mediate general repression of gene transcription.

The non-coding DNA that is closely associated with genes themselves, upstream and downstream flanking regions, are now known to be the major regulatory elements that modulate both gene transcription and the stability of mRNA; this will be considered in more detail in the following section.

Gene transcription

The upstream flanking DNA in most genes contains sequences involved in regulation of transcription. This stretch of DNA contains a number of specific sequences, known as *cis*-elements because they can only affect adjacent genes, that bind diffusible nuclear proteins (*trans*-elements) involved in transcription. The minimal upstream element necessary for transcription to occur is in many cases a clearly defined region of less than 30 base pairs of DNA and is termed the gene's 'promoter'. Additional upstream elements may stimulate or inhibit the process of transcription and are termed enhancers or repressors (Fig. 2.2). mRNA is transcribed from the genomic DNA by the enzyme RNA polymerase II, which starts the process at a point on the gene determined by specific sequences in the promoter region, such as a TATA motif (the TATA box). A complex of protein transcription factors (designated TFIIA, TFIIB, etc.) is established at this transcriptional start site, initiated by the binding of the factor TFIID, which binds to the TATA element itself. The cluster of TF proteins built up then allows RNA polymerase II to bind tightly as part of this transcriptional initiation complex (Fig. 2.3).

Upstream of the minimal promoter, enhancer elements may be extensive. These are often several thousand base pairs distant and contain a large number of characteristic sequences that serve as recognition motifs for other transcription factors. Enhancers have the ability to influence the rate of gene transcription at a variable distance and in either orientation relative to the promoter. Their transcription factors modulate the rate of transcription of the gene: some are specific to the cell type while others are ubiquitous but tightly regulated by intracellular signalling systems. The nature of their interaction

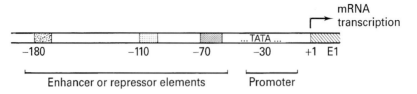

Fig. 2.2. Structure of the 5'-flanking DNA. Boxes represent DNA elements to which diffusible protein factors can bind. These occur at different points upstream of the transcriptional start site (right-angled arrow), which is known as nucleotide +1. Transcription of the exon occurs from +1. The non-coding region is numbered back from the start site with nucleotides numbered −1 upwards.

with the transcription initiation complex is not fully understood, but it probably involves looping of DNA in order to bring distant enhancer elements into proximity with the promoter to modulate the function of the transcriptional machinery (Fig. 2.3).

Transcription factors

A series of families of transcription factors have been described with distinct regions of the protein (domains) involved in DNA binding or in transcriptional activation. Several different classes of DNA-binding domains are now recognised, including 'zinc fingers', 'leucine zippers' and helix-turn-helix motifs; and more are being identified.

Zinc fingers.   These are found in many transcription factors, including steroid receptors, and consist of peptide loops in which an atom of zinc is tetrahedrally co-ordinated by cysteine and histidine residues at the base of the finger (Fig. 2.4*a*). Usually there are several zinc fingers in transcription factor proteins, and the tips of the fingers (containing basic amino acids) are thought to contact the acidic DNA by poking into the major groove of the double helix.

Leucine zippers.   These domains have been identified in several transcription factors, for example Jun, Fos and Myc, and are regions in which every seventh amino acid is leucine. In an α-helical structure, the leucines occur every second turn, and their long side chains can interdigitate with those of an analogous helix in a second protein like a zipper, allowing dimerisation of the two proteins (Fig. 2.4*b*). Leucine zippers are important not only for transcription factor dimerisation but also for DNA binding; they allow the formation of either homo-or heterodimers among related proteins, for example Jun–Jun, and Jun–Fos.

Helix-turn-helix motifs.   These comprise two α-helices separated by a β-turn. One of the helices, the 'recognition helix' lies in the major groove of the DNA and provides the DNA sequence specificity of binding, while the second lies across the major groove and probably stabilises the DNA contact (Fig. 2.4*c*). An example of this type of transcription factor is the pituitary-specific factor Pit-1/GHF-1.

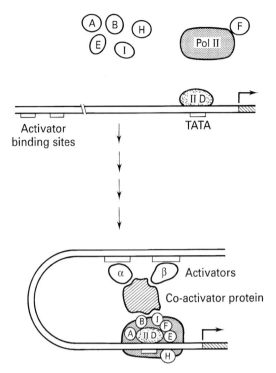

Fig. 2.3. Simplified model of the transcriptional initiation complex. Transcription factors TFIID, TFIIA, TFIIB, etc. sequentially bind at the TATA box and stabilize RNA polymerase II (Pol II) attachment. Upstream DNA -bound transcription factors (α, β) may interact directly or indirectly (via a co-activator) with the transcriptional complex. This probably involves some form of DNA looping.

Activation domains. These are less clearly defined in transcription factors than the DNA-binding structures but may contain characteristic acidic domains, or proline- or glutamine-rich domains. Their function has been confirmed by 'domain-swap' experiments in which chimaeric factors are constructed with the DNA-binding region of one factor linked to the activation domain of another. The mechanism of transcriptional action is still not well understood but may involve direct contact between the activation domains and the components of the transcription initiation complex (e.g. TFIID, TFIIB, or RNA polymerase II itself), or in some cases indirect contact via intermediate adaptor proteins.

Repression. Although most transcription factors seem to be activators, in some cases they can *repress* gene transcription, and several mechanisms are possible. For example, a negatively acting factor can simply interfere with the effect of an activator by occupying the activator protein's binding site (or a closely adjacent site) on the target DNA. In other cases, two factors may interact such that a positively acting factor is sequestered by dimerisation. For example, the glucocorticoid receptor can be prevented from trans-activating target genes by becoming complexed with the factor AP-1.

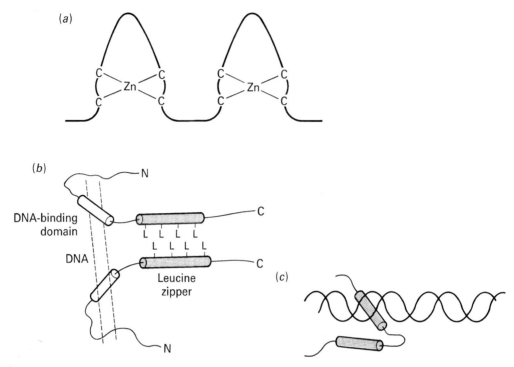

Fig. 2.4. Transcription factor structures.(*a*) Zinc fingers. (*b*) Leucine zipper, allowing dimerisation of two factors. (*c*) Helix-turn-helix motif orientated against a DNA helix.

Regulation of gene transcription by intracellular signalling systems is an important aspect of transcriptional control and this is one of the best characterised systems. Most of the steps between an external stimulus and a cellular response have been defined. This will be discussed in more detail later in this chapter.

Control of transcription: tissue specificity

Differentiation of tissues with a variety of distinct phenotypes requires the expression of particular genes in a cell type-specific manner, and recently a number of tissue-specific transcription factors have been identified in addition to those that are ubiquitous. For example, the factor MyoD is a transcription factor expressed only in differentiating myoblast cells, and artificial expression of MyoD alone in undifferentiated fibroblast cell lines can induce this differentiation process. MyoD can either form transcriptionally active homodimers or it can heterodimerise by helix-loop-helix interaction with other proteins with varying effects. One such protein, Id, is a negative regulator that lacks a DNA-binding domain and so prevents MyoD from binding to DNA. Levels of Id decline during differentiation; therefore, the overall effect of the tissue-specific factor MyoD will depend on its interaction with changing levels of other factors, such as Id, that determine its transcriptional activity.

Another tissue-specific transcription factor is Pit-1/GHF-1, which is expressed in the

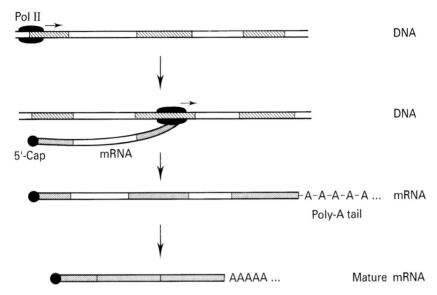

Fig. 2.5. Formation of mature mRNA. Double-stranded DNA is transcribed by RNA polymerase II (Pol II) and the mRNA is modified at its 5'-end by the addition of a G residue with a triphosphate bond (Gppp) that is methylated (5'-cap). Splicing removes intronic sequences and a poly-A 'tail' is added.

differentiating fetal pituitary gland. This factor is necessary not only for pituitary-specific expression of the peptide hormones prolactin and growth hormone but also for the development of the respective lactotroph and somatotroph cell types. Recently, a number of cases have been described of loss-of-function mutations of Pit-1/GHF-1 in which patients are hypopituitary, with pituitary hypoplasia as well as prolactin and growth hormone deficiency.

mRNA and protein synthesis

The process of gene transcription occurs by complementary base pairing from the genomic DNA template from to a primary transcript of heterogeneous nuclear RNA (hnRNA), which contains both exonic and intronic sequences. This RNA forms the pre-cursor to mRNA, whose message is carried in the genetic code of nucleotide triplets (codons), each specifying one of the usual 20 amino acids. The hnRNA is then processed to form mature messenger RNA (mRNA) by a series of steps (Fig. 2.5).

(1) A methylated guanosine residue (m^{7}Gppp) is added at the 5'-end (the 5'-cap) at the start of the first exon's untranslated leader sequence; the end of this untranslated region is marked by an AUG initiation codon encoding the first methionine residue of the protein.

(2) Intronic regions are removed and the exons spliced together by a 'spliceosome' complex of small ribonucleoproteins, the splice sites being marked by characteristic GU and AG splice donor and acceptor sites at the beginning and end of intron transcripts.

(3) A long tract of 100 or more A residues (the 'poly-A tail') is added at the 3'-end, signalled by characteristic polyadenylation sequences (such as AAUAAA) downstream of the stop codon (UGA, UAA or UAG) that terminates protein translation.

These features of mature mRNA are important for stability and translocation. In particular the structure of the 5' and 3' untranslated regions appears to be significant, with secondary structures such as hairpin and cruciate loops affecting the rate of peptide translation in the ribosome. The process of splicing also appears to have a significant function, allowing the cell to select which exons will be represented. Therefore, alternative splicing of the primary transcript can generate alternative gene products, as in the case of calcitonin and the calcitonin gene-related peptide (CGRP), which are encoded by one gene. The gene encoding the transcriptional repressor CREM (cyclic AMP-response element modulator, see p. 31) similarly can be alternatively spliced to produce two forms of the factor with different DNA-binding domains.

Protein synthesis: mRNA translation

mRNA is translated into protein in the cytoplasm by a complex process of matching nucleotide sequences to amino acids. These are polymerised to form the polypeptide chain at the ribosomes.

Ribosomes.   These are large multimolecular complexes of many different proteins associated with several structural RNA (ribosomal RNA, rRNA) molecules. These complexes act to position transfer RNA (tRNA) molecules sequentially to match the triplet code of mRNA. Each ribosome comprises two subunits, one large and one small. The small 40S subunit contains a single (18S) rRNA molecule with over 30 proteins, and the large 60S subunit contains three different rRNAs and over 40 proteins. The overall assembly has a molecular weight of 4.5 million and forms a particle that is visible by electron microscopy. The three-dimensional structure allows this molecular machine to engage both a strand of mRNA and a growing peptide chain (Fig. 2.6).

tRNA.   Molecules of tRNA are essentially adaptors that recognise both a mRNA nucleotide sequence *and* an amino acid sequence. They are single polynucleotide chains, 70–90 bases in length, that undergo internal base pairing to form a complex with exposed nucleotide loops. One such loop contains the 'anticodon' that can base pair with the corresponding codon in mRNA, while the exposed 3'-end of the tRNA molecule is attached covalently to a specific amino acid (Fig. 2.6).

Translation.   The process of translation is rapid, a single ribosome taking only 1 minute to polymerise over 1000 amino acids. The ribosome binds to a specific site on the mRNA, allowing the first 'initiator tRNA' to bind to the AUG initiation codon and start the peptide chain with the initial methionine residue. Subsequently, the ribosome moves along the mRNA translating codon by codon with a series of tRNAs adding amino acids

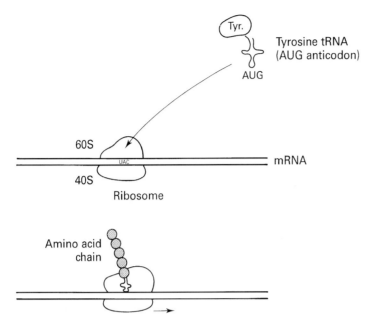

Fig. 2.6. Translation of mRNA. tRNAs enter the ribosome and bind to the mRNA by matching of their anticodons. Peptide bonds are formed between the amino acids to give a growing amino acid chain with its sequence defined by the nucleotide sequence of the mRNA.

to the growing peptide chain. When the end of the message is reached at the stop codon, the ribosome subunits are released along with the newly made peptide.

Protein secretion

The fate of the protein product of mRNA translation depends upon the nature of the protein and the cell type. For proteins such as peptide hormones that are exported by the cell into the extracellular fluid, specialised secretory processes are involved. Cells can secrete hormones 'constitutively', in a continuous manner unaffected by external stimuli and dependent only on the rate of transcription and translation, or via a 'regulated' pathway using secretory granules to package and store hormone until an external or internal stimulus causes exocytosis.

Secreted proteins are synthesised on ribosomes attached to rough endoplasmic reticulum. They then enter the lumen of the endoplasmic reticulum by the binding of a hydrophobic leader sequence of the peptide with a 'signal recognition particle' to a docking protein on the endoplasmic reticulum surface. The proteins are then transported to the Golgi complex where they undergo post-translational modification, such as glycosylation, before being concentrated into granules which are pinched off from the Golgi membrane (Fig. 2.7). Finally, under the influence of secretory stimuli, the granules 'marginate' and fuse with the cell membrane, allowing their contents to be released into the extracellular fluid, the process known as exocytosis.

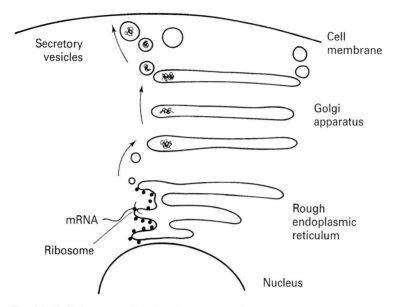

Fig. 2.7. Cellular organelles involved in protein synthesis. Ribosomes attached to rough endoplasmic reticulum synthesise peptide chains that contain signals allowing entry to the endoplasmic reticulum. These leader sequences are later cleaved off and the protein is routed through the Golgi apparatus to secretory vesicles or other cellular destinations.

Post-translational processing

Post-translational processing of proteins is an important regulating process that modifies the biological activity of many proteins. It occurs largely in the endoplasmic reticulum, the Golgi apparatus and the cytoplasm, but it can also occur within the secretory granule.

An important initial modification is the *three-dimensional folding* of the new polypeptide chain, which is largely determined by the array of hydrophobic or hydrophilic amino acid side chains. Particular patterns of protein folding have been confirmed by X-ray crystallography to occur in many different proteins, namely the *α-helix*, a rigid cylinder formed by a spiral of amino acid residues, and the *β-sheet*, formed by alignment of antiparallel or parallel straight chains of amino acids.

The folded protein conformation may be stabilised by the formation of covalent bonds between or within chains by *disulphide bridges* between nearby cysteine-SH groups.

Further covalent post-translational modifications include *phosphorylation*, catalysed by protein kinases that transfer a high-energy phosphate group from ATP to specific amino acid sequences in proteins, and *glycosylation*, the addition of complex carbohydrates to particular residues, often asparagine (N-linked oligosaccharides) or the hydroxy groups of serine or threonine (O-linked oligosaccharides). Other modifications include the aggregration of protein subunits to form multimers, the attachment of co-enzymes such as biotin to some enzymes, and acetylation and hydroxylation of certain amino acids.

Cellular signalling and growth regulation

Cells respond to a series of extracellular stimuli such as hormones, growth factors and neurotransmitters. Some agents, such as steroid and thyroid hormones, are able to enter the cell and bind to intracellular receptors that in turn bind to DNA as transcription factors, directly altering the transcription of target genes. However, many other factors (such as peptide hormones) are unable to enter the cell and instead must stimulate a receptor on the cell membrane to trigger an intracellular 'second messenger'. This then generates a cellular response. This process is termed signal transduction, and a variety of intracellular signalling processes have been discovered.

The systems are complex and can be viewed as molecular cascades comprising receptors, transducing proteins (G-proteins), effector proteins, second messenger molecules, protein kinases and kinase substrates. The complexity of these systems allows for great amplification within the cell of an initial extracellular signal, and also for interaction and co-regulation of parallel signalling pathways. The corollary is that the genes for some of the many proteins involved are subject to mutations that result in human disease, including tumour formation. Indeed these genes are in many cases known as 'proto-oncogenes', the normal cellular homologues of viral 'oncogenes' that cause cancers (see pp. 31–33 and Chapter 12).

Membrane receptors

Peptide hormones, catecholamines, growth factors and neurotransmitters bind to specific cell surface receptors, which are coupled to intracellular signalling pathways in a variety of ways.

G-protein-linked receptors

A very large number of membrane receptors are coupled to second messenger-generating systems via intermediate *transducers*, 'G-proteins' (see below), which in turn are linked to *effector* molecules that generate the intracellular second messenger. Molecular cloning has shown that these G-protein-linked receptors belong to a super family of proteins that have similar structures. They are characterised by seven hydrophobic α-helices traversing the membrane, with an extracellular amino-terminal and an intracellular carboxy-terminal, three intracellular loops that are thought to couple to the G-proteins and three extracellular loops that are involved in ligand binding (Fig. 2.8). The G-protein-linked receptors in general operate to initiate the generation of diffusible small molecules such as cyclic AMP, which in turn activate protein kinases.

G-protein-independent receptors

Not all receptors are linked to G-proteins, and a number of transmembrane receptors possess intrinsic intracellular effector domains without intermediate transducing proteins. Some such receptors, such as the epidermal growth factor (EGF) receptor, have a

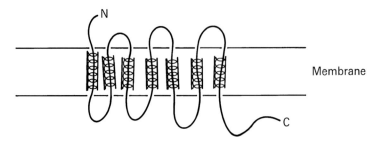

Fig. 2.8. A membrane receptor with seven α-helical transmembrane domains.

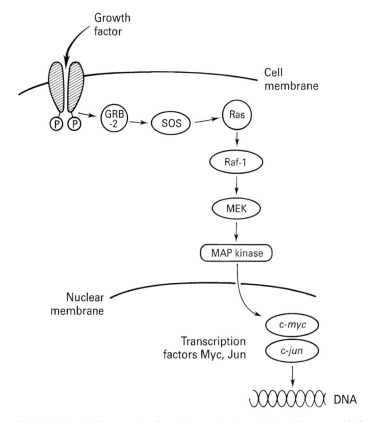

Fig. 2.9. A typical cascade of protein activation induced by growth factor binding to a transmembrane receptor.

single polypeptide chain, while others such as the insulin receptor have linked α- and β-subunits. Some of these receptors possess intrinsic tyrosine kinase activity, allowing them to phosphorylate (and hence activate) target intracellular proteins, while others are closely associated with separate tyrosine kinase proteins, for example the 'Janus kinases' such as Jak-2 linked to the erythropoietin and growth hormone receptors. Thus, these receptors are able directly or indirectly to initiate a cascade of protein phosphorylation as their mechanism of action, without necessarily generating intermediate second messengers. A typical phosphorylation cascade of this sort is illustrated in Fig. 2.9.

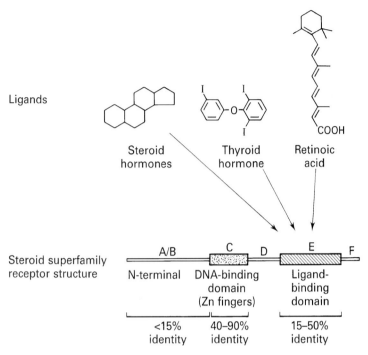

Fig. 2.10. Nuclear receptors. Widely differing hormonal ligands bind to conserved members of the steroid receptor superfamily; the conservation of structure resides in the DNA-binding domain.

Nuclear receptors

Steroid and thyroid hormones, vitamin D and retinoic acid are small lipophilic molecules that are membrane soluble and interact directly with intracellular receptor proteins. These receptors exist in the cytoplasm complexed with 'chaperone' molecules (for example heat shock protein 90, hsp-90), from which they dissociate on activation by the hormonal ligand. After dissociation they change conformation and translocate to the nucleus.

Again, molecular cloning has shown that there is a large superfamily of nuclear receptors that function as ligand-activated transcription factors. Some of these receptors have no identifiable ligand and have been termed 'orphan receptors'. Nonetheless, despite having widely differing ligands, the nuclear receptors have remarkable structural similarity, with six identifiable domains (A–F), including conserved DNA-binding domains with two zinc finger motifs (see above), and a hormone-binding domain (Fig. 2.10).

The receptors for oestrogen and glucocorticoid activate gene transcription as homodimers bound to short, palindromic DNA response elements (for example a typical oestrogen response element would be 5'-GGTCAnnnTGACC-3', the palindrome being apparent on the complementary strand in the reverse direction). The other members of the family form heterodimers with a different protein, the retinoid X receptor (RXR),

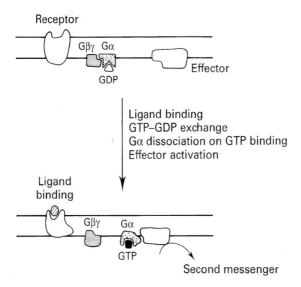

Fig. 2.11. Model for activation of an effector molecule by an activated receptor via a G-protein. The heterotrimer (Gα/Gβ/Gγ) dissociates such that Gα, binding GTP, will activate (or inhibit) the production of an intracellular signal by the effector protein (for example, the production of cyclic AMP by adenylate cyclase.

whose ligand is 9-*cis*-retinoic acid, and the nature of the complexes that form on DNA is determined by the arrangement of the response elements in the enhancer regions of gene promoters, usually as short direct-repeat or inverted-repeat sequences with variable spacing of one to five nucleotides.

G-proteins

G-proteins are a large family of membrane-associated transducing proteins that are linked to transmembrane receptors, as described above. G-proteins are so named because they bind guanosine triphosphate (GTP) and are themselves members of a larger superfamily of GTP-binding proteins (that includes the *ras* proto-oncogene product p 21) whose general function in cells is proposed to be one of molecular switching. The receptor-associated G-proteins fulfil exactly this role, conveying an 'on-signal' from a newly occupied receptor to switch an intracellular effector protein into its activated state.

G-proteins are heterotrimers, consisting of α-, β- and γ-subunits. The β- and γ-subunits are tightly associated and function as a single βγ complex; the α-subunit binds GTP and possesses intrinsic GTPase activity (Fig. 2.11). Hormone activation of a G-protein-linked receptor allows the α-subunit to exchange a GDP molecule for GTP; this results in its dissociation from the βγ-complex and enables the α-subunit to change to its active configuration to switch on or off the effector protein to which it is coupled. In some cases the βγ-complex appears to have a signalling function in its own right.

Different types of G-protein are coupled to different intracellular signalling systems:

for example G_s is the stimulatory G-protein that activates adenylate cyclase to form cyclic AMP (3′, 5′-cyclic adenosine monophosphate); G_i inhibits adenylate cyclase; G_q stimulates phospholipase C to hydrolyse phosphatidylinositol bisphosphate; while other proteins are linked to ion channels. In some cases, a particular type of receptor can be linked to different intracellular effectors via different G-proteins; for example, the dopamine D_2 receptor can be linked either to adenylate cyclase via G_i or to phospholipase C via G_q.

Second messengers: the cyclic AMP/protein kinase A system

Cyclic AMP

Cyclic AMP is one of several small diffusible molecules that are produced as a result of receptor–G–protein activation of effector proteins. The production of these small molecules allows for amplification and diffusion of the initial signal.

The formation of cyclic AMP from ATP (adenosine triphosphate) is catalysed by the enzyme adenylate cyclase, whose activity is modulated by extracellular signals via receptor-associated G-proteins. Levels of cyclic AMP are tightly controlled, rising within seconds of activation of the cyclase enzyme, and the cyclic AMP signal is also rapidly terminated by cellular phosphodiesterases, which hydrolyse cyclic AMP to inactive 5′-adenosine monophosphate (5′-AMP).

Protein kinase A

A number of protein kinases are activated by cyclic AMP, but the best understood is protein kinase A. This is an inactive holoenzyme complex comprising two regulatory (R) subunits and two catalytic (C) subunits: the C subunit is highly conserved, but the R subunit varies among different cell types. Binding of cyclic AMP to the R subunit allows dissociation and activation of free C subunits, which rapidly translocate to the cell nucleus where they phosphorylate substrate proteins such as the CREB (cyclic AMP response element-binding protein) transcription factor (see below) (Fig. 2.12).

Second messengers: the phospholipid/calcium signalling system

Phosphatidylinositol 4,5-bisphosphate (PIP_2) is a minor component of membrane phospholipids which nonetheless has a crucial role in intracellular signalling. It is formed by the phosphorylation of phosphatidylinositol (PI) and is rapidly turned over in the membrane after stimulation by certain hormones and growth factors. A large number of membrane receptors are coupled via the G-protein G_q to *phospholipase C*, which hydrolyses PIP_2 to form two important second messengers: namely the membrane lipid *diacylglycerol* (DAG) and a hydrophilic sugar phosphate molecule *inositol 1,4,5-triphosphate (IP₃)*. DAG remains in the membrane and activates protein kinase C, while IP_3 is released into the cytoplasm and mobilises calcium from intracellular stores (see Fig. 2.13).

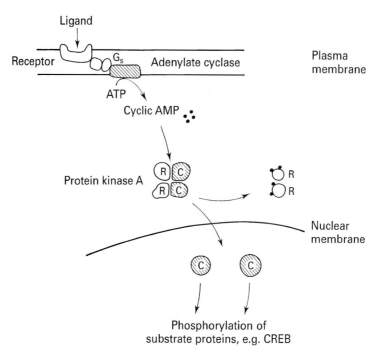

Fig. 2.12 Activation of protein kinase A by cyclic AMP. The kinase holoenzyme complex dissociates so that free catalytic subunits can diffuse into the nucleus to phosphorylate proteins such as the CREB transcription factor.

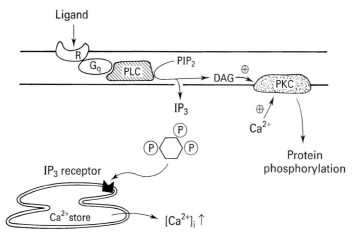

Fig. 2.13. The phosphatidylinositol signalling system. Activation of phospholipase C (PLC) results in the hydrolysis of the membrane lipid PIP_2 to form DAG and IP_3. DAG is a lipid and remains in the membrane to activate protein kinase C (PKC); IP_3 is water soluble and diffuses into the cytoplasm to mobilise calcium from intracellular stores.

Protein kinase C and DAG

DAG formed in the cell membrane directly activates the phospholipid-dependent calcium-activated kinase protein kinase C. There is, in fact, a family of protein kinase C molecules, derived from alternative splicing of several different genes. DAG increases the affinity of protein kinase C for calcium, rendering the kinase highly active. The effect of DAG may be mimicked pharmacologically by tumour-promoting phorbol esters such as 12-O-tetradecanoylphorbol-13-acetate (TPA); this allows detailed studies of the role of protein kinase C. It has a wide range of effects in different cell types, including regulation of hormone secretion, modulation of ion channels and gene transcription; though only in the last have the mechanisms been dissected in detail, as described below.

DAG may be metabolised to generate further second messenger lipid molecules including arachidonic acid, which in turn may be metabolised to yield active substances such as prostaglandins, leukotrienes and thromboxanes.

IP_3, intracellular calcium and calmodulin

IP_3 binds to a specific tetrameric protein receptor located on the endoplasmic reticulum, which is the major store of intracellular calcium. The IP_3 receptor is homologous to the ryanodine receptor found in muscle cells, and both are calcium sensitive, so that an initial release of calcium induced by IP_3 may promote further calcium release, thus amplifying the initial signal. Ryanodine receptors are thought to be activated by cyclic adenosine diphosphate-ribose (cyclic ADPR), which may prove to be an important second messenger parallel to cyclic AMP in certain cell types.

Measurements of single cell intracellular calcium concentrations using fluorescent dyes and high-resolution microscopy have shown that calcium levels fluctuate rapidly in response to stimulation by extracellular signals. Calcium concentrations rise rapidly in one part of the cell and this calcium 'spike' propagates across the cell as a wave. The frequency of the calcium spikes is proportional in many cases to the concentration of the agonist, suggesting that the calcium signal is frequency modulated not amplitude modulated (Fig. 2.14).

The initiation of a full calcium spike depends on *calcium entry* as well as mobilisation from intracellular stores, and calcium entry occurs through a series of membrane calcium channels, which may be voltage-operated (VOCs, opened by cell depolarisation) receptor-operated (ROCs, opened by agonist binding to membrane receptors) or second messenger-operated (SMOCs, affected by other intracellular signals such as cyclic AMP).

Calcium within the endoplasmic reticulum is released from calcium-sequestering proteins such as calreticulin and calsequestrin in a quantal manner, which can be visualised using fluorescent dyes in muscle cells as localised 'calcium sparks'. The frequency of this localised sparking is increased by entry of extracellular calcium until a critical point is reached, and a full calcium wave is irreversibly triggered.

Calcium exerts its intracellular effects through binding to one or more calcium-binding proteins, the best known of which is calmodulin. Calmodulin is a highly con-

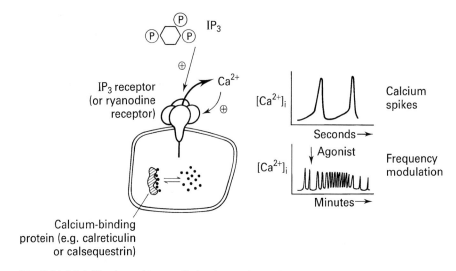

Fig. 2.14. Mobilisation of intracellular free calcium by IP_3. Activation of the tetrameric IP_3 receptor allows efflux of free calcium from intracellular organelles, where it exists in equilibrium with protein-bound calcium.

served protein found in all mammalian cells: it is a single chain peptide with four calcium-binding sites and activates a number of calcium/calmodulin-dependent protein kinases such as CaMK-II (calmodulin dependent kinase-II), myosin light chain kinase and adenylate cyclase itself.

IP_3 is removed from the cytoplasm by progressive dephosphorylation to form free inositol, which is recycled to form phosphatidylinositol. In some cases, IP_3 is further phosphorylated to form inositol 1, 3, 4, 5-tetrakisphosphate, which has been implicated in calcium influx into the cell and the replenishment of calcium stores.

Effects of signalling pathways on gene transcription

The end-points of the signalling cascades described above have been defined most completely in terms of the regulation of gene expression. The techniques of molecular biology have been used first to locate signal-responsive elements within regulatory regions of DNA that control gene transcription and then to use these DNA sequences to isolate and characterise the protein transcription factors that are activated by signalling pathways. Two of the signal transduction pathways described above, namely the cyclic AMP–protein kinase A pathway and the DAG–protein kinase C pathway, have been analysed in such a way, leading to the identification of the CREB and AP-1 transcriptional regulators.

Cyclic AMP and CREB

Analysis of the promoters of cyclic AMP-regulated genes has revealed that their cyclic AMP responsiveness could be attributed to short DNA sequences, termed 'cyclic

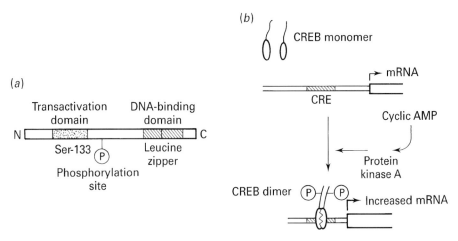

Fig. 2.15. CREB: the binding protein that modulates genes responsive to cyclic AMP levels by binding to cyclic AMP response elements (CREs). (*a*) structure of CREB showing the phosphorylation site at Ser-133. (*b*) Activation of transcription by CREB phosphorylation and dimerisation at the CRE.

AMP response elements' (CREs). The classical CRE contains a conserved 8 bp palindromic sequence (5'-TGACGTCA-3'), and its identification led to the discovery of a 43 kDa CRE-binding protein termed CREB. CREB is a transcription factor and contains a typical leucine zipper allowing it to form homo- and heterodimers. It is phosphorylated by protein kinase A, which promotes its dimerisation and increases its transcriptional activity (Fig. 2.15). In fact, CREB has proved to be one member of a large family of related factors, including a series of activating transcription factors (ATFs 1–8), and CRE-modulator proteins (CREMs) that repress transcription.

In summary, the complete cyclic AMP signalling pathway can now be described in which an external hormonal stimulus can trigger a molecular cascade (receptor–G_s-protein–adenylate cyclase–protein kinase–CREB), with the final end-point of post translational modification of a transcription factor altering the transcriptional rate of a target gene.

Protein kinase C and activator protein-1

Activation of protein kinase C increases the transcription of a number of genes; the mechanism of this activation has been analysed using phorbol esters such as TPA as specific pharmacological activators of protein kinase C. Promoter analysis revealed that the TPA responsiveness of these genes could be attributed to a specific 7 bp 'TPA-response element' (TRE) very similar to the CRE (5'-TGAGTCA-3'). This TRE binds a transcription factor complex of 44–47 kDa termed activator protein-1, or AP-1, which contains the protein *jun*.

Jun is the protein product of the cellular *proto-oncogene* c-*jun*, which is the normal cellular homologue of the *oncogene* v-*jun* found in avian sarcoma virus (ASV-17). Like CREB, Jun is a 'bZip' transcription factor, containing both a conserved basic domain and

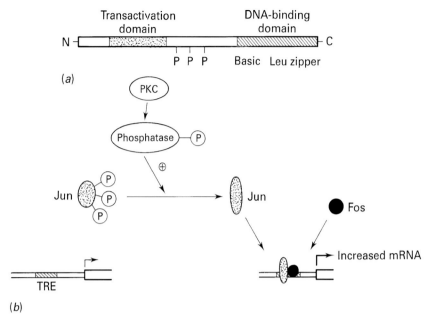

(a)

(b)

Fig. 2.16. Activator protein 1 and c-*jun*. (a) The structure of Jun. (b) Jun is activated by dephosphorylation. This is catalysed by a phosphatase which is itself activated by protein kinase C (PKC). The activated Jun can form a heterodimer with FOS at a phorbol ester response element (TRE) which activates gene transcription.

a leucine zipper that allows dimerisation. Therefore, Jun can heterdimerise with Fos, the product of the c-*fos* proto-oncogene (again a normal cellular homologue of an oncogene, v-*fos*, found in the FBJ murine sarcoma virus). Jun–Fos heterodimers bind to TREs with high affinity, but their activity depends on intracellular signalling pathways (Fig. 2.16).

Jun is activated both by amino-terminal phosphorylation (induced via other proto-oncogenes such as *ras*) and by carboxy-terminal dephosphorylation, probably by phosphatases activated by protein kinase C. c-*jun* mRNA levels are normally low in unstimulated cells but rise rapidly after exposure to growth factors and in response to several 'transforming' proto-oncogenes such as *src*, *ras* and *mos*.

In summary, it is now clear that signalling pathways can interact at the level of transcription factors themselves. A variety of signals converge on Jun transcription factor in addition to its activation by the classical protein kinase C pathway. Furthermore, the composition and activity of heterodimers is variable, Jun interacts not only with Fos (which is cyclic AMP regulated) but also with CREB.

Alterations of signalling pathways in human disease

The complex cascades of signalling molecules are susceptible to alteration, and many components have been identified as responsible for a series of human diseases. A whole cascade may be activated or blocked by abnormal stimulation of a receptor (for example by immunoglobulins that bind to a hormone receptor), or any one of the proteins involved in the cascade may be mutated with damaging consequences. Indeed, many of the proteins have been identified as 'proto-oncogenes', which may be susceptible to oncogenic mutation that can either impair or enhance their function and lead to tumour formation. Examples are shown in the box.

Cancer development linked to changes in the DNA of proto-oncogenes

Proto-oncogene	Role in signalling system	Human neoplasm
myc	DNA-binding protein	Burkitt's lymphoma
ras (K and N)	G-protein	Melanoma
abl	Protein kinases	Chronic granulocytic leukaemia
erbB	EGF receptor	Squamous cell carcinoma
sis	Growth factor (β-chain of PDGF)	Astrocytoma

Membrane receptors

G-protein-coupled membrane receptors are the largest family of membrane receptors, and some examples illustrate the potential for activating of these proteins by mutations. The receptor for thyroid-stimulating hormone (TSH) controls thyroid cell function and growth, and activating mutations affecting the structure of its third intracellular loop produce functioning *thyroid neoplasms* and hyperthyroidism. Activating mutations in the gene for the receptor for the pituitary gonadotrophin luteinising hormone (LH) are responsible for abnormal sensitivity of the testis to LH, resulting in *precocious puberty*. In the hereditary disease *retinitis pigmentosa*, which leads to blindness, germ cell mutations have been found that constitutively activate rhodopsin, a light-responsive retinol-binding receptor in the human retina.

G-protein-independent receptors such as growth factor receptors may also be constitutively activated by mutation, and several viral oncogenes represent tumour-inducing counterparts of normal cellular proteins; for example the c-*erbB* product is the EGF receptor, while v-*erbB* is responsible for avian erythroleukaemia.

Loss-of-function mutations may affect the insulin receptor, giving severe *insulin resistance*, and the growth hormone receptor is disrupted in *Laron-type dwarfism*, which explains the failure of these patients to respond to therapy with growth hormone.

G-proteins

The G_s α-subunit of the heterotrimeric G_s-protein complex coupled to the cyclic AMP system has been found to be mutated in several human tumours, notably endocrine tumours. These '*gsp*' oncogenic mutations occur in somatic cells after embryogenesis and result in constitutive activation of adenylate cyclase. The high levels of intracellular cyclic AMP stimulate not only differentiated cell function but also cell proliferation: for example in some cases of *acromegaly* growth hormone hypersecretion occurs from a pituitary tumour.

A major example of a related GTP-binding protein involved in human disease is that produced by the *ras* proto-oncogene. This protein is part of the signal transduction pathway linked to several growth factor receptors such as the EGF receptor. Oncogenic mutations result in permanent activation of Ras and are commonly found in human cancers.

Kinases

The role of spontaneous kinase mutations in human disease is less clear, though mutations of protein kinase C have been detected in certain endocrine tumours. However the c-*src* proto-oncogene is the cellular homologue of the v-*src* oncogene, found in the Rous sarcoma virus and responsible for sarcoma formation in chickens.

The c-*abl* proto-oncogene produces a cytosolic tyrosine kinase (see below for its involvement in apoptosis) and this has been found to be involved in a chromosomal translocation that results in *chronic myeloid leukaemia*. The translocation on the 'Philadelphia chromosome' results in part of the coding region of c-*abl* (chromosome 9) being spliced onto part of the *bcr* gene on chromosome 22. The Bcr–Abl fusion protein is oncogenic, possibly because Bcr is able to autophosphorylate and activate the Abl portion of the hybrid oncogene.

Nuclear receptors and transcription factors

Mutations in genes for intracellular receptors have been found in a series of hormone-resistance syndromes. For example, single base substitutions can result in impaired ligand binding to the androgen receptor, and the resulting resistance to androgen action in a genetic male can result in a spectrum of effects, from the profound changes of a female phenotype (as in the *'testicular feminisation'* syndrome) to mild infertility.

Similar mutations have been identified in the genes for the vitamin D receptor (leading to vitamin D-resistant rickets), the thyroid hormone receptor (giving thyroid hormone resistance) and the glucocorticoid receptor (giving cortisol resistance), all with major phenotypic consequences. In many cases, these mutations are in the area coding for the hormone-binding domain, but in some cases they may affect the zinc fingers in the DNA-binding domain or produce truncated mRNAs. Pit-1 is an example of a tissue-specific transcription factor that may have loss-of-function changes in the DNA-binding domain; these are responsible for loss of development of certain pituitary cell types, resulting in hypopituitarism and growth failure.

Summary: signalling, proto-oncogenes and oncogenes

A series of proteins are involved in intracellular signalling, and they are mutated in many different types of human disease (see the box). In some cases, loss-of-function

Examples of diseases linked to changes in signalling pathways

Role in signalling system	Component	Disease
G-protein coupled membrane receptor	TSH receptor	Hyperthyroidism
G-protein-independent membrane receptor	Insulin receptor	Insulin resistance
Adenylate cyclase activation	G, α-subunit	Acromegaly
Nuclear receptor	Vitamin D receptor	Vitamin D-resistant rickets
Transcription factor	Pit-1	Hypopituitarism

mutations generate hormone-resistant states, while in others, gain-of-function mutations give rise to tumours. In the latter case, many of the proteins involved have come to be termed 'cellular proto-oncogenes' because of their homology with tumour-generating viral oncogenes. These include receptors, G-proteins, kinases, intracellular receptors and transcription factors (see Fig. 2.17). Oncogenes may be derived from proto-oncogenes by gain-of-function mutations that increase activity or level of expression. Oncogenic viruses either carry oncogenes or, in some cases, activate normal cellular proto-oncogenes.

Cell cycle and growth regulation

Normal mammalian cells undergo a 'cell cycle' of replication, with protein synthesis, DNA synthesis and mitosis occurring in defined phases. *Mitosis* (M phase) of a somatic cell generates two daughter cells, each with a full genetic complement of chromosomes. After mitosis, cells enter G_1 *phase*, representing a 'gap' during which RNAs and proteins are synthesised, and then enter *S phase*, when DNA synthesis (i.e. replication of the genome) starts. Finally there is a further 'gap', termed G_2 *phase*, before the cell enters mitosis. Cells may withdraw from the cycle during the G_1 phase into a non-cycling state termed G_0 (Fig. 2.18).

The cell cycle is subject to control by a series of cell cycle genes (best characterised in yeasts) whose activity is affected by phosphorylation and dephosphorylation. Homologues for some of these genes have been found in humans, and a series of *cyclin* proteins have been cloned that appear to have important evolutionarily conserved functions, with sequential activation through different stages of the cell cycle.

Tumour suppressor genes

Tumour suppressors are identified by the fact that loss-of-function mutations give rise to increased cell proliferation.

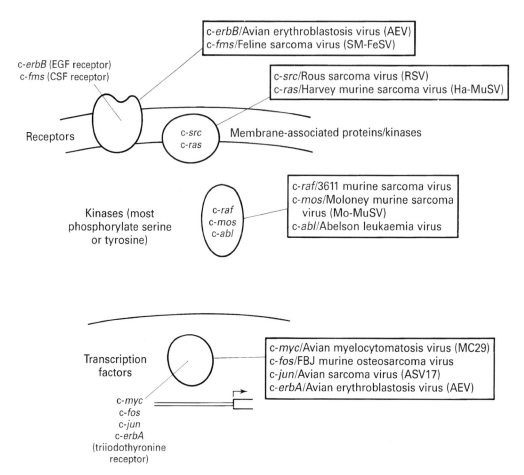

Fig. 2.17. Examples of cellular proto-oncogenes whose products are involved in different steps in signal transduction. The viral oncogenic homologues are shown in the boxes and the protein products in parentheses.

p 53.   The best known example is p 53, which was originally thought to be an oncogene because mutations were associated with cancers. In fact these mutations are largely mis-sense, i.e. loss-of-function mutations, inhibiting the action of normal p 53 produced by the unaffected allele. p 53 is a nuclear phosphoprotein, whose mechanism of action is still not known though it is a DNA-binding protein capable of activating transcription from some promoters. Mutant p 53 molecules are unable to bind the SV40 virus large T tumour antigen: normal p 53 binds to T antigen and prevents it from replicating the SV40 genome. Therefore, it has been proposed that normal cells contain a homologue of the large T antigen, and that this function is lost in cells with mutant p 53, allowing uncontrolled cell growth.

The retinoblastoma gene (Rb).   This is another tumour suppressor gene. It was first identified in the childhood retinal tumour retinoblastoma, where both copies of the gene are inactivated or deleted; however, Rb gene deletions have now been demon-

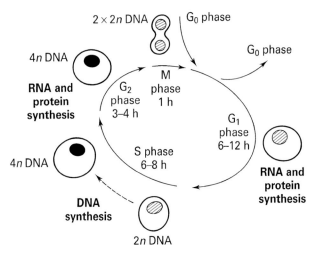

Fig. 2.18. Stages of the cell cycle. The normal diploid complement of genetic material is given as $2n$ DNA; $4n$ is the tetraploid content just before mitosis.

strated in a series of human tumours apart from retinoblastoma, for example small cell lung cancer. The tumour itself contains no Rb protein, usually because of a loss of gene expression rather than point mutations affecting protein function. Rb is a nuclear phosphoprotein that is unphosphorylated in resting (G_0 phase) cells but undergoes phosphorylation at the end of the G_1 phase, probably by a cyclin E-dependent protein kinase. The Rb protein is once again dephosphorylated at the end of mitosis. The unphosphorylated protein is able to bind several cell cycle proteins, such as the E2F transcription factor and cyclin D, and this places a block on the cell entering the cell cycle by preventing these proteins from being released.

Apoptosis

Cell population number is affected not only by proliferation but also by cell death. Apoptosis is an active, regulated form of cell death, unlike necrosis, and it is central to embryogenesis and development as well as homeostasis of adult tissues. Abnormally regulated apoptosis has recently been implicated in several human diseases including cancer and neurodegeneration.

Apoptosis was first identified microscopically as a distinctive reduction in cell volume and condensation of nuclear chromatin. The nucleus then breaks into smaller fragments, but other organelles remain intact. Eventually the endoplasmic reticulum fuses with the plasma membrane, and round apoptotic bodies are released and rapidly phagocytosed. Intracellular events accompanying apoptosis include characteristic internucleosomal fragmentation of DNA resulting from regulated endonuclease activity. A number of genes have been identified that control the initiation of these processes, notably *ced-3* and *myc*, which promote apoptosis, and *bcl-2* and c-*abl* (see above), which can suppress it *in vitro*.

Molecular biology: methods of investigation

Studies of the molecular basis of disease depended initially on identifying an abnormal product, such as a protein. The development of techniques to manipulate DNA made it possible to utilise information from characterised proteins to clone and identify genes, from which further information about the disorder could be found. A further development is the isolation and cloning of genes likely to be involved in a disease and using these to produce and identify abnormal proteins (see the box).

Disorders studied by cloning

1. Knowledge of abnormal protein allowed mapping and cloning of the gene, e.g. haemophilia, the factor VIII gene.
2. Knowledge of a disease allows a marker or 'candidate' gene to be identified and its linkage to the disease to be examined, e.g. genes for the muscle proteins actin and myosin were candidate genes for the disease of heart muscle familial hypertrophic cardiomyopathy.
3. When the underlying defect in a disease is unknown, polymorphisms known to be linked to the disease can be used to identify the gene(s). Cloning of the genes then allows identification and characterisation of the protein product, e.g. the dystrophin protein in Duchenne muscular dystrophy (see Chapter 3, p. 83).
4. Random testing can find DNA polymorphisms linked to the disease phenotype, e.g. in Huntington's disease.

Enzymes

The development of modern molecular biology was made possible with the discovery of a series of enzymes that allowed specific (usually sequence-specific) manipulations of DNA and RNA. This made it possible to produce DNA fragments reproducibly from a variety of tissues, and in particular allowed the generation of new DNA molecules by recombining fragments from different sources.

Endonucleases (restriction endonucleases). These are bacterial enzymes that cleave double-stranded DNA at specific symmetrical (palindromic) sequences leaving fragments with characteristic patterns, either blunt-ended or with overhanging ends of specific bases ('sticky ends') (Fig. 2.19a). A huge number of enzymes is now available. Each one recognises and cleaves at a specific DNA sequence usually 4–6 bp in length. Using different endonucleases, specific DNA fragments can be produced and then cloned by inserting them into plasmid or bacteriophage vectors for propagation in bacteria, as described below.

Ligases. These enzymes catalyse the formation of a DNA molecule from two fragments with compatible termini (as shown in Fig. 2.19b).

(a)

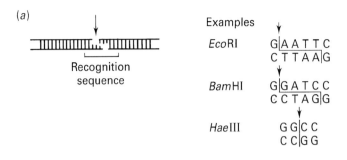

(b)

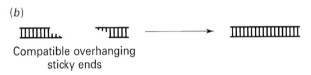

Compatible overhanging
sticky ends

Fig. 2.19. Examples of DNA-modifying enzymes. (*a*) Endonucleases. (*b*) Ligases.

Polymerases. Polymerases catalyse the generation of a new DNA or RNA molecule by assembling nucleotides linearly along a pre-existing DNA or RNA template. This property can be used to incorporate radiolabelled nucleotides into a molecule, for example in the production of labelled DNA or RNA probes and for sequence analysis.

Reverse transcriptase. This enzyme can be used to transcribe mRNA to produce a complementary DNA (cDNA) molecule that can be used for direct cloning or for polymerase chain reaction (PCR) amplification as described below.

cDNA synthesis

One of the most powerful uses of endonucleases and other enzymes is the synthesis of DNA molecules that are complementary to a DNA or RNA template. cDNA can be produced from a template of unknown or only partly known mRNA, propagated in bacteria and then sequenced and its function analysed in detail. This process is summarised in Fig. 2.20. Essentially, polyA-rich RNA (i.e. mRNA) is extracted from a suitable tissue or cell line, and a synthetic DNA sequence is added that contains a series of T residues. This 'oligo-dT primer' anneals to the poly-A tail of the mRNA, and then the enzyme reverse transcriptase can be used to snythesise a new DNA molecule by base pairing of nucleotides with the mRNA template. A second strand of DNA can be made from the first strand using DNA polymerase. The final product is a new double-stranded DNA molecule that can be inserted into a vector for cloning, as outlined below.

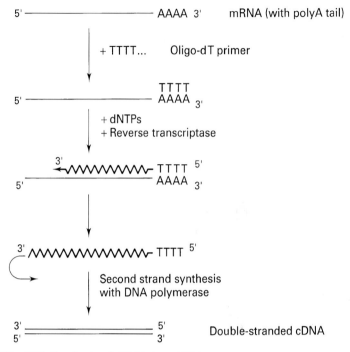

Fig. 2 20. Synthesis of cDNA from RNA.

Cloning

Vectors

The discovery of specific enzymes for DNA and RNA manipulation has allowed the cloning of recombinant DNA fragments such as cDNA in *vectors* that can carry such foreign sequences in host bacteria. Bacterial plasmids have been widely used as vectors: they are circular double-stranded DNA molecules that are normally found in bacteria, and although not an integral part of the host genome, they can replicate within the bacterium. The plasmids can be isolated and artificially introduced into special strains of bacteria developed for experimental use that are unable to grow outside of laboratory conditions, and in this way the bacteria can be used to propagate large amounts of DNA. Plasmids were originally discovered because they conferred resistance to antibiotics, and this property can be used to select only those bacteria that have successfully taken up the plasmid DNA. The principles of cloning are summarised in Fig. 2.21.

The technology of using vectors for cloning has advanced rapidly, and a great variety of tools is now available, including plasmids with synthetic sequences incorporating multiple restriction endonuclease recognition sites ('polylinkers', or multiple cloning sites). Plasmid vectors have been developed to incorporate promoter sequences to allow *in vitro* transcription of the cloned DNA, or *in vivo* expression of the protein product in living cells. Other types of vector also include bacteriophage lambda (λ), a bacterial virus that multiplies rapidly within its host and can carry large amounts of DNA.

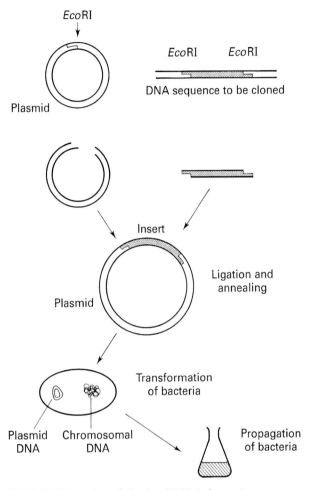

Fig. 2.21. Principles of cloning DNA in bacteria.

The specialised techniques used in cloning large eukaryotic genes are discussed more fully in Chapter 3 (p. 80).

Libraries

Using cloning techniques, it is possible to prepare DNA from a human tissue, digest it into fragments using one or more endonucleases, insert the fragments into a vector and propagate them as a 'library' in bacteria. Total genomic DNA can be prepared in this way, in which case the transformed bacteria will carry a 'genomic library'; alternatively, cDNA prepared from the mRNA expressed by a given cell type can be used to generate a 'cDNA library'.

Nucleic acid libraries contain many millions of sequences, and in order to identify bacteria bearing specific DNA fragments of interest, a series of screening procedures are used.

In the case of genomic libraries, fragments of DNA can be screened, for example, to identify upstream regulatory elements of specific genes for studies of transcriptional regulation. cDNA libraries can be screened to identify sequences encoding newly discovered proteins.

Library screening

Recombinant bacterial clones in a cDNA library can be screened with antibodies or with DNA probes. Antibody screening requires that the library is constructed in an *expression vector* that contains promoter sequences to direct transcription and translation of the cloned DNA in the bacteria. The bacteria are lysed to expose the intracellular protein and transferred to a membrane that is then incubated with the antibody. Positive colonies can be selected from the bacterial cultures for selective propagation and further rounds of screening. Screening of cDNA libraries with small known sequences of DNA – probes – is simpler because it does not require synthesis of an immunoreactive peptide, but it does require some prior knowledge of the DNA sequence being sought.

Subtractive hybridisation

A number of approaches have been developed to enrich cDNA libraries for sequences that are specifically found in certain tissues or that are associated with differentiation. Two cDNA libraries are prepared, a [+]cDNA from a tissue that expresses the factor of interest, and a [−]cDNA from a tissue that does not. The [+]cDNA is prepared with specific restriction endonuclease recognition sites at each terminus so that it can be cloned, and it is then allowed to hybridise with the [−]cDNA. Those [+]cDNAs that fail to hybridise with [−]cDNA represent species that are only present in the [+] tissue; they can be selectively cloned, resulting in a library that has been enriched by the 'subtraction' of irrelevant [−] clones.

Nucleic acid analysis

Gel electrophoresis

DNA and RNA molecules can be separated by electrophoresis through gels of agarose or polyacrylamide, migrating towards the anode because of the negatively charged phosphates along the DNA backbone. As the charge/mass ratio of DNA of different lengths is the same, the rate of migration through a gel is determined by the size of the molecule (up to about 50kb) (Fig. 2.22). However the conformation of DNA alters its electrophoretic mobility, so that molecules such as supercoiled closed circular plasmids migrate faster than linear DNA of the same base length because of their different hydrodynamic radii. The concentration of gels can be adjusted to give optimal separation of fragments varying in length from 20bp to 20000bp.

Larger molecules (25000 to over 150000bp) can be separated by more complex tech-

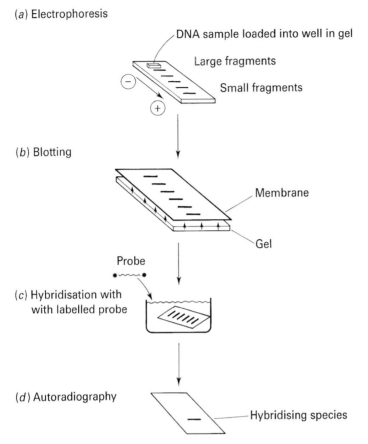

(a) Electrophoresis

DNA sample loaded into well in gel

Large fragments

Small fragments

(b) Blotting

Membrane

Gel

Probe

(c) Hybridisation with
    with labelled probe

(d) Autoradiography

Hybridising species

Fig. 2.22. Principles of nucleic acid analysis. (*a*) Electrophoresis separates DNA by fragment size and shape. (*b*) Blotting techniques allow the separated fragments to be transferred to a membrane for analysis (*c*). The fragments are labelled by hybridisation with probes. (*d*) Autoradiography indicates the position of positive fragments where probe has bound to target DNA.

niques such as *pulsed field electrophoresis* (PFGE). In this technique, an electrophoretic gel is subject to alternating-angle electric fields. This discriminates between the differing abilities of very large DNA molecules to alter their conformation rapidly on changing the electric field (which varies with size); this determines their speed of migration.

Blotting techniques

DNA or RNA, once separated in a gel, may be transferred to a membrane for easier analysis by a number of 'blotting' techniques. The first technique to be widely used was developed by E. M. Southern and involving the transfer of DNA from gels onto nitrocellulose membranes by capillary blotting; this has become known as Southern blotting (Fig. 2.22). Various processes of macromolecule transfer from gels to membranes have since been applied to RNA (non-eponymously called Northern blotting) and to protein (usually for analysis with antibodies, Western blotting). Once transferred, nucleic acids can be fixed covalently onto nitrocellulose or nylon-based membranes by baking or ultraviolet cross-linking and subjected to analysis.

Labelling nucleic acids

DNA and RNA, once separated by electrophoresis, can be visualised directly by incorporation of the dye ethidium bromide. This intercalates between the stacked bases of the nucleic acid and fluoresces orange under ultraviolet light. Analysis of specific DNA or RNA sequences relies on labelling of a known sequence – a 'probe' – and allowing it to hybridise with separated nucleic acids that have been transferred onto a membrane. Probe labelling is commonly achieved with radioactive phosphorus (^{32}P), though non-radioactive methods are becoming popular.

Short sequences of DNA, such as oligonucleotides of 20–40bp can be end-labelled by transfer of a ^{32}P-labelled γ-phosphate group from ATP to the 5'-hydroxyl terminus of a DNA molecule using the enzyme T4 polynucleotide kinase. Longer DNA molecules require 'body-labelling', and a widely used method uses random-sequence hexamer primers to prime synthesis of a new DNA strand from a single-stranded DNA or RNA template: the primers anneal at multiple sites on a long DNA template and can prime second-strand DNA synthesis, incorporating radiolabelled nucleotides, in the presence of DNA polymerase.

Identification

The fragments of DNA and RNA that have hybridised with the probes are identified by autoradiography.

Sequencing

DNA sequencing relies on the separation of a series of radiolabelled oligonucleotides that differ by a single base using high-resolution denaturing polyacrylamide gels (sequencing gels). A set of single-stranded oligonucleotides is generated that all have one fixed end but which terminate in each successive base of the template DNA sequence. Four separate reactions are used to generate oligonucleotides that terminate in A, T, G or C. The reaction products are resolved on the gel such that four 'ladders' are seen, and the sequence can be read directly from the autoradiograph (see Fig. 2.23).

Two techniques are used in most sequencing reactions, namely the dideoxy or enzymatic method, originally developed by Sanger, and the chemical method developed by Maxam and Gilbert. These techniques form the basis of rapid sequencing equipment that has dramatically reduced the time involved in sequencing DNA fragments. The complementary development of computer programs to store, examine and compare sequences has allowed the ambitious genome projects, to define genomes from major species groups, to be attempted.

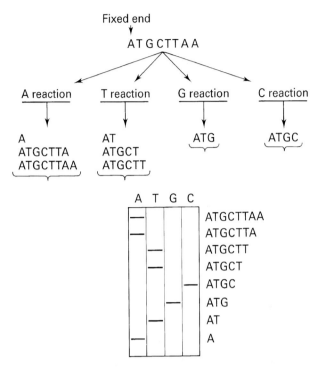

Fig. 2.23. DNA sequencing. A set of radiolabelled oligonucleotides is generated in four different reactions, resulting in a terminal A, T, G or C, respectively. The DNA fragments are separated on a gel and the sequence of the substrate DNA is read directly from the autoradiograph.

In the dideoxy method, 2', 3'-dideoxynucleotide triphosphates are used to terminate the elongation of a newly synthesised DNA molecule made from a synthetic primer annealed to the template DNA under study. Thus, ddATP can be utilised by DNA polymerase to extend a DNA chain, but further deoxynucleotides cannot be added and so random stops in the extension occur, depending on the ddNTP used. Four different ddNTPs are used to generate the four reactions whose products are visualised on the gel.

In the chemical method, a labelled single-stranded DNA molecule is subjected to a set of base-specific cleavage reactions: again the reaction results in a set of oligonucleotides, all labelled at one end, but with different termini (A, T, G or C) according to the chemical cleavage, and the products are visualised in the same way as a set of ladders on a gel.

Polymerase chain reaction

Since its first description in 1986, the polymerase chain reaction (PCR) has revolutionised the practice of molecular biology by allowing rapid enzymatic amplification of specific DNA fragments in large amounts from very small amounts of starting material, even single cells. RNA can be amplified by converting it first to DNA using reverse transcriptase. A huge variety of applications has been found for PCR, including direct

cloning of genomic DNA or cDNA, engineering of new recombinant fragments, forensic analysis of small tissue samples, prenatal diagnosis and detection of pathogenic DNA
from microorganisms (such as viruses and mycobacteria) in diseased human tissues.

The technique requires a double-stranded DNA template and a pair of single-
stranded oligonucleotide primers that are complementary to sequences flanking the
region of interest, so defining the ends of the region. The template DNA strands are denatured by heating, and the primers, added in large excess, anneal, on cooling, to the
respective opposite strands of DNA. New DNA synthesis is then catalysed by DNA
polymerase in the presence of deoxynucleotide triphosphates (dNTPs). The resulting
new double-stranded molecules are in turn denatured and in turn form new templates
for the next round of DNA synthesis, again using the oligonucleotide primers (Fig. 2.24).

The technique relies on successive cycles of denaturation, annealing and DNA synthesis, and exponential amplification of DNA is possible such that, in principle, 30 cycles
would result in almost 270000000-fold (2^{28}-fold) amplification. With the discovery of
thermostable DNA polymerases (such as that from the thermophilic bacterium *Thermus
aquaticus*, Taq polymerase), and technological advances in the development of thermal
cycler machines, it is possible to perform multiple simultaneous PCR reactions in just a
few hours.

The specificity of PCR can be increased by using 'nested' primers, which are complementary to sequence between the two original primer sites. This technique is used to
prevent closely related DNA sequences being amplified along with the desired
sequence.

Application of molecular techniques

Analysis of gene transcription

The techniques of nucleic acid analysis described above have been extensively applied
to studies of gene expression, and this has led to a detailed understanding of transcriptional control, as outlined in the first section of this chapter. Here, some of the approaches
currently used will be briefly illustrated.

mRNA analysis

RNA can be isolated for analysis by a variety of methods. In general, strict precautions
must be taken to avoid degradation of the mRNA by ribonucleases, and it must be
separated from contaminating DNA and proteins. Either total RNA (which comprises
more than 90% ribosomal RNA) or polyA-enriched RNA (i.e. mRNA) is purified and
subjected to hybridisation analysis with labelled probes. Membrane blotting of electrophoresed RNA (Northern blotting) is commonly used before hybridisation, but alternative techniques involve solution hybridisation followed by electrophoresis of
RNA–probe hybrid molecules (for example ribonuclease protection assays). In some
cases, the mRNA species under study are rare transcripts and may be reverse transcribed (using reverse transcriptase) to make cDNA, which is then amplified by PCR

(*a*) Denature (heat for 60 s)

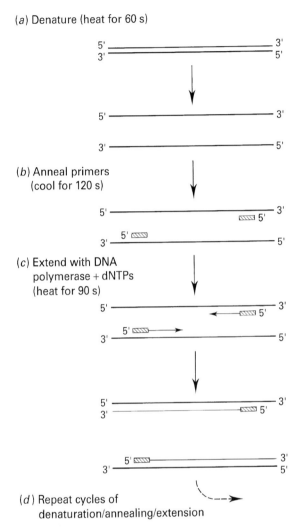

(*b*) Anneal primers
(cool for 120 s)

(*c*) Extend with DNA
polymerase + dNTPs
(heat for 90 s)

(*d*) Repeat cycles of
denaturation/annealing/extension

Fig. 2.24. The principle of PCR. A single cycle consists of three steps (*a–c*) at the end of which there is twice the amount of target DNA. Repeating the cycle once gives four times the DNA and so on.

to provide amounts of material sufficient for more detailed analysis (reverse transcription PCR, or rt-PCR).

This type of mRNA analysis has led to detailed definition of the patterns of gene expression in different tissues, and it has become clear that this expression involves tissue-specific mechanisms as well as regulation by external stimuli such as hormones.

Mechanisms of regulation: gene promoter analysis

Analysis of the mechanisms of mRNA regulation has required detailed investigation of the function of genomic DNA associated with a series of coding genes, and a typical approach will be outlined here as an example of the molecular dissection of genetic control.

In principle, alteration in the level of mRNA in a cell may depend either on changes in the rate of gene transcription, or on altered stability of the mRNA. Both mechanisms have been found to operate, but most progress has recently been made in our understanding of transcriptional control, which in most cases is a function of upstream (5′) elements in the gene's promoter and enhancer regions.

Genomic DNA libraries are commonly used as the starting material from which a stretch of putative upstream regulatory DNA can be isolated. This DNA is first sequenced and the sequence searched for typical consensus motifs to which known transcription factors may bind, such as the TATA and CAAT boxes, and for recognition sequences for other factors such as AP-1 and steroid hormone receptors. In addition, sequencing is useful for defining potential endonuclease sites that may be valuable for engineering new DNA constructs for functional studies. In this way, a physical map of the promoter is built up, but the significance of particular sequences now requires direct experimental confirmation.

In order to determine whether a given stretch of DNA really functions as transcriptional regulator, it may be isolated from its genomic context and linked to a 'reporter gene' in a new synthetically engineered plasmid; the new plasmid construct is then introduced into a living cell. Systems include the *Xenopus* oocyte, bacterium or yeast cell or mammalian cell lines. A reporter gene is one that encodes a protein product which is easily measured in living cells, usually a protein not normally produced by those cells. For example, the firefly luciferase gene encodes a protein not found in mammalian cells that catalyses the production of light from the substrate luciferin. If a plasmid containing the luciferase gene is introduced into a cell by a process of 'transfection', then the amount of luciferase produced is determined by the activity of the promoter element to which it is linked. Then, when cell extracts are made and incubated with luciferin and ATP, the amount of light produced is a measure of promoter activity.

A series of techniques is now available for the introduction of DNA into mammalian cells, including calcium phosphate transfection and DEAE-dextran transfection (which each promote DNA attachment to the cell surface allowing endocytotic uptake), liposome-mediated transfection and electroporation. In each case, the cell type for study must be carefully chosen and the actual transfection procedure carefully optimised (see Fig. 2.25).

Using these techniques, a functional map can now be produced of the important control elements that modulate transcription of a given gene. DNA elements responsible for conferring cell-type-specific transcription or intracellular signal-mediated transcription can be closely defined, and those sequences can then in turn be used as tools with which to identify the protein transcription factors to which they bind. For example, double-stranded synthetic oligonucleotide probes containing multimers of a critical DNA sequence can be used to screen a cDNA expression library for DNA-binding proteins and hence characterise new factors (see Latchman, 1995).

(*a*) Isolate putative regulatory DNA

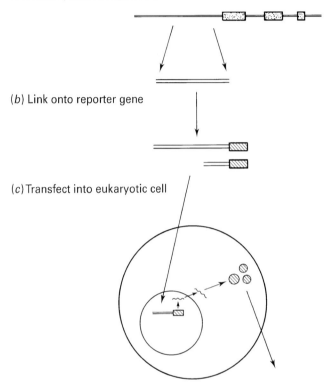

(*b*) Link onto reporter gene

(*c*) Transfect into eukaryotic cell

(*d*) Analyse cell for expression of reporter gene product

Fig. 2.25. Gene promoter analysis. The segment of putative regulatory DNA is isolated (*a*) and linked to a reporter gene (*b*). Deletions may be introduced into the regulatory DNA to define critical regions involved in transcriptional control. After transfection (*c*), the cell is analysed to assess the level of expression of the reporter gene. This is a function of the activity of the promoter under examination.

Transgenic animals

Gene function can be studied by genetic manipulation of whole animals using a series of 'transgenic' approaches. Essentially, transgenic animals are produced by incorporation of an exogenous 'transgene' into the genome of an early stage embryo. This routinely involves microinjection of the exogenous gene construct of interest into a pronuclear stage embryo where it integrates into the host DNA of the fertilised oocyte. The foreign DNA is integrated at random in the recipient genome, which may result in loss of expression of host genes, changed expression patterns of the foreign DNA because of its modification by host gene-controlling elements or its control by a strong constitutive host promoter, or no expression of the foreign DNA because it integrated into a transcriptionally quiet region. If possible, the inclusion of as much as is possible of the human gene's controlling elements will avoid these problems.

The alternative approach to the production of transgenic animals involves

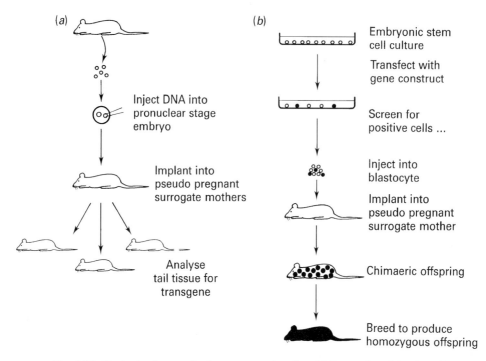

Fig. 2.26. Strategies for producing transgenic mice. (*a*) Pronuclear injection. (*b*) Embryonic stem cell transfection.

transfection of embryonic stem (ES) cells. These cell lines are derived from the inner cell mass of an early blastocyst embryo, which are transfected with the exogenous gene construct of interest: those cells positive for the transgene can be identified, and the mutant clones are then microinjected into a normal blastocyst to produce chimaeric animals.

The resulting modified embryonic cells produced by either approach are capable of differentiation into any tissue, including germ cells in the gonads, and hence animals that are chimaeric in their germ-line can be bred to produce offspring that are heterozygous for the transgene throughout their somatic cells. These animals can in turn be interbred to produce homozygous offspring if desired (see Fig. 2.26).

The pronuclear injection approach has been widely used to study the tissue-specific activation of promoter regions by examining the expression of reporter genes, and also to study the targeted expression of specific proteins using well-characterised promoters. For example, the activation of homeodomain gene promoters in embryonic development has been studied using the β-galactosidase reporter gene the expression of which is easily detected in whole embryos. If a tissue-specific promoter is used, expression can be targeted to a certain cell type. For example, pituitary-specific promoters have been used to target high-level expression of mutant CREB to the pituitary, in order to demonstrate the role of CREB in pituitary cell development and function. Other applications of the latter technique include achieving the targeted expression of the herpes virus 1 thymidine kinase (HSV-TK) gene in specific tissues, which then become uniquely sensitive to drugs whose metabolites kill dividing cells (a 'TK obliteration system') (see the box).

The use of transgenic animals

1. Disease models
     cystic fibrosis: the transmembrane regulator protein (CFTR)
     DiGeorge syndrome: *hox-1.5* gene
2. Gene function
     thymus development: various genes
     tumour suppressor genes: Rb, p 53
3. Drug and hormone effects
     wound healing: the role of keratinocyte growth factor (KGF)

Gene targeting by homologous recombination

Transgenic mice have been used recently to produce animals with mutations in any desired gene (see cystic fibrosis, p. 83). This involves gene targeting by homologous recombination to completely inactivate the target gene (often called gene 'knockout'). Different types of targeting gene construct are used, but commonly they will consist of two regions of homology with the target normal gene that are separated by an intervening DNA segment (Fig. 2.27). This intervening segment is generally a drug-resistance gene that will both interrupt and mutate the target gene and also allow ES cells to be selected according to whether the construct has been integrated or not. This approach has been widely used to study the functions of candidate genes in thymus development, and recently the role of tumour suppressor genes such as Rb and p 53 (see p. 36).

Targeted dominant negative receptor mutants

Finally, transgenic animals have recently been used to study effects of hormones or drugs on specific tissues in intact animals by interfering with normal receptor function. Dominant negative receptors (see p. 54) may occur in disease states or may be deliberately engineered: they are themselves inactive but have the effect of blocking the effect of the normal receptors in a cell. Dominant negative growth factor receptor cDNAs can be linked to a strong tissue-specific promoter in transgenes such that the transgenic animal will express the mutant receptor only in a specified cell type. In such a way, the role of keratinocyte growth factor (KGF) in skin development and wound healing has been determined using a construct linking the KGF receptor dominant-negative mutant to a skin-specific gene promoter, providing unique new information about skin differentiation and wound re-epithelialisation.

Analysis of abnormal DNA

A number of molecular techniques have been used to identify genetic abnormalities associated with disease. These will be illustrated in specific sections elsewhere

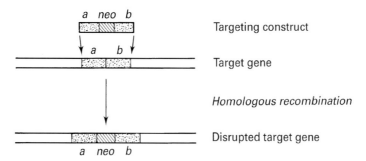

Fig. 2.27. Gene targeting by homologous recombination. A transgenic 'knock-out' animal is created by replacing a segment of the target gene with a construct that includes a selectable marker gene, such as *neo*, a drug-resistance gene.

(particularly in Chapter 3); here a brief summary will be given of the rationale for some of the standard approaches.

Southern blotting: gene deletions

In the simplest case, some diseases are known to be caused by the total absence of a known gene product, suggesting a single gene deletion. For example, in type 1A isolated growth hormone deficiency, growth hormone production is completely absent, and deletion of a large part of the growth hormone gene cluster in these patients was demonstrated directly by Southern blotting. Genomic DNA (obtained from peripheral blood leucocytes) was digested with an endonuclease that was known to yield a characteristic pattern of DNA fragments within the growth hormone gene, then the digestion products were electrophoresed and transferred by Southern blotting onto a membrane for hybridisation with a radiolabelled growth hormone cDNA probe (see Fig. 2.28).

Southern blotting: restriction fragment length polymorphisms

In other conditions, a candidate gene has not been identified, and here Southern blotting has been used in a less direct way to determine disease associations with chromosomal locations, and hence progressively localise an unknown abnormal gene linked with the disorder. This technique uses natural inherited polymorphisms (variations) in DNA sequence among different individuals to track the segregation of disease in families with particular chromosomal markers. Polymorphic DNA sequences can create or destroy restriction endonuclease sites, resulting in characteristic fragment lengths when given pieces of genomic DNA are digested with certain endonucleases. These restriction fragment length polymorphisms (RFLPs) have no disease significance in themselves but are simply markers that can be identified by using a series of chromosomal probes. They may or may not be close to a disease locus. As RFLPs are polymorphic, this type of analysis requires a set of family members affected or unaffected by the disease in order to determine whether a particular locus really segregates with the disease through the

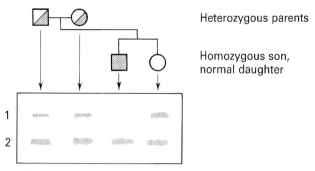

Fig. 2.28. Deletion of the growth hormone gene shown by Southern blot analysis in type 1A isolated growth hormone deficiency. Both heterozygous parents show reduced intensity in band 1, which is completely absent in the homozygous son but normal in the unaffected daughter.

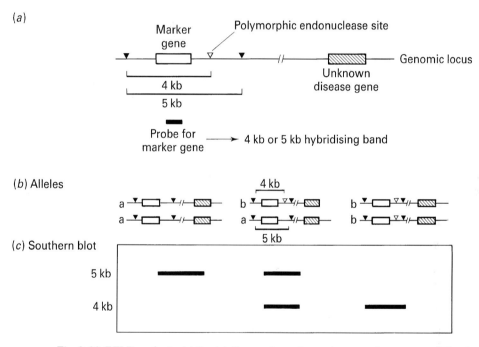

Fig. 2. 29. RFLP analysis. (*a*) Restriction endonuclease sites may be constant (▼) or be created by polymorphic variation in the DNA sequence (▽). (*b*) A probe for a marker gene will hybridise to variable fragment lengths of genomic DNA depending on the presence or absence of the restriction site. (*c*) The appearance on a Southern blot of the three potential combinations of alleles. A pedigree analysis within a family where a disease occurs will show whether the marker gene segregates with the disease phenotype.

generations. The principles are illustrated in Fig. 2.29 and discussed in more detail in Chapter 3 (p. 75). Once a sufficiently small region of chromosomal DNA has been localised, direct genetic analysis by sequencing becomes feasible, and a disease gene can be firmly identified and characterised. RFLP analysis linked early onset familial Alzheimer's disease with chromosome 21 in the area involved in Dolon's syndrome.

Patients with Dolon's syndrome also show Alzheimer's disease in middle age. RFLP analysis has also been used to detect fragile X syndrome.

Disease genes: mutation analysis

In many cases of human disease, a particular gene is known to be abnormal. This gene may be subject to mutational change (deletions or point mutations with single-base changes), giving either loss of function of the protein product or, in some cases, gain of function.

Analysis of DNA sequence is normally undertaken using genomic DNA (usually from leucocyte DNA) in cases of germ-line mutations (e.g. inherited diseases) or cDNAs from affected tissues in cases of somatic mutations that have been acquired since conception (e.g. tumours). Mutational change may be heterozygous, affecting only one allele, or homozygous affecting both alleles, and a number of different types of mutation are found. Point mutations (changes affecting a single base) include substitution of a base with an abnormal base, which may change the amino acid sequence or may encode a premature stop codon, which will terminate translation. Single-base deletions or insertions result in a frameshift, disrupting the reading frame of triplet codons so that a non-sense non-coding mRNA sequence is produced downstream of the mutation. Point mutations are the molecular defect in the β-thalassaemias. In some cases, several bases may be deleted, as in cystic fibrosis, where a deletion of three nucleotides results in loss of a phenylalanine residue in the ATP-binding domain of a transmembrane protein.

As mentioned above, some diseases are associated with expansion of repetitive DNA sequences, such as triplet repeats within coding regions or untranslated regions of disease genes, and these mutations may have general transcriptional repressive effects. For example, myotonic dystrophy results from an unstable trinucleotide repeat $(AGC)n$, with disease severity parelleling the number of repeats. Larger-scale chromosomal deletions or rearrangements have more or less drastic effects on the coding genes, but in some cases can lead to one gene's coding sequence coming under the control of another gene's promoter, giving rise to abnormally regulated protein synthesis. An example is the Bcr–Abl hybrid oncogene caused by a chromosome 9 to 22 translocation and responsible for chronic myeloid leukaemia (p. 34).

Point mutations giving rise to amino acid substitutions may have a variety of effects. Some lead to loss of protein function: for example, mutations of tumour suppressor genes, such as p53, in many different cancers. Others cause abnormal activation: for example, the $G_s \alpha$-subunit gene mutation *gsp* is a constitutive activator (that is, no longer regulated) of adenylate cyclase that is found in various benign endocrine tumours. Some point mutations give rise to a profound change in phenotype even though they occur on only one allele, which implies that they over-ride the function of the normal protein, termed a *'dominant negative'* effect.

Functional effects of mutations such as these have been investigated in two different ways: (i) by cloning the mutated sequence the abnormal protein can be expressed in transfected cells and its transcriptional effects determined using promoter–reporter gene constructs (see cystic fibrosis, p. 83); (ii) transgenic mice can be produced in which the phenotypic effects of particular mutations can be analysed in more detail than may be possible in humans.

A variety of screening techniques have been developed to enable large numbers of clinical cases to be studied for mutations; in most cases, these techniques rely on PCR amplification of genomic DNA. Direct analysis of known mutation 'hot-spots' can be made by hybridisation with wild-type (natural) or mutant sequences using specially made oligonucleotide probes. Other methods such as *single-strand conformational polymorphism* (SSCP) screen for potential unknown mutations in larger regions of DNA by detecting small changes in electrophoretic mobility of mutant DNA strands compared with wild-type fragments.

Gene therapy

The amazing speed of molecular biology's advances since the early 1980s will be obvious from the preceding sections. It means that gene therapy has moved from being an exciting but speculative possibility to a practical reality in modern medicine. The scope for gene therapy is obvious and would include not only replacing defective or absent genes with normal ones but also engineering new genes to inhibit expression of deleterious disease genes. Techniques will vary depending on whether the therapeutic gene must be introduced into every cell (e.g. replacing a defective tumour suppressor gene in cancer) or whether less than 100% replacement will rectify the clinical phenotype (e.g. cystic fibrosis, p. 90).

The essential problem of gene therapy is one of drug delivery: that of transporting a large highly charged molecule to the nucleus. A series of strategies have been developed, mostly involving virus-based vectors but also including other approaches such as molecular conjugates (for example DNA–protein complexes), using ligands for cell targeting and using liposomes. Viral vectors include retroviruses, adenovirus and adeno-associated virus (AAV); these can be used to package the DNA construct and infect human cells so that the DNA is taken up into the nucleus. The use of vectors in gene therapy is discussed in more detail in Chapter 3 (p. 90).

Example: homozygous familial hypercholesterolaemia

A recent successful example of gene therapy is the experimental treatment of homozygous familial hypercholesterolaemia. This disease results from a mutation of the receptor for low-density lipoprotein (LDL), which prevents clearance of LDL from plasma. The heterozygous form of the disease is common, affecting 1/400 people in Britain, and it results in early onset of ischaemic heart disease. The very severe homozygous form usually results in death from heart disease before 30 years of age. This severe, single gene disease was, therefore, a good candidate for gene therapy, and early successes have been reported.

Gene therapy here has involved resection of a portion of the patient's liver, using the patient's hepatocytes to generate primary cell cultures that are then infected with retrovirus containing the LDL receptor cDNA. Virus particles are removed, and the transfected cells are reintroduced into the patient via a catheter in the hepatic portal vein to allow seeding in the host liver. After pilot studies in rabbits and then primates to establish feasibility and safety, a number of patients have been treated, with clinically useful, though only partial, reductions in circulating LDL-cholesterol for over one year.

Antisense gene therapy

A number of candidate diseases have now been proposed for development of 'replacement' gene therapy approaches, but the more challenging cases will be those that require interference with endogenous gene function. A number of experimental examples have suggested that this too is feasible and practicable. 'Antisense therapeutics' is being developed on the basis that antisense RNA will bind (by complementary base pairing) to mRNA and prevent its translation into protein, or in some cases may generate a triple helix with double-stranded DNA to prevent transcription. One of several exciting recent examples of experimental uses of this therapy is the suppression of Philadelphia chromosome-positive human leukaemia cells in immunodeficient mice by systemic administration of a 26-mer antisense to the B2A2 breakpoint junction of the *bcr–abl* fusion gene (see p. 34).

A variety of modified antisense molecules have been developed, including modified oligonucleotides that are resistant to ribonuclease digestion, and 'peptide nucleic acids' in which the entire deoxyribose phosphate backbone is replaced by a polyamine backbone. Ribozymes are naturally occurring 'RNA enzymes' that can be modified to cleave specific RNA sequences, and these have been targeted against oncogenes such as *ras*, and also against the human immunodeficiency virus (HIV).

Further examples of gene therapy approaches are being developed. For example, there is *in vitro* evidence that it is possible to correct a malignant phenotype by insertion of normal tumour suppressor genes, and trials are in progress in which the normal Rb gene is inserted intravesically in bladder cancer, and in which bronchoscopic application of the normal p 53 gene is made in lung cancer. More common diseases may also be susceptible to these new therapies: in the case of vascular disease, excessive smooth muscle cell proliferation can be reduced with locally applied gene therapy (for example antisense c-*myb* DNA) using carefully targeted intra-arterial catheters; by comparison, vascular endothelial growth factor (VEGF) cDNA can be applied locally to induce angiogenesis in ischaemic limbs. For many of these new applications, gene therapy may prove to be both cheaper and more effective than alternative treatments with recombinant proteins.

Cell biology: methods of investigation

Cell culture

Detailed analysis of the principles of cell biology became possible with the advent of techniques for growing individual cell types in isolation from the whole animal, a technique known as cell culture (see Fig. 2.30).

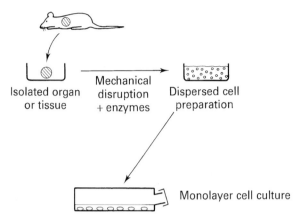

Fig. 2.30. Primary cell culture. A suspension of isolated cells is prepared and forms a monolayer that is maintained in nutrient culture media.

Primary culture

In its simplest form, primary culture entails preparing a suspension of cells from a tissue and using enzymes to break down the intercellular matrix. The isolated cells can then be maintained *in vitro* as a primary culture using a nutrient growth medium of essential amino acids, sugars, vitamins and salts, usually supplemented with animal sera to provide essential growth factors. Primary cultures can readily be maintained for several weeks, and certain cell types will proliferate, allowing much longer-term cultures to be established. Cells in primary culture re-establish cell–cell interconnections, and they have the advantage of being closely representative of the cells present in the intact tissue *in vivo*. However, such cultures often include several different cell types, and for this reason clonal cell lines may be preferred.

Clonal cell lines

Clonal cell lines are cell cultures that represent the progeny of a single cell, and in general these cells are characterised by unlimited proliferative potential, defined as being capable of subcultivation at least 70 times. Such cell lines may be derived by selecting clones that arise in primary cultures under the influence of hormones or growth stimuli or, for some tumour cell lines, by alternate culture and transplantation in animals. They have the advantage that they contain a single cell type that is immortalised and able to survive indefinitely in culture conditions, avoiding the need to obtain tissue repeatedly from living animals. They can grow as monolayers, adherent to a plastic substratum or, in the case of 'anchorage-independent' cells such as haemopoietic cells or transformed or malignant cells, as suspension cultures. However clonal cell lines may have some disadvantages: the cells may be 'transformed', implying some genetic alteration that allows unrestrained growth, and they may lose certain differentiated characteristics, acquiring abnormal morphology and karyotype.

Immortalisation of cells

Immortalisation of cells can be valuable as a way of generating new cell lines from primary cell cultures. A standard approach has been to use the SV40 virus, whose large T antigen can be transfected into quiescent non-proliferating cells to induce growth. Temperature-sensitive mutants of SV40 have become popular, such that large T antigen will be expressed at 33°C but not at 37°C: thus, the cells can be induced to proliferate at the lower temperature but become quiescent (and potentially express their differentiated characteristics) at 37°C.

A huge range of very well-characterised cell lines from human and animal tissues is now available, and these have provided a fundamental resource for the cell biological and molecular biological studies outlined earlier. Cell culture requires special dedicated facilities, including humidified 37°C incubators, laminar flow hoods and meticulous technical care to minimise contamination by bacteria and fungi. Nonetheless, it has come to be centrally important in many different disciplines, including the study of the cell cycle itself, the control of tumour growth, regulation of gene expression and developmental biology.

Protein detection

Antibody production: monoclonal antibodies

Proteins can be identified in tissue extracts on the basis of their chemical properties, using gel electrophoresis, but much modern protein detection relies on their immunological properties. Thus, proteins can be detected by their ability to react with highly specific antibodies that have been labelled with radioactivity or colour-generating reagents.

Antibodies can be raised in an animal in response to injected foreign protein, and the animal's serum may then be purified to yield the immunoglobulin fraction. These antisera are *polyclonal* in that they contain many different antibodies of differing specificity and affinity for different parts of the injected protein. Another disadvantage is that antibody production is limited to the lifetime of the immune animal. Nonetheless, their properties have been exploited to form the basis of much of the protein detection system that has developed since the early 1970s.

An alternative approach is to produce monoclonal antibodies. These are antibodies of single specificity secreted by hybrid cell lines *in vitro*. The mice immunised with the foreign protein are used as the source of antibody-producing splenocytes that are fused with myeloma cell lines to confer immortality on the resultant hybrid cells. The hybridoma cells are cloned to separate different antibody-secreting cells, which are then selected on the basis of their production of antibody reactive with the target protein. The technique of monoclonal antibody production was a major advance in immunology, allowing almost limitless production of individual well-characterised antibodies from clonal cells grown in suspension culture.

Immunocytochemistry

The proteins expressed within or on the surface of intact cells can be identified immunolog-ically using either monoclonal or polyclonal antibodies coupled to a visualisation system. This approach is particularly applicable to tissues from a whole animal but can equally be applied to cultured cells. Tissues are fixed, sectioned and processed for microscopic analy-sis as for routine histology, but with special steps taken to allow adequate penetration of antibody into the section. Antibodies may be coupled to detection reagents such as fluo-rescent dyes (e.g. fluorescein or rhodamine) without destroying their specificity, and these conjugates are able to bind to antigen present in a tissue section. Fluorescent dyes require the use of a fluorescence microscope but have a particular advantage over other detection systems in that more than one fluorochrome may be simultaneously detectable in the same cell: thus, two or more specific antibodies may be linked to different fluorochromes and exposure of the same tissue to light of different excitation wavelengths will produce differ-ent colours, allowing studies of co-localisation of different peptides.

Flow cytometry and fluorescence activated cell sorting

Antibody binding to cells can have a number of applications apart from direct visualisa-tion of protein expression. The amount of fluorescent antibody bound to each cell can be quantified by *flow cytometry*. Cells stained with fluorescent antibody can be dispersed and made to flow past a laser beam of a chosen wavelength: a first light detector is arranged to measure the amount of fluorescent light emitted, while a second light detector measures cell size by 'forward light scatter'. This technique generates a two-dimensional plot of antigen expression against cell size, giving quantitative data about different cell populations within a whole tissue.

Cells can be specifically selected, using fluorescent antibodies, according to the antigen expressed on the cell surface in a technique termed *fluorescence activated cell sorting* (FACS). A dispersed preparation of single cells can be arranged to flow in a stream as for flow cytometry: the stream is broken into droplets each containing one cell, which are charged according to whether or not they give a fluorescent signal. The charged droplets are diverted by an electric field so that these cells can be separately collected, resulting in a sorted subpopulation of cells (Fig. 2.31).

Immunoassay techniques

Proteins (and other small molecules) can be detected immunologically in complex bio-logical fluids or cell extracts using a series of different immunoassay techniques. These assay methods have amazing sensitivity and specificity and rely on quantifiable interac-tions between the protein antigen and the antibody that has been conjugated with a label. A series of labels is now available, from the traditional ^{125}I radioactive label to enzyme-linked reactions and chemiluminescent reagents that avoid the use of radioactivity. Two classical techniques, immunoassay and immunometric assay, are illustrated in Fig. 2.32 and described below.

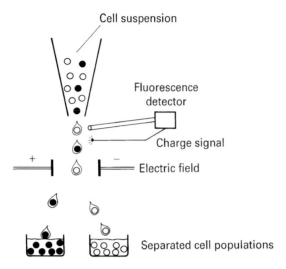

Fig. 2.31. Fluorescence activated cell sorting. A suspension of individually dispersed cells, some labelled with fluorescent dye, is separated by charging the fluorescent cells and diverting these charged cells with an electric field.

Immunoassay.   The principle involved in immunoassay is the competition between radioactively labelled antigen and the unlabelled antigen in a biological fluid for a fixed and limited amount of antibody. Various methods can be used to separate complexes of antigen–antibody from excess labelled protein, and the amount of label in the complexes is then inversely proportional to the amount of unlabelled protein, allowing a calculation to be made of its concentration. This technique was first developed in the 1960s and is still routinely used to detect very small quantities of protein, routinely down to the picomolar range (10^{-12} mol/l).

Immunometric assays.   These assays have proved even more sensitive and robust than immunoassay and have been widely developed as commercial kits for rapid measurement of antigens, including peptide (and steroid) hormones, immunoglobulins and drugs. Essentially, a first monoclonal antibody is coated onto a solid phase such as plastic, the unknown antigen solution is added and allowed to bind and, after washing, the amount of antigen bound to the solid-phase first antibody can be estimated by adding an excess of labelled second antibody. In this case, the more antigen that is present, the more labelled second antibody will be bound to the solid phase. With high-affinity monoclonal antibodies that can recognise different parts of a protein molecule, two-site immunometric assay has become highly specific and sensitive, and many automated assays can be performed simultaneously in as little as 1 hour in diagnostic laboratories.

Future perspectives

The explosion of knowledge of cell and molecular biology since the early 1970s has at times seemed abstruse and unconnected with clinical practice, yet already the practice of medicine, both diagnostic and therapeutic, has been transformed by this knowledge.

(a)

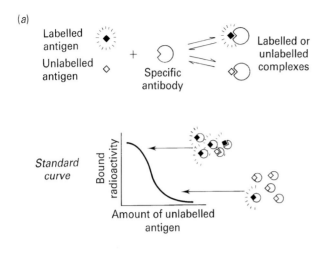

(b)

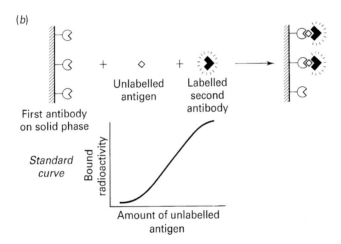

Fig. 2.32. Immunoassay techniques. (*a*) In immunoassays, competition between labelled and unlabelled antigen for limited amounts of antibody result in varying amounts of radioactivity in the antigen–antibody complexes formed. (*b*) In immunometric assays, labelled second antibody is only able to bind to the solid phase via the antigen. As a result, bound radioactivity is proportional to the amount of antigen present.

Therapeutic agents are now produced by recombinant DNA techniques, including insulin, growth hormone, erythropoietin and coagulation factor VIII, avoiding the risks and limitations of extracting these substances from human tissues. Recombinant vaccines are also becoming available, and drug design is able to look to new targets such as transcription factors. Gene therapy is already practicable for a number of diseases and is likely to make a major impact in the developed world very soon. For the practice of medicine in the Third World, too, molecular biology is now relevant to a series of issues: not only are the techniques becoming cheaper and more robust for diagnostic purposes, but the more immediate medical priorities of food supply and vaccine development are major targets for the new technology.

Summary

This chapter has reviewed key elements of molecular and cell biology that are relevant to our current understanding of some mechanisms of human disease. The aim has been to describe normal cell function, with some illustrations from specific diseases, but later chapters will have fuller accounts of pathogenetic mechanisms of different types of disease.

Analysis of gene structure has led to a clear understanding of the mechanism of gene transcription, and to the identification of many different transcription factors. In some cases, these factors are actually hormone receptors, while in others they are nuclear proteins that are activated by extracellular stimuli. Mutations in these proteins may lead to loss of function and lack of target gene expression, for example the hypopituitarism seen with mutations in the pituitary-specific factor Pit-1, while mutations in steroid and thyroid hormone receptors cause typical hormone-resistance syndromes.

Cell membrane receptors are linked to intracellular signalling systems, which are made up of chains of cellular proteins. The complexity of the signalling systems is important to enable cells to integrate many different signals from the environment. Many of these proteins may be susceptible to mutation, with loss of function or increased function, and the normal cellular proteins have been identified as the proto-oncogene counterparts to viral oncogenic proteins that commonly cause cancer.

The techniques of DNA and RNA manipulation and gene transfer have been fundamental to the dissection of normal and abnormal cellular function but have also been developed to the point where gene therapy is being applied to human diseases that are otherwise often untreatable, such as homozygous familial hypercholesterolaemia and some cancers.

FURTHER READING

Alberts, B., Bray, D., Lewis, J. *et al.* (eds.) (1994). *Molecular Biology of the Cell*, 3rd edn. New York: Garland.

Ausubel, F.M., Brent, R., Kingston, R.E. *et al.* (eds) (1995). *Current Protocols in Molecular Biology.* New York: Wiley.

Brock, D. (1993) *Molecular Genetics for the Clinician.* Cambridge: Cambridge University Press.

Brown, T.A. (1990). *Gene Cloning, An Introduction,* 2nd edn. London: Chapman & Hall.

Latchman, D.S. (1995). *Gene Regulation – A Eukaryotic Perspective,* 2nd edn. London: Chapman & Hall.

Lewin, B. (1994). *Genes V.* Oxford: Oxford University Press.

Morgan, S.J. & Darling, D.C. (1993). *Animal cell culture.* Oxford: ßIOS Scientific.

Pinkert, C.A. (1994). *Transgenic animal technology.* London: Academic Press.

Rapley, R. & Walker, M.R. (1994). *Molecular Diagnostics.* Oxford: Blackwell Scientific.

Roitt, I.M. (1994). *Essential Immunology,* 8th edn. Oxford: Blackwell Scientific.

Weatherall, D.J. (1991). *The New Genetics and Clinical Practice,* 3rd edn. Oxford: Oxford University Press.

3

Hereditary disease

G. ANDERSON, J. F. J. MORRISON AND A. F. MARKHAM

- Molecular genetic techniques enable the genetic basis of many diseases to be defined.
- Inherited disease can result from single gene changes, polygenic multifactorial causes, mitochondrial disorders or gross chromosomal disorders.
- Linkage analysis enables disease phenotypes to be correlated with inheritance of a marker region of DNA.
- Some diseases, e.g. ankylosing spondylitis, are associated with the MHC alleles.
- Cystic fibrosis is an inherited multisystem disease that has been analysed by genetic techniques.
- A mutated protein involved in chloride channels, the cystic fibrosis transmembrane conductance regulator (CFTR), has been identified and its function assessed in gene expression systems and transgenic mice.
- Gene therapy is a potential strategy to correct genomic malfunctions by introducing replacement functional DNA.
- The human genome project is intended to define the whole human genome and will provide a basis for identification and manipulation of malfunctioning genes.

Molecular genetics

The discipline of genetics involves understanding the pattern of transmission of characteristics from parent to offspring and generation to generation. The characteristics studied may be biochemical, physical or behavioural and are termed traits. The unit of inheritance is the gene. Genes are arranged in a linear fashion along chromosomes, which are composed of both coding (exons) and non-coding (introns) genetic material along with associated supporting proteins (histones). The complete set of chromosomes of an organism is called its genome and the position of an individual gene on a chromosome within the total genome is termed a locus.

The characteristic banding pattern seen on human (and other) metaphase chromosomes is produced by Giemsa staining. It is currently believed that the light bands are relatively GC rich and contain an excess of genes compared with the dark bands. Genes produce their effect largely through the production of protein molecules (Chapter 2, p. 20).

An international standard defines how the positions of genes on the chromosomes are described. The centromere is the constricted part of the chromosome where the chromatids are joined. This divides each chromosome into a short arm (p) and a long arm (q). Each arm is divided into regions that comprise one or more bands. These are numbered from the centromere out. Further reduction can give sub-bands. So the cystic fibrosis gene on chromosome 7 at sub-band 3 of band 1 of region 3 of the long arm is given as 7q31.3.

In humans there are 22 pairs of autosomes and two sex chromosomes (two X chromosomes in females and an X and Y in males), in total containing approximately 3×10^9 bp DNA, encoding between 50 000 and 100 000 different protein molecules. On average, therefore, a typical gene occupies some 30 000 bp of the human genome. In practice, human genes show an enormous variation in size from a few hundred base pairs (e.g. the β-globin gene) to several million base pairs (e.g. the dystrophin gene mutated in Duchenne muscular dystrophy). This is not necessarily reflected in the sizes of the corresponding proteins. A diploid human cell contains about 5pg (5×10^{-12} g) DNA.

Different forms of a gene at a locus are called *alleles*. Each person will carry two alleles, one on each of the pair of chromosomes. An individual is *homozygous* if both alleles are identical and *heterozygous* if they are different. The *genotype* is the genetic make-up of an organism; the *phenotype* is the characteristics of the organism (determined by its genotype and the environment) and a *haplotype* is a set of DNA markers at one locus that is inherited as a unit.

Not surprisingly, mistakes are occasionally made in this huge human lexicon containing three billion bits of information, especially when it is replicated for cell division. Hereditary disease occurs when such errors appear in germ-line (haploid) cells and are passed to the offspring. An enormous range of genetic abnormalities is found that cause disease. Problems with whole chromosome segregation at meiosis (germ cell formation) lead to monosomy or trisomy in children and cause a spectrum of conditions (Turner's syndrome, XO; Down's syndrome, trisomy 21; Edward's syndrome, trisomy 18; Patau syndrome, trisomy 13; Klinefelter's syndrome, XXY, etc.) that are lethal with most other chromosomes. Gross rearrangements of chromosomes (translocations) may occur that lead to altered numbers of many genes (gene dosage effects) so that one or three rather than two copies are present. Where translocations occur within genes, as is often the case in leukaemias and lymphomas, specific gene functions may be lost, or juxtaposition of two genes may lead to the production of a new hybrid protein with deleterious effects on the cell. For example where the immunoglobulin heavy chain or kappa or lambda light chain promoters drive c-*myc* oncogene expression as a result of a 8–14, 8–2 or 8–22 translocation, respectively, in Burkitt's lymphoma.

As well as the gross macroscopic errors, subtle microscopic mistakes at the level of individual genes have equally devastating clinical effects. Small deletions of all or part of a gene will result in loss of function and 50% reduction in gene dosage. In some circumstances, this will cause disease in a 'dominant' fashion. Where a 50% level of gene function is adequate (because the remaining functional gene makes enough protein to do its job) a heterozygote 'carrier' state arises that will lead to 'recessive' disease in a subsequent generation where two such individuals each pass their mutant gene copy to a

Table 3.1. *Examples of the ways in which small mutations alter gene function*

Site of mutation in a gene	Possible effects
Promoter	No transcription into mRNA
	Not recognised by transcription factors or RNA polymerase
	Altered transcriptional control with uncontrolled gene expression in inappropriate cells or tissues
	Transcription from alternative promoters with proteins made with altered amino-termini and different activities
Exons	Change an individual amino acid with variable, unpredictable effects on protein function
	Change a codon to a stop codon so a truncated protein is made.
	Change the real stop codon to a translated codon so that a protein with a carboxy-terminal extension is synthesised
	Small deletion or insertion mutation changes protein sequence or creates a frameshift and a premature termination codon
	Destroys a splicing site so that intronic sequence is left in processed mRNA and translated into aberrant protein
Introns	Destroys a splicing site as above
	Creates a spurious splicing site so that again intronic sequence is left in mRNA
mRNA 5′-untranslated region	Destroys ribosome recognition site
mRNA 3′-untranslated region	Destroys polyadenylation signal
	Alters an mRNA stability element leading to inappropriately long- or short-lived mRNA species and altered protein concentrations

child, who has zero gene function as a result. As a very crude rule-of-thumb, mutations in the genes for metabolic enzymes tend to be recessive whereas mutations in structural proteins tend to be dominant, either because insufficient protein is made or because the mutant protein itself interferes in some way with the proper functioning of its normal partner.

As well as rearrangements and deletions, even smaller mutations are just as damaging. Table 3.1 illustrates some of the many ways in which single point mutations or small insertions/deletions of a few base pairs can completely or partially interfere with gene function. The vast range of possible changes that can arise explains to some extent the very wide range of clinical phenotypes and disease severity observed in many inherited diseases.

Given the disastrous consequences to the organism of any of these different types of genetic damage, human cells have developed a very extensive repertoire of mechanisms to protect against such events and to repair them should they occur. Mechanisms such as programmed cell death (apoptosis) are thought to be activated after gross chromosomal damage, to ensure that the mutant cell does not divide. A wide range of processes is designed to repair damage to DNA that alters its coding capacity (e.g. where chemical carcinogens or ultraviolet light cause chemical reactions at DNA bases that change their Watson–Crick hydrogen-bonding patterns). Another subtle underlying mechanism by which hereditary diseases arise is, therefore, damage to the genes that encode the very proteins involved in protection against genome damage. Individuals with such mutations are particularly prone to additional, progressive somatic mutation, and malignancy is frequently part of the clinical picture they present. This spectrum of disease ranges from Li–Fraumeni syndrome (loss of p53 function and apoptosis capability) through chromosome fragility states (such as Bloom's syndrome) to hereditary non-polyposis colon cancer, where an inability to repair DNA mismatches is present.

Developments in molecular genetics

The study of the molecular basis of inheritance and genetics is now a mature scientific discipline and one in which there has been an astonishingly rapid acceleration in the knowledge base since the 1950s (Table 3.2).

The development of molecular genetics has benefited from advances in the associated fields of biochemistry, physical and organic chemistry, medical genetics and microbiology, which have allowed real progress to be made in the study of mechanisms of inherited disease.

The origin of modern genetics is generally agreed to be 1866 when the Austrian monk Gregor Mendel published his work on the transmission of physical characteristics in plants, outlining the first principles of inheritance. Traits were inherited independently (law of segregation) and the offspring had a pair of elements (genes) controlling the observed traits, one inherited from each parent. Mendel's studies suggested the presence of elements that could be expressed when occurring as a single copy (dominant genes) and others that required double copies (recessive genes.) His work remained neglected for many years until rediscovered by the Danish botanist Wilhelm Johannsen in 1901.

The structure and function of genes

The next major advance in the study of genetics occurred when Walter Sutton, then a medical student working with Edmund B. Wilson at Columbia University, proposed in 1902 that the traits described by Mendel were carried on chromosomes. Their work was extended by Thomas Hunt Morgan, an experimental zoologist also at Columbia University. These studies, with the fruit fly *Drosophila* again suggested that the chromosomes were carrying the genes accounting for the inherited characteristics described by Mendel. They compared the transmission of chromosomes (of which *Drosophila* had four) from parent to offspring with the Mendelian theories of gene segregation and random assortment. It was shown that genes were arranged in a linear fashion along the corresponding chromosomes and that genes on the same chromosome were linked together in transmission to offspring. However, it was noticed that this phenomena of linkage was rarely absolute and that alleles could be reassorted during meiosis when homologous chromosomes paired-up. This concept of alleles 'crossing over' was termed recombination and occurred at random, with a probability of recombination occurring

Table 3.2. *Advances in molecular biology: datelines*

Year	Advance
1866	Gregor Mendel describes a mechanism to explain the inheritance of characteristics of peas
1877	Chromosomes observed inside cells
1900	Mendel's work rediscovered independently by Danish botanist Wilhelm Johannsen
1901	Alkaptonuria described by Garrod who proposed that the enzyme defect was caused by an inherited aberrant gene; expanded theory as 'inborn errors of metabolism'
1902	Chromosomes proposed as carriers for Mendel's hereditory factors, by Sutton and Wilson at Columbia University
1905	Sex chromosomes described by Stevens and Wilson at Columbia
1908	Hardy–Weinberg law of population genetics
1911	First gene ascribed to a chromosome: Wilson at Columbia proposes that the gene for colour blindness resides on the X chromosome
1910–15	Thomas Hunt Morgan's work using the fruit fly (*Drosophila* sp.) leads to postulations that genes are arranged in line along the chromosome and that such linkage of genes was incomplete because of recombination during meiosis
1926	Muller and Stadler discover that X-rays enhance the rate of mutation in genes
1928	Griffith reports that extracts of heat-killed pathogenic strains of *Streptococcus pneumoniae* transform non-pathogenic strains into pathogenic type
1944	Avery, McCarty and Macleod show that DNA was the transforming factor in Griffith's study of *Streptococcus pneumoniae*
1952	Hershey and Chase show conclusively that DNA is the genetic element, in studies using bacteriophages
1953	Watson and Crick's studies, along with Franklin and Wilkins's work, culminate in the proposal of a double-helix model for DNA structure
1957	Ingram shows that sickle cell anaemia is the result of substitution of valine for glutamic acid at position 6 on the β-globin chain
1960	Marmur and Doty show that the two strands of the double helix can be made to separate by extremes of pH or temperature and that renaturation can be achieved by reversing these conditions
1961	Brenner and Crick propose that the genetic code for amino acids is carried by three consecutive base pairs: the 'triplet codon'
1961–66	Nirenberg, Matthaei and Khorana elucidate the codons of the genetic code
1967	DNA ligase discovered by Gilbert
1970	The restriction enzyme *Hind*III discovered by Hamilton Smith
1972	Boyer, Cohen and Berg develop techniques of cloning and creation of recombinant DNA molecules using plasmids
1975	Southern publishes report establishing the technique of blotting nucleic acid separation gels onto nitrocellulose filters and probing with labelled DNA sequences to identify specific DNA fragments (later called Southern blot)
1975–77	Novel methods for rapid DNA sequencing developed by Sanger and Barrell, and Gilbert and Maxam.
1983	RFLP identified linked to Huntington's disease gene locus on chromosome 4 by Gusella and colleagues
1985	RFLP identified linked to cystic fibrosis gene locus on chromosome 7 by Lap Tsui and colleagues
1985	Polymerase chain reaction described by Mullis
1989	Cystic fibrosis gene identified by positional cloning`
1992	A transgenic model for cystic fibrosis created
1994	Trials begin of gene therapy for cystic fibrosis using adenovirus vector

between two genes proportional (approximately) to their distance apart on the chromosome.

At around the same time (1908), the study of population genetics was advanced by the work of Hardy and Weinberg, who independently reported the association between the frequencies of alleles of genes in a given population. They stated that if a gene exists with two alleles whose frequencies are p and q then $p + q = 1$. If mating occurs at random, then the gene frequencies in the offspring will be $p^2, 2pq$ and q^2. The frequencies of the alleles will remain constant in subsequent generations in a closed population where there are no survival advantages or disadvantages for a particular genotype, except where new mutations occur or within small populations, which may lose an allele by chance.

One of the first steps towards identifying the mechanism of action of genes was taken by George Beadle and Edward Tatum investigating the production of mutants of the mould *Neurospora* by X-ray and ultraviolet irradiation. They found that the resultant mutants, which required additional nutritional factors for survival, lacked active enzymes that in the wild type produced these factors naturally. This suggested that genes produced their effects through the production of proteins. Subsequent studies defined the nature and replication of DNA, and many of the mechanisms that control the transcription and translation of genes are now being described. See Chapter 2 (p. 16) for further details. The ability of small stretches of DNA to bind to DNA of complementary sequence allows translocation of pieces of DNA from one strand to another and replication of DNA to give repeat sequences. It is likely that the families of related genes found in humans have arisen as a result of duplication and divergence during evolution from a common ancestor gene and these gene families share related functions and their products have many similarities (common domains).

Recombinant DNA

A series of discoveries and innovations at the end of the 1960s paved the way for the manipulation of DNA sequences in artificial systems, which is commonly referred to as 'genetic engineering'. The study of simple unicellular bacterial organisms provided the basis for these discoveries. The bacterial plasmid was identified as a source of transmitted antibiotic resistance in bacteria in 1965. Early attempts at sequencing DNA fragments were hampered by the lack of specific nucleases that would cut the DNA into reproducible fragments. At the time, proteins could be fragmented for sequencing more easily than DNA, using various chemical reagents or sequence-specific protease enzymes. Restriction enzymes were detected in the late 1960s by Linn and Arber; these enzymes recognise specific symmetrical (palindromic) base pair sequences and cut both the strands to generate blunt ends or overlapping 'sticky' ends (see Chapter 2, p. 38).

DNA cloning techniques were developed in the wake of the discovery of plasmids and restriction enzymes. The first hybrid DNA molecules were constructed in 1972 at Stanford University and the University of California at San Francisco in work led by Herbert Boyer, Stanley Cohen and Paul Berg, which spawned the modern 'Biotechnology' industry. The techniques involved in characterising and manipulating genes are described in Chapter 2 (p. 38). By the early 1980s, these technical achievements had set the stage for the great advances that have occurred in understanding human hereditary disease.

Basic patterns of inherited disease

Genetic approaches allow construction of models of the inheritance of traits within family groupings and within the population at large. The pattern of transmission and level of expression (penetrance) of an allele causing a disease trait defines the mode of inheritance. This approach provides information for diagnosis, dictates appropriate clinical management, predicts prognosis for affected individuals, allows counselling of parents and relatives about the probability of disease recurrence in the pedigree and generates resources for research into the molecular basis of a disease.

The prevalence of a gene in a population may be of importance in deciding the practicalities and economics of screening, either for asymptomatic persons at risk of developing a particular disease or for carriers at risk of producing affected offspring. Establishing the pattern of transmission is of critical importance in the search for the aberrant gene at the molecular level. Clinical genetics involves the management of conditions caused by a variety of genetic changes (Table 3.3):

- single gene (monogenic, Mendelian) changes
- some polygenic multifactorial conditions
- mitrochondrial disorders
- gross chromosomal disorders

The single gene disorders represent the majority of specific inherited diseases, with well over a thousand examples recorded. Given that there are 50–100 000 human genes, there are probably many more rare monogenic diseases to be characterised. However, the individual incidence of these disorders is very rare. Common clinical problems with a genetic component but with multifactorial aetiology (e.g. asthma, coronary artery disease, some forms of cancer, Alzheimer's disease, manic depression and schizophrenia) have proved very difficult to analyse because of the complex range of factors influencing pathogenesis and expression of the phenotype and also because different aetiological agents result in indistinguishable clinical pictures.

Mendelian disorders

In studies of families with a disorder passed from generation to generation (pedigree), a pattern of disease expression may be attributable to the passage of a single gene from parent to offspring. The pattern of inheritance reflects random assortment of the chromosomes and hence genes in the gametes of the parents, the presence of two homologous chromosomes each with a single copy of the gene and the possibility of recombination events. The extent of disease expression resulting from a mutant gene in an individual may be variable both in terms of incidence in those inheriting a mutant disease allele (*penetrance*) and in terms of severity (*expressivity*). The mode of inheritance of a disease,

Table 3.3. *Basic patterns of inherited disease*

Type	Examples
Whole chromosome disorders	Down's syndrome (trisomy 21)
Translocations of DNA	Burkitt's lymphoma
Amplification of triplet repeats	Myotonic dystrophy
Single gene changes	
Autosomal dominant	Huntington's disease
Autosomal recessive	Cystic fibrosis
X-linked	Haemophilia A
Multifactorial polygenic disorders	Diabetes mellitus
Disorders of the mechanisms protecting against *genome damage*	Hereditary non-polyposis colon cancer
Mitochondrial DNA disorders	Familial mitochondrial encephalomyopathy

i.e. recessive, dominant or X-linked, does not necessarily imply a particular molecular mechanism but simply mutation at a single genetic locus. Diseases linked to the non-sex chromosomes are termed autosomal.

Autosomal dominant diseases

Autosomal dominant inheritance implies that possession of a single copy of a mutant gene is sufficient for full expression of the disease phenotype. The specific characteristics of a dominant mode of inheritance are that disease occurs in the heterozygote state and that 50% of offspring will be affected from a mating with one parent affected (unless there is incomplete penetrance or expressivity or where there has been a new mutation in a child). The other important discriminating features are equal male/female incidence and usually equal male to male/female and female to male/female transmission (Fig. 3.1).

An autosomal dominant disorder with a severe effect on reproductive ability would rapidly disappear from the population, so it is not surprising that in many of these conditions the age of disease onset is typically delayed until later in life (e.g. Huntington's disease). Alternatively, there may be incomplete penetrance/expressivity of the gene (myotonic dystrophy) or a significant number of new mutations may occur (Duchenne muscular dystrophy, Marfan's syndrome, retinoblastoma and tuberose sclerosis). Overall, the frequency of mutant genes in the population (all in affected individuals) will be relatively low (Table 3.4). Other interesting phenomena that may be seen are an increasing severity of a disease as it passes through several generations, termed 'anticipation' (e.g. myotonic dystrophy) and an increased severity of a disease when inherited from a particular sex of parent. For example, father to son transmission in Huntington's disease seems to result in expression earlier in life. The reverse is true for myotonic dystrophy, with earlier onset when the gene is inherited from the mother.

Although traditional dogma states that for a disease to be labelled dominant full disease expression only requires a single mutant copy of the gene, there are certain

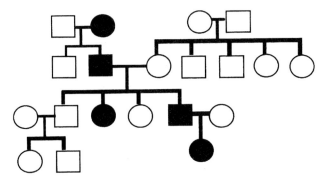

Fig. 3.1. Autosomal dominant pedigree: □, unaffected male; ■, affected male; ○, unaffected female; ●, affected female.

Table 3.4. *Autosomal dominant diseases*

Disorder	Approximate incidence
Adult-onset polycystic kidney disease	1:1250
Huntington's disease	1:3000
Familial polyposis coli	1:8000
Myotonic dystrophy	1:8000
Marfan's syndrome	1:20 000
Tuberose sclerosis	1:100 000

exceptions. Familial hypercholesterolaemia is the result of a defect in the low density lipoprotein (LDL) receptor leading to reduced numbers of receptors available for the endocytosis of these cholesterol-transport particles. Inheritance of a single copy of the defective gene is common, affecting around 1 in 500 people in Caucasian populations and resulting in a twofold or greater increase in plasma cholesterol. Diagnosis may be made at birth through a sample of umbilical cord blood taken for measurement of cholesterol levels and the ratio of LDL to high density lipoprotein (HDL). The clinical sequelae of this persistently elevated serum cholesterol level include accelerated atherosclerosis with premature coronary artery disease in the fourth and fifth decades and tendon xanthomata, xanthelasma and corneal arcus. Two copies of a defective LDL receptor gene result in homozygous affected individuals with an exaggerated disease severity, a massive increase in serum cholesterol and extremely accelerated artherosclerosis, with death from myocardial infarction in the late teens if the disease is left untreated. Treatment is usually with drugs to block endogenous cholesterol synthesis (hydroxymethyl glutaryl coenzyme A (HMG-CoA) reductase inhibitors) or sometimes by liver transplantation in homozygotes. Very recently, *ex vivo* gene therapy has been attempted with retroviruses used as vectors to introduce functional LDL receptor genes to biopsied patient hepatocytes. These transformed cells have been reinfused into patients and have been shown to lower cholesterol levels.

Autosomal recessive diseases

In autosomal recessive diseases, the presence of two copies of the mutant gene trait on homologous chromosomes is required for disease expression, i.e. a homozygous state. Although these disorders tend to be uncommon, the frequency of mutant genes in populations may be relatively high. As inherited diseases of this type frequently have an onset in infancy and a marked effect on reproductive fitness, the number of affected children born to affected parents is relatively low. Most patients will be the offspring of unaffected 'carrier' parents. The most common example in Caucasian populations is cystic fibrosis, which for unknown reasons has a high carrier incidence of up to 1 in 20 people in northern Europe. Presumably this reflects some reproductive advantage for heterozygotes. It has been suggested that this may have been resistance to cholera in the past because the cystic fibrosis gene encodes a membrane protein, the cystic fibrosis transmembrane regulator protein (CFTR), with properties of a chloride channel. Excessive chloride loss with diarrhoea is a distinctive feature of cholera. The comparable disease in populations of African origin is sickle-cell anaemia. Here the carrier rate for this mutation in the β-globin gene is as high as 1 in 12 in some populations, with resulting disease incidences of around 1 in 600. Heterozygotes are thought to be at a survival advantage because of a relative resistance to carriage of malaria parasites in their red blood cells. In this type of inherited disease, the characteristics are that the parents are commonly unaffected, and from a mating of two heterozygotes 25% of the offspring are homozygous for the normal gene, 50% are heterozygotes and 25% are homozygous for the mutant gene and, therefore, express the disease phenotype (Fig. 3.2). Other important discriminatory features include an equal male:female incidence, skipping of generations and an increased occurrence rate after consanguineous marriages.

The molecular basis for many autosomal recessive disorders has been determined at the protein level, as exemplified by the known biochemical defects resulting in the various inborn errors of metabolism. Individually, these range from rare to vary rare disorders, but collectively they may be present in 1 in 500 to 1 in 1000 live births. In these diseases, the loss of function of an enzyme, either as a consequence of a decreased quantity of protein synthesised or as a result of impaired enzyme specific activity, results in blockage of a metabolic pathway and build-up of potentially toxic metabolic intermediates with resulting side-effects.

Amongst the most common of such conditions is *phenylketonuria*, caused by a deficiency of phenylalanine hydroxylase, which catalyses the conversion of phenylalanine to tyrosine. This arises from mutations in the phenylalanine hydroxylase gene on chromosome 4. The result is elevated serum and urine levels of phenylalanine and its neurotoxic by-products (phenylpyruvate, phenylacetate, phenyllactate and phenylacetylglutamine). The incidence is approximately 1 in 10000 births and all new-born babies are routinely screened using the Guthrie test so that treatment can be initiated within the first 30 days of life. Avoidance of phenylalanine by means of a carefully prepared diet during the critical period when the CNS is developing prevents the development of the devastating clinical sequelae of mental retardation, hyperactivity, seizures, skin hypopigmentation and eczema.

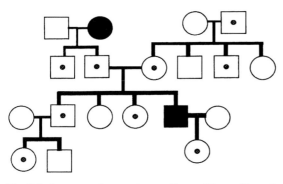

Fig. 3.2. Autosomal recessive pedigree: □, unaffected male; ■, affected male; ⊡, carrier male; ○, unaffected female; ●, affected female, ⊙, carrier female.

These features of autosomal recessive disorders have many practical implications. In most families, a single affected child is the only afflicted member of the pedigree. This makes accurate clinical diagnosis essential for genetic counselling and also makes research into the location and nature of the underlying defect more difficult. By the same token, a cluster of individuals in a pedigree all affected by a rare recessive inherited disease may suggest the possibility of a consanguineous mating (Table 3.5).

X-Linked disorders

X-linked transmission occurs when the mutant gene locus is on the X chromosome. Disease expression varies between the sexes because of the presence of two X chromosomes in the female and a single X in the male. The Lyon hypothesis (single active X chromosome) states that in the female one of the two X chromosomes in each cell is randomly inactivated early in development. This results in an organism that is mosaic in terms of X chromosome expression. Males inheriting a copy of the mutant X-linked gene on their single X chromosome will express the disease phenotype. The Y chromosome does not behave as a homologous chromosome. The discriminating features for X-linked transmission include absence of transmission of disease from father to son and skipped generations of female carriers between generations of affected males. Rarely, X-linked recessive conditions may present in homozygous female offspring of an affected father and carrier mother or in XO females (Turner's syndrome) (Table 3.6, Fig. 3.3).

Multifactorial/polygenic disorders

Diseases in which there is familial clustering are common. In these disorders, the frequency of disease in a pedigree is higher than can be explained by chance or by apparent exposure to common environmental factors. Incidence is higher than in the population as a whole, but the pattern does not conform to a recognised form of single gene (Mendelian) transmission. The majority of common diseases in adults have been noted to occur in familial clusters, to a greater or lesser degree, for example diabetes mellitus, essential hypertension, coronary artery disease, schizophrenia, manic depressive

Table 3.5. *Autosomal recessive diseases*

Disorder	Approximate incidence
Haemochromatosis	1:300
Cystic fibrosis	1:2500
Sickle cell anaemia	Wide variation (approximately 1:600) depending on ethnic origin
Thalassaemias	Wide variation depending on ethnic origin
Alpha-1 antitrypsin deficiency	1:3500
Phenylketonuria	1:13 000
Wilson's disease	1:30 000

Table 3.6. *X-linked diseases*

Disorder	Approximate incidence
Colour blindness	1:10 males
Duchenne and Becker's muscular dystrophy	1:3500 males
Fragile-X syndrome	1:1500 males
Glucose 6-phosphate dehydrogenase deficiency	Common
Haemophilia A	1:7000 males
Hypophosphataemic rickets	Rare
Testicular feminisation	Rare

psychosis, Alzheimer's disease, atopy, asthma and various cancers (colon, breast, ovary, uterus, prostate, etc.) It is apparent from epidemiological studies that both a genetic predisposition and factors from the environment, such as smoking, diet, exercise, air pollution and occupation, etc., may combine to produce disease. However, dissecting out their relative contributions has been impossible to perform with confidence until recently. The genetic component of these disorders can be thought of as the cumulative effect of a number of genes that interact to increase the risk of disease expression if the appropriate environmental conditions are present.

Another possibility is that common polygenic diseases represent collections of different single gene disorders that all share a clinical phenotype. Unfortunately, there are complicating factors such as the situations when the same genotype produces different phenotypes and when different genotypes produce an indistinguishable phenotype (phenocopies). The degree of disease expression (penetrance) is frequently variable and this will hamper investigators who lack unified criteria for diagnosis in epidemiological and genetic studies. Asthma, for example, is largely a symptom-based diagnosis, and coronary artery disease may be asymptomatic until very advanced and may present as sudden unexplained death. The relative risk for an individual in an affected pedigree is difficult

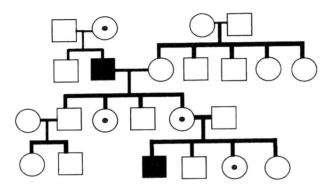

Fig. 3.3. X-linked recessive pedigree: □, unaffected male; ■, affected male; ○, unaffected female; ⊙, carrier female.

to judge but may often best be estimated by examining the pedigree and comparing this with previously established recurrence risks for other similar pedigrees. The degree of genetic contribution to particular diseases can be estimated most effectively by comparing the relative risk between identical (monozygotic) and non-identical (dizygotic) twins. Concordance rates should be significantly higher in the former group. Unlike single gene disorders, the recurrence risk for first-degree relatives of patients with polygenic disorders is typically considerably less than the 25 or 50% expected in Mendelian traits.

Linkage analysis

Linkage studies are used in pedigrees to study diseases with unknown biochemical defects by detecting linked transmission of a marker region of DNA on one chromosome with possession of the disease phenotype. A genetic marker is simply any feature of the human genome that can be discriminated between and within individuals, e.g. the ABO blood groups. Polymorphisms, those regions of DNA that can occur in more than one form, are markers that can be detected by the occurrence or lack of a restriction endonuclease site (restriction fragment length polymorphism (RFLP), see Chapter 2, p. 52) (Fig. 3.4). Nowadays, polymorphic sequence variations occurring randomly in human DNA can be examined rapidly by a variety of PCR techniques (p. 45). The closer a marker DNA sequence is to the disease gene itself, the less frequently the two will be separated by homologous recombination occurring at meiosis. The recombination rate between genetic marker and disease phenotype can give an estimate of their physical separation. The unit of recombination is the morgan. A recombination rate of 1 in 100 matings (1 cM) will occur when the genes are approximately 1000 kb (10^6 bp) apart. The whole human genome is approximately 3000 cM (3×10^9 bp). At a recombination distance of 50 cM, with a 50% chance of recombination, the co-segregation rate of 'linked' loci is reduced to that arising by random assortment of the paired chromosomes. The use of sophisticated statistical methods to determine the relevance of an observed segregation of markers in affected and unaffected individuals is vital to ensure that the results have not arisen by chance alone.

The two most common methods used to assess linkage are the LOD score and sib-pair

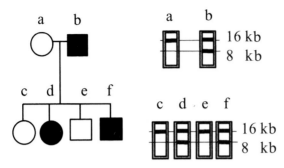

Fig. 3.4. The inheritance of a physical trait in a family may be associated with the inheritance of a genetic characteristic, e.g. the presence or absense of a restriction enzyme site. RFLPs with DNA markers close to the site of a disease locus may show linkage and permit the inherited disease to be tracked within a family. In the above case, the disease phenotype is associated with the presence of an extra band on the DNA blot at 8 kb on the southern blots.

analysis. The LOD score stands for logarithm of the odds that linkage is present as against it having arisen by chance. A score of 3 or more is usually taken to be significant. This score means that the odds of an observed linkage of a polymorphic marker to the disease phenotype occurring by chance alone rather than reflecting genuine linkage are at least 1 in 1000 against. Similarly, a LOD score of 4 implies that the odds against linkage are 1 in 10 000, and so on. Sib-pair analysis examines whether two or more siblings from a pedigree have inherited the same allele along with the disease phenotype. Linkage is implied if a particular allele segregates with disease more frequently than would be expected by chance. Often in this method, only affected individuals are studied and, therefore, the penetrance of the disease is not a confounding variable as it can be in linkage analysis.

Polymorphic markers

A large number of genetic loci are polymorphic in humans. It has been estimated that between 0.1 and 1% of all base are variable. Such genetic markers are usually dimorphic (one of two possibilities is found). This type of polymorphism, the basis of RFLP, is of limited value because many individuals will be uninformative, especially where the frequencies of the two forms are unequal. An RFLP is no use in a pedigree if obligate carriers are not heterozygous. In practice, this meant that many of the families initially collected for linkage analysis could not be used (they were 'uninformative'). The result was that very large numbers of pedigrees were needed for linkage studies, an unrealistic proposition in rarer conditions. The level of 'informativeness' anticipated is reflected in a factor termed the 'polymorphism information content' (PIC) value, which is greatest for any RFLP when the frequencies of each allele in the population are 0.5.

Minisatellites (VNTRs)

A major advance in human genetics was the discovery of very highly polymorphic genetic markers. The first type discovered was called minisatellites or VNTRs (for variable number of tandem repeats). A few thousand of these markers are found scattered throughout the human genome, with some concentration near the telomeres at the ends of chromosomes. To a first approximation, there may be a minisatellite once every million base pairs in human DNA. The variability of these sequences is caused by the fact that they comprise large numbers of repeated sequence blocks of approximately 10–30bp. The numbers of such blocks at each locus in individuals is extremely variable. Therefore, when analysed using this class of genetic marker, the vast majority of individuals are fully informative at every minisatellite locus and all affected pedigrees are useful in linkage studies. The number of families needed for a linkage study falls proportionately.

Microsatellites

Nowadays, a new generation of highly polymorphic genetic markers termed microsatellites are routinely used in molecular genetic analysis. The simple practical explanation for this is that the microsatellites can be easily examined using PCR (see Chapter 2, p. 45). Microsatellites are similar to minisatellites except that the allele size is smaller, consisting of repeats of di-, tri- and tetranucleotides; the number of such repeats is again highly variable and microsatellite markers are highly informative. Furthermore, there are estimated to be 30 000 microsatellite sequences in the human genome, which means that one occurs approximately every 10^5bp in human DNA. Therefore, highly informative genetic markers are now available in very close proximity to all human genes. This is the basis of the current genetic map of the human genome and represents a major achievement of the international Human Genome Mapping Project.

Linkage analysis techniques have been developed that can estimate the number of genetic loci associated with polygenic disorders and their relative contributions to disease expression. The growing number of recognised human polymorphisms allows complementary approaches to be taken. Polymorphism in or close to candidate genes (genes with a putative role in the disorder) can be used to detect linkage in some of the affected pedigrees. Examples include a polymorphism in an intron of the angiotensin converting enzyme (ACE) gene, which segregates as one of the many independent risk factors for myocardial infarction; the glucokinase gene on 7p 13 and hepatocellular nuclear factor gene on chromosomes 12q24 and 20q13 in maturity-onset diabetes of the young (MODY), a rare autosomal dominant form of non-insulin-dependent diabetes mellitus (NIDDM). Microsatellite markers can also be used to assess linkage to a number of loci simultaneously. Combined with computerised statistical analysis, this may provide evidence for involvement of a number of disease genes and their approximate location in the genome. For example, in insulin-dependent diabetes mellitus, there are at least 18 separate genetic loci associated with an increased relative risk of developing the condition, presumably secondary to exposure to an environmental agent that triggers pancreatic islet cell autoimmunity. To overcome the confounding variables of environmental factors and genetic heterogeneity, study design is, of necessity, extremely complex.

The classification of disease is frequently imprecise in clinical practice, and absolute

Table 3.7. *HLA alleles and disease*

Disorder	Allele
Addison's disease	B8
Ankylosing spondylitis	B27
Chronic active hepatitis	B8
Coeliac disease	B8
Haemochromatosis	A3/B14
Insulin-dependent diabetes	DR3/4
Narcolepsy	DR2
Rheumatoid arthritis	DR4
Seronegative spondyloarthropathies	B27

diagnostic accuracy in pedigrees is really required for the study of inherited conditions. The probability of identifying groups of patients and families with a homogeneous genetic make-up may be increased by choosing only those with the most severely affected phenotype, only those with early age at onset or by confining analysis to discrete isolated populations and ethnic groupings. To overcome environmental contributions, analysis may be limited to affected individuals only, on the assumption that whatever environmental factors predispose to disease, they have then already acted and the genetic predisposition is undoubtedly present. To allow the potential contributions of the vast number of permutations of inherited gene variations to be examined, individual comparisons can be directed at (affected) siblings who will share a more similar overall genetic background: the sib-pair approach.

The major histocompatibility complex and disease susceptibility

In the study of multifactorial disease, it has been found that some diseases can be associated with the presence of certain alleles within the genes of the major histocompatibility complex (MHC, also known in humans as HLA, the human leucocyte antigen complex). The MHC is a genetic region on the short arm of human chromosome 6, where genes encoding the class I and class II surface antigen-presenting proteins are located. The MHC class I locus expressed on all cells consists of four separate loci, A, B, C and D, concerned with the functioning of the immune system. The locus is involved in the presentation of peptides to immune effector cells, allowing the identification of self and the recognition of foreign antigens. Neighbouring regions are involved in the regulation of the immune response. The individual MHC loci have a number of distinct alleles encoding immunologically discrete proteins. Certain of these individual alleles have been found to confer susceptibility to disease in discrete populations (Table 3.7).

The best known example is the association of the *HLA-B27* allele and *ankylosing spondylitis*, a disease of unknown aetiology characterised by inflammation affecting the axial skeletal joints, with extra-articular manifestations such as aortitis and aortic regurgitation, pulmonary fibrosis (with a predilection for the upper zones) and uveitis. There is a strong association between *HLA-B27* and disease, with the presence of this antigen in 95% of affected individuals. However, the *HLA-B27* allele occurs in 6–14% of the population and only 10% of these will go on to develop ankylosing spondylitis. The incidence rises to 30% in those with affected relatives and to 50% in those with an affected parent. This indicates the necessity for additional factors in disease expression, including both environmental effects and alleles at different genetic loci: the pathogenesis remains obscure but a number of findings suggest involvement of the B27 antigen directly in the disease process. A transgenic model of the human disease has been produced, with animals containing the human *HLA-B27* allele spontaneously developing spondylitis.

These diseases with a strong association to alleles of the MHC represent a different example of linkage analysis, where the alleles of genes with known function rather than anonymous DNA markers are used. When alleles are present in association with a disease phenotype more frequently than expected by chance in a given population the marker allele is described as being in *linkage disequilibrium* with the disease locus. The implication of this finding is that the distance separating the two loci is small and that, since the original mutation occurred to produce the disease gene, this minimal separation has resulted in few recombination events, with alleles at the two linked genetic loci inherited together at a frequency greater than that predicted from their prevalence in that population. A example of such a phenomenon is the inherited disorder *haemochromatosis*, which has been found to be closely linked to the *HLA-A3* locus. Haemochromatosis is a disorder of iron storage with excessive intestinal absorption and accumulation of iron, resulting in damage to various tissues including liver, heart, pancreas, pituitary and the joints. The disease is typically inherited in an autosomal recessive manner with variable penetrance. The disease gene(s) occurs at high frequency in the population, with about 10% carriers and 0.25% homozygotes who are susceptible to develop the disease.

A similar range of diseases shows an association with HLA class II gene alleles, as revealed by significantly increased relative risks in individuals with particular genotypes. A number of these associations are striking, including pemphigus vulgaris (*DR4*), narcolepsy (*DRB1*1501*), Goodpasture's syndrome (*DR2*) and Sjogren's syndrome (*DQB1*0201*).

In summary, it is now well appreciated that many diseases have a genetic component in terms of both predisposition to occurrence as well as age of onset and severity. Only relatively few individuals with inherited diseases have conditions with clear cut single gene Mendelian inheritance. Most are polygenic or multifactorial in aetiology, with a significant environmental component. In many disease states a common clinical phenotype conceals a multifactorial aetiology and may encompass a number of less frequently encountered subsets, each with a single gene pattern of inheritance. There are a number of well-defined examples of this in clinical medicine, including Alzheimer's disease (the common cause of senile dementia, where approximately 10% of cases are thought to be monogenic-familial Alzheimer's disease (FAD). FAD is further subdivided into FAD-1, FAD-2, FAD-3 and FAD-4 depending on whether the mutation present is in a gene on chromosome 21q21, 19q13, 14q24 or 1q31, respectively). Further examples are non-insulin-dependent diabetes mellitus (where MODY constitutes a set of clinically indistinguishable autosomal dominant diseases arising from mutations in several independent genes, as discussed above) and coronary artery disease (where different subsets are associated with familial hypercholesterolaemia, apolipoprotein B or E abnormalities and lipoprotein Lp(a) variants). These are all obviously complicated by multiple environmental factors. Therefore, separate but complementary approaches must be used to elucidate the mechanisms of inherited disease. Population studies are used to identify patterns of disease and determine common alleles predisposing to, or modifying, disease expression in polygenic disease. Single gene disorders are studied, which, by defining the fundamental biochemical and genetic defects involved, may shed light on related complex multifactorial disorders. In the next section, the specialised tools of the molecular geneticist are explained followed by a description of their use in the investigation of inherited diseases.

Specialised techniques

Vectors

Vectors are used to carry segments of DNA into a cell where it can be identified and pro-duced in larger amounts. The large size of eukaryotic genes was an obstacle for many years when probing the aetiology of inherited disease. The development of improved DNA cloning vectors such as cosmids and yeast artificial chromosomes has greatly facil-itated the search for inherited disease loci and the characterisation and manipulation of the genes involved.

Cosmids.   Cosmids are derived from bacteriophage vectors and will allow the integration of up to 50 000 bp of foreign DNA between the phage vector arms, this being the maximum possible to allow successful viral particle packaging. The large size of cosmids permits the construction of maps of chromosome regions using overlapping, adjoining (contiguous) cosmid clones, which are termed *contigs*. In the search for an inherited disease, it is possible to move rapidly along the chromosome from a DNA marker to the disease locus itself in jumps of approximately 50 000 bp by analysing con-secutive cosmid clones. A knowledge of the direction travelled along the chromosome is required and the process is simplified if flanking markers are available, so demarcating the region of interest and allowing genome 'walking' inwards from both flanks towards the disease gene.

Yeast artificial chromosomes (YACs).   These are constructed from sections of yeast chromosomes that are required for autologous replication of these chromosomes within the yeast cell. The constructs contain two telomeres (one at each end), a centromere (for attachment to the mitotic spindle) and a yeast DNA replication origin along with the inserted foreign DNA fragment. Selectable markers are also incorporated to allow recombinant yeast clones containing a YAC to be grown in media lethal for untrans-formed yeast host cells. The capacity of this class of vector for exogenous DNA is vast (over 1000 kb) and this has allowed cloning and characterisation of genes at a very much faster rate than was previously attainable. However, this technique would not have been so useful without the development of methods to separate such very large DNA sequences for analysis without fragmenting them. DNA molecules of over a million base pairs are extremely long and are easily broken physically by shear forces in solution. For this reason, very large DNA fragments are usually handled in the solid phase by immobilising them in blocks of agarose (Chapter 2, p. 43).

Positional cloning

The combination of YAC cloning with PFGE (see Chapter 2, p. 43) for manipulating large DNA fragments allows the construction of long-range physical maps of chromosomes. This is extremely helpful in the task of determining the location of an inherited disease gene when a marker closely linked to the disease is available but the molecular defect is unknown. The process is known as *positional cloning* (originally called reverse genetics). When a disease is mapped (i.e. linkage is established between a disease gene and a marker locus), the physical distance between them can be estimated by the frequency at which they become separated in meiosis: the recombination rate. As this is reduced, to say 1 cM, the disease gene in physical terms is usually within about 1000 kb of the linked marker (the recombination rate varies throughout the genome). The closer the markers are to the gene of interest, the larger the size of the study population required for detection of recombination events. The key to localising disease genes is, therefore, to identify two closely linked DNA markers flanking the area of interest followed by the construction of a physical map, which will remove the dependence on the detection of recombination events. The fragment of DNA defined by both flanking markers is the starting point for further chromosome walking and sequencing in towards the disease gene itself.

PCR

The development of PCR (see Chapter 2, p. 45) has revolutionised molecular genetics as a whole, including positional cloning exercises and RFLP analysis. PCR prior to restriction digestion allows RFLP analysis to be performed on much smaller quantities of starting DNA. This is particularly advantageous, for example, in prenatal diagnosis where PCR permits the presence or absence of RFLPs to be detected rapidly.

PCR can also be used to amplify satellite elements by using primers complementary to sequences flanking the microsatellite or minisatellite repeats. The size of the PCR product then reflects the number of repeats. This procedure has dramatically increased the speed and power of molecular genetics in pedigree linkage analysis. In addition, it has also been discovered that a number of human diseases are caused by spontaneous increases in the copy number of trinucleotide repeats at certain locations, which can be detected by PCR. This list of these disorders now includes myotonic dystrophy, Huntington's disease, fragile X syndrome, spinocerebellar ataxia I, dentatorubral pallidoluysian atrophy, fragile X 'E' and Machado–Joseph disease.

DNA sequencing can now be performed without the need to obtain a clone to generate a reasonable quantity of single-stranded DNA. Rapid sequencing can be achieved using PCR to extend the template DNA in the presence of oligonucleotide primers and

chain-terminating dideoxynucleoside triphosphates. Routine detection of known mutations is also now possible using PCR. Cystic fibrosis carriers are now detected employing this technique and minute sample size requirements allow accurate prenatal testing.
The most frequently used approach is the amplification refractory mutation system
('ARMS'). In this method, at least one of the pair of reaction primers is designed so that
its 3′-terminal residue lies precisely at the disease-causing point mutation site. Two parallel tests are usually run together. In the first, the allele-specific primer is complementary to the normal sequence. In the second, it is complementary to the mutant
sequence. A product is obtained only when the 3′-residues form base pairs so that the
oligonucleotide can prime synthesis correctly. The products obtained in the 'normal' and
'mutant' reactions allow normal and mutant homozygotes as well as heterozygote carriers (where a product is obtained with both primers) to be rapidly and accurately identified.

Finding genes for inherited diseases

The new strategies in molecular genetics have allowed the discovery of genes causing
inherited diseases without any prior knowledge of their biological function. Up to the
early 1980s, our best approach was to determine the biochemical aberration peculiar to
that disease. An abnormal protein (e.g. haemoglobin S in sickle cell anaemia), an absent
protein (e.g. lack of α- or β-globin in thalassaemias), the presence of inactive forms or
complete lack of a functional enzyme (e.g. phenylalanine hydroxylase in phenylketonuria) are examples where the biochemical abnormality was identified. Once an
understanding was gained of the metabolic basis of the disease, attention was focused
on partially sequencing the aberrant protein and using the genetic code to produce a
degenerate series of 'best guess' oligonucleotide probes to screen cDNA and genomic
DNA libraries for matching clones. Positive clones were sequenced to confirm that they
encoded the responsible protein. Genes were then cloned and sequenced from affected
individuals to demonstrate the presence of mutations. This was invariably a difficult and
time-consuming process.

Despite numerous short-cuts and innovations to facilitate this overall procedure
(even including PCR), it remains a laborious business and obviously the approach
cannot be used if the primary biochemical defect is uncertain. Positional cloning is used
to overcome this problem. Linkage of a disease locus to a genetic marker, either a protein
or more commonly a DNA polymorphism, can be established by demonstrating co-
segregation of disease and marker in affected families as discussed above. There must
be a large number of marker loci covering the genome evenly to allow all regions of the
chromosomes to be screened with markers no more than about 10cM apart; above this
distance recombination events make the markers less powerful. The polymorphic
markers must be straightforward to use and detect and we have described the types that
have been used: protein polymorphisms (greatly restricted by their small number and
limited polymorphism), RFLPs and (by far the most useful) microsatellite markers.

Since the late 1980s, positional cloning has achieved major breakthroughs (Table 3.8).
The use of the techniques described above to elucidate the genetic basis of an inher-

Table 3.8. *Genes identified by positional cloning*

Disorder	Altered product
Duchenne muscular dystrophy	Dystrophin protein
Cystic fibrosis	Cystic fibrosis transmembrane conductance regulator protein (CFTR)
Myotonic dystrophy	DM gene with unstable $(AGC)_n$ triplet repeats (disease severity parallels n)
Huntington's disease	Huntingtin protein
Retinoblastoma	p 105–RB protein
Fragile X mental retardation	Fragile site in the X chromosome caused by (CCG) triplet amplification
Chronic granulomatous disease	Electron transport protein

ited disease and the result of those gene changes is exemplified in the study of cystic fibrosis.

CYSTIC FIBROSIS

Cystic fibrosis (CF) is a common, life-threatening, inherited multisystem disease usually with onset in early childhood. Although death was usual in the second decade, advances in clinical management with improved physiotherapy, antibiotic regimens and treatment for malabsorption problems with pancreatic digestive enzyme supplements mean that an increasing proportion of patients are surviving into adulthood. The disease occurs in all geographical regions and populations, but the incidence varies considerably between different ethnic groups, being greatest in those of northern European ancestry. In these northern European populations, CF occurs at a frequency of about 1 in 2500–3000 live births and represents the most common life-threatening autosomal recessive genetic disease.

   CF is characterised clinically by obstruction of exocrine glands, with viscid secretions. This leads to chronic airways infection, bronchiectasis with eventual respiratory failure, and functional failure of the exocrine pancreas resulting in food malabsorption and growth failure. Additional features include biliary cirrhosis, chronic sinusitis and infertility in males. The first full description of the clinical syndrome of CF was reported in the 1940s and was followed by the realisation that it followed an autosomal recessive pattern of inheritance (Table 3.9). Thereafter, despite much research into the underlying biochemical defects, the aetiology of CF remained obscure. By the early 1980s, a number of groups of researchers were trying to determine the cause of CF by circumventing biochemical studies and looking directly for the disease gene.

Identifying the disease gene

The task of finding a particular genetic locus within the vast human genome has often been compared to hunting for a needle in a haystack. The gene in question must be

Table 3.9. *Cystic fibrosis: datelines*

Year	Advance
1938	First description of CF as a distinct clinical entity by D.H. Anderson in New York
1940s	Suggestion that CF is typified by failure of exocrine glands to empty their mucous secretions, causing damage to the pancreas and lungs
	Antibiotics introduced as treatment for lung sepsis.
	Autosomal recessive inheritance pattern recognised.
1950s	Excessive loss of salt demonstrated in children with CF, leading to development of the pilocarpine iontophoresis sweat test for the diagnosis of CF
1960 and 1970s	Improved supportive care resulting in markedly increased survival of affected individuals
1980s	The genetic locus of CF is tracked down to the long arm of chromosome 7
	First linkage detected with the locus of the genetic determinant of serum paroxonase activity
1985	Then using anonymous informative RFLP DNA markers to screen for linkage in affected pedigrees, a flurry of papers detailing DNA markers with linkage to the CF locus appeared: Lap-Chee Tsui and co-workers
1989	Putative locus and mutations described after 'walking and jumping' along chromosome 7
	Characterisation of the CF gene: cystic fibrosis transmembrane conductance regulator (CFTR)
	Early studies showed reversal of defective chloride channel regulation in CF airway epithelial cells following expression of normal CFTR but not the mutant gene
	Transgenic mouse models of CF were created by gene targeting, producing mice homozygous for disrupted CFTR genes; these mice showed pathological changes in a number of organs similar to those found in human CF
1990s	Gene therapy for CF pursued. Animal and phase I clinical trials in humans (safety). Using recombinant CFTR DNA, trials examining the safety and efficacy of administration using liposomal and adenovirus vectors
	Trials of prenatal genetic screening for CF, addressing the practicalities, efficacy and cost–benefit of a routine service

detected in a genome containing 3×10^9 bp DNA, coding for between 50 000 and 100 000 genes. Much of the DNA is not transcribed and has no apparent function. It has often been called 'junk' DNA, although perhaps we currently lack the insight to understand its role. Trying to find a 30 000 bp sequence of DNA (the size of the average gene) within the human genome is difficult enough. Pinpointing a single point mutation in these 30 000 bp is even more daunting. Therefore, identifying the disease gene at a specific locus appears an almost impossible task. However, with a systematic approach and using a number of ingenious short-cuts, finding single base pair mutations in the human genome has now become possible. Having some pointer towards chromosomal localisation is always a major advantage. For example, the chromosome may be known from cytogenetic analysis (e.g. fragile X syndrome, retinoblastoma, Wilm's tumour, etc.) or because of sex-linked inheritance (e.g. Duchenne muscular dystrophy).

The initial step is to localise a given disease gene to a single chromosome and specific subregions; nowadays the most commonly used linkage markers are polymorphic di-, tri- or tetranucleotide 'microsatellite' repeats (see p. 77). Since its development in the late 1980s as a method of determining genetic linkage, the microsatellite analysis technique has been progressively enhanced by using fluorescence-based technology with auto-mated reading and improved genome coverage. In the mid-1990s, there are thousands of marker loci available, providing coverage at an average separation of less than 3 cM. Using microsatellite markers, linkage can be established between the disease locus and two flanking markers, so demarcating the sequence of DNA of interest.

The next step in identifying a disease gene is the construction of a physical map of the area flanked by the linked markers, as discussed above. Long-range physical maps have become a possibility with the development of the techniques for the manipulation of large fragments of DNA (in the range of 1 million base pairs): PFGE to separate large DNA fragments, rare-cutting restriction enzymes to produce these fragments of DNA and YACs to clone them. The YACs used in this process can either be constructed *de novo* or be obtained from clone libraries already in existence, such as those produced by the Généthon group in Paris, which are cross-indexed with their microsatellite marker system. A number of YAC clones may be necessary covering the region of interest to establish a set of clones spanning the locus. This set of contiguous clones is called a 'contig'.

Recognising genes in the area of interest

Within any stretch of DNA, which in this situation may be several million base pairs long, there will be many expressed genes and potentially unexpressed 'pseudogenes'. A number of techniques have been developed to focus the search for the affected gene by homing in on expressed sequences only. *CpG island selection* detects regions at the 5'-ends of many expressed genes. Regions of DNA that are rich in hypomethylated cytosine next to the base guanine (CpG) are frequently found 5' to vertebrate genes, often in the vicin-ity of the promoter and first exon of the gene. The CpG dinucleotide is prone to methyl-ation in vivo (to 5-methyl cytosine), leading to deamination and mutation to TpG. The sequence CpG, therefore, tends to be underrepresented in the human genome as a whole. Genes with CpG islands can be selected using affinity purification to separate them from other methylated CpG-containing DNA fragments.

Using mRNA (cDNA) to screen for genes in a region of genomic DNA is a common method but relies on the availability of cDNA from an appropriate source, i.e. a tissue in which the gene is exclusively or heavily expressed. In the search for the gene causing cystic fibrosis, such a technique employing cDNA libraries from a variety of epithelial tissue sources eventually enabled researchers to find a gene with characteristics consis-tent with those predicted from the clinical picture.

The presence of coding regions may be inferred by the detection in a DNA sequence of the splice sites associated with RNA processing, in which introns are removed from exons to produce a full-length mRNA transcript. Exon amplification or trapping also takes advantage of this mechanism. Using a specialised cloning vector that gives any eukaryotic cell transformed with it particular growth characteristics *only* when the exogenous human DNA cloned in it harbours a natural splice site enables the DNA from within exons to be selected. Cloned exons are then further characterised by identifying the corresponding full-length transcripts in cDNA libraries and sequencing.

Zoo blots are used to detect regions of DNA conserved between species. Using small fragments of DNA as probes, cross-hybridisation is assessed between the piece of human DNA and the genomes of a variety of other species. The occurrence of cross-hybridisation frequently corresponds to regions of transcribed DNA because these are most conserved between species. Although this technique has been useful in isolating the genes mutated in a number of human conditions, including CF, the technique is laborious and can produce many false–positive hybridisations because of repetitive non-coding DNA sequences in closely related species.

Pinpointing the mutation

The final hurdle to overcome in defining the molecular mechanism underlying an hereditary disease is characterisation of the actual mutation. Once the area of interest has been reduced to a small area of genomic DNA containing a limited number of genes, then a number of strategies can be used to attempt to find the mutation accounting for the inherited disease. As discussed above, cytogenetic abnormalities (deletions and rearrangements), if present, can be invaluable in helping to localise and identify the disease gene itself, where the chromosome break points occur consistently within a specific gene in patients. Unfortunately, gross changes in cytogenetic structure are relatively infrequent. Less conspicuous changes at the molecular level include point mutations, insertions and deletions of varying length, which will alter the amino acid composition of the protein or produce shifted open reading frames (a base sequence that has no stop codons and so is open to translation) and usually premature stop codes. The subtlety of these changes requires extremely sensitive techniques for detection and, ultimately, DNA sequencing of the gene in numbers of normal individuals and in those affected by disease to prove that the changes found represent disease-causing mutations. A mutation may be detected by differing sizes of restriction fragments on a Southern blot when either insertions and deletions or a mutation affect a restriction site. A different example of expanding DNA fragments is found in myotonic dystrophy and those other dominant conditions in which a trinucleotide repeat is greatly expanded compared to normal. Ultimately, direct sequencing of the gene is required to establish the nature of the mutation.

To prove that a given collection of base pair changes are the cause of the disease phenotype, a number of basic criteria can be applied. First, a putative mutant allele must be consistently associated with all observed cases of disease. It is vital to exclude polymorphic variations that have no impact on protein function. Unfortunately, as mentioned above in relation to polygenic inheritance, both genetic heterogeneity (single distinct genes at different loci) and allelic heterogeneity (different mutant alleles at the same locus) that still cause an identical clinical phenotype may obscure the simple one-to-one relationship between mutations and a disease. An example of allelic heterogeneity is found in CF where the ΔF508 mutation, a 3 bp deletion in exon 10 resulting in omission of a phenylalanine amino acid residue from the CFTR, accounts for 65–85% of mutations in Caucasian populations. The remaining 15–35% of CF alleles are made up of a further 200 different disease-causing mutations.

The CFTR is a 170kDa protein and consists of five distinct domains. Two putative membrane-spanning domains comprise an ion channel pore, and two intracellular nucleotide-binding domains bind ATP to control channel function. A single regulatory domain acts as a plug for the channel and is controlled by phosphorylation, itself regulated by cyclic AMP levels. Mutations in the CFTR cause CF by a number of molecular mechanisms. The common ΔF508 mutation (in nucleotide-binding domain 1, NBD-1) causes defective processing of CFTR in the endoplasmic reticulum rather than affecting protein function *per se*. A stop codon at amino acid residue 542, also in NBD-1, prevents protein production. A glycine to aspartic acid mutation at residue 551, yet again in NBD-1, causes defective ATP binding and channel function. Mutations in the membrane-spanning domains frequently generate channels with altered conduction properties. Therefore, the molecular mechanisms at work in the single gene that is mutated in CF are many and varied. Patients may be either homozygotes or compound heterozygotes. Not only does this heterogeneity make correlation of a mutation with a disease phenotype more complicated, it also makes the implementation of genetic diagnosis and carrier screening less precise unless all alleles in the population have been identified.

To return to the question of proving that a given set of genetic changes are causing a disease, a number of strategies can be adopted to determine the function of the putative gene and to study the effect of a mutation *in vitro* and *in vivo*. The mutant gene product's structure and function may be predicted from the genetic code and by searching through databases of known proteins for homology either with entire proteins (suggesting membership of superfamily of molecules, e.g. immunoglobulins) or with domains within the protein. Homology may be found within the protein sequence with functional domains or secondary structure motifs, for example DNA-binding motifs or the trans-membrane domains and nucleotide-binding domains found in the CFTR. The predicted biological effects of malfunction of a protein of the type found should then be consistent with the observed clinical phenotype.

Gene expression systems

Gene expression systems can be used to establish the functional impact of abnormal proteins from mutant genes. Although sequence comparisons may help to suggest a function for a novel protein, an expression system is required to eventually test the hypothesis. The role in the cell or entire organism of both the 'normal' and the 'mutant' gene products can then be defined. Single cell systems such as the *Xenopus* oocyte allow microinjected or transfected mRNA to be translated into protein. Other simpler expression systems in bacteria, yeast strains or baculovirus allow large-scale production of the protein for biochemical studies, to raise antibodies or even for therapeutic use. Mammalian cell lines and cells cultured directly from tissue samples are used in an attempt to model more accurately the role of the gene in health and in inherited disease, as all the intracellular machinery for exon splicing and for post-translational processing should be present. Such systems were used in the characterisation of the CFTR, with a patch clamp technique to monitor flux through chloride channels and a fluorescence microscopic assay to assess intracellular cyclic AMP production. Primary cultures of cystic fibrotic and normal airway epithelial cells and also a CF epithelial cell line were transfected with recombinant plasmids containing either normal or the mutant ΔF508 CFTR. Transfection with the normal CFTR but not the mutant corrected both the chloride channel defect and the cyclic AMP increase in response to isoprenaline, suggesting that CFTR was a chloride channel or functions to regulate such channels.

Transgenic animals as models

The introduction of foreign genetic material into mouse embryos and the subsequent stable integration of this DNA into the mouse genome represents an extremely powerful and flexible system for investigation of the actions and interactions of genes and their controlling elements in higher animals – the transgenic mouse (see Fig. 2.26, p. 50). Transgenic models of inherited diseases have also been established in which to evaluate potential interventions (including gene therapy) in human disease. This has been a major motivation for the development of CF transgenic mice.

The two basic approaches are microinjection of foreign DNA into the pronucleus of a single cell embryo and modification of mouse embryo stem cells in culture by transfection with vectors in which the mouse gene to be targeted is mutated or grossly disrupted. The process of homologous recombination or gene targeting thus creates 'knockout' mice where the target gene is no longer functional. This loss of function mirrors the situation in most inherited human diseases. The technique has been used in the investigation of the genetic defect found in CF, producing mouse models with a number of pathological similarities to the human disease (Fig. 3.5). The CFTR gene was targeted in mouse ES cells and the sequence disrupted in a number of ways. Disruption of exon 10 (the site of the ΔF508 mutation in humans) produced a variable phenotype depending on whether low levels of normal CFTR mRNA were generated by unexpected splicing artefacts. Duplication of exon 3 leading to premature stop codons produced a severe phenotype with a high incidence of neonatal deaths.

Homozygotes for a truncated CFTR message displayed a number of pathological changes reminiscent of those seen in humans with CF. These included the presence of inspissated secretions in various glands and changes in the respiratory tract, such as increased numbers of goblet cells, dilatation of the gland ducts and destructive changes in the upper airway epithelium. The CFTR homozygous knockout mouse also demonstrated a shortened lifespan, mainly as a result of gastrointestinal obstruction that is probably secondary to these inspissated secretions.

The creation of animal models for CF holds great promise as a guide to the spectrum of tissue expression of CFTR in development and the involvement of CFTR mutations in the pathogenesis of CF. These models are also critical in assessing potential strategies for intervention, including gene therapy. They will be invaluable in defining its efficacy and safety. This example also points to the future as precise transgenic models of many inher-

Pancreas: enlargement of the acini and inspissation with eosinophilic material

General features: increased perinatal mortality and decreased lifespan; premature death caused by gastrointestinal obstruction

Gall bladder: abnormal distension and gall bladder wall inflammation

Liver: histologically normal, unlike human CF patients

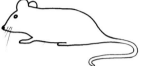

Respiratory tract: minimal changes in distal airways, mostly nasal sinuses (atrophy of serous glands)

Intestinal tract: loss of weight, intestinal obstruction, plugging of the lumen by viscous mucus/faeces

Fig. 3.5. Transgenic mouse model for CF: 'knockout' mice homozygous for the mutant CFTR have been created.

ited and acquired human diseases will allow therapeutic manoeuvres to be investigated more safely and expeditiously.

Gene manipulation in clinical management

Gene therapy

Gene therapy was devised as a strategy to correct genomic malfunction by introducing new recombinant sequences to replace the absent or aberrant function of the mutated gene in specific human diseases. The current objective in human gene therapy is the manipulation of genetic material in somatic cells but not germ-line cells in an attempt to correct inherited or acquired (e.g. mutations in cancer cells) gene damage in life-threatening human diseases for which no acceptable alternative treatment is available. At present the manipulation of germ-line DNA is not considered appropriate for ethical reasons. As well as the ethical considerations, the safety of germ-line engineering is unknown. There must be a finite risk that serious diseases, including potential malignancy, may present many years or generations after the time of the initial gene insertion. Until there is greater experience with somatic gene therapy and appreciation of its risks, germ-line therapy will remain shrouded in uncertainty. The ethical issues surrounding both forms of gene therapy, somatic and germ-line, extend beyond the medical profession, and public debate and education will be critical to the development of a consensus on the place of this type of treatment in routine clinical practice.

Gene tracking

In addition to replacing inactive genes with functional genes by gene therapy, the technique of inserting genetic markers into selected cell types has been used to probe their function and behaviour in disease states. An example is the monitoring of autologous bone marrow transplant cells after they have been given back to the host to determine the source of the residual leukaemic cells that cause relapse in acute myelogenous leukaemia (AML). In one study of children suffering from AML, a gene marker was used to monitor reconstitution of the bone marrow and the reason for relapse. In first remission, the children received autologous bone marrow transplants after the marrow had been purged (purified in an attempt to remove any residual leukaemic cells) and the cells transfected with the β-galactosidase gene as a marker. The presence of marked blast cells was confirmed in patients following relapse, indicating that leukaemic cells were present in the purged marrow, remained viable and contributed to the relapse. This suggests that to reduce the likelihood of relapse in AML more efficacious marrow purging methods will be more effective than increasing the severity of bone marrow ablative chemotherapy immediately prior to transplantation.

Vectors for introduction of exogenous DNA into cells ex vivo

Gene therapy requires a gene delivery system to introduce the desired replacement gene into the appropriate tissues and cell lineage(s) with acceptable efficiency but without damage to these cells or any bystanders (other tissues or cell types) (see Chapter 2, p. 55). If gene expression needs to be limited to a specific tissue and cell type or is only required at a particular stage of development, then promoters that only function to drive gene expression in the correct circumstances are essential. The choice of vector system is also influenced by whether it is essential to introduce a therapeutic gene into every cell (e.g. in cancer when replacing a defective tumour suppressor gene) or whether expression in less than 100% of the cells in an organ may correct the disease phenotype (e.g. CF where a proportion of cells handling chloride correctly may rectify the overall clinical phenotype).

Two basic vector systems are currently available: the *viral vectors* (including retroviruses and adenoviruses) and *cationic liposomes*. Both have a range of practical and theoretical advantages and many shortcomings. Viral vectors are useful because of their unique tropism for certain tissues and the high efficiency with which they achieve gene delivery. The basic function of viruses is to deliver genetic material to cells and they have evolved to perform this task very effectively. More particularly, viruses are capable of delivering DNA not just to the cell but targeting it to the nucleus where it will be functional. Retroviral vectors also provide the machinery to allow integration of a recombinant gene into the recipient cell's genome. A disadvantage of retroviral vectors is that they require cell division to achieve integration of their genome and are, therefore, less useful *in vivo* in differentiated tissues. Although integration of therapeutic genes is advantageous in that the functional gene will be passed on to daughter cells in future cycles of cell division (e.g. in the bone marrow), the danger is that random insertion of viral genes may disrupt host genes with an increased risk, for example, of cancer resulting from oncogene activation or tumour suppressor gene disruption. A serious practical limitation of retroviral vectors is that they are difficult to grow in high yield on production scale. The importance of this point is that as little as 1g tissue contains approximately 10^9 cells, so that a billion viral particles are required to transform every cell even at 100% transformation efficiency. A further serious potential drawback with retroviral vectors is the possibility that they can undergo spontaneous rearrangements to generate replication-competent viruses (gene therapy retroviruses are crippled by removal of key genetic elements so that in theory infectious virus cannot be regenerated). These have the potential to cause infections in recipients and, equally worryingly, to be transmitted with their recombinant genes to other individuals.

A number of other viruses are being studied as potential vectors. Most experience has been gained with adenovirus. In recent small-scale trials of gene therapy for CF, a modified adenovirus that shows natural tropism for respiratory epithelial cells was used to achieve successful expression of recombinant human CFTR mRNA and protein, albeit at low levels and for a short time. A general observation in most gene therapy studies attempted to date has been that it is unexpectedly difficult to maintain expression of the introduced genes for protracted periods. The reasons for this are still not fully understood. When using viral vectors, consideration must be given to preventing host cell damage by the cytopathic effects of viral gene products and especially viral replication. Therefore, viral vectors have been engineered lacking genes critical to replication or to the process of causing host injury. Viruses with deleted DNA sequences may not remain stable indefinitely and common species such as adenoviruses may be prone to recombination with wild-type viruses to produce replication-competent virions containing a recombinant gene. Again, this may lead to infection of both the recipient of gene therapy and also bystanders, raising safety concerns that need to be quantified.

Attention should also be paid to the potential of the viral vector to produce an immunological response in the host. This limits the efficacy of repeated exposure to the vector, which is destroyed by the immune system and may also produce acute inflammation following repeated exposures. This has been a problem in CF gene therapy attempts using adenoviral vectors. The population is widely exposed to adenoviruses and most individuals have some level of immune responsiveness to them. One patient receiving an inhaled adenoviral CFTR delivery vector developed acute inflammation of the respiratory epithelium necessitating termination of gene treatment. The requirement for repeated treatments in somatic gene therapy where gene expression does not persist makes understanding the biology of viral vectors essential. It is vital to minimise host responses while maximising tissue specificity and persistence of gene expression. It is to be hoped that with greater experience, other cytopathic and immunogenic viral genes can be identified and removed from future vectors.

A second approach is the use of cationic liposomes as vectors for gene therapy. Liposomes are constructed from a phospholipid bilayer. The theoretical advantage of this form of vector is its greater safety in terms of the decreased risk of both a host immune response and production of infectious recombinant virions capable of autologous replication. Liposomes are less efficient than viral vectors, which represents a major drawback. Whilst they may achieve a reasonable degree of overall cell transfection, they are not specifically adapted to ensure that encapsulated DNA then finds its way to the recipient cell nucleus and avoids lysosomal degradation.

Prospects for gene therapy

At present a number of gene therapy projects are ongoing at various centres around the world. The major initiatives are concerned with treatments for cancer, AIDS, CF, familial hypercholesterolaemia (see p. 55), adenosine deaminase deficiency (severe combined immunodeficiency) as well as a variety of gene marking studies. Initially only diseases of accessible tissues such as the lungs (to aerosolised vectors) or components of the haemopoietic system (to *ex vivo* modified bone marrow stem cell transplants) were viewed as suitable targets. Recent studies using hepatocytes transfected *ex vivo* with the LDL receptor in the treatment of familial hypercholesterolaemia have shown that some genetic defects in solid organs may be amenable to therapy. The prospects for gene therapy are indeed encouraging. However the temptation to allow such therapy into regular practice without careful scrutiny of safety aspects, its efficacy and the economics of the process compared with conventional treatments should be resisted.

The human genome project

The human genome initiative arose in the late 1980s as a reaction to the fragmented approach that was the consequence of competitive research in the field of human gene mapping and molecular genetics. This was in marked contrast to the success of multicentre collaborative projects to map the genomes of lower organisms. The objective of sequencing the entire human genome of 22 autosomes and the sex chromosomes, or 3×10^9 bp, is daunting. However with modern automated sequencing, powerful information technology and a systematic co-ordinated approach, it should be achievable. This multinational project is progressing through a number of intermediate stages using several complementary approaches.

The first step towards defining the human genome has been the creation of a high-resolution map of highly informative genetic markers, which allows researchers to use linkage studies to determine the genetic locus of any inherited disease. The development of the Généthon genetic linkage map and various others is of enormous value to investigators attempting to identify mutant genes, as described above (p. 85). The present coverage of the genome, although extensive, remains incomplete in some chromosome regions. The first objective was a map of the genome at a resolution of 10–20cM, which had been achieved by the early 1990s. The next step is to narrow the separation of markers further to give a resolution of about 1–5cM, the distance at which the intervening segments of DNA may be incorporated into single YACs for cloning.

A distinct but complementary approach is to produce a map showing where expressed genes (and hence the encoded proteins) are situated on the chromosomes. The strategy uses a straightforward technique of taking random cDNA clones from all available tissue sources and sequencing these, at least in part. The partial sequences generated are called expressed sequence tags (ESTs) and these can be positioned on the chromosomes physically either by FISH (fluorescence *in situ* hybridisation) or by using somatic cell hybrids. Even though full-length cDNA clones may not be available for characterisation, the provision of limited cDNA sequence is enormously valuable. Over

50 000 such ESTs are already known and the task of accurately mapping them individually onto chromosomes proceeds apace. This means that genetic mapping of an inherited disease will immediately point to a small number of candidate genes by virtue of their chromosome location. Already there are many examples where the function of anonymous ESTs becomes apparent because they show sequence homologies to known genes in other species or in humans. It is hoped that by unravelling the information in the human genome, a complete knowledge of our genes, their control elements and the protein products will provide unprecedented insights into function in normal and abnormal cells.

Summary

The pace of research advances in molecular genetics is frenetic. The characterisation of all the common single gene inherited disorders is well under way. Although the actual genes and the specific base pairs mutated are now known precisely for many Mendelian diseases, the mechanisms resulting in the biochemical and pathological consequences are often obscure and always complex. The stream of advances in molecular genetics became a flood with the development of the PCR technique in 1985 and its application in identification, cloning, sequencing and, latterly, mapping genes (with microsatellite markers) has produced remarkable savings in the time and manpower required for laboratories to undertake this kind of research. Additional techniques for the investigation of human genetic disease, such as the use of PFGE and YAC cloning to facilitate the manipulation of large megabase DNA sequences, are now well established.

For the clinician, the steps from understanding the genetic aberration and its effect on protein function to the clinical manifestation of an inherited disease remain long. In a number of inherited diseases, such as the inborn errors of metabolism, the consequences of a lack of an enzyme activity are well-defined and predictable. In the majority of others, however, there is often no clear cut reason why the diseases have the spectrum of pathology that is found. Why does a defect in a chloride channel in CF result in mucous impaction in exocrine glands and lead to respiratory tract infections, bronchiectasis, respiratory failure, pancreatic exocrine failure and eventually complete or partial pancreatic endocrine failure? These questions are now being addressed by a variety of means: immunohistochemistry and *in situ* hybridisation to correlate gene function with the progression of pathology *in vivo* in normal and diseased specimens, and expression systems including cell lines and, more recently and excitingly, transgenic animals for functional genetic analysis. These approaches allow the consequences of gene expression to be studied at the cellular, tissue and whole animal levels and will provide great additional insights into the mechanisms of inherited human disease. They will also allow the testing of novel therapeutic manoeuvres and encourage better stratification of patients in clinical trials of new treatments for specific conditions.

Gene therapy is in its infancy. The promise is great but many hurdles need to be overcome before its role in therapeutics is established. The efficacy of gene replacement as proved by a subsequent improvement in clinical course needs to be demonstrated. The safety of both the patients and the staff involved in administering the treatments needs to be carefully monitored.

At present, molecular genetics makes a direct contribution to clinical practice in a number of ways including the ability to make an accurate diagnosis of presymptomatic affected individuals and carriers in inherited diseases, the ability to detect cryptic infection or minimal residual disease in leukaemia patients and the use of recombinant DNA technology to produce limitless supplies of polypeptide hormones, growth factors and vaccines for direct therapeutic use. At the end of the twentieth century, the major practical clinical issue to be addressed is the role of genes in complex multifactorial diseases such as asthma, coronary artery disease and schizophrenia. The public understanding of molecular genetics and its unique potential in medicine lags significantly behind the point it might ideally have reached, which implies that widespread education programmes are essential before the ethics of many of its possible applications can be fully debated.

FURTHER READING

Molecular biology

Alberts, B., Bray, D., Lewis, J. *et al.* (1994). *Molecular Biology of the Cell*, 3rd edn. New York: Garland. A textbook containing a wide range of topics mostly in basic cell and molecular biology; well referenced.

Watson, J.D. (1987). *The Molecular Biology of the Gene*, 4th edn. Wokingham, UK: Benjamin/Cummingham.

Watson, J.D., Gilman, M., Witkowski, J. & Zoller, M. (1992). *Recombinant DNA*, 2nd edn. New York: Scientific American Books. A treatise covering topics in basic and applied molecular biology; well referenced.

Molecular genetics

Collins, F.S. (1995). Positional cloning moves from the positional to the traditional. *Nature Genetics*, 9, 347–350. Reviews current state of the art in the genome project.

Caskey, C.T., Pizzute, A., Fu, Y.H., Fenwick, R.G. & Nelson, D.L. (1992). Triplet mutations in human disease. *Science*, 256, 784–789. A review of this novel form of inherited disease.

Emery, A.E.H. & Mueller, R.F. (1992). *Elements of Medical Genetics*, 8th edn. Edinburgh: Churchill Livingstone. General textbook covering aspects of genetics directly of interest to the physician in concise and accessible format.

Lander, E.S. & Schork, N.J. (1994). Genetic dissection of complex traits. *Science*, 265, 2037–2047. A comprehensive review of the strategies available to the molecular geneticist to analyse the inherited component of multifactorial/polygenic disorders.

Reed, P.W., Davies, J.L., Copeman, J.B. *et al.* (1994). Chromosome-specific microsatellite sets for fluorescence-based, semi-automated genome mapping. *Nature Genetics*, 7, 390–396. A review of the latest incarnation of microsatellites for the genome navigator.

Cystic fibrosis

Sferra, T.J. & Collins, F.S. (1993). The molecular biology of cystic fibrosis. *Annual Reviews in Medicine*, 44, 133–144.

Tsui, L.C. & Buchwald, M. (1993). Biochemical and molecular genetics of cystic fibrosis. *Advances in Human Genetics*, 20, 153–166.

Gene therapy

Alton, E. & Geddes, D. (1994). A mixed message for cystic fibrosis gene therapy. *Nature Genetics*, 8, 8–9.

Various authors (1995). Gene therapy. *British Medical Bulletin*, 51, No. 1. A collection of reviews covering a wide range of practical and theoretical aspects of gene therapy. Includes reviews of progress in treating CF and severe combined immune deficiency and adenosine deaminase deficiency.

Wetherall, D. (1993). Heroic gene surgery. *Nature Genetics*, 6, 325–326.

4

Autoimmune mechanisms

A. P. WEETMAN

- Most autoreactive T and B cells are removed or inactivated during fetal development; several mechanisms normally control the remainder. Disorders in these mechanisms cause autoimmune disease.

- Susceptibility to most autoimmune disease is dependent on both genetic and environmental factors. Genes in the major histocompatibility complex, called HLA in humans, have an important role in determining whether an immune response (including autoimmunity) occurs.

- Autoimmune disease is produced by humoral (antibody) or cell-mediated (T cell-dependent) mechanisms.

- There is a spectrum of autoimmune diseases ranging from organ-specific disease, such as those conditions affecting the endocrine system (see also Chapter 7), to non-organ-specific diseases, such as rheumatological disorders.

- Autoimmune thyroid disease may result in hyperthyroidism (Graves' disease), caused by TSH receptor-stimulating antibodies, or hypothyroidism (Hashimoto's thyroiditis or primary myxoedema), caused mainly by antibodies against thyroid peroxidase and by T cell-mediated injury to thyroid follicular cells.

The immune system has evolved to protect the organism against infection and, probably later, against malignancy (see Chapter 12). The devastating effects of congenital or acquired immunological deficiency states, resulting infection and neoplasia, are proof of this central role. Protection must be effective against the vast array of infectious agents likely to be encountered, and it operates via two flexible recognition systems: the T cells and B cells. These recognise foreign antigens by specific cell surface receptors: the T cell receptor (TCR) and surface-bound immunoglobulin or antibody. By recombination events, dealt with below, a vast array of antigens can be recognised by these receptors, but such huge diversity brings the penalty that, occasionally, self or autoantigens will be targets for the immune response.

At the beginning of the twentieth century, it was generally believed that the body was incapable of reacting against itself, a property termed *horror autotoxicus* by Paul Ehrlich. The reasons for this were not understood, and much of the study of immunology for the next 50 years was devoted to the immunochemistry of antigens and antibodies. Then, however, the investigation of transplantation and rejection by Medawar, Owen and others, and the demonstration of autoimmune disease in animals and humans by Witebsky, Rose, Doniach and Roitt marked a new era in which immunobiology and its application to clinical problems became dominant. Thanks to the ideas of Jerne and Burnet, attention focused on selection of antibodies by antigen as a means of ensuring a restricted and yet appropriate response by particular clones of B cells. By comparison, 'clonal abortion' was postulated as a mechanism whereby autoreactive cells were destroyed by their contact with self antigens at a critical stage of fetal development: failure of clonal abortion would cause autoimmune disease.

Since the early 1960s, these initial precepts have been expanded to include T cells, which lie at the heart of the immune response. The recent application of molecular techniques has led to spectacular developments in our understanding of how the T and B cells most likely to be beneficial are selected, and how tolerance to self antigens is imposed on potentially dangerous cells recognising these autoantigens. The same methods have greatly increased our knowledge of how cells of the immune system communicate with each other, through an enormous array of receptor–ligand pairs and soluble mediators called cytokines.

The normal immune response

Autoimmune mechanisms of disease can only be understood by reference to the normal immunological response to an exogenous antigen. A brief outline follows, taking in sequence the steps of antigen presentation, activation of T cells and B cell stimulation (Fig. 4.1).

Antigen presentation

Extracellular bacteria, viruses and proteins are taken up by endocytosis (via binding to receptors on the cell surface) or phagocytosis and processed by the antigen-presenting cell (APC) before presentation to the T cell. This processing occurs in acidic endosomes or lysosomes, resulting in short peptide fragments of around 20 amino acid residues. These peptides then associate with one of a particular group of polymorphic molecules encoded by the class II region of the MHC genes. This complex is termed HLA in humans and three types of class II gene product are expressed: HLA-DR, HLA-DQ and HLA-DP (Fig. 4.2). The intracellular association between antigenic peptide and class II molecule stabilises the latter; this association occurs predominantly in distinct vesicles following the synthesis of class II molecules in the Golgi apparatus. Antigen binding to class II molecules on the APC surface is not a major pathway, because class II molecules bind processed peptides with high affinity and are, therefore, already complexed when expressed.

The peptide sequence of an antigen recognised by a T cell is termed the *epitope*. Each epitope constitutes around 10 amino acid residues that lie in an antigen-binding groove of the class II molecule during presentation; the ends of peptide that are not part of the epitope protrude from either side of the groove (Fig. 4.3). The polymorphic structure of class II molecules ensures that only certain peptides fit each particular groove, account-

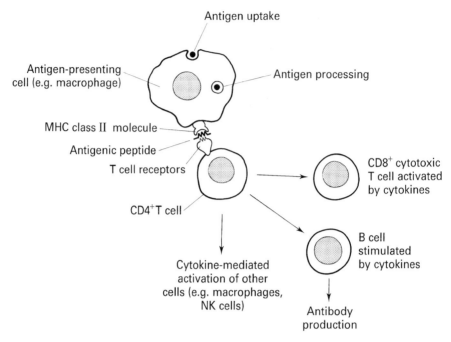

Fig. 4.1. Antigen presentation to a CD4$^+$ T cell induces helper activity for CD8$^+$ T cells or antibody production and is mediated by cytokines. Such cytokines can also activate other cells for example natural killer (NK) cells.

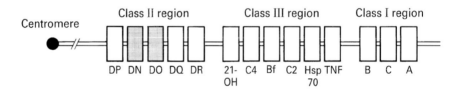

Fig. 4.2. Sequence of the major loci in the HLA complex on chromosome 6. The entire complex covers over 300 kb and is not drawn to scale. Shaded gene loci are not expressed. TNF, tumour necrosis factor; hsp, heat shock protein; 21-OH, A, B loci encoding 21-hydroxylase; C4, Bf and C2 are complement components.

ing for the influence of class II genes in determining immune responses. Selection is also imposed during the next step in the immune response, because the peptide–class II molecule complex is recognised by a specific TCR. If a suitable TCR is not available, no response to this particular epitope is possible. Most foreign antigens contain several T cell epitopes, and, therefore, a response can be mounted by genetically diverse individuals.

T cell stimulation

The major class of TCR is a heterodimer composed of an α- and β-chain (Fig. 4.4), each with a constant (C) and variable (V) region, joined by junctional (J) and diversity (D)

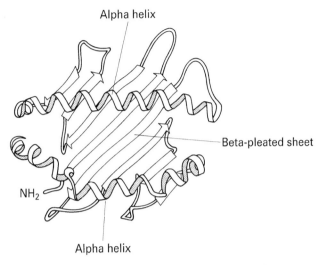

Fig. 4.3. Model of the antigen-binding groove on the HLA-A2 molecule (after Bjorkman *et al.* (1987). *Nature*, 329, 506). Class II molecules have a similar structure. The most polymorphic residues line the groove, either on the α-helices or the β-pleated sheet floor.

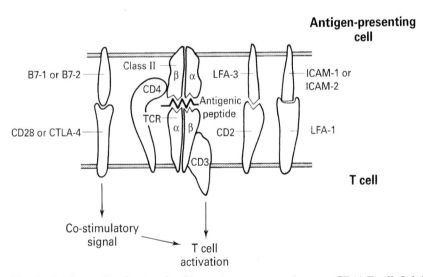

Fig. 4.4. Major molecules involved in antigen presentation to a CD4$^+$ T cell. Soluble cytokines (e.g. IL-1) are also involved. LFA, lymphocyte function-associated antigen; ICAM, intercellular adhesion molecule.

generating sequences. Epitope recognition is primarily determined by the V region and, to a lesser extent, the D and J sequences. A minor population of T cells expresses a TCR comprising a γ- and δ-chain; the exact function of these cells is not clear. The structure of the TCR is similar to the immunoglobulin molecule. There are around 100 different $V\alpha$ and $V\beta$ gene segments in humans and these can pair with over 50 Jα and 13 Jβ segments, as well as two D regions in the case of the β-chain. In addition, nucleotides can be added between the *V–J*, *V–D* and *D–J* regions during gene rearrangement, a process not encoded in the germ-line. The result is a vast repertoire of different TCRs, only a small fraction of which is ever used. Many TCRs formed during development will, by chance, recognise self antigens and such T cells will (hopefully) be deleted.

The trimolecular interaction between an αβ TCR and MHC class II–peptide complex results in T cell activation through signal transduction mediated by CD3, a complex of proteins non-covalently associated with the TCR (Fig. 4.4). This leads to the production of interleukin-2 (IL-2) and the IL-2 receptor by the T cell, which in turn promote prolife-ration and further activation. However, several other accessory molecules are required for the interaction of the TCR and the APC to occur efficiently: T cells at different stages of development require varying combinations of accessory molecules (Fig. 4.4). Foremost amongst these are:

1. Adhesion molecules; these allow binding between the cells: some of these inter-actions partially activate the T cell. Some adhesion molecules contribute to the binding of T cells to any APC; others are restricted to interactions with certain types of cell.

2. The CD4 and CD8 glycoproteins; these recognise cells carrying MHC class I and II molecules, respectively. The T cell CD4 molecule stabilises the interaction between the class II molecule–peptide complex and the TCR by binding to a non–polymorphic region on the MHC molecule. As CD4 is expressed only on a subset of T cells, these alone can interact with class II molecule–peptide com-plexes. The reciprocal T cell subset expresses CD8, which binds to class I MHC molecules. These present endogenous antigens (such as viral proteins syn-thesised within a target cell) rather than antigens of exogenous origin. Therefore, a major role for the $CD8^+$ subset is recognition (and destruction) of virally infected cells.

3. Co-stimulatory molecules, particularly B7-1 and B7-2; these are present on APCs and provide an essential second signal to $CD4^+$ cells by binding to CD28 and CTLA-4 on these T cells. In the absence of this co-stimulatory signal, CD4 T cells are not stimulated by the class II molecule–peptide complex and, in many cases, instead become inactivated. This process is called *anergy*. Anergic T cells are paralysed, failing to respond to antigen subsequently even if this is presented with the correct second signals.

$CD4^+$ T cells are often called helper (T_H) cells. Once a $CD4^+$ T cell has been activated, it can proliferate and express a number of different cytokines. Two broad patterns of cytokine production can be identified (Table 4.1.), which correspond to the main effector functions of $CD4^+$ T cells, namely producing an inflammatory or *delayed-type hyper-sensitivity* response (T_H1 cells) and providing help for antibody production by B cells (T_H2 cells). The cytokines produced by each $CD4^+$ subset reciprocally inhibit the other, resulting in either a predominantly delayed-type hypersensitivity or a humoral response, mediated by whichever subset is initially activated. Cytokines released by stimulated $CD4^+$ T cells are also essential to the activation of $CD8^+$ T cells, which can then mediate cytotoxicity against antigen-specific targets.

Table 4.1. *Profile of cytokines produced by the two main CD4⁺ T cell subsets, T_H1 and T_H2, in humans. Naïve T cells may only secrete IL-2 after initial stimulation and some activated cells have cytokine profiles that do not fall into these two categories*

	T_H1	T_H2
γ-IFN	++	0
TNF	++	+
Lymphotoxin	++	−
IL-2	++	+
IL-4	−	++
IL-6	−	++
IL-10	+	+
Function	Macrophage activation, producing delayed-type hypersensitivity responses	B cell stimulation leading to antibody formation, eosinophil and mast cell production

Note:
IL, interleukin; γ-IFN, γ-interferon; TNF, tumour necrosis factor.

B cells and antibody production

Antibodies are the second type of molecule involved in specific antigen recognition. Each comprises two heavy and two light chains. The amino-terminus in both sets of chains contains a V region domain, analogous to the TCR and also responsible for antigen binding. The V region determines the antibody specificity, that is what antigen the antibody will recognise. Unlike the TCR, antibodies usually recognise conformational determinants on an antigen that depend on its tertiary structure.

Antibody diversity is generated by recombination events similar to those responsible for TCR diversity, with the important addition of somatic mutation (see also Chapter 5). An enormous number of different immunoglobulin molecules can be generated by (i) the large number of genomic immunoglobulin *V* gene segments whose mRNA can be spliced with different *D* and *J* segments; (ii) nucleotide addition at the regions coding for the heavy chain VDJ and light chain VJ junctions; (iii) pairing between the different types of heavy and light chain; and (iv) somatic mutation, which changes nucleotides coding for the key parts of the immunoglobulin V region involved in antigen recognition, resulting in slightly different V regions derived from a primordial *V* gene segment. The last mechanism is particularly important in determining fine specificity, and most B cells express V regions that have undergone somatic mutation.

Antibodies are synthesised by B cells after antigen-specific triggering of the TCR induces T cell activation and the provision of cytokines that cause B cell activation (Fig. 4.2). However, B cells can also serve as APCs to amplify the immune response. The presence of specific antibodies on the B cell surface allows them to focus on a particular antigen, which can be taken up and processed. This leads to a close collaboration between the T and B cell, resulting in amplification of the immune response (Fig. 4.5).

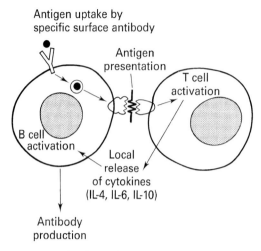

Fig. 4.5. Role of B cells in antigen presentation. Surface immunoglobulin allows presentation of specific antigen: close contact with the T cell permits local delivery of non-specific cytokines to the appropriate B cell.

Discrimination between self and non-self

The best way to prevent autoimmune disease is not to generate T cells and B cells that recognise self. However, the random events of recombination for both TCRs and antibodies, which are necessary to generate diversity, ensure that autoreactive cells *will* be produced. A hierarchy of defences has evolved to deal with this threat (Table 4.2); different autoantigens evoke different control mechanisms.

Clonal deletion of T cells

Two kinds of experiment have supported Burnet's hypothesis of clonal abortion or deletion. The first utilised the knowledge that a particular kind of TCR, encoded by the V gene segment termed $V\beta17a$, recognises the MHC class II molecule I-E, which occurs in some strains of mice. Strains of animals not expressing I-E have $V\beta17a^+$ T cells, but crossing these mice with a strain expressing I-E results in the near absence of $V\beta17a^+$ T cells in the offspring. Sequential study of these animals revealed that $V\beta17a^+$ T cells were present in the thymus early in T cell development, at a stage when CD4 and CD8 are both expressed. However, these cells were deleted as they matured into the distinct $CD4^+$ and $CD8^+$ populations, following recognition of I-E at a critical stage in their development. The second kind of experiment used transgenic mice to demonstrate clonal deletion (Fig. 4.6) with similar results.

The thymus can also positively select T cells, again shown most elegantly in transgenic experiments. Such selection occurs at an earlier stage of T cell development than negative selection and ensures that the T cell repertoire contains T cells that react appropriately with self MHC molecules. T cells with an absent or very high affinity for MHC molecules (the latter, therefore, likely to be dangerous) die. Although the molecu-

Table 4.2. *Hierarchy of defence mechanisms normally preventing autoimmune disease: clonal deletion of autoreactive T cells is the most secure, sequestered autoantigen the least*

Mechanism	Comment
1. Clonal deletion	Some T cells inevitably escape
2. Clonal anergy	Can be bypassed, e.g.. if excessive IL-2 is provided
3. Functional ignorance	Certain self antigens may not be susceptible to processing by APCs; exact importance unknown
4. Active suppression	Requires active and continuing suppression of autoreactive T cells and, therefore, is likely to become defective with time
5. Lack of T cell help	Autoreactive CD8$^+$ T cells and B cells are only harmful if specific CD4$^+$ T cells are stimulated
6. Sequestered autoantigen	Accidental exposure to antigen will rapidly induce an autoimmune response

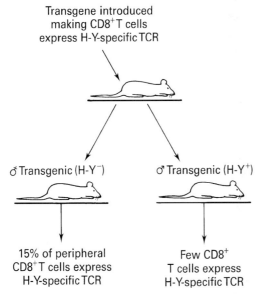

Transgene introduced
making CD8$^+$T cells
express H-Y-specific TCR

♂ Transgenic (H-Y$^-$)

♂ Transgenic (H-Y$^+$)

15% of peripheral
CD8$^+$T cells express
H-Y-specific TCR

Few CD8$^+$
T cells express
H-Y-specific TCR

Fig. 4.6. Demonstration of intrathymic clonal deletion in transgenic mice. Male mice constitutively expressing the male transplantation antigen H-Y delete the majority of CD8$^+$ T cells bearing the transgenic H-Y-specific TCR during intrathymic development. Those that escape deletion have low levels of CD8, which may limit their pathogenicity.

lar events causing positive and negative selection are only now becoming clarified, it seems certain that the developing T cell must encounter appropriate adhesion molecules, cytokines and co-stimulators as well as self MHC to mature: inappropriate or inadequate recognition of self MHC leads to deletion by programmed cell death (apoptosis).

These experiments clearly show the importance of clonal deletion in eliminating the bulk of autoreactive T cells, but they also show that deletion is not complete, even for self antigens that are in abundance. The huge number of potential autoantigens, which may not be expressed at the appropriate time for deletion to occur, poses one limitation on this mechanism. It is also difficult to envisage the intrathymic expression of all self antigens, such as tightly regulated cell surface receptors and intracellular enzymes. This is because only soluble or cell-bound antigens in the blood are likely to enter the thymic medulla where they can be presented to T cells by dendritic cells and epithelial cells.

The failure to delete T cells capable of reacting with tissue-specific autoantigens may not be a problem providing the antigen remains sequestered. Autoreactive CD8$^+$ T cells can also be permitted, provided CD4$^+$ T cells with the same specificity are firmly controlled or *tolerised*, as the CD8$^+$ subset will not respond unless appropriate help is provided for their activation. Both of these are rather dangerous strategies to prevent autoimmune disease, because infections and local inflammation in an organ may lead to release of hitherto hidden self antigens or provide indiscriminate cytokine-mediated help, resulting in an autoimmune response. Therefore, additional mechanisms have evolved to control autoreactive T cells that have escaped intrathymic deletion.

Anergy and T cells

Anergy is an incompletely understood process by which autoreactive T cells are not deleted but are somehow disabled so that they no longer respond to autoantigen. As long as an anergic T cell continues to ignore an autoantigen, no danger of autoimmune disease exists, but there is always a potential risk that anergy may be reversed. Anergy may occur in the thymus or in the periphery. As an example, *intrathymic tolerance* imposed during development can be demonstrated in mice for T cells reactive with endogenous Mls (minor lymphocyte-stimulating) antigens. The Mls-1^a autoantigen is recognised by T cells expressing a TCR that includes the Vβ6 element. If a strain of mouse that possesses the Mls-1^b rather than the Mls-1^a autoantigen is immunised with Mls-1^a cells, the animal does not mount a response against Mls-1^a, but also it does not delete the Vβ6$^+$ T cells, which can still be detected in the recipient. By using a chimaeric animal in which the bone marrow and thymus are derived from different strains, it can be shown that anergy is induced in the thymus.

Peripheral tolerance has been most clearly demonstrated in transgenic animals. For example, if I-E$^-$ murine β cells (in the islets of Langerhans of the pancreas) express an I-E transgene they become I-E$^+$, and it might be predicted that Vβ17a$^+$ T cells (discussed above) present in these otherwise I-E$^-$ mice would recognise and attack the β cell. However, this is not the case, nor are the Vβ17a$^+$ T cells absent, showing that insufficient I-E finds its way into the developing thymus of the transgenic mice to delete those 'self-reactive' T cells (Fig. 4.7). Instead the T cells become anergic, ignoring the β cells (although it must be said that this anomalous expression of I-E class II molecules by the β cell alters intracellular processes, which ultimately leads to β cell death and diabetes).

Intrathymic and peripheral anergy both occur because an antigen-specific TCR encounters a class II molecule–antigen complex in the absence of a co-stimulatory signal, particularly B7-1 and B7-2. This results in a fundamental change in intracellular tyrosine

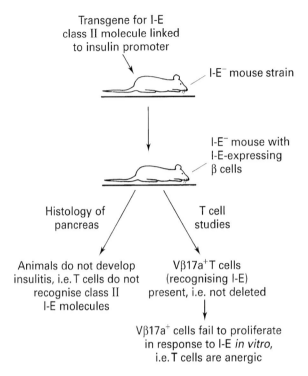

Fig. 4.7. Demonstration of peripheral tolerance in transgenic mice. Mice expressing the MHC class II molecule I-E normally delete T cells with the Vβ17a TCR; these cells are only found in I-E⁻ animals. If the I-E molecule is expressed by pancreatic β cells in I-E⁻ mice, Vβ17a⁺ T cells are not deleted but become anergic beacused the β cells fail to express the necessary co-stimulatory signal

kinase activation by the TCR, together with an alteration in inositol phosphates and intracellular free calcium. These changes prevent the T cell from producing IL-2. In the thymus, it is likely that thymic epithelial cells that do not express co-stimulators are responsible for anergy, particularly for those T cells specific for epithelial cell peptides not expressed by thymic dendritic cells.

However, under normal circumstances, pancreatic β cells (and most other cells in the body) do not express class II, which is largely a property of 'professional' APCs such as macrophages, dendritic cells and B cells. At first sight, therefore, peripheral tolerance hardly seems important, but class II expression can be induced by cytokines, particularly γ-interferon (γ-IFN). As these cytokines are released locally in inflammation, the resulting capacity to induce anergy could prevent autoimmune attack at the exact time and place when it is likely to occur. It is also now known that T cell deletion can occur in the periphery as well as in the thymus. This could be an extreme outcome of the same mechanisms that result in anergy. The affinity of interaction between the TCR and MHC class II molecule–peptide complex may determine the ultimate fate of the T cell both within the thymus and in the post-thymic environment.

T cell suppression

Anergy only operates on certain T cells, depending mainly on their maturational state. There are also theoretical problems with anergy as an explanation for control of all auto-reactive T cells. First, it is hard to imagine how thymic epithelial cells can both positively select and anergise T cells, but this may depend on different properties of medullary and cortical epithelial cells and on the stage of T cell development. Second, anergy could be bypassed, for instance by conditions that supply sufficient IL-2 to overcome the anergic state. Finally, 'professional' APCs are present in most tissues, and these might be expected to deliver appropriate co-stimulatory signals if self antigens are processed, thus overcoming peripheral tolerance.

The concept of suppressor T cells has been controversial, but there are now many examples which suggest that self-reactive T cells that have escaped deletion or anergy are prevented from causing autoimmune disease by active suppression (although the term immunoregulation is perhaps more appropriate, as the way 'suppression' is achieved is not clear). It is very unlikely that suppression is mediated by a distinct T cell subset or by a single mechanism. Suppression can be demonstrated crudely by the trans-fer of T cell subsets, often from animals that have recovered from an autoimmune dis-order, to a recipient with the condition, resulting in amelioration of the disease. Both $CD4^+$ and $CD8^+$ populations can mediate such effects.

In more refined experiments in which an autoantigen is recognised by a specific TCR, vaccination with fragments of this TCR can prevent disease, probably through the activation of T cells whose TCRs recognise these peptides (Fig. 4.8). This is an example of a network between idiotypes (the disease-associated TCR) and anti-idiotypes (the induced TCR), terms originally applied by Jerne to a control network of antibodies. Stimulation of one part of the network (e.g. an increase in idiotype) results in compensation in another part (increase in anti-idiotype), and the balance is restored. Other possibilities also exist to account for suppression (Fig. 4.8), including release of suppressive cytokines that either reduce the immune response generally or cause inhibition of an ongoing T_H1 or T_H2 response by the reciprocal inhibition mentioned previously.

B cell tolerance

In the absence of T cell help, autoreactive B cells will not produce high-affinity IgG class autoantibodies. Therefore, the need for T cell tolerance is of key importance, but B cell tolerance is also necessary to prevent the emergence of self-reactive B cells as a result of somatic mutation. In addition, the accidental supply of B cell help arising, for instance, from a T cell responding to a microbial antigen that cross-reacts with a self antigen, could be disastrous. As with T cell tolerance, transgenic mice have been used to show that auto-reactive B cells are subject to both deletion and anergy.

In the first such experiment, the offspring from two transgenic mice were studied, the parents expressing either hen egg lysozyme (HEL) or antibodies against HEL (anti-HEL). In this situation, the mice treat the transgenic HEL as a self antigen. The doubly

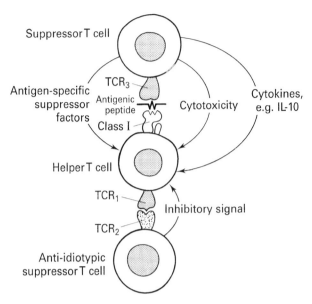

Fig. 4.8. Possible mechanisms to explain T cell-mediated suppression of autoreactive T cells. The importance of these remains to be determined, although it is now clear that T_H1 and T_H2 cells can inhibit each other by cytokines. Anti-idiotypic T cells may react with fragments of the TCR on the helper cell (TCR_1) presented by MHC class I or II molecules.

transgenic progeny did not delete anti-HEL-expressing B cells, which could readily be detected using a specific marker on this particular antibody. However, the B cells did not produce anti-HEL even after stimulation *in vitro*, indicating that they were anergic. Such cells had reduced levels of IgM but still expressed IgD on their surface. Clonal deletion has also been demonstrated in doubly transgenic mice expressing both a novel MHC class I gene in their liver and antibodies against the class I product. These animals delete almost all of the B cells synthesising class I antibody in the spleen and lymph nodes and neither make such antibodies nor have detectable transgene-expressing B cells.

Multivalent antigens on cell surfaces seem particularly good at inducing deletion, whereas soluble, univalent antigens induce anergy. This presumably reflects an important role for the affinity of the antigen binding to the surface immunoglobulin on the immature B cell in determining outcome. The maturational state of the B cell is also important, with antibody-producing plasma cells being very resistant to deletion and anergy.

Initiation of autoimmune disease

Given these complexities, and the realisation that even more levels of control probably operate in the intact animal, it hardly seems surprising that autoimmune diseases arise through a breakdown in tolerance. The following are the most likely points at which the control of autoreactive lymphocytes may be disturbed.

1. Autoreactive lymphocytes are not deleted. This may arise in particular strains of animal where particular MHC molecules cannot present self antigen. Failure of deletion could occur in all members of a species if an organ-specific auto-antigen does not appear in the thymus at the requisite time; autoimmune disease then arises in those individuals who fail to control such T cells subsequently.
2. Failure of intrathymic anergy. For T cells, this may result in autoimmune disease if sufficient IL-2 or other signals are supplied to overcome the anergic state. Anergic B cells may also be activated by sufficient help in the form of T cell-derived cytokines.
3. Failure of peripheral tolerance and suppression. Drugs and thymectomy may alter an animal's capacity to provide active T cell suppression, or local APCs may provide co-stimulatory signals to overwhelm peripheral tolerance.
4. Cross-reactivity. If an immune response is mounted against a foreign antigen that is by chance sufficiently similar to self (i.e. *cross-reactive*), then autoimmunity may result. The participating T cells are not tolerised, perhaps because they have a relatively low affinity for the self antigen, but their activation by foreign antigen leads to a strong response that is then sufficient to cause problems.
5. Exposure of sequestered autoantigens. Certain antigens, such as lens protein, may never gain access to the immune system under normal conditions and, therefore, do not induce tolerance of any kind. This is usually trouble-free, but leakage and exposure of the antigen in adult life results in a severe autoimmune response. With lens protein, this causes sympathetic ophthalmitis, which damages the intact eye when the other eye is injured.

Whether or not autoimmune disease appears in an individual depends on one or more of these malfunctions occurring. The chances of this happening are related to exogenous and endogenous factors: the simplest example is the eye trauma just mentioned. However, most autoimmune diseases are the result of a complex interplay between genetic susceptibility and non-genetic influences, which operate on the (imperfect) state of self-tolerance, making it more or less likely that such conditions will arise.

Immunogenetics and autoimmunity

Genetic susceptibility is demonstrated in many of the more common autoimmune diseases by the increased frequency of these disorders in family members. Inheritance does not follow a clear pattern and, even in genetically identical monozygotic twins, there is only 30–50% concordance (i.e. disease occurring in both individuals) for disorders such as type I diabetes mellitus, rheumatoid arthritis and Graves' disease. There are two explanations for this. First, the random nature of immunoglobulin and TCR gene rearrangements means that each family member, including twins, generates a unique T and B cell repertoire, which can modify disease expression. Second, and of greater importance, non-genetic factors also contribute to susceptibility. As a result, auto-

Table 4.3. *Effect of MHC-encoded immune response genes in guinea pigs immunised with synthetic peptide antigens. Strain 2 (but not strain 13) guinea pigs were known to respond to the antigens DNP-PLL and glutamyl alanine co-polymer; strain 13 (but not strain 2) animals respond to glutamyl tyrosine co-polymer. Macrophages from two strains and one hybrid were used to present antigen to T cells from immunised animals. The T cell proliferative response determines whether the antigen has been presented. The results show that strain governs the ability of macrophages to present antigen. Because the responses were blocked in separate experiments by antibodies against strain-specific MHC class II molecules, these molecules must determine whether antigen presentation occurs*

Peptide antigen	Response of strain 2 T cells with macrophages from strain			Response of strain 13 T cells with macrophages from strain		
	2	13	$(2\times13)F_1$	2	13	$(2\times13)F_1$
DNP-PLL	+	0	+	0	0	0
Glutamyl alanine co-polymer	+	0	+	0	0	0
Glutamyl tyrosine co-polymer	0	0	0	0	+	+

Note:
$(2\times13)F_1$ is the first generation hybrids from strain 2 and strain 13 matings. +, T cell response; 0, no T cell response.

immune diseases show incomplete penetrance, and a susceptible individual without the disease is at continued risk of developing it, depending on exposure to appropriate environmental factors. It is also now clear that several genes are involved in determining whether an individual develops an autoimmune disease, and some of these are (apparently) protective, making analysis of the complex roles of different genes very difficult.

The role of MHC class I and II genes

Autoimmune responses are not uniquely influenced by genetic factors; the production and strength of all immune responses are in part determined by the genetic background of the individual. This can be studied far more readily in inbred laboratory animals than in humans, and the results have provided vital information about the genes contributing to autoimmunity. In the seminal experiments performed by Rosenthal and Shevach in 1973, immune responsiveness to synthetic antigens in guinea pigs was shown to be linked to MHC loci encoding products expressed by macrophages, now known as class II molecules (Table 4.3; see also Chapter 3, p. 78). At about the same, Zinkernagel and Doherty demonstrated the role of MHC class I molecules in the genetic restriction of cytotoxic Tc cells (Fig. 4.9). These results focused attention on the critical role of the MHC in immunogenetics, although there is still incomplete understanding of the organisation and function of this huge complex (Fig. 4.2).

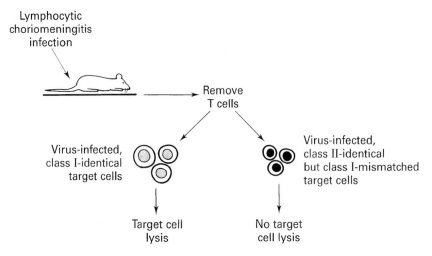

Fig. 4.9. Demonstration of MHC class I restriction of CD8$^+$ cytotoxic T cells in mice infected with a virus. A variety of class I molecules exist that present different viral antigens.

The basic structure of MHC class I and II molecules is similar. For class I molecules, a large polymorphic α-chain is non-covalently linked to the invariant β$_2$-microglobulin, whereas two polymorphic chains, α and β, associate for a class II molecule. In both cases, this structure results in an antigen-binding groove composed of two α-helices with a β-pleated sheet floor (Fig. 4.3). The groove is surrounded by the most polymorphic residues in the MHC molecule, encoded by the different class I or II alleles and creating a series of different grooves. Whether a peptide epitope can bind to a particular groove and be presented to a T cell, therefore, depends on the fit, which in turn is determined by the MHC alleles the individual has inherited.

The class I and II MHC genes may control immune responsiveness by a combination of the following mechanisms.

1. Determinant selection. The various MHC alleles inherited by an individual determine which antigenic peptides can be presented to T cells. If a particular peptide cannot bind to the range of grooves in an APC, the individual will not mount an immune response against that antigenic determinant.

2. Clonal selection. By a similar process but operating during T cell development, certain MHC molecules may tolerise particular T cells by deletion or anergy and positively select others. The MHC alleles, therefore, shape to the individual's T cell repertoire.

3. Immune suppressor genes. Certain MHC class II loci may operate as immune suppressor genes, influencing the behaviour of antigen-specific T cells that modulate the immune response. For complex antigens, there are many potential T cell epitopes and some may induce suppression rather than help. Thus, an individual may fail to respond to an antigen because particular MHC alleles can present these epitopes to induce suppression.

Other MHC genes

There are several other MHC genes that can influence immune responsiveness. One product, tumour necrosis factor (TNF), is a cytokine that is encoded in the MHC and has many important immunological effects; cytotoxicity against tumour cells is actually not its major property. Genetic variation in TNF levels could contribute to the strength of an immune response. Certain components of complement are also encoded in the class III region (Fig. 4.2), including C4. In individuals with deficiency of C4, caused by the presence of one or two null alleles of the gene for C4A, there is impaired complement activation that prevents the normal clearance of immune complexes. These may be deposited in various tissues, giving rise to the autoimmune disorder systemic lupus erythematosus (SLE).

This example is also important as it illustrates an important feature of MHC loci, *linkage disequilibrium*, by which certain alleles are found together more frequently than would be expected by chance. Linkage disequilibrium arises because recombination within the MHC is not random, being particularly restricted to sites called 'hot spots'. The loci between such hot spots are, therefore, inherited in a block, and selection has allowed certain combinations of alleles (termed a *haplotype*) to become frequent in the population. In Caucasians, the *HLA-A1*, *HLA-B8*, *HLA-DR3* haplotype is common and this haplotype also includes a C4A null allele. SLE is apparently associated with these particular class I and II alleles, but the likely mechanism is through the C4 class III allele in linkage disequilibrium.

Non-MHC genes

The role of these is at present unclear, but there is no doubt that several non-MHC loci determine immune and autoimmune responses. Likely candidates include genes encoding the TCR and immunoglobulins, as these are critical in antigen recognition, and also genes encoding cytokines and their regulators. Recently a gene on murine chromosome 19 has been discovered which encodes the Fas antigen that plays a fundamental role in negative selection in the thymus. Mice with a defective *fas* gene fail to delete autoreactive T cells and develop a condition resembling SLE.

Non-genetic factors in autoimmunity

Females are more prone to autoimmune disease and this is owing to female sex steroids, because the sex difference only becomes apparent after puberty, and oestrogens confer enhanced susceptibility in animal models of autoimmunity. Oestrogens generally enhance any immune response. In contrast, testosterone given to female animals reduces their risk of developing autoimmunity. Stress may precipitate autoimmunity via neuro-endocrine effects on the immune response. Glucocorticoids are particularly important, having suppressive effects that may impair regulation of autoreactive T cells. However, lymphocytes possess receptors for many hormones and for other regulatory molecules whose levels are altered by stress, and the sympathetic innervation of lymphoid organs can mediate effects of central nervous system stimulation.

Infections have been proposed as precipitating agents in many autoimmune diseases, but good evidence exists for only a few conditions. Possible mechanisms are as follows.

1. Direct infection of a cell by a virus leads to release of relatively hidden auto-antigens or modifies cell surface molecules making them immunogenic.
2. Infection affects the cells of the immune system, enhancing incipient auto-immune responses indirectly.
3. Amino acid sequences within endogenous proteins of the infecting organism sufficiently resemble self antigen that an immune response against the infection leads to recognition of the cross-reactive autoantigen. This is termed *molecular mimicry*. It accounts for the myocardial damage (rheumatic heart disease) that results from streptococcal infections in some individuals, as there is cross-reactivity between antigens in this organism and the heart.

Infections do not always precipitate autoimmunity. In some experimental models, autoimmune diseases occur more frequently if the animal is raised in a germ-free environment. Presumably non-specific immune stimulation from commensal organisms is required to maintain immunoregulation of autoreactive lymphocytes. Drugs can also induce autoimmune diseases by molecular mimicry or by combining with a self antigen to create novel antigens to which tolerance does not exist. Environmental toxins may likewise be involved.

Effector mechanisms

It is usual to consider the effector mechanisms in autoimmune disease as cell-mediated and humoral (i.e. antibody mediated) and the various possibilities are shown in Table 4.4. However, both types of response occur in most autoimmune diseases, and deciding which is the most important in initiation can be difficult (Table 4.5). In some cases, autoantibodies arise after the tissue is injured, but even in this secondary phase, they may be important determinants of disease outcome. The presence of circulating autoantibodies can be assessed by a number of immunoassays and the results of these are extremely valuable in diagnosis. Several tests are available to determine cell-mediated autoimmune responses but these tend to be used for research purposes only as their clinical relevance is not established. The results are often difficult to interpret, in part because the lymphocytes that can be most easily tested come from the circulation, but it is usually inaccessible T cells infiltrating the target organ that contain the major autoreactive population. The target organ also contains B cells making auto-antibodies, but these also secrete antibodies into the circulation, making serological testing feasible.

Treatment of autoimmune disease

Many autoimmune diseases require no immunological treatment as the condition is mild or simple treatment is sufficient (for instance, hormone replacement in some auto-immune endocrine disorders). Other conditions are more serious and an immunothera-

Table 4.4. *Effector mechanisms in autoimmune disease*

Antibody-mediated mechanisms
Complement fixation
Antibody-dependent cell-mediated cytotoxicity (ADCC): NK cells bind to antibodies on the target
  cell via Fc receptors and kill it
Direct effects, e.g. enzyme inhibition
Receptor stimulation or blockade

Cell-mediated mechanisms
CD8[+] T cell-mediated cytotoxicity
Release of cytokines with direct effects on the target cell
Indirect effects of cytokines, stimulating bystander lymphocytes and macrophages, which then
  exacerbate tissue injury

Table 4.5. *Features distinguishing between humoral and cell-mediated autoimmune disease*

	Humoral	Cell mediated
Antibodies against a specific autoantigen in all patients	Yes	No
T cells reacting against a specific autoantigen in all patients	Yes[a]	Yes
Autoantibody detectable in target organ	Yes	No
T cells present on target organ	Possibly	Yes
Disease in neonates of mothers with disease	Yes	No
Disease transferred to animals by T cells	No	Yes
Disease transferred to animals by serum	Yes	No
T cell removal improves disease	Yes[a]	Yes
Antibody removal (e.g. plasma exchange) improves disease	Yes	No

Note:
[a] Autoantibody production requires T cell help.

peutic solution would be optimal, yet at present the risks outweigh the benefits. For example, type 1 (insulin-dependent) diabetes mellitus causes considerable late morbidity, yet intensive insulin replacement provides the best current option (Chapter 7). Finally, some disorders are so pressing that immunological treatment is justified, although current regimens are relatively crude and non-specific (Table 4.6).

Glucocorticoids have a number of non-specific immunosuppressive actions and are used in several autoimmune disorders; however, they cause severe side effects when given at high dosage for a prolonged period. Other agents, like penicillamine and gold, have been found empirically to modify the immune response in rheumatoid arthritis, while newer immunosuppressive agents, such as cyclosporin A and tacrolimus, have been developed as successful treatment for transplantation rejection; their non-specific effects also make them useful in severe autoimmune disorders. Plasma exchange aims to remove circulating antibodies and immune complexes, but these recur unless immunosuppressive therapy is also started. All these treatments can suppress beneficial

Table 4.6. *Current treatments commonly used for autoimmune disease*

Treatment	Comment
Glucocorticoids	Anti-inflammatory and, at high dosage, immunosuppressive
Cytotoxic drugs (e.g. azathioprine, cyclophosphamide, methotrexate)	Non-specifically inhibit cell proliferation, particularly rapidly dividing lymphocytes
Disease-modifiying treatment (gold, penicillamine, chloroquine, sulphasalazine)	Diverse agents found to influence the course of rheumatoid arthritis and other non-organ-specific disorders; they have a variety of immunological effects
Cyclosporin A; tacrolimus	Non-specifically inhibit T cell function; also used in transplantation
Plasma exchange	Useful for severe antibody-mediated disease (e.g. myasthenia gravis) but only temporary effects if used alone
Intravenous immunoglobulin	Pooled normal immunoglobulin may contain naturally occurring anti-idiotypic antibodies that restore immunoregulatory networks

as well as harmful immune responses, so the complications of infection and certain malignancies are not surprising with prolonged usage.

Exciting preliminary results in non-organ-specific autoimmune disorders (Table 4.7) have been obtained using monoclonal antibodies to delete or block certain T cell populations. This is becoming more acceptable as mouse or rat monoclonal antibodies can be engineered to contain human C region sequences, thereby preventing an immune response to these animal proteins. Monoclonal antibodies against key cytokines like TNF may also suppress autoimmune responses. Long-term results are not yet available and such studies have only involved small numbers of patients. However, in some cases, lasting remission has occurred. This suggests that correcting only a single component in the complex sequence of events causing autoimmune disease is sufficient for innate immunoregulatory mechanisms to restore and maintain control over autoreactive lymphocytes.

More specific immunotherapy is possible, based on the results from animal models of autoimmunity (Fig. 4.10). These treatments require further advances in our understanding for their application to humans. In particular, it will be important to identify individuals at risk of developing autoimmune disease to enable early treatment to commence, as autoimmune responses diversify with disease duration. By the time a disease becomes clinically apparent, the number of autoantigens and TCRs involved is usually too great to make specific therapy feasible. Furthermore, target organ destruction may be irreversible. Immunogenetic markers could be of key importance in predicting those at risk, particularly if combined with markers of an early phase in the autoimmune response. Of course, if some of these approaches to restoring tolerance turn out to be

Table 4.7. *Major examples in the spectrum of autoimmune disease*

Spectrum	Disease	System affected
Organ-specific disease		
	Hashimoto's thyroiditis	Thyroid
	Type 1 diabetes mellitus	Pancreatic β cells
	Pernicious anaemia	Gastric parietal cells
	Addison's disease	Adrenal (sometimes ovary)
	Graves' disease	Thyroid, orbit (sometimes skin)
	Myasthenia gravis	Skeletal muscles
	Pemphigus vulgaris	Skin, mucous membranes
	Primary biliary cirrhosis	Intrahepatic bile ducts[a]
	Chronic active hepatitis	Liver[a]
	Sjögren's syndrome	Salivary and lacrimal glands[a]
	Rheumatoid arthritis	Joints[a]
	Scleroderma	Skin, joints, kidney, gut, lungs
Non-organic specific disease	Systemic lupus erythematosus	Widespread

Note:
[a] Associated with other features in some patients.

innocuous (e.g. orally induced tolerance), they could be universally applied, but considerable effort will be needed to ensure that such strategies do not actually cause disease in certain individuals.

The spectrum of autoimmune disease

The range of autoimmune disease is often considered as a spectrum, with organ-specific conditions at one end and non-organ-specific conditions at the other (Table 4.7). The various organ systems involved depend on the tissue distribution of the autoantigen, an ubiquitous autoantigen inducing non-organ-specific disorders. The organ-specific conditions tend to be associated with each other and there is quite extensive overlap in the autoimmune responses seen in the non-organ-specific disorders, to the point that a definite diagnostic label cannot be attached to certain patients. Shared immunogenetic susceptibility may be partly responsible for these associations, and the consequences of tissue injury in non-organ-specific disease can also result in a diverse autoimmune response.

AUTOIMMUNE THYROID DISEASE

The exemplar condition in this chapter is autoimmune thyroid disease, which includes both destruction of the thyroid (autoimmune hypothyroidism) and hyperthyroidism (Graves' disease). Some patients show a transition from one extreme to the other, and immune responses against the same thyroid autoantigens can be

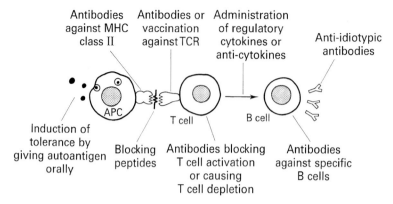

Fig. 4.10. Sites of action for novel forms of immunotherapy in autoimmune disease. These have been explored generally in animal models so far.

detected in both conditions. Autoimmune hypothyroidism is usually divided into two forms: Hashimoto's thyroiditis, in which there is a goitre (enlargement of the thyroid gland), and atrophic thyroiditis, in which the gland is smaller than normal. The goitre results from pronounced lymphocytic infiltration, whereas there is predominantly fibrosis in atrophic thyroiditis. Some cases of Hashimoto's thyroiditis can develop atrophy and fibrosis, so that these two forms of autoimmune thyroiditis may be a continuum.

Autoimmune hypothyroidism

Autoimmune hypothyroidism is common, affecting about 1% of women and 0.1% of men; it is an example of a predominantly cell-mediated autoimmune disease. However, in keeping with many autoimmune conditions, autoantibodies against thyroid antigens can easily be detected in these patients: antibodies against thyroglobulin (TG) were the first clear example of an autoimmune response to be described in humans. TG is a large protein that stores thyroid hormone in the colloid filling thyroid follicles. Antibodies to TG and other thyroid autoantigens are diagnostically useful, but their role in causing tissue injury is uncertain (see below). The major clinical features of autoimmune hypothyroidism are shown in Fig. 4.11.

   The condition is caused by destruction of thyroid cells so that few thyroid follicles remain. The remaining thyroid epithelial cells may show hyperplasia because they are stimulated by excessive thyroid-stimulating hormone (TSH) (Fig. 4.12). Some also show a vacuolated, eosinophilic cytoplasm because of an increase in mitrochondria and are termed Hurthle or Askanazy cells. Fibrosis predominates in atrophic thyroiditis, whereas lymphocytic infiltration, with the formation of germinal centres (like in lymph node cortex), is prominent in Hashimoto's thyroiditis. Both elements are present to varying degrees in most affected thyroids.

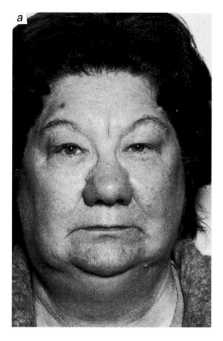
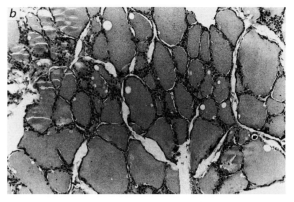
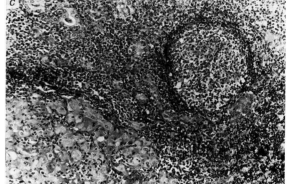

Symptoms
  Weight gain but poor appetite
  Loss of energy and depression
  Dry skin and hair
  Feeling cold
  Constipation
  Altered period (menorrhagia, oligomenorrhoea)

Signs
  Cool dry skin
  Slow pulse (bradycardia)
  Slow relaxing tendon reflexes
  Obesity
  Diffuse hair loss
  Goitre (in Hashimoto's thyroiditis)

Diagnosis
  Elevated TSH, low free T$_4$
  Thyroglobulin and thyroid peroxidase antibodies
  (detected by immunofluorescence,
  haemagglutination or ELISA methods)

Fig. 4.11. Major clinical features of autoimmune hypothyroidism. (*a*) Facial appearance of a patient with Hashimoto's thyroiditis. (*b*) Thyroid section from a normal thyroid. (*c*) Thyroid section from a patient with Hashimoto's thyroiditis. Note that destruction of thyroid follicles and the lymphocytic infiltration. (Original magnification ×200; photomicrographs courtesy of Dr T. J. Stephenson, Sheffield.)

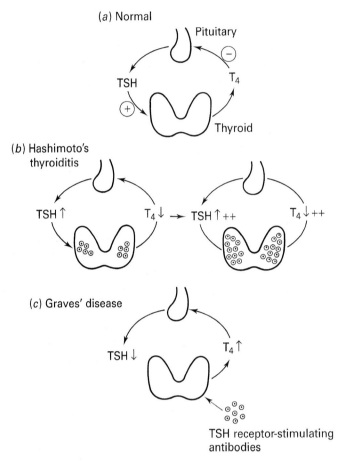

Fig. 4.12. Effect of autoimmune thyroid disease on the pituitary–thyroid axis. (*a*) The normal feedback loop. (*b*) In the early stage of Hashimoto's thyroiditis (left), a decline in thyroxine (T$_4$) production leads to an increase in TSH. This can stimulate the remaining thyroid cells to make sufficient T$_4$ to maintain values within the normal reference range. After months or years of continuing destruction (right), the TSH can no longer compensate and the T$_4$ levels become sub-normal. (*c*) In Graves' disease, there is production of TSH receptor-stimulating antibodies by B cells within and outside the thyroid. The antibodies induce hyperthyroidism and pituitary TSH secretion declines.

Lessons from experimental autoimmune thyroiditis

Experimental autoimmune thyroiditis (EAT) is the archetypal animal model of auto-immune disease. In 1956, the same year that TG antibodies were described in Hashimoto's thyroiditis, Rose and Witebsky showed that immunisation of rabbits with rabbit TG induced thyroid lymphocytic infiltration (i.e. thyroiditis) and TG antibody formation. To do this, TG had to be given with an adjuvant, a mixture of substances empirically found to enhance the immune response to an antigen. In this case, the adjuvant was a mixture of mineral oil and killed mycobacteria (called complete Freund's adjuvant), which probably enhances immunogenicity because the oil allows persistence of the antigen and the mycobacteria produce non-specific stimulation of a wide variety of immune responses, increasing the likelihood of specific antigen recognition.

These experiments showed that self-reactive T and B cells exist in healthy normal animals and, under extreme circumstances, can be provoked into responses against tissue-specific autoantigens. Subsequently, EAT was induced in a variety of species by the same technique, with most work being performed using mice. As a result of the availability of inbred mouse strains, it was soon appreciated that the autoimmune response to TG was influenced by MHC class II genes, which determined whether an animal was a good responder or a poor responder. This distinction presumably reflects the ability of certain class II molecules to bind TG epitopes and to influence the T cell repertoire. Other genes may also contribute to susceptibility. In particular, MHC class I genes may operate by determining whether or not a particular TG epitope, recognised by CD8$^+$ cytotoxic T cells, is expressed with class I molecules on the thyroid cell surface.

Using monoclonal antibodies to deplete T cell subsets, it can be shown that both CD4$^+$ and CD8$^+$ T cells are essential for the development of EAT after immunisation. TG-specific CD4$^+$ T cells can be cloned from diseased animals and grown in tissue culture: small numbers of these cells will produce EAT when transferred to a healthy recipient. TG- and MHC class I-specific CD8$^+$ T cells are responsible for thyroid cell killing, whereas TG antibodies have little effect on thyroid cells *in vitro* or *in vivo*. Therefore, this is clearly a T cell-mediated disease, with CD4$^+$ T cells being involved in initiation and CD8$^+$ T cells in tissue injury.

The central role T cells play in EAT is further demonstrated by manipulating the T cell repertoire without TG immunisation. In certain strains of mice and rats, removing the thymus at a critical stage in T cell development can induce severe EAT, with TG antibody formation and lymphocytic thyroiditis. Two mechanisms contribute to this. Thymectomy may result in the persistence of autoreactive T cells due to be deleted later in development and may also deplete the animals of critical immunoregulatory T cells that keep non-tolerised TG-specific T cells in check. The latter possibility is supported by transfer experiments: EAT gets better in animals receiving T cells from healthy donors, whose immunoregulatory network is intact. Thymectomy and other forms of T cell depletion will induce other autoimmune diseases, such as pernicious anaemia, oophoritis and type 1 diabetes mellitus, depending on the strain of the animal as well as on environmental factors. Given the influence of MHC genes in shaping the T cell repertoire, this genetic component is not surprising.

A third type of EAT arises spontaneously in certain animal strains and, therefore, most closely resembles autoimmune hypothyroidism in humans (Table 4.8). In one such example, the obese strain (OS) chicken, three separate genetic elements determine susceptibility. One lies within the MHC, another controls T cell regulation and the third determines the thyroid response to autoimmunity. The exact loci involved have not been delineated, but the idea of genetic susceptibility being in part target-organ specific is appealing as an explanation for the striking specificity of many autoimmune disorders.

The development of thyroiditis in OS chickens is critically dependent on T cells, although thyroid antibodies may also be important effectors of tissue damage by

Table 4.8. *Animal models of spontaneous autoimmune thyroiditis*

	Obese strain (OS) chicken	Buffalo strain rat	BB strain rat	Non-obese diabetic mouse
Thyroiditis (incidence, %)	>90	<25	Variable: up to 60	Variable: up to 90
TG antibodies	Yes	Yes	Yes	Yes
T cell dependent	Yes	Yes	Yes	Probably
Female preponderance	No	Yes	Yes	No
Dietary iodine exacerbates disease	Yes	Yes	Yes	Not tested
Hypothyroid	Yes	No	No	Not tested
Autoimmune diabetes also present	No	No	Yes	Yes

complement fixation and by antibody-dependent cell-mediated cytotoxicity (ADCC). TG is a heavily iodinated molecule because of the need for iodine in thyroid hormone synthesis. TG antibody formation in OS chickens depends on how much iodine is present in the diet: TG with a low iodine content does not induce antibody formation, presumably because the iodine is crucial to epitopes recognised by both T cells and B cells. Furthermore, murine EAT induced by TG immunisation results in T cell recognition of an epitope containing iodine at a critical site in the TG molecule where thyroid hormones are formed. Therefore, dietary iodine is an example of an environmental factor operating with genetic susceptibility to determine whether autoimmune thyroid disease is induced.

Immunogenetics of autoimmune hypothyroidism

In Caucasians, autoimmune hypothyroidism is associated with the class II specificity HLA-DR3, which can now be divided by molecular techniques into two alleles, DRB1*0301 and DRB1*0302. So far it is not clear whether one or both of these alleles is responsible for the association, and in certain Caucasian populations there are additional HLA-DR associations. The simplest way of determining whether an allele contributes to genetic susceptibility is to measure the frequency in patients and healthy subjects and determine the relative risk (Table 4.9), which gives some idea of how important a factor is for the individual. An alternative figure, the aetiological fraction, indicates how much of a disease may be attributed to the genetic factor. By both measures, the contribution of HLA-DR3 to the development of autoimmune hypothyroidism is quite small and does not explain the entire genetic contribution to susceptibility.

Furthermore, different class II alleles are associated with autoimmune hypothyroidism in non-Caucasian populations and, in Caucasians, only a small proportion of individuals with the HLA-DR3 specificity develop the disease. These facts show that HLA-DR3 itself cannot be responsible for autoimmune hypothyroidism, acting instead as a risk factor whose impact will be determined by other, unknown genes influencing the autoimmune

Table 4.9. *Measuring the strength of an association between an allele (HLA-X) and a disease. Data are obtained on N_1 plus N_2 patients and N_3 plus N_4 healthy controls, divided according to the presence or absence of* HLA-X

	$HLA\text{-}X^+$	$HLA\text{-}X^-$
Patients	N_1	N_3
Control subjects	N_2	N_4

Note:
The relative risk is $(N_1 \times N_4)/(N_2 \times N_3)$.

response, and by environmental factors. It is, therefore, not surprising that autoimmune hypothyroidism in juveniles shows a much stronger tendency to be inherited than the same condition in adults. If a potent combination of genes is inherited, autoimmune disease will result early in life without much need for an environmental contribution, whereas a mild immunogenetic susceptibility will only cause disease in combination with the appropriate non-genetic factors, which requires time for the exposure to occur.

The mechanism by which *HLA-DR3* increases susceptibility is not known, but a number of other autoimmune diseases are also associated with *HLA-DR3*, particularly the *DRB1*0302* allele. This is in linkage disequilibrium with *HLA-A1*, *HLA-B8* (and other MHC alleles) and forms a common haplotype in Caucasians. A number of non-specific immunological functions are altered in healthy *HLA-A1*, *HLA-B8*, *HLA-DR3*-positive individuals, including enhanced TNF production (as a result of a TNF allele also in linkage disequilibrium), and some survival advantage is probably conferred by this haplotype. Although heightened immune responsiveness against foreign, microbial antigens may have been a beneficial result, the same non-specific enhancement exacerbates any autoimmune response, explaining the frequent association of this haplotype and autoimmune diseases.

An alternative way to assess genetic contribution is to measure linkage. If a marker is associated with a disease, then it should segregate with the disease in a family with multiple affected members. The presence of disease in a family member without the marker is compelling evidence against its importance. Recently, linkage analysis has shown little evidence for HLA markers determining susceptibility to autoimmune thyroid disease. This is still in keeping with a role for *HLA-DR3* in *exacerbating* the autoimmune response but suggests that other genes outside the MHC are of key importance in disease *initiation*. The location of these other genes is unknown. By analogy with the OS chicken (in which MHC genes also make a relatively minor contribution) loci controlling T cell and target organ responses could be involved.

Non-genetic factors

The clearest non-genetic factor is the influence of hormones on the autoimmune response (although of course an individual's hormone profile is in part genetically determined). Autoimmune hypothyroidism is 4–10 times more common in women, this sex

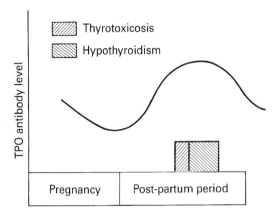

Fig. 4.13. Post-partum thyroiditis in a woman with thyroid peroxidase (TPO) antibodies before conception. TPO antibody levels, reflecting the severity of autoimmune thyroiditis, decline during pregnancy but rise in the post-partum period. At the peak of this rise, there may be sufficient thyroid injury to release stored thyroid hormones, causing transient thyrotoxicosis. If the injury continues, the stores are depleted and the patient becomes hypothyroid. When the antibody levels fall, the normal thyroid function is restored but the patient is at risk of autoimmune thyroid disease in the future.

difference beginning after puberty. Experiments in EAT show that disease can be prevented by giving testosterone to female animals and is exacerbated by oestrogens or castration in males, indicating that sex hormones are the important factors in this. Pregnancy also alters the autoimmune response, with a decline in disease activity during pregnancy and a post-partum rebound in the year after delivery (Fig. 4.13). Although it is not entirely clear yet why these changes occur, they seem likely to be related to the variations in sex and other hormones with pregnancy. In the majority of women, immunoregulatory mechanisms lead to recovery from the disease with few effects, but in some patients the post-partum exacerbation of pre-existing mild autoimmune thyroiditis may be severe enough to result in permanent clinical hypothyroidism. Therefore, pregnancy is a risk factor for the development of autoimmune hypothyroidism, further increasing the proportion of women with this disorder.

As in EAT, iodine intake is another factor determining susceptibility. An increase in dietary iodide in the West has been blamed for an apparent rise in Hashimoto's thyroiditis, but exact figures are not available to confirm this. There is no clear evidence that infection is important. Viral (or subacute) thyroiditis is not usually followed by autoimmune hypothyroidism and viruses have not been detected in affected thyroid tissue. However, it is possible that a viral (or bacterial) infection may trigger autoimmunity months or years before the condition becomes apparent clinically. At this stage, the absence of an infecting organism would be expected.

Autoimmune responses against thyroid autoantigens

There are three major thyroid autoantigens: TG, thyroid peroxidase (TPO), the key enzyme involved in thyroid hormone synthesis, and the TSH receptor, which transmits the stimulatory signal from pituitary-derived TSH to the thyroid cell (Fig. 4.12). The immune response to the TSH receptor is discussed in the next section. T cells recognising and reacting to TG and TPO can be detected in patients with autoimmune hypothyroidism and, occasionally, in much lower frequency, in healthy controls. This suggests that some thyroid-specific T cells escape thymic tolerance but are normally kept under control by immunoregulatory networks. Whether a primary defect in control contributes to the initiation of thyroid autoimmunity is unknown, as it is difficult to examine patients at the initiation of the autoimmune response.

By the time of clinical presentation, a number of different TG and TPO epitopes are recognised by polyclonal T cells expressing heterogeneous TCRs. This may represent *determinant spreading*, following the response to only a single dominant epitope in the initial phase of the illness. Once an autoimmune response starts, it spreads to involve other (cryptic) epitopes because the localised inflammation brings together activated APCs and T cells releasing cytokines, which overcome any tolerance to these cryptic determinants. As a consequence, attempts to limit immune damage by using modified epitopes or influencing specific TCRs is unlikely to succeed by the time disease becomes apparent. Fortunately, this is not necessary in autoimmune hypothyroidism, as thyroxine replacement is sufficient treatment, but similar diversification occurs in some serious autoimmune disorders where such treatment would be beneficial.

The B cell response to TG and TPO is also polyclonal. Antibodies to TG in particular are frequent in healthy subjects, but these are generally IgM class and of low affinity and specificity, so-called *natural* autoantibodies. During the autoimmune process, the B cell response matures because specific B cells are stimulated by thyroid-reactive T cells. These autoantibodies are IgG and have high affinity and specificity. They are also present at high concentrations and their presence is useful in determining that autoimmunity is the cause of hypothyroidism in a newly diagnosed patient (Fig. 4.12). TG antibodies do not fix complement, because the B cell epitopes are too widely spread to allow complement fixation, which requires two or more immunoglobulin Fc regions in proximity. TPO antibodies do fix complement and can also mediate antibody-dependent cell-mediated cytotoxicity (ADCC) and inhibit the enzymatic activity of TPO *in vitro*.

These antibodies, therefore, contribute to the development of autoimmune hypothyroidism, but it also seems likely that cytotoxic T cells play an important role in thyroid cell damage (Fig. 4.14). In addition, the cytokines released by the infiltrating T cells and macrophages (especially γ-IFN (gamma-interferon) and TNF) have a number of adverse effects on thyroid cells, directly inhibiting function and inducing expression of MHC class II molecules and adhesion molecules such as intercellular adhesion molecule-1 (ICAM-1). The role of this 'aberrant' class II expression in thyroid autoimmunity is not yet clear. Although it was originally suggested that class II-positive thyroid cells would present autoantigens to T cells, exacerbating the autoimmune response, there is no evidence that these cells can provide a second, co-stimulatory signal. Therefore, thyroid cell class II expression may result in peripheral tolerance. The appearance of ICAM-1 on thyroid cells stimulates the adherence of lymphocytes expressing LFA-1 (lymphocyte function-associated antigen 1) (Fig. 4.4) and *in vitro* experiments show that this increases the killing of thyroid cells by cytotoxic T cells.

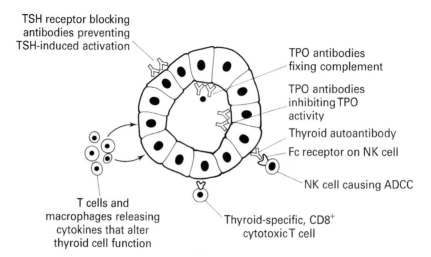

TSH receptor blocking
antibodies preventing
TSH-induced activation

TPO antibodies
fixing complement

TPO antibodies
inhibiting TPO
activity

Thyroid autoantibody

Fc receptor on NK cell

NK cell causing ADCC

T cells and
macrophages releasing
cytokines that alter
thyroid cell function

Thyroid-specific, CD8⁺
cytotoxic T cell

Fig. 4.14. Mechanisms causing thyroid cell injury and hypothyroidism in autoimmune hypothyroidism.

Graves' disease

In contrast to most cases of hypothyroidism, this is an example of a predominantly antibody-mediated autoimmune disease; TSH receptor autoantibodies bind to and stimulate the receptor, leading to hyperthyroidism (Fig. 4.12). The excessive production of thyroid hormones results in the main clinical features of the disease (Fig. 4.15). Graves' disease is frequently associated with a number of eye signs and symptoms, called ophthalmopathy, and this complication is discussed below. There is no animal model yet of Graves' disease.

The Graves' thyroid is enlarged as a result of hypertrophy and hyperplasia of the thyroid follicles, which have tall columnar epithelium with little colloid. There is also widespread lymphocytic infiltration and occasional germinal centre formation. Antibodies to TG and TPO are found in most patients with Graves' disease. In view of the shared autoimmune response against these two autoantigens, it is not surprising that some patients may have autoimmune hypothyroidism and then develop Graves' disease, and *vice versa*. Indeed, spontaneous hypothyroidism may occur in up to a quarter of Graves' patients followed for 20 years.

Precipitating factors

Graves' disease occurs in around 1% of women and 0.1% of men. There is a 30–50% concordance for Graves' disease in monozygotic twins, compared with around 7% concordance in HLA-identical siblings. These facts indicate the importance of both genetic and non-genetic factors in susceptibility and tell us that non-HLA genes make an important contribution. As in autoimmune hypothyroidism, *HLA-DR3* is associated with Graves' disease but the location of the other susceptibility genes is unknown.

Pregnancy and sex hormones, as well as dietary iodide, are important non-genetic

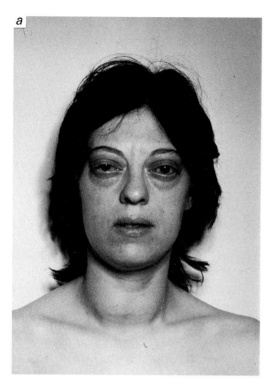 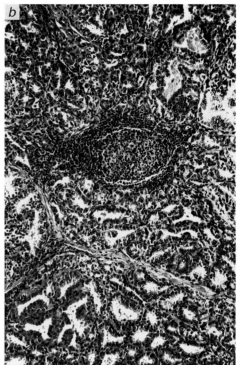

Symptoms
  Weight loss and increased appetite
  Irritability
  Feeling the heat; excessive sweating
  Tremor
  Palpitations
  Altered periods (oligomenorrhoea)

Signs
  Hot, sweaty palms
  Fine tremor of hands
  Fast pulse (sinus tachycardia, sometimes atrial fibrillation)
  Thin
  Diffuse firm goitre
  Eye signs (ophthalmopathy) in 60%

Diagnosis
  Suppressed TSH, elevated free T_4 and T_3 (triiodothyronine)
  TG and TPO antibodies in 75%
  TSH receptor antibodies in >95% (research assays;
  not in general clinical use)

Fig. 4.15. Major clinical features of Graves' disease. (*a*) Facial appearance of a patient with Graves' disease. Note the prominent eyes (proptosis) and swelling around the eyes (periorbital oedema), which are features of thyroid-associated opthalmopathy. (*b*) Thyroid section from a patient with Graves' disease (normal thyroid section is shown in Fig. 4.11*b*). Note the lymphocytic infiltration (centre). (Original magnification ×200; photomicrograph courtesy of Dr T. J. Stephenson, Sheffield.)

factors in precipitating Graves' disease. Stress, as measured by the frequency of adverse events such as divorce, bereavement and difficulties at work, can also initiate the condition. The effects of stress probably depend on altered neuroendocrine input into the immune system, altering regulation of the autoimmune response. There have been suggestions that infection may induce Graves' disease, although the evidence so far is fragmentary. Certainly *Yersinia* and other microorganisms contain proteins that cross-react with the TSH receptor, making molecular mimicry a possibility. If this does occur, it can only be a factor in a small proportion of patients, as most have no evidence of such infections. Nonetheless, it is important to appreciate that several different combinations of susceptibility factors, genetic and non-genetic, may induce the same clinical disorder.

TSH receptor antibodies

Several lines of evidence show that TSH receptor antibodies cause Graves' disease. First, they are detected in almost all Graves' patients, and when TSH receptor antibody levels fall, there is remission of the disease. Those without such antibodies have mild disease; therefore, the antibody level may be below the current level of detectability or the antibodies may be being made in the thyroid itself but do not appear in the serum. Second, thyroid stimulation can be produced by administration of the antibodies. Adams and his colleagues demonstrated in 1956 that radioiodine could be released from the thyroid gland of animals by administration of Graves' serum. Purified Graves' IgG stimulates thyroid cells *in vitro* and, using recombinant TSH receptors transfected into mammalian cells, can be shown to operate exclusively via this receptor. Finally, the babies born to mothers with high levels of TSH receptor-stimulating antibodies have transient thyrotoxicosis, produced by the placental transfer of maternal IgG. The severity of this neonatal thyrotoxicosis correlates well with the activity of TSH receptor antibodies in the mother's serum.

The production of TSH receptor antibodies is T cell dependent. Like the response against TPO and TG, this T cell response is polyclonal. The TSH receptor antibodies that cause Graves' disease bind to the extracellular domain of the TSH receptor and activate it, leading to an increase in intracellular cyclic AMP. This is the same pathway used by TSH, but the effects of TSH receptor antibodies may be longer lasting because of the high affinity of antibody binding to the receptor. Not all TSH receptor antibodies cause thyroid cell stimulation, however. Some bind to a different epitope on the receptor, which does not activate it but instead prevents TSH from doing so. These blocking antibodies, therefore, have the opposite effect to the stimulating antibodies, yet both may occur in the same patient, so that thyroid function is determined by the balance between the two. TSH receptor-blocking antibodies also occur in patients with goitrous and atrophic autoimmune hypothyroidism, in whom they may contribute to the impaired thyroid activity. Transient hypothyroidism can occur in babies born to such mothers, again because the antibodies cross the placenta.

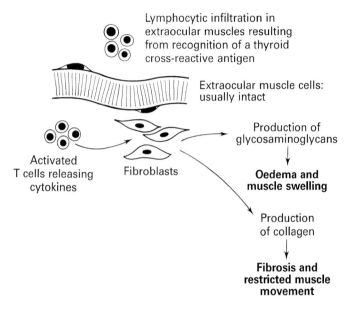

Fig. 4.16. Possible mechanisms involved in thyroid-associated ophthalmopathy. The nature of the shared autoantigen in thyroid and extraocular muscle is not known.

Thyroid-associated ophthalmopathy

Eye signs can be found in around two-thirds of Graves' patients (Fig. 4.15) and occasionally appear in Hashimoto's thyroiditis. These changes are caused by enlargement of the extraocular muscles, which are infiltrated by activated lymphocytes. As a result of cytokine production, fibroblasts in the muscles are stimulated, leading to increased production of glycosaminoglycans and collagen (Fig. 4.16). Using imaging techniques like CT scanning, it is apparent that almost all Graves' patients have some extraocular muscle enlargement and hence thyroid-associated ophthalmopathy. This suggests that the tissue-infiltrating lymphocytes in the thyroid and extraocular muscles may be recognising a similar (but unidentified) cross-reactive antigen present in the two sites. One obvious candidate is the TSH receptor, and recent preliminary experiments have shown the presence of a truncated form of the receptor in extraocular muscle. Smoking is a risk factor for the development of severe ophthalmopathy in Graves' disease, but the mechanism responsible is not known.

Summary

Autoimmune thyroid disease is important because it is common, and because research has elucidated basic mechanisms that apply to many other organ-specific (and, to a lesser extent, non-organ-specific) autoimmune conditions. It illustrates the occurrence of autoreactive T and B cells even in healthy individuals and the interaction of genetic and environmental susceptibility to induce these non-tolerised cells to produce autoimmune disease. Several different mechanisms could be involved, including the failure of patients to delete or anergise critical T and B cell populations, and disordered regulation of untolerised cells. The pathogenic mechanisms causing hypothyroidism and hyper-thyroidism are known and show how cell-mediated and antibody-mediated disease can be produced.

Treatment directed against the immune system is not required in autoimmune hypothyroidism or Graves' disease. Even if excessive destruction of the overactive thyroid results from radioiodine or surgical treatment of Graves' disease, thyroid hormone replacement restores normal function. However, in severe ophthalmopathy, which fortunately occurs in only around 5% of all Graves' patients, there can be major morbidity, as a result of disfiguring eye signs and compression of the optic nerve by the swollen extraocular muscles. Non-specific immunosuppressive agents such as corticosteroids and cyclosporin A have some beneficial effect but cause generalised immunosuppression and other side effects. Further understanding of the pathogenesis of ophthalmopathy may improve its treatment, and similar approaches are being exam-ined in many other severe autoimmune diseases, such as type 1 diabetes mellitus, rheumatoid arthritis and mul-tiple sclerosis.

FURTHER READING

General
Coutinho, A. & Kazatchkine, M.D. (eds.) (1993). *Autoimmunity Physiology and Disease*. New York: Wiley Liss.

Lachmann, P.J., Peters, D.K., Rosen, F.S. & Walport, M. (eds.) (1993). *Clinical Aspects of Immunology, 5th edn*. Oxford: Blackwell Scientific.

Paul, W.E. (ed.) (1993). *Fundamental Immunology, 3rd edn*. New York: Raven Press.

Roitt, I.M., Brostoff, J. & Male, D. (eds.) (1993). *Immunology, 3rd edn*. London: Mosby-Year Book Europe.

Talal, N. (ed.) (1991). *Molecular Autoimmunity*. London: Academic Press.

Theofilopoulos, A.N. (1995). The basis of autoimmunity. Parts I and II. *Immunology Today*, 16, 90–98; 150–159.

Specific topics
Burch, H.B. & Wartofsky, L. (1993). Graves' ophthalmopathy: current concepts regarding pathogenesis and management. *Endocrine Reviews*, 14, 747–793.

Kendall-Taylor, P. (ed.) (1995). Autoimmune Endocrine Disease. *Baillière's Clinical Endocrinology and Metabolism*, 5, 1–202.

Lanzavecchia, A. (1993). Identifying strategies for immune intervention. *Science*, 260, 937–944.

Lehmann, P.V., Sercarz, E.E., Forsthurber, T., Dayan, C.M. & Gammon, G. (1993). Determinant spreading and the dynamics of the autoimmune T-cell repertoire. *Immunology Today*, 14, 203–208.

Ramsdell, F. & Fowlkes, B.J. (1990). Clonal deletion versus clonal anergy: the role of the thymus in inducing self tolerance. *Science*, 248, 1332–1340. (There are several other excellent reviews in this issue of *Sc.. .ce*.)

Special Issue (multiple authors) (1993). Life, death and the immune system. *Scientific American*, September, 52–144.

Weetman, A.P. (1991). *Autoimmune Endocrine Disease*. Cambridge: Cambridge University Press.

Weetman, A.P. & McGregor, A.M. (1994). Autoimmune thyroid disease: further developments in our understanding. *Endocrine Reviews*, 15, 788–830.

5

Allergy

A. J. FREW, P. BRADDING, S. L. JOHNSTON, P. LACKIE, A.
SEMPER, J. SHUTE, A. F. WALLS AND S. T. HOLGATE

- Immediate hypersensitivity depends on IgE antibodies directed against external antigens. When relevant antigens bind to IgE molecules on the surface of mast cells, degranulation occurs with release of histamine and other mediators, which cause the symptoms of an acute allergic response.

- The tendency to make IgE antibodies is inheritable, but environmental factors are also important. Switching of B cells to make IgE is regulated by T lymphocytes, through focused production of IL-4 and contact through the CD40 receptor.

- Specific IgE antibodies can be detected by skin testing or blood tests.

- In allergic rhinitis and asthma, acute inflammation leads to the recruitment of eosinophils and T cells, which create a more chronic form of inflammation and cause epithelial damage.

- Respiratory virus infection may also be important in inducing and exacerbating allergic diseases.

- Possible future targets for intervention include: preventing B cells from switching over to IgE production; rendering tolerant the T cells that recognise allergens; inhibiting the actions of cytokines involved in the allergic response; blocking the effects of mast cell mediators (e.g. leukotrienes); preventing recruitment and activation of eosinophils.

Allergy and type I hypersensitivity

The ability to mount immediate or type I hypersensitivity responses is dependent on the production of IgE antibodies directed against environmental antigens. IgE binds to high-affinity Fc receptors (FcεRI) (one of two forms of Fc receptor, see below) on mast cells and basophils; when cross-linked, these cells release a range of chemical and protein mediators that initiate the allergic tissue response. The term *atopy* describes conditions that depend on type I hypersensitivity. These include conjunctivitis, rhinitis, asthma, urticaria and generalised anaphylaxis. Atopic eczema is also associated with high serum levels of IgE, although the precise role of IgE in eczema is less certain than in the other atopic conditions. The presence of antigen-specific IgE antibodies can be detected by skin testing with allergen extracts, and, depending on the population studied and the definition of reactivity, between 30 and 50% of a Caucasian population will show one or more positive responses. Positive skin tests mean that the subject is sensitised but do not automatically confirm the presence of clinical allergic disease. Atopic individuals with positive skin tests but no history of disease may be sensitised to allergens that they rarely encounter, or have target organs that are relatively insensitive to the inflammatory mediators released during mucosal allergic responses.

Family studies indicate that about 37% of the interindividual variation in total serum concentrations of IgE is determined by genetic factors, with the remaining 63% attributable to environmental factors and biological 'noise'. In 1989, Cookson and Hopkin presented a simple model for the genetics of atopy. Using a relatively broad definition of atopy and studying a total of 17 markers by RFLP analysis, they identified a single major autosomal dominant 'atopy gene' linked to D11S97 on chromosome 11q13. Building on this in a further sib-pair analysis, they proposed that the 'atopy gene' may be active preferentially when inherited from the maternal side, possibly by maternal modification of the infant's IgE response through the placenta or breast milk. In further studies, this group have shown that the β-chain of the FcεRI is within 10cM of D11S97, and variations in functional expression of FcεRI may influence the total serum or allergen-specific IgE levels. These preliminary findings need confirmation, however.

An alternative location for genes regulating the expression of atopy is the cluster of cytokine genes on chromosome 5, which includes the genes for IL-3, IL-4, IL-5, granulocyte-macrophage colony-stimulating factor (GM-CSF) and IL-13. As discussed below, these cytokines have been implicated in the regulation of IgE and of eosinophil numbers and function. It is easy to see how dysregulation of these genes might lead to increased ability to mount IgE responses and develop eosinophilic tissue inflammation. Polymorphisms have been identified in the 5' promoter regions of the IL-4 gene that have been tentatively correlated with high total IgE concentrations.

IgE antibodies and their receptors

IgE is one of five classes or *isotypes* of immunoglobulin, the others being IgM, IgG, IgA and IgD. IgE antibodies are a key element in the mechanism by which environmental allergens cause asthma. IgE molecules bind to isotype-specific Fc receptors (FcεR) on the surface of leucocytes, platelets and mast cells and, when cross-linked by antigen, induce the activation and degranulation of the FcεR-bearing cell with release of a range of stored and newly generated chemical mediators. There are two distinct forms of FcεR that are found on different cell types. The classical high-affinity receptor FcεRI is found on mast cells and basophils and is implicated in anaphylactic responses as well as atopic allergy. FcεRI consists of a tetrameric structure with a 45 kDa α-chain, a 33 kDa β-chain and two disulphide-linked γ-chains. IgE binds with high affinity to the α-chain via the distal portion of the IgE heavy chain. Signal transduction occurs through the β- and γ-chains. Cross-linking of two FcεRI molecules triggers activation of phospholipase C-γ and hydrolysis of inositol phospholipids, leading to degranulation with release of histamine and other performed chemical mediators, together with the generation of several newly formed mediators including leukotrienes and prostaglandins (Fig. 5.1).

More recently, a lower-affinity Fc receptor (FcεRII) has been described. Unlike most

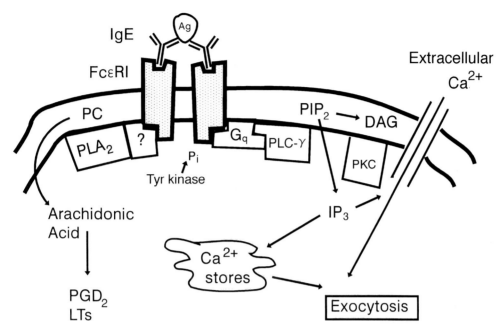

Fig. 5.1. IgE-dependent activation of the mast cell. Ag, antigen; PC, phosphatidyl choline; PLA_2, phospholipase A_2; G_q, G_q-protein; PLC-γ, phospholipase C-γ; PKC, protein kinase C; PIP_2, phosphatidyl inositol bisphosphate; IP_3, inositol trisphosphate; DAG, diacylglycerol; PGD_2, prostaglandin D_2; LTs, leukotrienes.

immunoglobulin Fc receptors, FcεRII, or CD23, is not a member of the immunoglobulin supergene family but has a lectin-like extracellular domain (Fig. 5.2). *Lectins* are proteins that bind carbohydrates and may induce proliferation of T or B cells. FcεRII is also unusual in that its carboxy-terminus is extracellular and the lectin domain is easily cleaved from the cell surface to form soluble CD23 molecules. Two forms (a and b) of human CD23 have been identified, which are formed by alternative splicing of mRNA and differ only in their amino-terminal intracellular portion. FcεRIIa is constitutively expressed on B cells only, while FcεRIIb is inducible by IL-4 and is expressed on a wider range of cells, including B cells, eosinophils, platelets, macrophages and activated T cells. IgE-dependent eosinophil and platelet activation have been shown to be important mechanisms in the killing of metazoan parasites *in vitro*, and FcεRII-bearing alveolar macrophages from asthmatic subjects can be sensitised to release leukotrienes on sub-sequent *in vitro* stimulation with allergen. It is less clear whether these FcεRII-dependent mechanisms are important in clinical diseases such as allergic asthma and rhinitis.

Although a great deal is now known about the structure of the Fc receptors for IgE, surprisingly little is known about the IgE antibodies themselves or the B cells that are recruited into IgE production. Clearly, better knowledge of the antibody component of the allergic response is essential in attempting to understand the allergic response and in looking towards ways of manipulating antibody production for therapeutic purposes. One of the reasons for our current lack of knowledge is that the amount of IgE in normal or atopic serum is very low (usually < 1 μg/ml), making conventional immunochemical

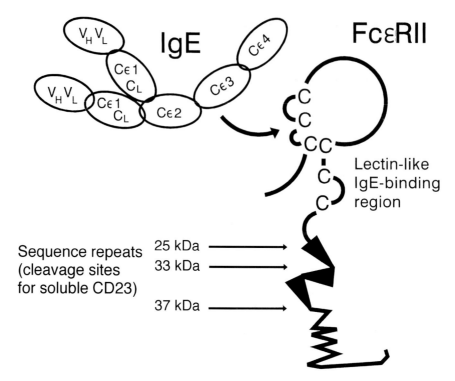

Fig. 5.2. Schematic representation of the structure of FcεRII and its attachment to IgE.

analysis difficult. Another complicating factor is the high susceptibility of IgE to proteolytic degradation. For IgG, IgA and IgM, a great deal of structural information has
been obtained from studying the monoclonal immunoglobulins secreted by neoplastic
plasma cells in patients with multiple myeloma. However, there are very few cases of
multiple myeloma in which the malignant plasma cells secrete monoclonal IgE. In fact,
most of our knowledge of the primary structure of human IgE has been obtained by
studies on just two myeloma proteins.

Recent advances in the techniques of molecular biology have made it possible to circumvent many of these analytical difficulties and have opened the way to probing not
only the general structural features of IgE but also the detailed amino acid sequences of
individual antibodies that interact with airborne allergens.

Antibodies bind to antigen via the variable regions of the heavy and light chains. The
'contact points' for interaction with antigen lie in the hypervariable or complementarity
determining regions (CDRs), of which there are three in each heavy and light chain. As
might be expected, these regions have immense variability in amino acid sequence,
which reflect the different specificities of individual antibodies. However, the framework sequences of the variable (*V*) regions, although less variable than the CDRs, are
also considered to have some influence on the binding of the antibody to antigen. During
the process of genetic recombination that gives rise to functional genes encoding the
heavy chains of antibody molecules, variable (V_H) region genes are juxtaposed to constant region genes (see Fig. 5.3). Initially, the constant region of the μ-chain is utilised so

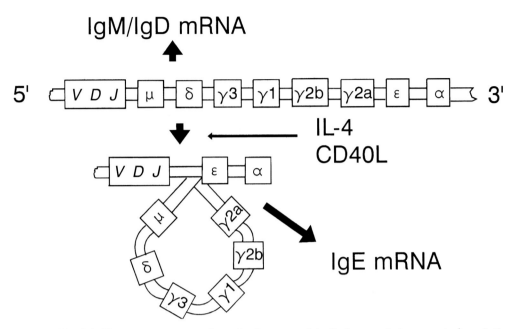

Fig. 5.3. The rearrangement of murine immunoglobulin heavy chain genes to form IgE: switching from IgM to IgE.

that IgM can be synthesised, but, under the influence of antigen and T cells, immunoglobulin class switching to IgG, IgA or IgE can occur. Specificity for antigen lies initially in the sequence of the *V* region chosen by recombination and, for the CDR3 region, in amino acids generated during nucleotide additions or losses during the recombination process. However, under the influence of antigen selection, further changes in amino acids also occur subsequently by somatic mutation, which result in altered amino acid sequences in CDR1 and CDR2 that can interact more efficiently with antigen. This means that the affinity of IgE antibody for allergen is affected first by the germline sequence of the *V* region chosen, second by the events of recombination and third by subsequent somatic mutations that occur particularly during isotype switching from IgM to IgE.

Altogether, there are about 100 V_H genes, which are divisible into six V_H families, with the genes in each family sharing similar sequences in their framework regions. It is becoming clear that some of these genes are used preferentially for antibodies against certain antigens, which suggests an influence of framework sequence on antibody activity. The largest studies so far have been concerned with autoantibodies, where there is asymmetric usage of V_H genes by B cells encoding rheumatoid factors and erythrocyte autoantibodies. Although there have been few studies of V_H genes used by antibodies to exogenous antigens, there is some evidence that these too show restricted V_H gene usage. Analysis of V_H gene usage in IgE antibodies has shown a higher than expected frequency of V_H5 gene usage and a high incidence of shared mutations in V_H transcripts from different individuals, which strongly supports a role for antigen in selecting particular antibody sequences.

The nature of allergens

Most allergens are proteins or glycoproteins, but IgE-mediated responses can also occur to a variety of drugs and carbohydrates. To be clinically relevant, an allergen must be capable of stimulating the immune system of susceptible individuals to make IgE antibodies directed against stable epitopes of the molecule and must then be encountered by an appropriate route in sufficient amounts to trigger an allergic tissue response. Therefore, pollen allergens are biologically important only if they are released in large amounts on respirable particles, from plants that exist in proximity to humans, and if the allergenic components are released from the pollen grains on contact with the respiratory mucosa. Similar considerations apply to mite antigens and animal danders. Low-molecular-weight allergens, such as drugs and various chemicals encountered in industry, are generally incapable of eliciting immune responses in their own right, but can act as *haptens* to trigger T cell-dependent responses by combining with host proteins (or carriers) and presenting altered hapten–carrier determinants to the immune system. Many allergens are enzymatically active and it has been proposed that protease activity may be important in facilitating access of the allergen to the immune system or in altering the way in which the allergen is handled by phagocytic cells and presented to the immunocompetent cells (T cells and B cells) that react specifically and generate the IgE directed against the allergen.

Other allergens may enter the body via the skin, e.g. hymenoptera venom, where phospholipase A_2 and other enzymes in the venom are the main elements recognised by IgE. The route of presentation is also important in the development of contact dermatitis, although this principally involves type IV (cell-mediated) hypersensitivity and will not be discussed further here. Immediate hypersensitivity can also develop against food allergens: IgE directed against cows' milk proteins is very common in infancy but generally remits with increasing age, whereas hypersensitivity against other food allergens (especially nuts, fish, shellfish, various fruits, chocolate, etc.) often arises later in life and tends to persist. Very little is known about the mechanisms responsible for these phenomena, although there is some evidence that immaturity of the infant gut mucosa may predispose towards the development of IgE antibodies against any ingested antigenic material.

Allergen extracts are complex mixtures of proteins. The precise number of components varies depending on the allergen source and on the extraction process. Multiple antigens have been identified in animal dander extracts (10–20 separate antigens), dust mite extracts (20–40 antigens) and pollen extracts (20–50 antigens). Crossed immunoelectrophoresis or immunoblot techniques can be used to determine which components of an extract bind IgE. Antigens that stimulate an IgE response and bind IgE are termed *allergens*, while antigens that bind IgE from more than 50% of a pool of allergic patients are regarded as *major allergens*. Potentially, all the antigenic components recognised by animal antisera may be allergens in humans. However, in practice 25–50% of the proteins in any allergen extract are allergens and one to three proteins will be major allergens.

Numerous major allergens have now been described and many have been sequenced at the protein and/or cDNA levels. It has been possible to map the B cell epitopes of some allergens, using competitive inhibition of binding of pairs of mouse monoclonal antibodies, or patients' sera. It has long been known that development of IgE responses is T cell dependent. The mechanisms controlling isotype switching are discussed in detail below. However, it has recently become clear that the antigen receptors of T cells and B cells have different recognition requirements (see Chapter 4). As a result, the epitopes recognised by T cells are distinct from those that are recognised by IgE antibodies. The ability to define immunodominant T cell epitopes could have major clinical implications as it opens up the possibility of using peptide fragments to induce T cell tolerance to allergens without exposing the patient to the risk of injecting IgE-binding epitopes, which might trigger local or systemic adverse reactions.

Cells involved in allergic reactions

Antigen-presenting cells and T cells

As discussed above, in atopic individuals, allergen-specific IgE is present both in the circulation and bound via FcεR to cells resident in mucosal tissues, particularly mast cells. Upon subsequent exposure, the allergen binds to surface IgE, leading to receptor cross-linking, mast cell degranulation and release of inflammatory mediators. However, allergen exposure also induces other events that maintain IgE levels and hence contribute to the chronicity and perpetuation of the allergic disease. These events are mediated by interactions between APCs, T cells and B cells (see Chapter 4).

To be effective, an APC must be capable of endocytosing potential antigens, of proteolytically digesting them and of associating the resulting peptides with MHC molecules before transporting the complex to the cell surface. Furthermore, the APC must provide accessory molecules for co-stimulation of T cells. Classical APCs fulfilling these criteria are the dendritic cell, cells of the monocyte/macrophage lineage and the B cell. Dendritic cells constitutively express a range of accessory molecules that other APC types usually only express upon activation.

In the lung, inhaled antigen is delivered to the luminal surface of the airways where it may be taken up by alveolar macrophages or by intraepithelial dendritic cells. *In vitro* studies have shown the alveolar macrophage to be a poor APC, whereas the dendritic cell is a potent activator of T cells. Since all known allergenic molecules are soluble, they could penetrate into the submucosa for uptake and presentation by 'professional' APCs such as the interstitial macrophage and the parenchymal B cell. For technical reasons, few *in vitro* studies have compared the function of putative APC populations derived from the lungs of asthmatics and normals. However, there is evidence that alveolar macrophages may actually suppress T cell responses, and those derived from asthmatics are less inhibitory to T cell activation than those from normal subjects.

The activation of CD4$^+$ T cells and their classification according to cytokine secretion have been considered in Chapter 4. Cytokines of major importance in asthma are shown in Table 5.1. In asthma, T cells derived from the peripheral blood or from the lung by bronchoalveolar lavage or bronchial biopsy have been cloned *in vitro* in the presence of

Table 5.1. *The principal activity and cell sources of cytokines that have been implicated in the pathogenesis of asthma*

Cytokine	Effects	Principal sources
IL-1	Lymphocyte activation	Macrophages, fibroblasts, epithelial cells
IL-2	T and B cell growth, eosinophil chemotaxis	T cells
IL-3	Eosinophil growth and activation, basophil growth	T cells, eosinophils
IL-4	IgE regulation, VCAM-1 upregulation, T_H2 cell growth, fibroblast activation	T cells, mast cells
IL-5	Eosinophil growth, chemotaxis, activation, survival and adhesion	T cells, mast cells, eosinophils
IL-6	B cell differentiation, IgE synthesis	T cells, macrophages, mast cells fibroblasts, eosinophils
IL-8	Neutrophil, T cell and eosinophil chemotaxis	Neutrophils, macrophages, epithelial cells, mast cells
GM-CSF	Eosinophil growth, chemotaxis and activation	T cells, eosinophils, epithelium
TNFα	Endothelial cell adhesion molecule upregulation	Macrophages, mast cells, T cells, eosinophils
γ-IFN	Antagonises many actions of IL-4 eosinophil activation, ICAM-1 upregulation	T cells
TGFβ	Fibrosis	Fibroblasts, macrophages, eosinophils, epithelial cells

Note:
TGF, transforming growth factor; VCAM/ICAM, vascular cell/intracellular adhesion molecule.

mitogen or specific allergen; the resulting clones produce IL-4. *In vivo* studies of mild, atopic asthmatics have also suggested a T_H2-like pattern of T cell cytokine production.

The factors responsible for this preferential activation of T_H2 cells in asthma and other human diseases are poorly understood. T cells stimulated in the presence of exogenous IL-4 tend to develop a T_H2 phenotype, a mechanism that might operate in established disease. Another potential mechanism is the release of IL-4 from mast cells (see below). What determines the outcome of stimulation of a naive T cell is more controversial, but it is likely that the phenotypic fate of a T cell is determined by the nature of its interaction with an APC. It has been suggested that APCs lacking a full repertoire of accessory molecules or those expressing IL-1 could favour the development of T_H2 cells. At the subcellular level, this may result in the activation of a particular signal transduction network that determines the response of the T cell. For example, T cells that fail to produce the transcription factor NF–κB, which is required for IL-2 production, go on to develop a T_H2 profile.

The site and mechanisms of IgE regulation

Activated T cells of the T_H2 subtype are particularly relevant to the pathogenesis of asthma. In the context of IgE production, the T cell delivers both contact-mediated and soluble signals to B cells. IL-4 is essential for somatic recombination, which switches the immunoglobulin *VDJ* gene cassette to the ε-heavy chain constant gene region. A second cytokine product of activated T_H2 cells, IL-13, can also switch B cells to IgE production. FcεRII on follicular dendritic cells together with CD40 ligand (CD40-L) on the activated T cell are necessary co-stimuli directing a B cell that has undergone IgE switching to proliferate and become an IgE-secreting plasma cell.

It is likely that the initiation of a primary immune response occurs in local draining lymph nodes when antigen-bearing dendritic cells enter T cell-rich areas of the lymph node and present antigens for perusal by T cells. Activated T cells are then able to interact with follicular dendritic cells and B cells in the germinal centres of secondary follicles. However, on repeated exposure to allergen, the cellular interactions responsible for IgE production could occur in the periphery, such as the specialised areas of bronchus-associated lymphoid tissue.

The maintenance of IgE levels in chronic allergic diseases such as asthma probably results only in part from the preferential stimulation of T_H2 cells. Mechanisms exist for inhibition of IgE production, most notably by γ-IFN, a product not only of T_H1 cells but also of some $CD8^+$ T cells. Asthma could, therefore, also be partly attributed to a defect, either actual or functional, in suppressor cell populations, leading to reduced ability to inhibit IgE production.

Mast cells and their mediators

Mast cells are central to type I hypersensitivity reactions. These cells are widely distributed throughout most tissues of the body but they tend to be present in highest numbers at potential portals of entry in the mucosal tissues of the respiratory and gastrointestinal tracts and in the skin. Although frequently situated close to blood vessels, mature mast cells are not found in the circulation and they are not closely related to their blood-borne analogues, the basophils. Mast cell hyperplasia is not a consistent feature of the affected tissues in allergic disease. However, there is abundant evidence for an increased degree of mast cell activation, and immediate hypersensitivity reactions in the nose, lung or skin are invariably associated with elevated concentrations of mast cell products in the interstitial fluid.

Mast cell granules contain potent mediators of inflammation synthesised within the cell and stored in its granules. These include histamine, several unique proteolytic enzymes, proteoglycans and some relatively poorly characterised factors that attract and activate eosinophils and neutrophils. The extrusion of these stored products is usually accompanied also by the generation of lipid mediators, including prostaglandin D_2 (PGD_2) and leukotriene C_4 (LTC_4). Recent evidence indicates that mast cells may be an important source of inflammatory cytokines. Although several of these are stored in mast cells, some may also be generated and released subsequent to mast cell activation.

The explosive degranulation of mast cells is a cardinal feature of allergic reactions and classically is triggered by an allergen cross-linking specific IgE molecules bound at the cell surface to FcεRI. In addition, substance P, a neurotransmitter released from the terminals of certain peptidergic nerves, the anaphylatoxins C3a and C5a, derived from complement, natural degranulating agents such as mellitin in bee venom, some drugs (e.g. morphine and codeine), and other stimuli may induce mast cell activation. Mast cell populations show considerable heterogeneity in their responsiveness to these agents. For example, substance P is a potent activator of human skin mast cells but does not affect lung mast cells.

Preformed mediators

Mast cells are the principal source of histamine in tissues, whereas basophils are the chief source in circulating cells. Histamine has been the most extensively studied of the mast cell mediators and has been a major target for drug development. It is a spasmogen for smooth muscle of the respiratory and gastrointestinal tracts and can induce mucus secretion. Histamine facilitates the local influx of circulating cells by increasing venular permeability and causes itching and vasodilatation in the skin, eyes and nose.

The most abundant secretory product of the mast cell is neutral proteases. The trypsin-like enzyme tryptase is the major protease in all human mast cells. Chymase, a chymotrypsin-like protease, is restricted to a subpopulation and is a useful biochemical marker of mast cell heterogeneity. Relative numbers of each mast cell subset may be altered in disease, but normally those mast cells that contain both tryptase and chymase (MC_{TC}) are most numerous in the skin and in submucosal tissues of the airways and intestine; whereas those which contain tryptase but not chymase (MC_T) predominate in mucosal tissues.

Increased concentrations of mast cell tryptase have been detected in lung lavage fluid from patients with asthma, in nasal lavage fluid from patients with rhinitis and in the serum of patients undergoing anaphylactic reactions. An understanding of the role of mast cell proteases has lagged behind an appreciation of their value as biochemical markers for mast cells. However, tryptase has been shown to degrade certain regulatory peptides including the bronchodilator vasoactive intestinal peptide (VIP) and the potent vasodilator calcitonin gene-related peptide (CGRP). Tryptase may also act as a growth factor for several cell types, including fibroblasts, epithelial cells, smooth muscle cells and keratinocytes. Chymase can generate the vasoconstrictor angiotensin II from angiotensin I (more efficiently than angiotensin-converting enzyme itself), can degrade certain tissue components and by activating IL-1β and cleaving IL-4 may help to control cytokine bioavailability at sites of inflammation. Both tryptase and chymase have been found to induce microvascular leakage and neutrophil accumulation when injected into laboratory animals.

Newly generated mediators

Following mast cell activation, arachidonic acid is liberated from membrane lipids. This is processed either by the cyclo-oxygenase pathway leading to the production of PGD_2

or by the 5-lipoxygenase pathway leading to the production of LTC_4. Basophils lack the capacity to generate PGD_2, and because the mast cell appears to be a major source of this product, PGD_2 has attracted attention as a biochemical marker for mast cell activation *in vivo*.

When a quantity as low as 1 nM PGD_2 or LTC_4 is injected into skin, a wheal with erythema may be observed for at least 2 hours afterwards. Both PGD_2 and LTC_4 are also powerful bronchoconstrictor agents. PGD_2 is some 10 times more potent than histamine in inducing bronchospasm, while LTC_4 is about 1000 times more potent. The ability of some leukotriene receptor antagonists to attenuate allergen-induced bronchoconstriction provides evidence that leukotrienes may be of importance in allergic disease.

Cytokines

Inflammatory cytokines were originally considered to be derived predominantly from lymphocytes, but it is now clear that they may be generated by a variety of cell types. In the late 1980s, experiments with mouse mast cell lines established that IgE-dependent activation could result in the release of a range of cytokines, including IL-1,IL-2, IL-3, IL-4, IL-5, IL-6, GM-CSF, TNFα, γ-IFN and at least four members of the chemokine family. Human mast cells have been shown to contain TNFα, IL-4, IL-5, IL-6 and IL-8 and can certainly release TNFα, IL-4 and IL-8. The ability of mast cells to produce cytokines means that the mast cell should be seen not just as an effector cell but also as a cell that may play a key role in the initiation and modulation of inflammatory and immune reactions.

Eosinophil biology

The eosinophil is derived from bone-marrow progenitors closely related to the basophil, and eosinophilic myelocytes generally reside in the bone marrow. Eosinophil production outside the bone marrow occurs only in disease, nasal polyposis for example. Little is known of the mechanisms leading to production of committed eosinophil progenitors from pluripotent stem cells. However, their subsequent proliferation and differentiation is under the influence of the cytokines IL-3, IL-5 and GM-CSF. IL-3 and GM-CSF generate eosinophil myelocytes and metamyelocytes, while IL-5 supports the terminal maturation that follows cessation of proliferation. In addition, these three cytokines support the survival of mature eosinophils, and eosinophils chronically exposed to these cytokines in inflamed tissue may have a lifespan of several weeks. Mature cells enter the circulation from the bone marrow and rapidly marginate in venules prior to emigration into perivascular subepithelial tissues of the respiratory, gastrointestinal and genitourinary tracts. Their adhesion and migration is carefully regulated (see below).

The mature eosinophil has a bi-lobed nucleus and a cytoplasmic compartment filled with membrane-bound secretory granules. There are three types of cytoplasmic granule: specific, primary and small dense granules. The most prominent are the specific (also called secondary) granules, which contain a crystalloid core surrounded by an outer matrix that is bounded by granule membrane. The basic proteins eosinophil cationic protein (ECP), eosinophil-derived neurotoxin (EDN) and eosinophil peroxidase (EPO)

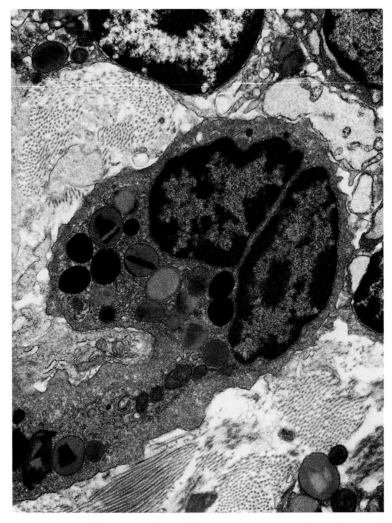

Fig. 5.4. Ultrastructure of an eosinophil in the bronchial mucosa of an asthmatic subject. Note the characteristic morphology of the cell granules, which show variable intensity of staining consistent with cellular activation.

are localised to the matrix of specific granules, while major basic protein (MBP) is found in the core (Fig. 5.4). Secretion of the basic proteins of the specific granules is central to the effector mechanisms of eosinophil-mediated cytotoxicity. These proteins are some of the most basic proteins in the human body, a property that is thought to be related to their cytotoxic activities. The focal secretion of the entire contents of specific granules during parasite killing is achieved by cumulative fusion of granules within the cytoplasm and subsequent compound exocytosis. The primary granules contain the Charcot–Leyden crystal protein, while the enzymes aryl sulphatase, acid phosphatase and catalase are found in the small dense granules. Eosinophils are a potential source of several cytokines, including IL-1α, IL-3, IL-5, GM-CSF, IL-6, MIP-1α, TNFα, TGFα and TGFβ.

Eosinophils possess both high- (FcεRI) and low-affinity (FcεRII) receptors for IgE. IgE-dependent activation of eosinophils from patients with allergic disease leads to selective release of EPO and MBP, but not ECP. Normal eosinophils are not responsive by this route. IgG and secretory IgA binding to receptors on eosinophils are also stimuli for the selective release of granule proteins. Other activating stimuli include complement factors and platelet activating factor (PAF). PAF is not only one of the most important activators of eosinophils but it is also synthesised and released by stimulated eosinophils. Responses to PAF include chemotaxis *in vitro* and *in vivo*, increased adherence to cultured human umbilical vein endothelial cells, respiratory burst, exocytosis and increased vascular permeability. The respiratory burst results in the generation of potentially toxic oxygen metabolites, including superoxide anions, O_2^- and hydrogen peroxide, H_2O_2. The stimulated production and release of H_2O_2, together with the release of EPO, generates tissue-damaging acids in the microenvironment of the cell. Thus, both pre-formed and newly generated mediators contribute to the tissue damage associated with eosinophil accumulation and activation in allergic disease.

Tissue and blood eosinophilia associated with atopic diseases, including asthma, is associated with the appearance of cytoplasmic vacuoles and loss of the dense core of specific granules, indicating secretion of granule contents. The increased capacity of these cells to generate LTC_4, superoxide and PAF, their greater adherence to endothelial cells and increased *ex vivo* survival indicates activation has occurred *in vivo*. These cells have a distinct membrane receptor profile. Fc receptors for immunoglobulins are upregulated and there is increased expression of adhesion molecules, which may contribute to eosinophil recruitment.

Eosinophil functions are upregulated *in vitro* by the cytokines IL-3, IL-5 and GM-CSF, leading to prolonged survival, enhanced degranulation and adhesion, and augmented LTC_4 and superoxide production. It seems likely, therefore, that the physical and functional phenotype of eosinophils within the inflammatory environment results from chronic exposure to these cytokines in allergic disease.

Cellular recruitment and adhesion molecules

Interest in the mechanisms of cellular recruitment in asthma has directed attention towards the vascular endothelium as a potential site for therapeutic intervention. Recruitment and activation of granulocytes and lymphocytes are mediated by a range of surface receptors and their corresponding ligands on endothelium, matrix proteins and other leucocytes. There are three main classes of leucocyte-endothelial adhesion molecule, which have been classified according to their structural similarities (Table 5.2): the selectins, the integrins and the members of the immunoglobulin supergene family. Under conditions of high shear flow, leucocytes use selectins to bind to the endothelium. Once bound firmly, members of the integrin and immunoglobulin supergene family come into play and are required for transendothelial migration (see Fig. 5.6, below).

Selectins contain an amino-terminal lectin-like domain that can bind to carbohydrate elements on the appropriate cellular ligand and are expressed on endothelial cells, platelets and some leucocytes. P-selectin is mobilised rapidly to the endothelial cell surface

Table 5.2. *Leucocyte-endothelial adhesion molecules*

Family	Structure	Name	CD	Distribution
Selectins	glycoprotein with lectin-like amino-termius	P-selectin E-selectin L-selectin	CD62P CD62E CD62L	Endothelium, platelets Endothelium Lymphocytes, monocytes, granulocytes
Integrins[a]	Heterodimers with common β-subunits			
β$_1$-Integrins	Common CD29 subunit	VLA-1 VLA-4	CD49a/CD29 CD49d/CD29	Activated T lymphocytes Eosinophils, lymphocytes
β$_2$-Integrins	Common CD18 subunits	LFA-1 Mac-1	CD11a/CD18 CD11b/CD18	All leucocytes Monocytes, granulocytes, NK cells
		p 150.95	CD11c/CD18	Monocytes, granulocytes
Immunoglobulin supergene family		ICAM-1	CD54	Endothelium (constitutive and inducible), some epithelia
		ICAM-2 VCAM-1	CD102 CD106	Endothelium, leucocytes Activated endothelium

within 5 minutes of exposure to inflammatory stimuli. Endothelial P-selectin is the principal selectin involved in the acute recruitment of granulocytes in the early phases of allergic inflammation. E-selectin (endothelial leucocyte adhesion molecule 1, ELAM-1) is an inducible endothelial adhesion molecule that is synthesised and expressed within 4 hours of exposure to the inflammatory stimuli, such as the cytokines IL-1 and TNF-α. E-selectin binds to the same determinants as P-selectin and its expression is usually transient, disappearing within 24 hours of the initial stimulus. L-selectin is a similar molecule expressed on most leucocytes; it serves as a non-specific ligand for granulocytes but in lymphocytes, a differentially glycosylated form is a tissue-specific homing receptor for lymphocytes. Lymphocyte L-selectin binds to a 50 kDa sulphated mucin-like endothelial glycoprotein that is selectively expressed on lymph node high endothelial venules.

The β$_2$-integrins are a family of three heterodimer proteins with a common β-subunit (CD18) and different α-subunits (CD11a, CD11b and CD11c). The β$_2$-integrins are only expressed on leucocytes: CD11a/CD18 (LFA-1) is found on all leucocytes, CD11b/CD18 is present on monocytes, granulocytes and NK lymphocytes, while CD11c/CD18 is largely confined to monocytes and granulocytes.The β$_1$-integrins are a similar family of heterodimer proteins with a common β-subunit (CD29), which is paired with one of a range of six different α-chains (identified by monoclonal antibodies: CD49a to CD49f). The β$_1$-integrins are widely distributed on most cell types, including lymphocytes, neurones and structural cells (fibroblasts etc.). The β$_1$-integrin that has attracted most attention in the context of allergy is VLA-4 (CD49d/CD29), which is expressed by activated

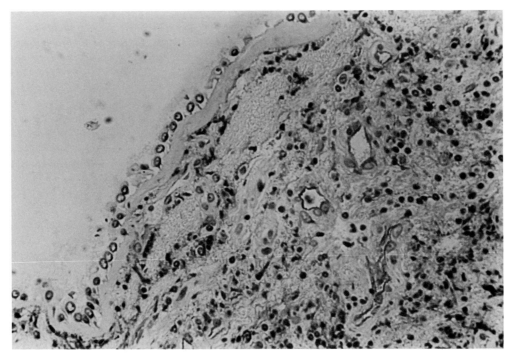

Fig. 5.5. Photomicrograph of bronchial biopsy stained by immunoperoxidase method to show expression of the adhesion molecule ICAM-1 on endothelium in asthma.

T cells and by eosinophils and seems to play a critical role in the binding of eosinophils to activated endothelium.

The principal cellular ligands for the β_2- and β_1-integrins are members of the immunoglobulin supergene family. Over 100 different members of this family have been described and although their primary structures are quite diverse, they all have a conserved tertiary structure consisting of a short cytoplasmic section, a hydrophobic transmembrane domain and a series of immunoglobulin-like looped domains cross-linked by disulphide bridges. ICAM-1 (CD54) is the principal ligand for CD11a/CD18 and CD11b/CD18. ICAM-1 is expressed constitutively at low levels on lymphocytes and a few other cells but is inducible on many different cell types following exposure to IL-1, γ-IFN or TNFα (Fig. 5.5). VCAM-1 (vascular cell adhesion molecule-1) is a 110 kDa molecular mass inducible endothelial molecule that is the principal cellular ligand for the integrin VLA-4 (CD49d/CD29). VCAM-1 is largely confined to endothelial cells and is not expressed on small blood vessels in non-inflamed skin, although it can be identified on up to 20% of small vessels in regional lymph nodes. VCAM-1 expression can be induced by the cytokines IL-4 and TNFα and has similar kinetics to the ICAM-1 expression induced by IL-1 and TNFα. The central importance of VCAM-1 in allergic inflammation is highlighted by the expression of VLA-4 on activated eosinophils and T cells, the role of IL-4 in inducing VCAM-1 expression and the recent demonstration that immunoreactive IL-4 is present in mast cells and is released upon immunological triggering.

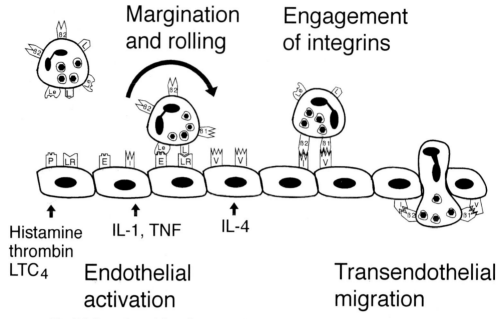

Fig. 5.6. Overview of the adhesion and migration of eosinophils. E, E-selectin; P, P-selectin; L, L-selectin; LR, L-selectin receptor; Le, sialyl-Lewis^x; I, ICAM-1; V, VCAM-1; β1 and β2, β_1- and β_2-integrins.

From the available *in vivo* and *in vitro* data, the following scenario can be derived (Fig. 5.6): after a local insult or inflammatory stimulus, endothelial cells become activated and express P-selectin. Leucocytes begin to marginate and roll along the vessel wall in a process that involves successive adherence and detachment of selectins and their counterligands (sialyl-Lewis^X). The transient nature of this adhesion is in part because of the low basal affinity of L-selectin for its ligand and partly because of the ability of endothelial products (e.g. PAF and IL-8) to terminate L-selectin-mediated adhesion. If the leucocyte is pre-activated, it is more likely to become tightly adherent, owing to increased affinity (and to a lesser extent increased numbers) of leucocyte surface adhesion molecules. The β_2- and β_1-integrins then engage their endothelial ligands (ICAM-1, ICAM-2 and VCAM-1) and initiate the process of transendothelial migration. As leucocytes move through the endothelial layer, they shed their surface L-selectin molecules and begin to migrate into tissue, possibly under the influence of local chemotactic gradients and probably using β_1-integrin–matrix binding to relate to structural tissue components.

Epithelial cell biology

The epithelial lining of the conductive airways is the first line of defence against airborne toxins, pathogens and allergens. It is frequently disrupted in asthmatics and is the major site of the mast cell and eosinophil-related mucosal inflammatory response. The epithelial cells are increasingly recognised as active participants in these responses and can produce cytokines and other mediators. This, combined with the ability to modulate cell adhesion, emphasises their potential significance in cellular responses in allergic asthma. A further important aspect of epithelial defence is the mechanical clearance of airborne agents by the mucociliary escalator, for which the epithelium provides mucus and the cilia to propel it. Disruption of this protective mechanism will render the epithelium more vulnerable to airborne challenge.

In the regions of the conducting airways primarily exposed to allergens, the epithelium is stratified, comprising basal cells with an overlying columnar cell layer. Epithelial cells require a range of intrinsic adhesion mechanisms to maintain the structural and barrier functions of this layer. These mechanisms can be divided into junctional and non-junctional mechanisms.

The tight junction complex found at the apex of the epithelial cells maintains the barrier function of the epithelium between cells. Below the tight junction, the zonula adherens junction mediates more dynamic processes, particularly during the formation and repair of the epithelium. Desmosomal contacts, formed between cells along lateral and basal aspects of the epithelium, are the major structural link between the epithelial cells. Also at the lateral margin of the cells are gap junctions, which facilitate cell–cell communication. Finally, at the base of the epithelium are hemi-desmosome contacts, which link cells in the epithelium to the basement membrane (Fig. 5.7).

In addition to junctional adhesion between cells, there are a wide range of non-junctional adhesion molecules that are found on epithelial cells in the airway. These adhesion molecules characteristically mediate more transient adhesive processes than those of junctional adhesion and include ICAM, E-cadherin (also involved in the zonula adherens), CD44 and various integrins. Many adhesion molecules, originally identified on endothelial cells, may have different functions in epithelium, which have yet to be fully investigated.

As the primary site of environmental or pathogen challenge, the epithelium is a target for infiltrating cells mediating the cellular and humoral immune responses. These cells migrate from the vascular system, after extravasation following endothelial cell adhesion. Migration to the epithelium is probably directed primarily by soluble factors, some of which (e.g. IL-8) may be derived from the epithelial cells themselves. Once infiltrating cells are in close proximity to the epithelium, cell–cell adhesion molecules are then involved in proximal signalling. Surface molecules such as ICAM, CD44, integrins and HLA-DR, which are expressed on epithelial cells, may be involved in modulating the response of infiltrating cells. In turn, infiltrating cells modulate cell adhesion molecule expression, as shown by the increased epithelial cell levels of ICAM-1 in response to γ-IFN and TNFα. Levels of ICAM, HLA-DR and CD44 are upregulated on epithelial cells in asthma.

Increased interepithelial cell spaces in asthmatics may facilitate cell infiltration. Loss of columnar epithelial cells is characteristic of asthmatic subjects and associated with exacerbation of the disease (Fig. 5.8). Such epithelial damage leads to increased smooth muscle sensitivity to bronchoconstrictive stimuli by increased accessibility. The mechanism for this loss is as yet unclear, although MBP and ECP derived from eosinophils are implicated. Epithelial cells have been shown to produce a variety of mediators includ-

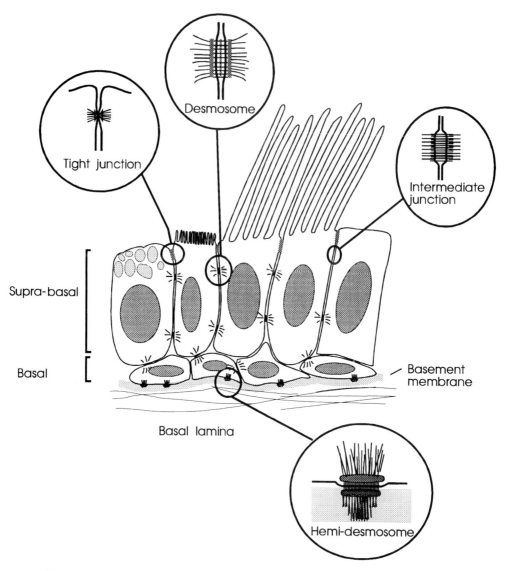

Fig. 5.7. Junctional adhesion in normal bronchial epithelium. The four major epithelial adhesion mechanisms that are localised as discrete junctions are shown in this figure. Gap junctions, which are not shown, may also provide some structural adhesion, although this is not thought to be their major function. *Tight junctions (zonulae-occludens)* prevent the movement of small molecules between cells and divide the epithelial cell membrane into apical and baso-lateral domains. There is no gap between the membrane of adjoining cells at tight junctions. *Desmosomes* are the major structural link between the cytoskeleton of adjoining cells. Desmosomes are characterised by a dense intercellular plaque and an increased gap between the cell membranes, which is bridged by desmoglein and desmocolins. *Intermediate junctions (zonulae-adherens)* are associated with α-actinin, vinculin and E-cadherin and are characteristically found below the tight junction. *Hemi-desmosomes* link the basal cell cytoskeleton to the basement membrane and underlying connective tissue. Hemi-desmosomes are not formed from the same molecules as desmosomes but also have a dense intercellular plaque when viewed by electron microscopy. *Non-junctional adhesion molecules* may be found on the baso-lateral cell surface of epithelial cells and can be clustered to form regions where the cell membranes of adjoining cells are closely apposed.

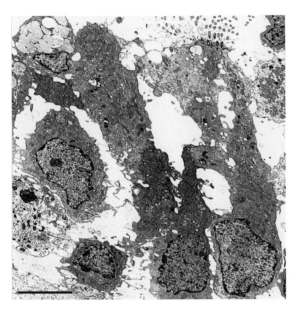

Fig. 5.8. Electron micrograph of bronchial epithelium. Electron microscope image of the disrupted bronchial epithelium of an asthmatic patient. Note the greatly reduced cell–cell contact, large intercellular spaces and lack of structural organisation. Ciliated cells and secretory cells are still present in this area but are often lost completely, leaving only basal cells (Scale bar 5 μm.)

ing cytokines (IL-1β, IL-6, IL-8 and GM-CSF), prostaglandins (PGE$_2$ and PGF$_{2\alpha}$) as well as 15-hydroxyeicosatetraenoic acid (15-HETE), and PAF. The sequence of cause and effect by which these factors interact to produce the exacerbation of symptoms in asthma remains to be determined.

The epithelial cell is the first barrier encountered by pathogens and provides a host for many successful viruses (e.g. rhinoviruses, respiratory syncytial virus, influenza). In the context of asthma, respiratory virus infection is often associated with exacerbation of symptoms (see below). The mechanism of this change is likely to involve upregulation of proinflammatory mediators produced by epithelial cells, such as IL-6, IL-8 and GM-CSF, and the selective recruitment of T cells.

Epithelial cells have a relatively rapid turnover and are able to repair normal damage caused by exposure to environmental factors. It is clear that the repair process has to be more active in asthma, especially in asthmatics with respiratory virus infections. It seems likely that the overall efficacy of repair will influence the level of chronic disease and this hypothesis is a major target for future study.

ASTHMA

The exemplar condition in this chapter is asthma (Fig. 5.9). Other diseases that may also be mediated by IgE are given in the box. The significance of IgE varies in these different conditions and not all cases of the disease will be caused by allergy. Bronchial asthma is a common clinical condition that is an important cause of respiratory morbidity and

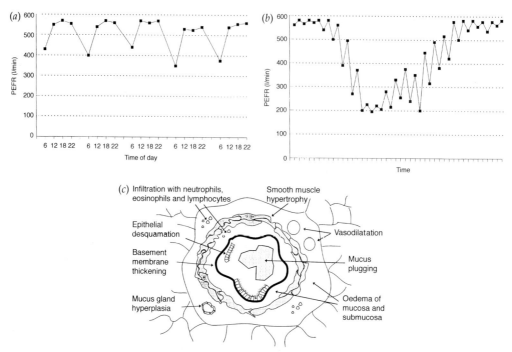

(c) Infiltration with neutrophils, eosinophils and lymphocytes

Smooth muscle hypertrophy

Epithelial desquamation

Vasodilatation

Basement membrane thickening

Mucus plugging

Mucus gland hyperplasia

Oedema of mucosa and submucosa

Symptoms
   Wheeze
   Early morning waking
   Breathless on exertion
   Cough (may be only symptom)

Diagnosis
   Excessive peak flow variability
   Response to bronchodilator
   Response to corticosteroid
   Non-specific bronchial hyper-responsiveness
   Specific allergen inhalation challenge

Fig. 5.9. Overview of asthma. (a) Peak expiratory flow rate: morning dips; (b) peak flow changes in exacerbations; (c) the principal features of the pathology of asthma.

IgE-mediated allergic diseases

Asthma
Rhinitis
Conjunctivitis
Urticaria
Anaphylaxis
Eczema

mortality. Recent epidemiological surveys suggest that the prevalence of asthma is steadily increasing, while death rates attributed to asthma have not improved since the 1960s. Possible causes of these temporal trends in asthma prevalence include increased environmental pollution from domestic allergens and motor vehicles, dietary changes associated with affluence and the increased use of bottle feeding in infancy. Much new information on the pathophysiology of asthma has been obtained since the early 1980s; in particular the recent advent of fibreoptic bronchoscopy as a research tool has allowed detailed examination of the respiratory tract in mild asthma. This has led to a fundamental reappraisal of the pathophysiological mechanisms of this disease and has provided a firm scientific basis for treatment strategies.

Epidemiology and genetics

Asthma can arise at any age, but there are peaks of onset in childhood and in middle life. Childhood asthma is usually associated with atopic allergy. When asthma arises in adult life, it may present reactivation of childhood asthma, in which case atopic allergy is usually demonstrable. Asthma arising *de novo* in adulthood is less frequently associated with atopy: the serum IgE concentration is usually within the normal range and skin tests to common airborne allergens are negative. Many individuals with late-onset asthma appear to develop the condition for the first time following upper respiratory tract infections. Others may develop asthma as a result of occupational exposure to a range of high- and low-molecular-weight sensitisers.

In atopic asthmatics, IgE-dependent mast cell activation is an important cause of episodic bronchoconstriction. More chronic asthma is associated with ongoing mast cell degranulation and the accumulation of eosinophils and T cells. Although the regulation of these cellular events is complex it is clear that IgE continues to play a role in maintaining the chronic inflammatory process, as shown by enhanced responsiveness to allergens and the observation that clinical improvement follows cessation of exposure to relevant allergens. Moreover, eosinophil activation is driven at least in part by leukotrienes and associated inflammatory mediators released from mast cells.

Both allergic and non-allergic asthma appear to have significant inherited components. However, the inheritance of asthma does not obey simple Mendelian laws and family studies suggest that at least two separate components are required before asthma becomes evident. In the case of allergic asthma, these are, first, the ability to make specific IgE antibodies against relevant airborne allergens and, second, possession of a susceptible airway that will develop chronic inflammatory changes when exposed to relevant allergens.

The pathology of asthma

Until quite recently, virtually all the available information on the histology of asthma was based on post-mortem studies. When individuals die from acute severe asthma, their lungs show widespread obstruction of the small airways with mucus plugs containing fibrin and eosinophils. Death in such patients is primarily caused by asphyxiation secondary to endobronchial plugging rather than bronchoconstriction. The bronchial epithelium is often damaged and may be shed into the airway. The basement membrane is thickened with subepithelial fibrosis and there is bronchial inflammation with oedema, vasodilation and a mixed cellular infiltrate consisting of eosinophils, neutrophils and T cells.

In the mid-1980s, it was thought that these changes reflected severe fatal asthma and were not present in milder forms of the disease. This view has radically changed following a series of studies that have used fibreoptic bronchoscopy to obtain biopsies from asthmatic airways for histological examination. It turns out that bronchial biopsies from mild asthmatics show inflammatory changes similar to those found in asthma deaths, with fragility of the bronchial epithelium and subepithelial fibrosis with deposition of types III and V collagen. Light and electron microscopy reveal mast cell degranulation and infiltration by eosinophils and mononuclear cells. The eosinophils present in such biopsies are activated, as shown by monoclonal antibody staining for the secreted form of ECP in their surface.

The lymphocyte content is slightly increased in bronchial biopsies from asthmatic subjects, but the principal difference from control subjects is increased expression of the T cell activation marker CD25 (IL-2 receptor) and the presence of mRNA for the cytokines IL-5 and GM-CSF. These changes are clinically relevant in that there is an association between eosinophil infiltration, T cell activation and the degree of bronchial hyper-responsiveness. Four weeks' treatment with inhaled corticosteroids leads to a reduction in all inflammatory markers, which parallels the reduction in non-specific bronchial responsiveness.

Histological studies of intrinsic, non-allergic asthma and occupational asthma show very similar findings to the biopsy appearances of allergic asthma. In fact, eosinophil and lymphocyte activation are, if anything, rather more prominent in intrinsic asthma, emphasising the importance of cellular inflammation as a common feature of all forms of asthma and raising the possibility that intrinsic asthma may represent a form of auto-immune disease. Taken together, these findings have led researchers to reclassify asthma as an inflammatory disorder of airways mucosa, and to regard bronchial hyper-responsiveness and other associated features as consequences of inflammation rather than as primary phenomena.

Non-specific and specific bronchial hyper-responsiveness

Asthma is characterised by marked variation in the calibre of the intrapulmonary airways over short periods of time. In addition, asthmatic individuals often report acute episodes of bronchospasm following exposure to non-specific irritants such as cold air, inorganic dusts, cigarette smoke, perfumes, paint, etc. These are not allergic responses but exaggerated responses of the airways to the non-specific irritant. This phenomenon is termed non-specific bronchial hyper-responsiveness and can be formally documented by showing increased responsiveness to non-specific bronchoconstrictors such as mechacholine or histamine. This increased non-specific responsiveness is characteristic of asthma and correlated with disease severity. Symptoms such as exercise-induced asthma, nocturnal asthma, cough and variability of peak flow measurement are largely manifestations of bronchial hyper-responsiveness.

Several mechanisms have been proposed to explain bronchial hyper-responsiveness. Originally it was thought that the abnormality might lie in the bronchial smooth muscle, but the accumulated evidence indicates that bronchial smooth muscle behaves no differently in asthmatics to that in normals when studied *in vitro*. Current thinking emphasises the importance of changes in the geometry of the airway on the response to bronchoconstriction. Thickening of the airways mucosa caused by inflammation and oedema has little influence on baseline airway resistance, but when the bronchial smooth muscle contracts, the swollen mucosa continues to occupy the same absolute volume and thus the lumen of the airways is decreased by a much greater proportion than if the mucosa was not swollen. Since resistance is inversely proportional to the fourth power of the radius (Poiseuille's law), a small increase in the thickness of the airway mucosa will have a marked effect on airway resistance in response to a given contraction of the bronchial smooth muscle. Intraluminal secretion of mucus and cells will also narrow the lumen and, like mucosal swelling, will have a disproportionate effect on airway resistance when the bronchial smooth muscle contracts. Finally, peribronchial oedema reduces the elastic recoil of the airway and this in turn allows a greater degree of narrowing of the airways to a given dose of a bronchoconstricting agonist.

As well as increased non-specific bronchial responsiveness (NSBR), many asthmatic patients are hypersensitive to airborne allergens (such as pollens, house dust mites, animal danders). This specific responsiveness results from the presence of IgE antibody directed against the relevant allergen, and in these individuals, acute exposure to allergens will lead to bronchoconstriction. When sensitised asthmatic subjects are exposed to allergen under standardised conditions, they show a characteristic pattern of physiological response as assessed by dynamic spirometry. Bronchoconstriction begins to develop within 5–10 minutes with measurable reductions in forced expiratory flow rates. Generally, this early asthmatic response (EAR) peaks at 15–20 minutes after allergen exposure and then resolves over 1–2 hours. Subsequently a proportion of subjects will go on to develop a secondary or 'late-phase' asthmatic response (LAR) with recurrence of their bronchoconstriction between 3 and 9 hours after exposure (Fig. 5.10). The LAR usually evolves slowly and can last a few hours or continue for several days. Subjects who experience LARs often report destabilisation of their asthma following challenge and will have increased non-specific bronchial responsiveness for up to two weeks after challenge, even though their spirometric values have returned to baseline. Patients who experience an isolated EAR do not usually show alterations in NSBR or destabilisation of their asthma. Interestingly, the propensity to develop LARs is associated with worse clinical status and patients with seasonal asthma are more likely to develop LARs during or after the natural pollen season than in the winter.

The magnitude of the EAR depends on the concentration of allergen-specific IgE and the degree of non-specific bronchial responsiveness. If all other factors are kept constant, it is possible to predict accurately the magnitude of response or, alternatively, to predict the dose of allergen that will induce an EAR of fixed magnitude. The factors that determine the magnitude of the LAR are less well defined. There are considerable difficulties

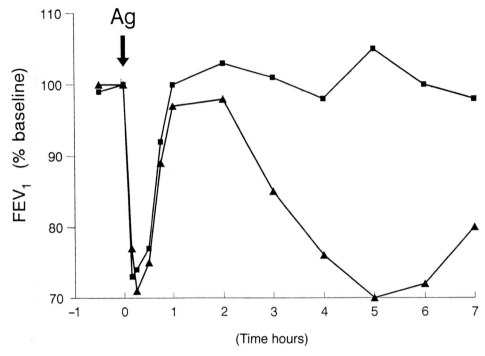

Fig. 5.10 Patterns of airways response to allergen inhalation; ■, single response; ▲, dual response. Allergen (Ag) is given at 0 hours and the forced expiratory volume (maximum in 1 second) is followed.

in comparing studies from different centres because of variation in the methodology and end-points used. In most instances, LARs are preceded by EARs, but there is no direct correlation between the magnitude of the EAR and the subsequent LAR. Similarly, there is only a very limited association between serum concentrations of allergen-specific IgE, bronchial responsiveness or cutaneous sensitivity to allergen and the magnitude of the LAR. Nevertheless, within individuals, LARs do appear to be dose-dependent phenomena in terms of the dose of allergen administered. The LAR is associated with the accumulation of neutrophils, eosinophils and other leucocytes. These cells augment the response by releasing additional proinflammatory mediators, especially those that activate endothelial cells and promote microvascular leakage.

Allergen challenge of the airways also leads to recruitment of T_H2-like cells. T cells in bronchoalveolar lavage (BAL) specimens and bronchial biopsies are generally more 'activated' than peripheral blood T cells, as shown by increased expression of the IL-2 receptor CD25. Further evidence supporting the importance of eosinophils and T cells in the pathogenesis of asthma comes from histological studies performed before and after a course of inhaled corticosteroids. This form of treatment is very effective for most forms of asthma and reduces both non-specific bronchial responsiveness and airway inflammation. When given over a six week period, beclomethasone dipropionate induces a 90% reduction in the numbers of eosinophils and a 60% reduction in activated T cells in asthmatic airways.

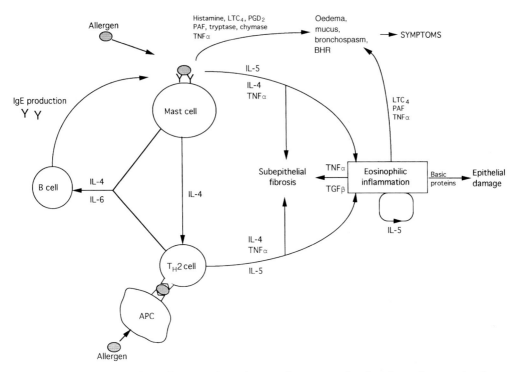

Fig. 5.11 An outline of potential cytokine pathways involved in the pathogenesis of asthma.

Cytokines and asthma

With the vast and rapidly expanding array of cytokines now identified, and the many cell types likely to be involved in allergic mucosal inflammation, it is clear that several cytokines may play a part in the pathogenesis of asthma. Their major effects are summarised in Table 5.1. To study the role of a cytokine in a disease process requires several investigational approaches. Although clues can be gained from *in vitro* experiments, *in vivo* observations are required in order to prove that a cytokine has an important disease effect. *In vivo* experiments include analysis of the effects of cytokine administration, the presence of the cytokine within a given tissue by identification of mRNA or protein and the effects of specifically blocking cytokine activity. However, with the vast overlap in the biological effects of many cytokines, it is unlikely that inhibiting any single cytokine is likely to make a significant impact on asthma, although IL-4, IL-5 and TNFα seem particularly important.

Many other cytokines also exert actions relevant to the pathogenesis of asthma and are produced *in vitro* by cells known to be present in the bronchial mucosa (Fig. 5.11). IL-1 upregulates endothelial cell adhesion molecules and activates T cells, while IL-2 is a major T cell growth factor. IL-6 is important for the terminal differentiation of B cells, whereas γ-IFN, IL-8 and IL-12 all antagonise IL-4 induced IgE synthesis. In fact γ-IFN antagonises many of the activities of IL-4 and may, therefore, be a particularly important regulatory cytokine. IL-8 is chemotactic for eosinophils after priming with IL-3, IL-5 or GM-CSF. Fibrogenic cytokines such as TGFβ (together with IL-4 and TNFα) may be important in the development of the sub-basement membrane collagen deposition that is characteristic of asthma.

Increased concentrations of IL-4 and IL-5 have been found in the BAL fluid of mild atopic asthmatic subjects compared with normal controls. Increased concentrations of IL-2 and IL-5, but not IL-4, are found in non-atopic asthmatics. Elevated concentrations of TNFα, IL-6 and GM-CSF have been observed in BAL fluid of symptomatic asthmatics compared with asymptomatic asthmatics. *In situ* hybridisation has shown the presence of cytokine mRNA in BAL cells as well as in bronchial biopsies. Increased proportions of BAL T cells expressing mRNA for IL-2, IL-3, IL-4, IL-5 and GM-CSF, but not γ-IFN, are found in allergic asthmatic patients compared with normal controls, providing evidence for the presence of T_H2-like cells in asthmatic airways. Increased numbers of cells expressing mRNA for TNFα occur in the BAL fluid of stable allergic asthmatic subjects – these may be eosinophils or T cells. BAL eosinophils also express mRNA for IL-5 and GM-CSF. Although the presence of mRNA for a protein does not necessarily mean that this is translated into protein product, these studies provide further evidence for cytokine upregulation in asthma.

When one looks for cytokine protein by immunocytochemistry, increased numbers of IL-4-containing cells are found in both the bronchial epithelium and the bronchial submucosa of mild perennial allergic asthmatic subjects compared with normal non-atopic controls. Cells containing IL-5, IL-6 and TNFα are identified in the bronchial submucosa, but only cells expressing immunoreactivity for TNFα are present in greater number in the patients compared with normal subjects. By staining sequential sections with specific cell marker and anti-cytokine monoclonal antibodies, IL-4, IL-6 and TNFα were all found to be localised predominantly in mast cells, while IL-5 was localised to both mast cells and eosinophils. These data indicate that, in addition to their production of spasmogenic mediators, mast cells may also contribute directly to the development of T_H2 cells and B cell isotype switching to IgE production. The failure to identify cytokine proteins in T cells probably reflects the limited capacity of T cells to store their products, giving values below the sensitivity of current immunohistochemical methods. To obtain a complete picture of cytokine expression within a tissue, it is, therefore, necessary to look for both mRNA and protein simultaneously.

Corticosteroids are very effective at reducing bronchial mucosal inflammation in many patients with asthma, and it is this effect that is thought to explain their clinical efficacy. However, the precise mode of action of corticosteroids in asthma is not yet fully understood. *In vitro* corticosteroids inhibit the production of many cytokines, although the response of individual cell types may vary. For example, corticosteroids inhibit the production of GM-CSF by human tracheal epithelial cells but not by endothelial cells. It is likely that at least part of the anti-inflammatory action of these drugs in asthma is related to their ability to inhibit cytokine production. Two weeks of treatment with oral prednisolone in symptomatic asthmatic patients leads to a significant reduction in the proportion of cells in BAL fluid expressing mRNA for IL-4 and IL-5, compared with symptomatic controls treated with placebo. In studies of the late asthmatic response, pre-treatment of subjects for 3 days with prednisone inhibits the appearance of cells expressing TGFα. Whether this reduction in cytokine expression is the result of inhibition of cytokine synthesis within the bronchial mucosa or simply reflects reduced numbers of cytokine-secreting cells remains to be determined.

In summary, there is considerable evidence for increased cytokine expression in asthma, particularly for the T_H2-dependent cytokines IL-4 and IL-5, and in view of their known biological activities, these cytokines may be particularly important in the pathogenesis of this disease. As yet there is little information on the effects of administering cytokines directly to the airways, or on specifically inhibiting individual cytokines. It is likely that the expression of many cytokines is suppressed by therapy with corticosteroids through effects on transcription and translation, and through a reduction in the numbers of cytokine-secreting cells. In the future, it may be possible to develop new compounds aimed at inhibiting the local effects of individual cytokines, which may permit dissection of the roles of individual cytokines in asthma and may provide a novel range of therapeutic agents.

Virus infections and asthma

Viruses have for a long time been thought to play a role in exacerbations of pre-existing asthma, and possibly also in the precipitation of asthma in previously healthy, susceptible children. Between 1960 and 1988, numerous studies addressed the role of viral infections in exacerbations of asthma, but these were largely inconclusive, and viruses were found in only 10–30% of exacerbations. The principal viruses sought in these studies were respiratory syncytial virus, influenza virus types A and B, parainfluenza virus types 1–4 and adenovirus. Standard virological techniques, such as cell culture, immunofluorescence microscopy and serological techniques, are reasonably successful at identifying these viruses. However, it is now appreciated that the majority of upper respiratory infections are caused either by rhinoviruses (approximately 50%) or by coronaviruses (approximately 15–20%). These viruses were only discovered in the late 1960s and the 1970s, and the identification techniques for these viruses have until recently been poor. Neither group grows well in standard cell cultures, and antibody-based detection is impractical because of serological diversity and the lack of specific antibodies or good quality antigens. As a result, the true role of respiratory viruses in the induction of asthma or in exacerbations of the disease has remained unknown.

In the late 1980s and early 1990s, complete genome sequences were determined for the two human coronaviruses and for several of the over 100 known rhinovirus serotypes. This information permitted the development of accurate and sensitive detection techniques, initially employing cDNA or oligonucleotide hybridisation techniques and, more recently, the polymerase chain reaction. Using these techniques, recent studies have demonstrated that 85% of exacerbations of asthma in school-age children are associated with respiratory viral infections (Fig. 5.12). In addition, respiratory virus infections are strongly associated with hospital admissions for asthma in both adults and children.

The mechanisms through which upper respiratory viral infections result in exacerba-

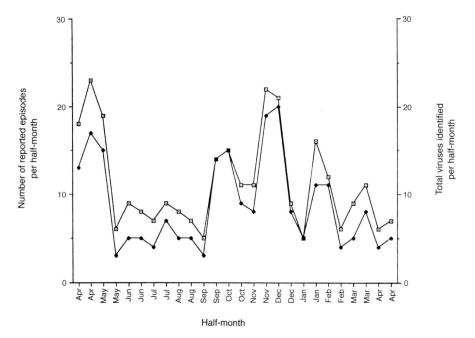

Fig. 5.12 The relationship of respiratory virus infections and exacerbations of asthma in cohort of children aged 10–11 years between April 1989 and April 1990. □, episodes; ◆, total viruses.

tions of asthma remain poorly understood. A number of mechanisms have been proposed, chiefly implicating effector cells and their pro-inflammatory products. However, no mechanism so far proposed is sufficient to explain the changes in respiratory physiology that are observed in patients with asthma. It is likely that the pathophysiological response to viral infections differs fundamentally in asthmatic and normal subjects, at an early point in the inflammatory cascade. This difference will then become amplified by subsequent events to result in the major pathophysiological differences observed.

Recent studies have shown that both normal and atopic subjects have increased numbers of eosinophils and $CD4^+$ T cells in the bronchial mucosa during experimental rhinovirus infections. However, in the asthmatic subjects, the eosinophil infiltrate was still present six weeks after infection, whereas in non-asthmatic subjects eosinophil numbers returned to baseline levels by this timepoint. These results suggest that the different pathophysiological response in asthmatics may be explained by a difference in the cytokine profiles of T cells activated by viral infections. Normal host immune defence against viral infections induces classical $CD8^+$ cytotoxic T cells (see Chapter 6). In addition, NK cells are also usually induced. $CD4^+$ T_H1 lymphocytes are thought to be important in the initial induction of this cytotoxic response through secretion of a range of cytokines that can activate many cell types, including endothelial cells and macrophages. T_H1 cytokines also downregulate B cell switching to the IgE isotype and inhibit T_H2 cells. If the asthmatic response to virus infection were to induce T_H2 cells instead, this might lead to a different pattern of epithelial injury, with eosinophilia. This hypothesis has not yet been tested in humans but has been explored in an animal model of respiratory syncytial virus infection in mice. Individual viral proteins were inserted into vaccinia viruses, which were then used to sensitise mice that were then challenged with native respiratory syncytial virus. Naive mice exhibited a neutrophilic lavage response and a T_H1 cytokine pattern, whereas mice sensitised to the G-protein of the respiratory syncytial virus showed pulmonary eosinophilia and a T_H2 pattern of cytokine release. If similar processes can be shown in human respiratory virus infection, the selective promotion of T_H2-type $CD4^+$ cells by viral infections in asthmatic subjects would provide a logical explanation for the ability of respiratory viruses to trigger exacerbations of asthma, while in non-asthmatic subjects the predominantly T_H1 response would result in elimination of the virus without triggering asthma.

Most rhinoviruses bind to epithelial cells using ICAM-1. This molecule has been cloned, and a soluble form is being produced in large quantities with a view to saturating viral receptors and preventing infection. Preliminary studies have shown some effect *in vitro*, but further studies are required to determine whether this will prove to be a useful treatment or not. Similarly, X-ray crystallography has now accurately defined the three-dimensional structure of rhinoviruses, and a canyon on the viral surface has been identified as the site where receptor binding occurs. Investigations are currently underway to design new drugs and antibodies to block the virus–receptor binding and thereby prevent infection.

Similar advances are to be expected in the other important respiratory viral infections, and these should lead eventually to a clear understanding of the role of viruses in exacerbating asthma and in inducing the disease *de novo*; ultimately this may lead to the development of effective acute and/or prophylactic intervention. Possible therapeutic options include (i) therapy with the appropriate counter regulatory cytokines; (ii) cytokine receptor blockade; (iii) computer-assisted development of drugs or peptides interfering with virus attachment or viral stages in viral replication; (iv) development of peptide vaccines that are sufficiently serotype cross-reactive to induce useful host immunity; and (v) vaccine enhancement by the use of cytokine adjuvants such as IL-12 to stimulate a T_H1-type response to viruses that might otherwise trigger a T_H2-type response and thereby exacerbate asthma.

Cellular adhesion molecules and asthma

Expression of adhesion molecules in allergic disease has been studied in several different contexts relevant to asthma. In atopic asthmatics, local allergen challenge induces infiltration by neutrophils, eosinophils and T lymphocytes within 6 hours. At the same time, ICAM-1 and ELAM-1 expression is upregulated on endothelial cells in the bronchial mucosa but there is no change in VCAM-1 expression, although this increases later. The degree of ICAM-1 and ELAM-1 expression correlates closely with the increase in submucosal and epithelial $CD11a^+$ leucocytes, and increased ICAM-1 expression is observed on bronchial epithelial cells in the allergen-challenged sites.

Only a limited number of reports have addressed adhesion molecule expression in clinical asthma. Sputum eosinophils of asthmatics express increased number of CD11b molecules and also express ICAM-1 and class II MHC (HLA-DR), reflecting the activated status of sputum eosinophils compared with blood eosinophils, but whether any of these adhesion molecules is critical to the process of accumulation of eosinophils in the sputum remains to be determined. Indeed, evidence from other *in vitro* studies has suggested that selective eosinophil recruitment may be driven by endothelial factors involved in transendothelial migration rather than a selective leucocyte–endothelial adhesion process. Cross-sectional studies of human asthma have shown constitutive expression of ICAM-1, E-selectin and VCAM-1 in allergic asthma, non-allergic asthma and normal control subjects, with no obvious difference between any of the three groups. Furthermore, six weeks of treatment with inhaled corticosteroids did not reduce the basal level of expression of these adhesion molecules, even though, *in vitro*, corticosteroids can rapidly and significantly reduce ICAM-1 expression on monocytic and bronchial epithelial cell lines.

In a primate model of asthma, ICAM-1 expression was found to be upregulated on the epithelium of the airways following allergen sensitisation. In further experiments, daily intravenous infusion of monoclonal antibody directed against ICAM-1 attenuated the allergen-induced rise in airway reactivity and the associated airway eosinophilia. Subsequent studies with this model have implicated E-selectin in the expression of acute and late-phase allergen-induced bronchoconstriction and in neutrophil recruitment, but not in the development of airway hyper-responsiveness. When an anti-ICAM-1 monoclonal antibody was given to animals with established inflammation of the airways, the inflammatory process did not resolve, although anti-ICAM-1 was effective in preventing recurrence of inflammation in animals treated with corticosteroids and then rechallenged. Taken together, these findings suggest that ICAM-1 is important in the recruitment of inflammatory cells including eosinophils into the airway, but targeting ICAM-1 alone may not be sufficient to switch off established inflammation of the airways.

This approach raises concerns about therapeutic specificity. For example, monoclonal antibodies directed against ICAM-1 might interfere with the proper functioning of ICAM-1 in the induction of immune responses to foreign pathogens. It is possible that short-term treatment with anti-ICAM-1 antibodies might be useful in acute episodes of asthma to combat the further accumulation of inflammatory cells, without adversely affecting long-term immunocompetence. It is also possible that different sites on the ICAM-1 molecule may be responsible for adhesion to different receptors or cell types, especially given the heterogeneity in size and glycosylation of ICAM-1. If confirmed, this might permit the development of specific interventions targeting particular ICAM-1β_2 integrin pairings.

Summary

Much has been learned in recent years about the cellular and molecular basis of atopic allergy and asthma. The challenge for clinical scientists is now to construct a rational framework from the many threads of information and to identify points at which therapeutic intervention is likely to be worthwhile. Recognition of the inflammatory basis of asthma has already led to a reappraisal of treatment strategies in asthma, with increased emphasis on anti-inflammatory treatment, even in very mild forms of the disease. The current rationale of treatment is to try to suppress the inflammatory component of asthma using prophylactic anti-inflammatory drugs. With the present state of knowledge, prospects for new developments in therapeutic intervention have become focused on a small number of likely targets. These include individual cytokines involved in IgE production (IL-4, IL-13), or in eosinophil differentiation and activation (GM-CSF, IL-5). Direct anti-TH2 cell strategies might also be logical if suitable target molecules can be identified and local forms of therapy could be made available. Cellular recruitment is another sensible target area and efforts are needed to delineate endothelial adhesion mechanisms that can be blocked without compromising essential elements of the immune system. At the same time, efforts are clearly needed to establish appropriate model systems in which to test these novel approaches to asthma therapy. The principal goal for the turn of the century must be to consolidate existing knowledge and translate research activity into improved health for our patients.

FURTHER READING

General
Busse, W.W. & Holgate, S.T. (eds.). (1994). *Asthma and Rhinitis*. Oxford: Blackwell.
Lachmann, P.J., Peters, D.K., Rosen, F.S. & Walport, M. (eds.) (1993). *Clinical Aspects of Immunology*, 5th edn. Oxford: Blackwell Scientific.

Specific topics
Bardin, P.G., Johnston, S.L. and Pattemore, P.K. (1992). Viruses as precipitants of asthma symptoms. II. Physiology and mechanisms. *Clinical and Experimental Allergy*, (1993). 22, 809–22.
Churchill, L., Gundel, R.H., Letts, L.G. & Wegner, C.D. (1993). Contribution of specific cell-adhesive glycoproteins to airway and alveolar inflammation and dysfunction. *American Review of Respiratory Disease*, 148, S79–S82.
Corrigan, C.J., & Kay, A.B. (1992). T cells and eosinophils in the pathogenesis of asthma. *Immunology Today*, 13, 501–507.
Devalia, J.L. & Davies, R.J. (1993). Airway epithelial cells and mediators of inflammation. *Respiratory Medicine*, 87, 405–408.
Djukanovic, R., Roche, W.R., Wilson, J.W. *et al.* (1990). Mucosal inflammation in asthma. State of the art. *American Review of Respiratory Disease*, 142, 434–457.
Dreborg, S. & Frew, A.J. (1993). Allergen standardisation and skin tests. *Allergy*, 48, (S14), 48–84.
Durham, S.R. (1990). Late asthmatic responses. *Respiratory Medicine*, 84, 263–268.
Gleich, G.J., Adolphson, C.R. & Leiferman, K.M. (1993). The biology of the eosinophilic leukocyte. *Annual Reviews in Medicine*, 44, 85–101.
Morton, N.E. (1992). Major loci for atopy. Editorial. *Clinical and Experimental Allergy*, 22, 1041–1043.
O'Hehir, R.E., Garman, R.D., Greenstein, J.L. & Lamb, J.R. (1991). The specificity and regulation of T-cell responsiveness to allergen. *Annual Reviews in Immunobiology*. 9, 67–95.

6

Infection

D. WILKS and J. G. P. SISSONS

- Microorganisms employ a wide range of pathogenic mechanisms to ensure their survival and transmission.

- Host factors play a major role in determining susceptibility to infections.

- The clinical manifestations of infectious disease are the result of the interaction of microbial and host factors.

- Antibiotic therapy has revolutionised medical practice, but resistant organisms develop rapidly after the introduction of a new antibiotic.

- New therapies based on new biological methods have yet to enter routine clinical practice.

The human body continually interacts with innumerable microorganisms, only a small proportion of which are pathogenic. Even so, organisms that do cause disease belong to many different phyla, ranging from insects whose larvae spend part of their life cycle under human skin, to viruses and subviral organisms that can only replicate within human cells. Within this multiplicity of infectious organisms, there exist many and varied strategies for replication, and multiple pathogenic mechanisms. As microbial agents, cell biology and the host immune response become understood at a molecular level, it becomes possible to explain pathogenesis in molecular terms. *Virulence* is the term used to describe the ability of an organism to cause disease in a particular host compared with other related members of its family. An increasing number of genes determining virulence are being described and sequenced for individual microbial agents. This information can be used in many ways: homology to other microbial agents can be used for identification and classification, homology to other microbial and cellular genes enables functions of products to be predicted and analysis of the genome by mutation and deletion becomes possible.

This chapter will concentrate on some areas in which modern biological techniques are changing our understanding of microbial pathogenicity or are contributing to diagnosis and therapy. In particular, it will concentrate on bacterial infections, which are responsible for the majority of clinically significant infectious illnesses in the developed world and which demonstrate how knowledge acquired through the application of modern biological techniques is already affecting the practice of medicine, for example in the design and use of antibiotic drugs.

Infectious organisms

Pathogenic organisms range in size from tapeworms, some of which may be many metres in length, to single prion molecules whose size is best expressed in terms of their molecular weight (Table 6.1). Pathogens cause damage to the host in three main ways.

1. They may cause direct tissue injury to cells they enter or contact, either mechanically or chemically, or by interfering with normal cellular metabolism, for example by subverting cellular protein synthesis machinery to produce new viral particles to such an extent that the cell becomes non-viable.
2. Microbial products may be toxic to host cells. Many bacteria secrete toxins and enzymes that are toxic to cells and cause tissue damage, in many cases at sites distant from the site of colonisation. The subject of exo- and endotoxins is discussed in greater detail in later sections of this chapter.
3. Pathogens may cause the host immune system to damage host tissue: a process that may be referred to as immunopathogenesis.

The extent to which these three mechanisms operate for different classes of organism will now be discussed briefly.

Viruses

All viruses are obligate intracellular parasites and their pathogenesis is often closely related to their intimate association with normal cellular processes. After binding to and entering host cells, viral particles are uncoated and the virus genome is transcribed and translated. Viral proteins may themselves be pathogenic. For example, expression of the envelope glycoprotein of human immunodeficiency virus (HIV) on host cell membranes causes fusion of cells, with the formation of non-viable multinucleate syncytia. Viral proteins involved in the regulation of gene expression may inappropriately activate cellular genes, with pathogenic consequences. In many cases, for example vaccinia, viral infection shuts off host protein synthesis completely, and this is frequently the principal cause of cell death in acute lytic infection.

Some viruses do not always cause acute lytic infection; instead they may establish chronic persistent infection, often with integration of the viral genome into the host chromosomal DNA. This may have pathogenic complications, for example if it occurs in a way that activates cellular genes such as oncogenes. Some viruses, notably the α-herpes viruses, herpes simplex and varicella-zoster, establish a state of latent infection during which no viral proteins are produced. Later the virus may reactivate and cause acute lytic infection and this may be associated with clinical disease, as in the case of herpes zoster where shingles is caused by reactivation of latent varicella-zoster virus in the dorsal root ganglion of the spinal cord.

Much of the tissue damage caused by viruses is mediated by immunopathogenic mechanisms. For example, the hepatocyte injury seen in acute hepatitis B virus infection is mainly caused by the effects of cell-mediated immunity, in particular MHC class I restricted CD8$^+$ cytotoxic T cells directed against virally infected cells.

Table 6.1. *Pathogenic organisms belong to many phyla ranging in size from molecular to macroscopic and employ a huge number of pathogenic mechanisms*

Group	Characteristics	Example organism	Order of magnitude of genome (kb)	Size	Examples of disease associations	Comments
Prions	'Infectious protein'	Scrapie protein	None	22 kDa protein	Scrapie in sheep	Pathogenicity remains under investigation
Viruses	Obligate intracellular parasites containing protein and DNA *or* RNA	Hepadnaviridae Herpesviridae	~5–400	42 nm 120–200 nm	Hepatitis A Herpes simplex stomatitis	Use host cellular apparatus for DNA/RNA and protein synthesis, often with direct cytopathic effects
Bacteria	Free-living, unicellular prokaryotes	*Escherichia coli*	~4000	4 μm	Wound, urinary and intestinal infections	Pathogenic mechanisms include extra/intracellular growth within host. toxin production, immunopathogenesis
Fungi	Free-living uni- or multicellular eukaryotes	*Candida albicans*	~40000	3 μm (yeast form)	Vaginal 'thrush'	Frequently important as opportunist infections; often saprophytic
Protozoa	Free-living unicellular eukaryotes	*Plasmodium falciparum* *Entamoeba histolytica*	~40000	1 μm (merozoite) 25 μm (trophozoite)	Malaria Colitis, liver abscess	Complex life cycles, often involving multiple host species and specific insect vectors
Helminths	Three major classes of worms: nematodes (roundworms) trematodes (flatworms) cestodes (tapeworms)	*Ascaris lumbricoides* *Schistosoma mansoni* *Taenia solium*	~100000	30 cm 1 cm up to 3 m	Intestinal parasite Schistosomiasis Intestinal parasite	Complex life cycles, often involving multiple host species

Bacteria

Bacteria, in particular the obligate intracellular parasites Rickettsiae and Chlamydiae and the facultative intracellular parasites, which include mycobacteria and salmonellae, may also damage cells by direct injury. Bacteria also produce exo- and endotoxins and may trigger immunopathogenic reactions. The methods evolved by bacteria to avoid destruction by host defences and ensure their own survival and propagation are discussed in detail in later sections of this chapter.

Protozoa

Many species of Protozoa, such as *Plasmodium, Trypanosoma cruzi* and *Toxoplasma gondii* are also obligate intracellular parasites. Others such as *Entamoeba histolytica* are free-living. They may cause direct tissue injury or elicit hypersensitivity reactions, but toxin secretion is not generally seen.

Fungi

Fungi produce disease in all three ways, although toxin production is uncommon. Several fungal mycotoxins are of clinical importance; aflatoxin, produced by the mould *Aspergillus flavus,* may contaminate corn and peanut crops and has been shown to be a cause of hepatocellular carcinoma. Although some fungal infections, notably candidiasis and cutaneous fungal infections such as ringworm, can occur in the immunocompetent, invasive fungal infection is more often seen as an opportunist infection in the immunodeficient patient, for example during episodes of neutropenia associated with chemotherapy.

Helminths

Helminths are large complex organisms with complex life cycles, often involving specific animal hosts. Most spend several stages of their life cycle within the human host and the pathological consequences are usually stage specific. In general, the most severe tissue damage arises by immunopathogenic hypersensitivity reactions. For example, ingested eggs of the roundworm *Ascaris lumbricoides* hatch into larvae in the human small intestine. The larvae penetrate the intestinal mucosa and migrate to the lungs where they break out of the alveoli and are swallowed. They enter the gut a second time and mature into adult worms, which live free in the intestinal lumen breeding and producing eggs. As the larvae pass through the lungs they may cause a hypersensitivity reaction that is clinically apparent with pulmonary symptoms. Histology shows a focal eosinophilic inflammatory reaction with granuloma formation. Later, as adult worms in the gut, they cause few symptoms and then only as a result of their physical presence and large size (typically about 30 cm in length).

Fundamental features of prokaryotic cells

Many of the topics that will be discussed in the following pages, such as the targets of antibiotic action and mechanisms of antibiotic resistance, depend on differences between the prokaryotic bacterial cell and the eukaryotic mammalian cell. Certain major features of prokaryotic cell biology are important to an understanding of what follows and these will now be discussed.

Prokaryotic cells lack organelles

Prokaryotic cells lack internal membranes isolating respiratory or photosynthetic enzymes in specific organelles, unlike the membrane-bounded mitochondria or choloro-plasts of eukaryotic cells. Cross-sectional electron micrographs of bacteria such as *Escherichia coli* reveal a relatively simple sac-like structure in which an external envelope surrounds a membrane-free granular cytoplasm, the cytosol, which contains a fibrous DNA component. The site of oxidative phosphorylation in the prokaryotic cell is the inner cytoplasmic membrane rather than the membranes of organelles as in eukaryotes.

Important features of the bacterial genome

The prokaryotic cell lacks a discrete nucleus and has no nuclear membrane, nucleolus or separate non-identical chromosomes. In all bacteria so far studied most of the bacterial genome is arranged in the form of a single circular double-standard chromosome, which is not associated with histone molecules. The chromosome of *Escherichia coli* comprises 3.8×10^3 kb and would be 1300 μm long fully extended but exists compacted into irregularly shaped bodies, nucleoids, lying free in the cytoplasm. Single bacterial cells growing exponentially generally contain two to four such molecules in the process of duplication, beginning at the origin of replication present at one unique site on each chromosome.

Genes coding for the regulatory and functional proteins related to a given metabolic pathway are often clustered together on the chromosome, regulated as one unit and transcribed as a single polycistronic mRNA. Thus the *lacZ* gene coding for the bacterial enzyme β-galactosidase, which is required for the cleavage of the disaccharide lactose, is clustered on the chromosome with three other genes involved in lactose metabolism: *lacI*, which codes for a regulatory repressor protein, *lacY*, which codes for a permease required for active transport of lactose into cells, and *lacA*, which codes for a transacetylase that reduces the toxicity of some galactosides. This functional unit, known as the *lac* operon, is usually inactive but is switched on in the presence of suitable substrates such as lactose.

Transcription of mRNA from the *lac* operon is usually prevented by the repressor protein produced by the *lacI* gene binding to the operator site upstream of the *lacZYA* complex (Fig. 6.1). Inducers such as lactose bind to the repressor rendering it unable to bind to the operator. This allows transcription of mRNA coding for the three enzyme products of the *lacZYA* complex. This arrangement ensures that all three enzymes are

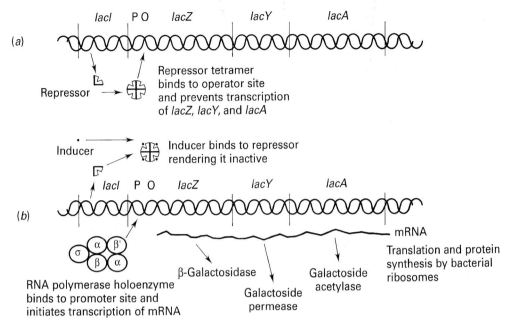

Fig. 6.1. The *lac* operon has been extensively studied as an example of the co-ordinate regulation of bacterial genes. (*a*) Constitutive expression of *lacI* produces a repressor protein. Tetramers of this repressor bind to *lacZ* at the operator site (O), preventing transcription, (*b*) Substrates for β-galactosidase, including lactose, act as inducers, binding to the repressor and preventing it from binding to the operator. This allows RNA polymerase to bind to the promoter site (P) and transcribe a single mRNA from the *lacZYA* complex. This is then translated to produce three enzymes required for the uptake and metabolism of galactosides.

regulated co-ordinately and that they are synthesised only when their substrate is available. In contrast to eukaryotic mRNA, bacterial mRNA molecules are relatively unstable, with a half life of 1 to 2 minutes. The *lac* operon has been studied in detail as a model of gene regulation and illustrates one way in which bacteria are able to respond rapidly and flexibly to their environment.

Bacterial RNA polymerase, the enzyme responsible for the transcription of bacterial DNA into mRNA, consists of two components. The core enzyme is a tetramer consisting of two α-subunits, a β-subunit and a β'-subunit. This is associated with another subunit, the σ factor. Core enzyme has the ability to synthesise RNA from a DNA template but cannot initiate transcription – this requires binding of the σ factor to the core enzyme to produce the holoenzyme ($\alpha_2\beta\beta'\sigma$). Core enzyme has high but non-specific affinity for DNA; binding of the σ factor to the core enzyme drastically reduces its affinity for non-specific binding but allows it to bind with high affinity to specific promoter sequences. The σ factor is, therefore, responsible for ensuring that mRNA initiation takes place at appropriate promoter sequences. After the mRNA chain has reached eight to nine bases in length, the σ factor dissociates. Major changes in bacterial physiology such as those involved in sporulation or the heat-shock response may involve the elaboration of alternative σ factors that direct the transcription of whole new classes of previously inactive genes.

The prokaryotic ribosome

The granular nature of the bacterial cytosol results from the very large number of ribosomes present. More ribosomes per unit mass are found in bacteria than in any other kind of cell, and this reflects the very high rates of protein synthesis needed to allow bacteria to divide every 20 minutes during exponential growth. The prokaryotic ribosome is smaller than its eukaryotic counterpart, consisting of 30S and 50S subunits, which together comprise the 70S ribosome (compared with 40S and 60S subunits in the 80S eukaryotic ribosome). These differences in structure are exploited by antibiotics that inhibit bacterial protein synthesis, and this is discussed in more detail in following sections. Unlike eukaryotic genes, prokaryotic genes do not have introns. Since the bacterial cell lacks internal divisions, the processes of transcription and translation proceed in the same cellular compartment; in fact multiple ribosomes may attach to nascent mRNA even as it is being transcribed. The association of multiple ribosomes with a single mRNA molecule creates a structure known as a *polysome* and these have been clearly visualised by electron microscopy.

Genes coding for ribosomal RNA (rRNA) are highly conserved among bacterial species and rRNA sequencing and DNA probes targeting ribosomal sequences have been used for typing, classification and identification of bacteria.

Transfer of DNA between bacteria

A change in the genome of a bacterial cell may arise by mutation or by the acquisition of additional DNA from an external source, and this may occur by three mechanisms: transformation, conjugation and transduction.

Transformation

Certain bacteria, notably pneumococci, *Haemophilus influenzae* and a number of *Bacillus* species are capable of taking up DNA released by lysis of cells of another strain. Such cells are referred to as 'competent'. In the laboratory, several methods are used to artificially render other species of bacteria competent and thus facilitate the transfer of recombinant DNA. This technique is important in many molecular biological methods.

Conjugation

Bacterial cells may carry one or more small circular extrachromosomal double-stranded DNA elements called plasmids. Plasmids replicate independently of the main chromosome and often carry information coding for beneficial properties (to the bacterium), such as resistance to antibiotics. Conjugation refers to the transfer of DNA between cells by direct contact. Certain plasmids, known as transfer or sex factors, carry the genes necessary for conjugation to take place, and only the cells that contain such plasmids can act as DNA donors. Not all plasmids can transfer themselves, but non-conjugative plasmids may be mobilised by other conjugative plasmids present in the same cell.

During conjugation, a 1–10 µm appendage termed a sex pilus develops on the surface of the donor cell and attaches to the membrane of the recipient. DNA can then be passed between the cells, although usually only the sex factor plasmid itself is transferred. One strand of the double-stranded DNA sex factor is nicked and transferred to the recipient. DNA replication proceeds in the donor to replace the transferred strand and in the recipient to reconstitute the double-stranded sex factor. Thus, the recipient becomes converted into a donor, able to conjugate with and convert other recipients.

The prototype sex factor is the F (fertility) factor of *Escherichia coli*. This is a 94 kb plasmid present in one copy per cell. About one-third of the plasmid is occupied by 19 transfer (*tra*) genes specifically involved in conjugation, including those responsible for the production of the sex pilus. Pair formation and F factor transfer occur very efficiently when F^+ and F^- cells are mixed, with all cells rapidly becoming F^+.

Transduction

Bacteria may also contain bacteriophages, which are viruses normally lethal to the bacterial host. In some instances, however, they can enter a long-term state of controlled replication called lysogeny, in which the phage chromosome is integrated into the bacterial chromosome (the 'prophage') and may thereby bestow additional properties on the host cell.

The lysogenic state is stable but not permanent. The prophage may be excised, phage proteins produced and the cell lysed as in normal lytic infection with the release of infectious phage particles. This process of phage induction occurs with low frequency spontaneously and phage excision is usually exact. However, occasionally the phage may pick up host DNA elements adjacent to the phage integration site and carry them to the new host. Since lysogenic phages usually have a specific insertion site on the bacterial chromosome, this process can only involve a short length of DNA on either side of the insertion site and is, therefore, referred to as *restricted* transduction. Other phages are capable of *generalised* transduction. In this instance, during lytic infection, a small fraction of new phage particles are packaged with host DNA rather than phage DNA, which they then transfer to new host bacteria. Phages of this type pick up host DNA at random and may, thus, transduce any part of the bacterial chromosome. Generalised transducing phages may also pick up plasmid DNA: for example, the penicillinase gene in staphylococci is located on a plasmid and may be transferred to other staphylococci by transduction.

The molecular biology of plasmids and phages has been heavily exploited in the *in vitro* manipulation of DNA, and these aspects are discussed in Chapter 2 (p. 40). The presence of phage DNA may also have profound clinical implications. For example, the diphtheria toxin, which is responsible for the clinical manifestations of diphtheria, is not coded for by the bacterial chromosome, it is coded for by the lysogenic phage β. Strains of *Corynebacterium diphtheriae* that have not been lysogenised are non-toxigenic.

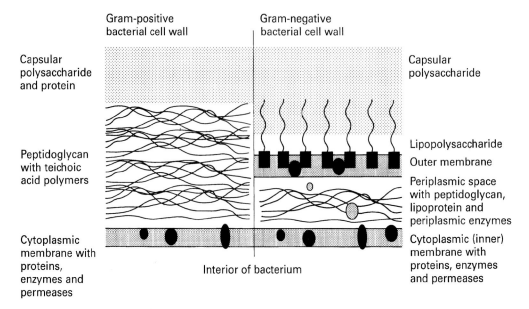

Fig. 6.2. A schematic representation of the cell wall components of Gram-positive and Gram-negative bacteria. The cell wall contains peptidoglycan: synthesis of this unique macromolecule is the target for penicillin action.

The prokaryotic cell wall

The prokaryotic cell has a rigid cell wall (except in the case of mycoplasmas) that contains a specific peptidoglycan substance not found in eukaryotes (Fig. 6.2). The basic structure of peptidoglycan consists of repeating disaccharide units of *N*-acetylglucosamine (NAG) linked to *N*-acetylmuramic acid (NAMA) (Fig. 6.3). Each NAMA residue bears a pentapeptide side chain that is cross-linked from its terminal *D*-alanine to the peptide side chain of an adjacent polysaccharide chain, either directly, as in Gram-negative bacteria, or via a short peptide, such as pentaglycine in Gram-positive bacteria. Peptidoglycan synthesis commences with the formation of NAMA–pentapeptide followed by alternate linkage to NAG to form peptidoglycan chains. These are cross-linked at the cell surface by bacterial transpeptidases.

Microbial pathogenicity

The capacity of microorganisms to cause disease depends on their ability to perform a number of tasks. They must be able to survive in the environment long enough to effect their transmission between hosts and they must be able to adhere to and gain access to new hosts. They must be able to survive and replicate within the new host. This section will consider some recent advances in our understanding of some of these aspects of pathogenicity. The survival advantage that has contributed to the evolution of these characteristics may bear little relationship to their role in the generation of human disease. For example, the production of exotoxins by bacteria has been well defined *in*

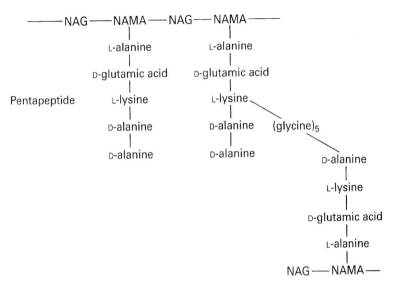

Fig. 6.3. The structure of peptidoglycan. Minor variations exist between bacterial species. The peptidoglycan of *Staphlycoccus aureus* is shown. The backbone consists of alternately linked molecules of *N*-acetylglucosamine (NAG) and *N*-acetylmuramic acid (NAMA). Each NAMA residue has a pentapeptide side chain. Pentaglycine links form between these side chains to connect adjacent molecules and produce a highly cross-linked and resilient structure.

vitro in many instances, but the role of individual exotoxins in the production of clinical disease and the way in which this benefits the bacterium has been defined in a much smaller number of examples.

Environmental survival

Environmental survival and transmission of organisms between hosts are closely related concepts. Organisms that are unable to withstand adverse environmental conditions must achieve transmission by routes that do not expose them to extremes of dessication, temperature and pH. For example, bacteria vary considerably in their ability to tolerate dessication. *Neisseria gonorrhoeae* dies rapidly in dry conditions whereas *Staphylococcus aureus* may survive for many weeks when dried in dust. These differences are reflected in the different routes of transmission of these two organisms and have implications not only for transmission in the natural history of infection but also for infection control in the artificial environment of a hospital.

Adherence

Pathogenic microorganisms show striking host specificity and tissue tropism. One of the many factors that determine these characteristics is the ability of an organism to adhere to host tissues.

In the case of many viruses, specific cellular receptors have been identified; these are usually host proteins that have specific physiological roles. Thus HIV attaches to human cells by a specific high-affinity interaction between the viral envelope glycoprotein gp 120 and the host CD4 molecule (see Chapter 2). Similarly, Epstein-Barr virus attaches to host cells by binding between its glycoprotein gp 350/220 and the human complement receptor type-2 (CR2 or CD21), which is expressed on mature B cells.

Most pathogenic bacteria begin host colonisation on a mucosal surface where they must overcome many non-specific defence mechanisms, including the action of cilia and desquamation of epithelial cells. In addition to host specificity, strains of bacteria may show strict preference for particular surfaces. Thus, strains of group A β-haemolytic streptococci isolated from throat culture adhere better to oral epithelial cells than to those of the skin; the converse is true for streptococci isolated from skin.

The surface of most bacterial cells carries a net positive electrical charge and contains protein and lipid components that render the surface hydrophobic. Non-specific electrostatic and hydrophobic forces may be important in the initial attachment of bacteria to prosthetic materials, but they are usually inadequate to enable bacteria to survive on mucosal surfaces. It is now clear that bacteria adhere to mucosal surfaces as a result of binding between specific membrane proteins (collectively referred to as *adhesins*) and host cell membrane components, which are frequently polysaccharide-rich structures. Many adhesins are associated with *fimbriae* (or *pili*) and the possession of adhesin-bearing fimbriae is often a determinant of virulence. Fimbrial adhesins may be encoded by transmissible plasmids; for example, some human strains of *Escherichia coli* possess adhesins referred to as *colonisation factors*, which are encoded by plasmids and which are associated with adhesiveness and virulence. The affinity between adhesin and receptor need not be enormously high since a single bacterium may bear several thousand adhesin molecules. Tissue tropism may, therefore, be defined by the distribution of a receptor for a given bacterial adhesin.

Adherence to prosthetic surfaces

As the practice of medicine changes, different organisms are given the opportunity to become pathogenic. In recent years, infections of implanted plastic devices, in particular intravenous cannulae, by coagulase-negative staphylococci have become a major cause of bacteraemia in hospital inpatients (discussed in more detail below). The causal bacterium is usually *Staphylococcus epidermidis*, which was considered for many years to be non-pathogenic. *In vivo, Staphylococcus epidermidis* grows as a biofilm adherent to solid surfaces, and the increased and widespread use of indwelling intravenous devices has led to renewed interest in this bacterial 'slime'.

Electron micrographs of staphylococcal biofilm show that the majority of organisms are not adherent to the solid surface but are held together by cell-to-cell aggregation. Colonisation of plastic surfaces is thought to occur by a two-stage process. Initial attachment to uncoated plastic is followed by slime production and the development of an accumulated mass of bacteria and extracellular material. Slime physically stabilises the bacterial colony and also protects it from elements of the host immune system and anti-biotics. The majority of these infections can, therefore, only be controlled by device removal. Despite advances in plastic technology, prevention depends very heavily on aseptic techniques during insertion.

Avoidance of humoral defences: antibodies and the complement system

To establish and maintain growth within the host, microorganisms must be able to evade the host immune system. The consequences of immunodeficiency are described in greater detail elsewhere in this chapter. This section will consider ways that bacteria have developed to avoid being killed by their hosts.

Bacterial cell wall

The cell wall of both Gram-positive and Gram-negative bacteria provides a resilient physical barrier but also has specific functions that subvert the immune system.

Gram-positive bacteria   The cell wall of Gram-positive bacteria is characterised by its thick peptidoglycan layer (Fig. 6.2). Other components of the cell wall, such as the M protein of group A β-haemolytic streptococci, interact specifically with the host immune system. M protein is one of the better understood virulence factors in Gram-positive bacteria; strains that lack it naturally or experimentally have reduced virulence. M protein is a membrane-anchored protein that demonstrates hypervariability in its 20–25 amino-terminal residues, which constitute the only part of the molecule exposed to interaction with macromolecules such as antibodies. Group β-haemolytic streptococci produce up to 75 antigenically distinct serotypes of M protein. M protein binds fibrin and fibrinogen, and at least one type has been shown to bind directly to a host negative complement regulatory molecule, factor H. M protein also interferes with the interaction of the complement fragment C3b with C3 receptors on phagocytes. In pathogenic strains of *Staphylococcus aureus*, a major component of the cell wall known as protein A binds to the Fc portion of IgG and thus may interfere with antibody-mediated phagocytosis, which depends on the binding of immunoglobulin to Fc receptors on phagocytic cells.

Gram-negative bacteria   Gram-negative bacteria have a different cell wall structure (Fig. 6.2), with an outer membrane, a thin layer of peptidoglycan and an inner membrane. The cell wall is protected by lipopolysaccharide (LPS) in the outer membrane, which forms a confluent and impermeable physical barrier, restricting access of lytic components of the complement cascade and antibodies. LPS is responsible for many of the features of endotoxic shock and its detailed structure is considered later. Many specific outer membrane proteins (OMPs) that are associated with virulence have been identified and in some instances their mechanism of action is known. For example in *Campylobacter fetus*, confluent fibrillar protein arrays known as S layers coat the organism and block antibody- and complement-mediated lysis.

Antigenic variation

Organisms can avoid the effects of antibodies directed against surface molecules by varying the structure and antigenic composition of such molecules during infection. For example, *Neisseria gonorrhoeae* (gonococcus) shows antigenic variation in both the outer membrane protein PII and in the pilin protein, which may vary from 16 to 24 kDa in size. The bacterial chromosome contains multiple pilin genes, but only one of these loci, *pilE*, encodes the complete gene sequence including the transcriptional start site and conserved amino-terminal portion. Multiple other loci, *pilS*, encode partial sequences consisting of the variable carboxy-terminal two-thirds of the molecule. Homologous DNA recombination between *pilE* and *pilS* loci results in the exchange of 'mini-cassettes': short variable sequences bounded by conserved amino acids, so that the *pilE* locus expresses an altered and antigenically different pilin protein. Variant pilin DNA may also be acquired by transformation from autolysed gonococci.

Eukaryotic pathogens have developed many sophisticated methods for avoiding humoral defence mechanisms, including antigenic variation. *Trypanosoma brucei*, the agent of African trypanosomiasis, produces a confluent glycoprotein layer (variable surface glycoprotein or VSG) that limits complement activation on the cell surface. The VSG also undergoes spontaneous, rapid and extensive antigenic variation. During the course of infection, the level of parasitaemia rises and falls cyclically every few days. Each new wave of parasites expresses a new antigenic variant of VSG, which is not recognised by host immune responses. The trypanosomal genome is estimated to contain over 1000 different VSG genes. Antigenic variation follows the activation of a new VSG gene: a process that frequently involves DNA rearrangement, with duplication of the new VSG gene at an expression site.

Antigenic variation is also important in the survival of viral pathogens. Influenza viruses are classified serologically into types A, B and C. The antigens that differentiate the three types are internal nucleoproteins, which are relatively stable and are not accessible to host antibodies. The virus also carries two major surface antigens, haemagglutinin and neuraminidase, which are variable and are important targets for host antibodies. All three types of virus may alter both haemagglutinin and neuraminidase gradually by mutation, a process known as antigenic drift. In addition, for influenza type A (but not types B or C) there exist at least 13 subtypes of haemagglutinin and at least nine subtypes of neuraminidase. The emergence of strains expressing different combinations of surface antigens is called *antigenic shift*. So far only H_{1-3} and N_{1-2} have been found in human influenza viruses. These two processes allow the virus to escape host immune responses; endemic cases occur continuously in most communities, but focal epidemics associated with antigenic drift occur every few years. Pandemics caused by antigenic shift occur every 10–20 years. For example, the severe pandemic of 1918 followed the replacement of H_1N_1 by H_2N_2 as the predominant strain. It is suggested that animal orthomyxoviruses may serve as a reservoir of antigenic variants. Human influenza viruses have a segmented RNA genome and may acquire new segments of RNA from these animal viruses, and thus undergo antigenic shift, by a process known as reassortment, which can occur when cells are infected by two viruses of different strains and their genomes reassort.

Phagocytosis

Phagocytic host cells such as neutrophils and macrophages recognise bacteria either through receptors for carbohydrate structures on the bacterial surface or after opsonisation by antibody or complement, for which they bear specific receptors. After phagocytosis, with invagination of the plasma membrane to form the phagosome and subsequent fusion with lysosomes, a number of microbicidal effector mechanisms come into action.

Oxidative killing

Binding of particles to the phagosomal membrane initiates a rapid increase in respiratory activity, the 'respiratory burst', which involves activation of a unique NADPH oxidase in the phagosomal membrane, and assembly of a multimolecular electron transport chain incorporating a unique phagosome cytochrome, b_{558}. NADPH is supplied by a sudden increase in anaerobic glucose metabolism via the hexose monophosphate shunt. Cytochrome b_{558} is the terminal electron donor to molecular oxygen producing reactive oxygen intermediates ($\bullet OH$, H_2O_2, $\bullet O$, $O2^-$). Each of these is highly toxic, and further toxic oxidants are formed by the interaction of H_2O_2 with halides such as chloride and iodide ions in the presence of myeloperoxidase.

Non-oxidative killing

The phagosome also contains numerous cationic proteins that are active at neutral pH. These include bactericidal/permeability-increasing protein (BPI) and the defensins, a family of small cysteine-rich bactericidal peptides. Both BPI and the defensins destabilise the bacterial cell membrane and render it permeable. Lysozyme is a well-characterised enzyme present in lysosomes that degrades peptidoglycan by cleaving the glycosidic linkage between *N*-acetylglucosamine and *N*-acetylmuramic acid. The pH within the phagolysosome falls to 3.5–4.0 partly as a result of the action of proton pumps in the membrane and partly as a result of protons produced during the respiratory burst. This low pH may itself damage some microorganisms; this is also the optimum pH for the activity of the majority of lysosomal enzymes, which act to break down the invading organism.

Avoiding or surviving phagocytosis

Pathogens have developed several means for avoiding being processed by this pathway.

Capsules   Bacteria such as *Klebsiella pneumoniae* and *Streptococcus pneumoniae* produce polysaccharide capsules that prevent opsonisation. Capsules are often relatively non-immunogenic. They may also be permeable to large proteins such as anti-bodies, permitting subcapsular deposition of antibody and complement at sites that are not accessible to receptors on phagocytic cells.

Evasion of the respiratory burst   Many intracellular pathogens of macrophages, such as *Leishmania donovani*, *Legionella pneumophila* and *Mycobacterium leprae* enter cells by binding to complement receptors. Unlike Fc receptors, these are not linked to activation of NADPH oxidase and, therefore, the respiratory burst is not triggered. Avirulent strains of *Legionella pneumophila* lack the ability to suppress the respiratory burst in neutrophils, unlike virulent strains. Microbes may also produce agents that block generation of the respiratory burst. The membrane lipophosphoglycan of *Leishmania donovani* inhibits protein kinase C, the central component in signal transduction leading to NADPH oxidase activation. Lipophosphoglycan, like many large microbial polysaccharide moieties, can also act as a non-specific scavenger of products of the respiratory burst. Most intracellular pathogens also produce enzymes such as catalase or superoxide dismutase, which inactivate hydrogen peroxide and superoxide, respectively.

Survival within the phagosome   Intracellular organisms have developed three general strategies for evasion of non-oxidative killing within cells. (i) Some organisms, such as *Toxoplasma gondii*, inhibit fusion of the phagosome with lysosomes. (ii) Another group of organisms rupture out of the phagolysosome into the cytoplasm, where replication can take place in a much less hostile environment. In *Shigella flexneri* this process has been associated with the production of a plasmid-encoded haemolysin. Once free in the cytoplasm, shigellae multiply, with subsequent inhibition of cellular protein synthesis. The ability of *Listeria monocytogenes* to escape from the phagosome has been shown by deletion mutagenesis to depend on listeriolysin. (iii) Some organisms, such as mycobacteria, are able to withstand and replicate within the hostile phagolysosomal environment. The mechanisms by which they resist inactivation in a location specifically designed to kill bacteria are not completely known but involve the bacteria in some way 'remodelling' the phagosome. Thus, phagosomes containing mycobacteria do not acidify and show a selective lack of the lysosomal proton-ATPase responsible for normal acidification of the lysosome.

Availability of nutrition

Bacteria must be able to take up nutrients from the host environment in order to replicate. Most bacteria can utilise a variety of substrates for energy production, and the enzyme system for their metabolism is often regulated by the presence or absence of the substrate in question. The regulation of the *lac* operon by lactose is an example.

Iron is required for the function of many bacterial enzymes, but the amount of free iron in tissue fluids is extremely low because it is chelated by high-affinity binding proteins such as transferrin and lactoferrin. Bacteria have evolved very efficient mechanisms of scavenging iron from mammalian iron-binding proteins. Some Gram-negative bacteria such as *Escherichia coli* and *Klebsiella aerogenes* secrete high-affinity extracellular iron chelators called siderophores. *Neisseria meningitidis* and *Haemophilus influenzae* have specific receptors for transferrin and lactoferrin on their surfaces,whilst some *Bacteroides* species remove iron by proteolytic cleavage of chelating proteins.

Toxin production

The term toxin is used to refer to either cell-associated endotoxin, the structure and effects of which are discussed below, or proteinaceous exotoxins, which are distinguished by their ability to cause severe damage to the host and the fact that they are often responsible for the clinical features of infection. Bacteria produce other less potent extracellular enzymes, such as proteases, nucleases, neuraminidase and hyaluronidase, which digest intercellular material and cause tissue damage, but these are not usually particularly potent and are not usually classified as toxins. Exotoxins are generally secreted and may, therefore, act at a distance from the site of colonisation. Broadly speaking, they fall into three main categories:

- intracellular enzymatic agents
- membrane active agents
- transmembrane active agents

Table 6.2 lists some of the known bacterial exotoxins.

Intracellular enzymatic toxins

Intracellular enzymatic toxins generally have an A–B subunit structure. The B subunit binds to the host cell via specific receptors and thus determines tissue tropism. The A subunit then enters the cell and produces toxic effects by its enzymatic action. For example, in diphtheria toxin, the A and B subunits form the amino- and carboxyl-terminal portions, respectively, of a single polypeptide. Attachment to the host cell is mediated by specific host receptors binding to fragment B, after which the polypeptide is cleaved and the A fragment enters the cell by endocytosis. The A fragment inhibits cellular protein synthesis by catalysing the attachment of adenosine diphosphate to the elongation factor EF2, rendering the EF2 inactive in the elongation of nascent polypeptide chains.

Other A–B toxins are assembled from non-covalently linked subunits, often products of the same operon. Cholera toxin and other related heat-labile enterotoxins, such as the shiga-like toxins of Enterobacteriaceae, are assemblies of six proteins in which a central A subunit is surrounded by five B subunits. The B subunit of cholera toxin binds to the ganglioside GM_1 on the cell surface of intestinal epithelial cells. The A subunit catalyses the ADP ribosylation of the membrane protein G_s, which is involved in the control of adenylate cyclase. This results in uncontrolled production of cyclic AMP and, in turn, in reduced sodium absorption and increased chloride secretion by the intestinal cell. As little as 5 μg cholera toxin has produced the features of cholera in volunteers; patients may pass up to 1 litre/hour of rice water stools, resulting in severe dehydration and circulatory collapse.

Table 6.2. *Examples of bacterial exotoxins and their actions*

Organism	Toxin	Effects mechanism	Disease association
Bacillus anthracis	Oedema factor Lethal factor Protective antigen	Adenylate cyclase Action unknown	Anthrax Tripartite toxin: oedema factor and lethal factor only active with protective antigen
Bacillus cereus	Enterotoxin Emetic toxin	Activates adenylate cyclase	Diarrhoea Vomiting
Bordatella pertussis	Pertussigen Adenylate cyclase Tracheal cytotoxin	ADP ribosylation of G_i Anti-phagocytic actions	Whooping cough
Clostridium botulinum	Neurotoxin (several serotypes)	Block acetylcholine release at neuromuscular junction	Botulism
Clostridium tetani	Tetanospasmin	Blocks release of inhibitory neurotransmitters in spinal cord	Tetanus
Clostridium difficile	Toxin A Toxin B	Main toxin *in vivo* Causes cytopathic effect *in vitro*	Antibiotic-associated diarrhoea and pseudomembranous colitis
Clostridium perfringens	Alpha toxin Enterotoxin Beta toxin Epsilon toxin Iota toxin Multiple less active toxins that are involved in the production of tissue necrosis	Phospholipase: disrupts host cell membranes Permease ADP ribosylation of actin	Gas gangrene Diarrhoea Necrotising enteritis ('pig bel') Tissue necrosis
Clostridium septicum, *Clostridium sordelli*	Several dermatonecrotising toxins		
Corynebacterium diphtheriae	Diphtheria toxin	ADP ribosylation of elongation factor 2	Diphtheria
Escherichia coli	Heat-labile toxin (LT) Heat-stable toxin (ST)	Similar to cholera toxin Activate guanylate cyclase	Diarrhoea Diarrhoea

Organism	Toxin	Mode of action	Disease/effect
	Shiga-like toxins (SLT-1, SLT-2, *syn.* verotoxin)	Inhibit protein synthesis (acts at 60S ribosomal subunit)	Diarrhoea, haemolytic uraemic syndrome
Pseudomonas aeruginosa	Exotoxin A	Inactivates elongation factor 2 by ADP-ribosylation	
	Leucocidin	Cytopathic for neutrophils	
	Protease, elastase, phospholipase	May promote invasiveness	
Shigella dysenteriae	Shiga toxin	Inhibit protein synthesis (acts at 60S ribosomal subunit)	Bacillary dysentery
Staphylococcus aureus	Enterotoxins A B C D and E	Pyrogenic enterotoxins; B toxin at least has effects like TSST-1	Diarrhoea and vomiting
	Epidermolysins	Cleaves epidermis	Scalded skin syndrome
	Alpha toxin	Membrane pore former	
	Beta toxin	Sphingomyelinase C	
	Delta toxin	Membrane pore former	
	Leucocidin	Degranulation and lysis of neutrophils	
	Toxic shock syndrome toxin 1 (TSST-1)	'Superantigen': T cell mitogen that promotes cytokine release	Toxic shock syndrome
Group A β-haemolytic streptococcus (*Streptococcus pyogenes*)	Erythrogenic toxin (three serotypes)		Scarlet fever / Wound infection
	Streptolysin O	Membrane pore former	
	Streptolysin S	Membrane pore former	
	Hyaluronidase	'Spreading factor': promotes invasiveness by digesting hyaluronic acid	
	Streptokinase	Catalyses plasminogen conversion to plasmin	
	DNAases, NADase, proteinase, amylase, esterase	Extracellular products which may enhance invasiveness	
	Toxic shock syndrome-like toxin	Similar to TSST-1	
Vibrio cholerae	Cholera toxin	ADP-ribosylation of G_s; activates adenylate cyclase	Cholera
Vibrio parahaemolyticus	Enterotoxin		Diarrhoea

Membrane-active toxins

A large number of cytolytic toxins, which damage cells by destabilising their membranes, have been characterised. Some are small peptides that disrupt membrane structure by direct interaction, such as staphylococcal δ toxin. This small peptide forms an amphipathic helical rod long enough to traverse the lipid bilayer; clusters of toxin molecules may form pores in the membrane preventing the cell from maintaining intracellular ion concentrations and ultimately resulting in cell lysis through the effects of osmotic pressure. Other membrane-active toxins are phospholipases that digest membrane lipids, such as the α toxin of *Clostridium perfringens*.

Transmembrane active toxins

A few bacterial toxins exert their effects by signalling across the intact cell membrane via transmembrane transducing systems, acting in many ways like peptide hormones. Thus the heat-stable enterotoxin of *Escherichia coli* (STa) is a small peptide that binds to the membrane of intestinal epithelial cells and causes an increase in the intracellular concentration of cyclic GMP. This results in changes in sodium and chloride transport and leads to a secretory diarrhoea. Other agents in this category include the neurotoxin of *Clostridium botulinum*, which is normally ingested pre-formed in contaminated food. It prevents the release of acetylcholine at the neuromuscular junction, producing flaccid paralysis.

Some transmembrane-active toxins have specific effects on cells of the immune system. The toxic shock syndrome (TSS) is an acute severe multisystem illness with fever, shock and a desquamating rash, most commonly associated with the use of high-absorbency tampons by menstruating women. The clinical manifestations of TSS are caused by toxic shock syndrome toxin 1 (TSST-1), produced by *Staphylococcus aureus*. The tampon provides a suitable environment for growth and toxin production by organisms colonising the cervix and vagina. Non-menstrual cases of TSS are less common and have occurred in a number of clinical situations including after surgical wound infection.

TSST-1 is thought to exert most of its effects by stimulating the release of cytokines, notably IL-2, γ-IFN and TNF, from lymphocytes. TSST-1 is a potent non-specific T cell mitogen; that is, it stimulates proliferation of a large subset of T cells, without regard for antigen specificity. This is because of its ability to bind directly to MHC class II molecules on antigen-presenting cells at a site distinct from the peptide-binding groove (p. 97). It will bind to most allelic forms of class II molecules, rather than to restricted alleles as do conventional peptide antigens. The TSST-1–MHC complex then reacts with the T cell receptor through the variable segment of the β-chain (Vβ) rather than with the normal antigen-binding site on the receptor, which is composed of both α- and β-chains. Molecules with this ability are referred to as 'superantigens'. Superantigens typically react with all T cells expressing a particular *V*β gene; there are approximately 50 different *V*β genes in humans, so a superantigen reacts with up to 1 in 50 T cells, whereas a conventional peptide antigen will react with 1 in 10^4 to 1 in 10^6 T cells. A number of other bacterial exotoxins are now known to act in this way.

Adaptive advantages of toxin production

Toxin production may benefit bacteria in many ways. In clinical terms, by producing diarrhoea, cholera toxin ensures the dissemination of *Vibrio cholerae* throughout the environment. At the cellular level, toxins may enhance the availability of nutrients such as iron by promoting cell leakage and death. Cell killing may also help bacteria such as *Clostridia* maintain an anaerobic environment within necrotic tissue. Many toxins are antiphagocytic. At high concentrations, staphylococcal α toxin kills cells, but at low concentrations it abolishes phagocytic function without causing cell death. Toxin production may only be appropriate in certain circumstances. It has been known for many decades that diphtheria toxin is only produced *in vitro* in conditions of low iron concentration – it may be that *in vivo* the toxin helps the bacterium to remedy an iron-poor environment. Toxin production is frequently regulated co-ordinately with other virulence factors. Thus, a single regulatory gene *agr* regulates the production of TSST-1, protein A and α toxin in *Staphylococcus aureus*.

Antibiotic action and resistance

Antibacterial agents depend for their action on the differences between bacterial and human cells. Table 6.3 lists the modes of action of many common antibiotics and the mechanisms of resistance commonly encountered. Most antibiotics are derived from naturally occurring substances, and it is, therefore, not surprising that bacteria have been able to evolve mechanisms of resistance. These fall into three broad categories.

1. Bacteria may develop altered target molecules that will no longer interact with antibiotics.
2. They may develop altered membrane proteins that reduce the permeability of the bacterial cell to antibiotic molecules.
3. They may acquire enzymes that inactivate antibiotics.

In molecular terms, bacteria acquire antibiotic resistance either by chromosomal mutation or by acquisition of new DNA, usually by plasmid transfer. Random spontaneous mutation occurs with low frequency in all bacterial populations, and in the presence of antibiotics, selective pressure may operate in favour of resistant organisms. Plasmids encoding resistance were first described in the late 1950s. They frequently encode resistance to multiple antibiotics and their prevalence has been of great clinical significance, as in the case of epidemic chloramphenicol-resistant typhoid fever in the early 1970s.

In some cases, it has been possible to chemically alter the structure of antibiotics to overcome developments in bacterial resistance, and this is illustrated by the development of the penicillins (Table 6.4).

Immunodeficiency

A full account of the functioning of the immune system is beyond the scope of this chapter. However, it is clear that the clinical picture of infectious illness results from the

Table 6.3. *Commonly used antibiotics, their mechanisms of action and common mechanisms of bacterial resistance*

Site	Class	Example	Mechanism of action	Mechanisms of resistance
Inhibition of peptidoglycan synthesis	Penicillin	Benzylpenicillin, ampicillin	Inhibition of bacterial transpeptidases, carboxylpeptidases ('penicillin-binding proteins')	Beta-lactamases, alterations in membrane permeability, altered pencillin-binding proteins
	Cephalosporins	Cefotaxime	Inhibition of bacterial transpeptidases, carboxylpeptidases	Modification of peptido glycan structure
	Glycopeptides	Vancomycin	Prevents polymerisation of polysaccharide chain	Altered ribosomal structure, modifying enzymes, alterations in membrane permeability
Inhibition of bacterial protein synthesis at bacterial ribosome	Chloramphenicol	Chloramphenicol	Inhibits peptidyl transferase at 50S subunit	
	Macrolides	Erythromycin	Acts at 50S subunit	
	Fusidanes	Fusidic acid	Binds to bacterial elongation factor 2	
	Tetracyclines	Oxytetracycline	Binds to 30S subunit preventing binding of aminoacyl-tRNA	
	Aminoglycosides	Gentamicin	Acts at 30S subunit	
	Lincosamides	Clindamycin	Acts at 50S subunit	
Inhibition of bacterial nucleic acid synthesis	Quinolones	Ciprofloxacin	Inhibition of DNA gyrase (α-subunit)	Mutation in DNA gyrase, alterations in membrane permeability
	Rifampicin	Rifampicin	Inhibits bacterial RNA polymerase (binds to β-subunit of core enzyme)	Mutation in β-subunit
	5-Nitroimidazoles	Metronidazole	Causes strand breakage in DNA	Reduces levels of pyruvate dehydrogenase, leading to reduced levels of active metabolite
	Nitrofurans	Nitrofurantoin	Causes strand breakage in DNA	
Inhibition of bacterial folate synthesis	Sulphonamides	Sulphamethoxazole	PABA antagonist	Mutation in dihydropteroate synthetase
	Diaminopyrimidines	Trimethoprim	Dihydrofolate reductase inhibitor	Mutation in dihydrofolate reductase

Table 6.4. *Overcoming bacterial resistance:*
(a) *Modifications to the side chain* (R) *of the penicillins have been introduced to improve antibacterial activity, stability in gastric acid and resistance to bacterial β-lactamases*

Basic structure of the penicillins: 1, β-lactam ring; 2, thiazolidine ring (6-membered in the cephalosporins)

Group	Examples (other group members in brackets)	Structure of R group	Comments
Natural penicillins	Benzylpenicillin (syn. penicillin G)		The first penicillin, sensitive to gastic acid
	Phenoxymethylpenicillin (syn. Pen-V)		Stable in gastric acid
Penicillinase-resistant penicillins	Flucloxacillin (methicillin, oxacillin, cloxacillin)		Resistant to staphylococcal penicillinases
Amino-penicillins	Ampicillin (amoxycillin)		Extended spectrum against Gram-negatives
Carboxy-penicillins	Carbenicillin		Wide spectrum including *Pseudomonas aeruginosa*
	Ticarcillin		Wide spectrum including *Pseudomonas aeruginosa*
Ureido-penicillins	Piperacillin (azlocillin, mezlocillin)		Very broad spectrum of activity including most Gram-negative bacilli and *Pseudomonas aeruginosa*

Table 6.4. (*b*) *Inhibitors of β-lactamases*

Examples	Structure	Comments
Clavulanic acid		Weak antibacterial activity only but are irreversible inhibitors of β-lactamases
Sulbactam		Used to extend the spectrum of amino- and carboxyl-penicillins

interaction of bacterial factors, some of which have been discussed above, and host factors, which include the functioning of the immune system. In clinical practice, secondary disorders of non-antigen-specific (natural) immunity, such as the damage inflicted on the epithelium of the respiratory tract by smoking or the increased incidence of urinary tract infection associated with the use of urinary catheters, are far more prevalent than those rare conditions in which one component of the immune system is absent or dysfunctional. However, these latter conditions have often allowed elucidation of the functioning of the normal immune system, and more recently the molecular basis of some of them has been determined. A characteristic feature of many forms of immunodeficiency is that while patients are at increased risk of infection from well-recognised pathogens, they are also at risk from organisms that in other circumstances would be unlikely to cause infection and which are, therefore, referred to as *opportunistic* pathogens.

Disorders of non-antigen-specific immunity

Damage to epithelial surfaces of the type referred to above accounts for a large proportion of clinical infectious disease but will not be discussed further. Disorders affecting the non-antigen-specific components of the immune system itself include complement deficiencies and disorders affecting neutrophils (Table 6.5).

Complement deficiency

The clinical phenotype of complement disorders varies. C3 occupies a central point in both the classical and alternative complement pathways. Congenital C3 deficiency occurs as an autosomal recessive disorder. Patients are at risk from a wide range of infections and in this respect present with similar clinical features to patients with hypo-

Table 6.5. *Disorders of natural immunity*

	Congenital	Acquired	Drug-induced	Common infectious complications
Neutrophil disorders				
Neutropenia	Infantile genetic agranulocytosis, autoimmune neutropenia, isoimmune neonatal neutropenia	Acute and chronic leukaemia: secondary to HIV infection, malignancy, alcoholism, nutritional deficiency, connective tissue disease; iatrogenic, e.g. after chemotherapy	Chloramphenicol, cyclophosphamide, carbimazole	Recurrent or severe infection with pyogenic bacteria (e.g. Gram-positive cocci, Enterobacteriaceae, *Pseudomonas aeruginosa*, *Haemophilus influenzae*) and fungi (e.g. *Candida albicans*, *Aspergillus* spp.)
Abnormal neutrophil function (e.g. abnormalities of chemotaxis, adherence, phagocytosis and microbial killing)	Chédiak-Higashi, lazy leucocyte, leucocyte adhesion deficiency, chronic granulomatous disease	Secondary to systemic illness, including diabetes mellitus, rheumatoid disease, chronic alcoholism, cirrhosis, renal failure	Steroids, aspirin, colchicine cyclophosphamide, phenylbutazone	
Complement disorders	Inherited deficiencies of C3, C5, C6, C7, C8, factor I, properdin	Splenectomy, sickle cell disease, systemic lupus erythematosus, protein–calorie malnutrition, burns		Severe recurrent infection with *Streptococcus pneumoniae*, *Neisseria meningitidis*, *Neisseria gonorrhoeae*

gammaglobulinaemia. In particular, they are susceptible to encapsulated bacteria such as *Streptococcus pneumoniae* and *Haemophilus influenzae*. By contrast, individuals who lack the later components of complement, which form the membrane attack complex, are particularly susceptible to systemic infection with *Neisseria meningitidis* and *N. gonorrhoeae*.

Neutrophil disorders

There are a number of rare inherited syndromes in which neutrophils are absent or defective. For example, chronic granulomatous disease is an inherited defect in the enzymes responsible for oxidative killing. Patients are highly susceptible to severe recurrent bacterial and fungal infections, in particular cellulitis and pneumonia caused by catalase-producing organisms such as *Escherichia coli*, *Serratia marscesens*, *Pseudomonas cepacia* and *Staphylococcus aureus*. However, neutropenia is usually acquired, most commonly as a result of cytotoxic chemotherapy for malignant disease. Patients rendered neutropenic represent a variety of clinical groups, such as patients receiving chemotherapy for solid tumours and others undergoing bone marrow transplantation. They differ in their susceptibility to different infections and a full consideration of these differences is beyond the scope of this chapter.

Patients with neutrophil counts below 500 cells/µl are at risk of bacterial and fungal infections, particularly if they have concomitant mucositis as a result of their chemotherapy. Patients are unable to mount an adequate inflammatory response and so the usual signs of infection may be absent. The organisms most likely to cause infection depend to a large extent on medical management. Gram-negative bacteraemia with gut-derived bacteria such as *Escherichia coli*, *Pseudomonas aeruginosa* and *Klebsiella* spp. is common, but its incidence can be reduced by the use of prophylactic antibiotics chosen to selectively kill intestinal Enterobacteriaceae. Staphylococcal infections, particularly with *Staphylococcus epidermidis* are particularly common in patients with indwelling central venous cannulae. Fungal pathogens include *Candida* spp., which may cause widespread disseminated infection, and *Aspergillus* spp., which more commonly presents as an acute pulmonary infection resistant to antibacterials.

The period of neutropenia may be shortened by the administration of recombinant granulocyte colony stimulating factor (G-CSF) which stimulates the differentiation of mature neutrophils from precursors. Clinical trials have demonstrated reduced morbidity from infection in patients treated with G-CSF.

Disorders of specific immunity

Disorders of specific immunity may affect humoral (antibody-mediated) immunity, cell-mediated immunity or both. Table 6.6 lists some primary disorders that affect lymphocyte function, in some instances the molecular basis of the defect is known. In many cases, these rare inherited conditions have helped to elucidate the mechanisms of immunity. For example, it has been shown that patients with the X-linked Wiskott–Aldrich syndrome (WAS) of thrombocytopenia, eczema and immunodeficiency have impaired expression of the CD43 glycoprotein on lymphocytes. The CD43 molecule negatively

Table 6.6. *Disorders of acquired immunity: primary diseases of lymphocytes*

	Comments	Common infectious complications
Deficiencies of humoral immunity		
X-linked hypogammaglobulinaemia	Development arrest at pre-B cell stage, occasionally associated with growth hormone deficiency	Chronic or recurrent bacterial infections, chronic disseminated enteroviral infection
Common variable immunodeficiency (CVID)	Heterogeneous group of patients with hypogammaglobulinaemia	Chronic respiratory and GI infection
IgA deficiency	Common, affecting 1:600 individuals, frequently asymptomatic	Chronic respiratory and GI infection
IgG subclass deficiency	Usually affects IgG2 or IgG2 and IgG4	Infection with encapsulated bacteria
Hyper-IgM syndrome	Failure of B cells to switch from IgM to IgG production	Recurrent pyogenic infection
Transient hypogammaglobulinaemia of infancy	May persist for many months	Diarrhoea, otitis media
Deficiencies of both cellular and humoral immunity		
Severe combined immunodeficiency (SCID)	Heterogeneous group of patients with deficient cell-mediated and humoral immunity. Variants include adenosine deaminase deficiency, purine nucleotide phosphorylase deficiency, MHC class II deficiency, reticular dysgenesis	Chronic recurrent bacterial, viral and fungal infections, often fatal in infancy
DiGeorge syndrome	Embryopathy of 3rd and 4th pharyngeal pouch resulting in thymic aplasia, hypoparathyroidism and congenital heart disease	Chronic and recurrent respiratory and GI infections
Wiskott–Aldrich syndrome	Thrombocytopenia, eczema and immunodeficiency, associated with impaired CD43 expression on lymphocytes	Bacterial and fungal infections, lymphoma
Ataxia telangiectasia	Cerebellar ataxia, oculocutaneous telangiectasia and immunodeficiency	Chronic sinopulmonary infection, lymphoma and lymphatic leukaemia also common
Chronic mucocutaneous candidiasis	Frequently associated with endocrinopathies and autoimmune disease	Also more susceptible to bacterial and viral infections
X-linked lympho-proliferative syndrome	Genetic inability to mount immune response to EBV infection	Chronic EBV infection with hypogammaglobulinaemia, pancytopenia and lymphoma

Note:
GI, gastrointestinal; EBV, Epstein–Barr virus.

regulates T-lymphocyte activation and probably has an important role in immune regulation. The gene for CD43 is located on chromosome 16. The *WAS* gene, which is mutated in individuals with this syndrome, is located on the X chromosome and encodes a protein thought to control CD43 expression.

Until recently, acquired immunodeficiency was restricted to haematological malignancy, intercurrent severe illness and immunosuppressive or cytotoxic drug therapy. However, the advent of the HIV has made the management of severely immunodeficient patients a far more common occurrence.

HIV and AIDS

Following infection with HIV, most patients remain asymptomatic, although some develop a flu-like illness with fever, myalgia, headache and a rash. This coincides with the development of specific antiviral antibodies and effector T cells, which unfortunately do not prevent viral persistence. Progression to AIDS, defined in the UK as development of one of the conditions listed in Table 6.7 in a patient with HIV infection, occurs after a median interval of about 10 years in adult patients in the developed world. Clinically, AIDS is associated with severe immunodeficiency and presents with a very wide range of opportunistic infections and malignancies, which vary depending on the population in question. Patients in the developed world typically presented either with Kaposi's sarcoma or with *Pneumocystis carinii* pneumonia, an unusual fungal infection that had previously been seen mainly in patients with severe iatrogenic suppression of cell-mediated immunity following organ transplantation, although this is much less common now that prophylactic therapy is instituted when signs of progression develop.

HIV infects a variety of cell types that express the CD4 molecule, including T and B lymphocytes, macrophages, promyelocytes, fibroblasts and epidermal Langerhan's cells. Infection of neural tissue has also been demonstrated and it appears that this may take place via CD4-independent means. HIV causes disease in three main ways. First, it produces profound suppression of cell-mediated immunity. Second, it is believed to cause direct tissue damage, particularly to nervous tissue, and third, it promotes a number of immunopathogenic phenomena such as immune thrombocytopenic purpura. A wide spectrum of immunological abnormalities has been reported in HIV-infected individuals, some of which are summarised in Table 6.8.

The interaction of HIV with the immune system is undoubtedly complex and the mechanism by which HIV causes depletion of CD4 cells remains controversial. It has recently been shown that HIV replication proceeds at high levels during the period of clinical latency between seroconversion and AIDS. Sensitive detection methods based on PCR have demonstrated high levels of virus in blood and lymph nodes, and mathematical modelling suggests a rapid rate of replication and destruction of virus particles, even during the latent period when patients remain asymptomatic. These observations have contributed to our understanding of the steady decline in $CD4^+$ lymphocytes, and the rapid development of resistance to antiviral drugs seen in patients treated with single agent regimens. Recently, combination therapy with two or three antiviral drugs has been shown to reduce dramatically viral replication and to be associated with improved survival.

Table 6.7. *An HIV-infected patient is defined as having AIDS if they have one of the following indicator diseases. In the USA a CD4 count below 200 cells/μl is also considered diagnostic of AIDS*

AIDS indicator disease	Comments and qualifications
Bacterial infections, recurrent or multiple	In a child less than 13 years
Candidiasis	Affecting oesophagus, trachea, bronchus or lungs
Cervical carcinoma	Invasive
Coccidioidomycosis	Disseminated or extrapulmonary
Cryptococcosis	Extrapulmonary
Cryptosporidiosis	With diarrhoea for greater than one month
Cytomegalovirus disease	Onset after age one month, not confined to liver, spleen or lymph nodes
Cytomegalovirus retinitis	
Encephalopathy (dementia) caused by HIV	HIV infection and disabling cognitive and/or motor dysfunction, or milestone loss in a child, with no other causes by CSF examination, brain imaging or post-mortem
Herpes simplex	Ulcers for greater than one month or bronchitis, pneumonitis or oesophagitis
Histoplasmosis	Disseminated or extrapulmonary
Isosporiasis	With diarrhoea for greater than one month
Kaposi's sarcoma	
Lymphoid interstitial pneumonia and/or pulmonary lymphoid hyperplasia	In a child less than 13 years
Lymphoma	Burkitt's or immunoblastic or primary in brain
Mycobacteriosis	Disseminated or extrapulmonary
Mycobacteriosis	Pulmonary tuberculosis
Pneumocystis carinii pneumonia	
Progressive multifocal leucoencephalopathy	
Recurrent non-typhoidal salmonella bacteraemia	
Recurrent pneumonia	Two episodes within 12 months
Toxoplasmosis of brain	Onset after age one month
Wasting syndrome resulting from HIV	Weight loss (over 10% of baseline) with no other cause, and 30 days or more of either diarrhoea or weakness with fever

Table 6.8. *Summary of the major immunological defects demonstrated in HIV infection*

Cell type affected	*In vivo* defects	*In vitro* defects
T cells	Increased susceptibility to infections and neoplasms, reduced delayed type hypersensitivity	Quantitative and qualitative defects in T cell function, absolute decline in CD4$^+$ T cells, reversal of the normal CD4/CD8 ratio
B cells	Polyclonal hypergammaglobulinaemia, hypogammaglobulinaemia in children, impaired responses to immunisation	Impaired responses in *in vitro* assays
NK cells		Cytoxic capability reduced
APCs		Impaired ability to present antigen to T cells, impaired monocyte chemotaxis

Immunopathogenesis

A central theme of this chapter has been that the clinical features of an infectious illness are caused by the interaction of microbial pathogenic mechanisms with host factors. The immune system has evolved to enable the host to resist and overcome infection, but it is clear that in many cases the immune response is responsible for almost all the clinical features of infection. This phenomenon is referred to as *immunopathology*.

Antibody-mediated immunopathology

Antibodies may mediate immunopathology in a number of ways. For example, in some circumstances, antibody can facilitate entry of viruses into cells that express Fc receptors. This process, known as antibody-dependent enhancement, was first described for dengue virus. Infection by dengue is often more severe, with the development of shock and disseminated intravascular coagulation, in patients who have had a previous infection by a dengue virus of a different serotype. It is hypothesised that non-neutralising antibodies from the first infection mediate enhancement, with more widespread infection of macrophages, greater release of inflammatory mediators and more severe shock.

Antibody-mediated immunopathology also occurs in bacterial infections. Chronic bacterial infection with release of antigens into the circulation may cause immune complex disease. The two classic examples in which this occurs in human disease are bacterial endocarditis and infected ventriculo-atrial shunts, where sustained release of bacterial antigen leads to formation of immune complexes and consequent glomerulonephritis. In many instances, infection triggers an autoimmune response that causes tissue damage at a site distant from the site of infection, discussed further in Chapter 4.

Cell-mediated immunopathology

Most bacteria are extracellular pathogens and T cells, therefore, play a less central role in their elimination than does antibody; however, they are important for the elimination of intracellular bacteria and may take part in immunopathological reactions to bacterial infection. Delayed type hypersensitivity reactions are a characteristic feature of mycobacterial infections and play an important part in their resolution. It has been suggested that the predominance of either T_H1 or T_H2 T cells (see Chapter 4) responding to infection by *Mycobacterium leprae* may determine the clinical course of leprosy infection. In the tuberculoid form of the disease, bacilli are very scanty and skin and nerves are infiltrated by lymphocytes and macrophages. Damage to nerves in this form of leprosy is thought to be caused by host cellular immune responses, and T cells present in these lesions are predominantly γ-IFN-secreting (T_H1-like). T cells isolated from lesions of lepromatous leprosy, where there are many intracellular organisms and poor or absent delayed hypersensitivity to *Mycobacterium leprae*, have been shown to be mainly IL-4 secreting (T_H2-like).

Immunopathological responses to bacterial infection may be associated with HLA haplotype. For example, reactive arthritis following infection with *Yersinia enterocolitica* and other diarrhoeal organisms is very strongly associated with possession of the MHC class I allele *B27*. Putative mechanisms for this association include molecular mimicry between bacterial antigens and the B27 molecule itself.

Animal models of viral disease clearly demonstrate T cell-mediated immunopathology, but human examples are few. It is likely, for example, that the hepatocyte injury seen in acute hepatitis B virus infection is mainly caused by the effects of cell-mediated immunity, in particular MHC class I restricted CD8$^+$ cytotoxic T cells directed against virally infected cells.

SEPTIC SHOCK

The exemplar syndrome for this chapter is septic shock. Microorganisms frequently enter the bloodstream but host defence mechanisms are usually sufficient to destroy them. If host immunity is weakened by intercurrent illness or age, or if the virulence or magnitude of the invading organisms is enhanced, for example after establishment of a focus of infection in the chest, abdomen or urinary tract, illness may result. Septic shock, broadly defined as the development of hypotension and organ failure as a result of severe infection, is an important cause of death in hospital patients, particularly on the intensive care unit. Variations in the definition of shock and the many antecedent causes make it difficult to establish true figures for incidence and mortality. The diagnosis of septic shock remains a clinical one (Fig. 6.4), confirmed by positive blood cultures in only a proportion of cases. Blood cultures may not yield a result for several days, and for these reasons, and to allow comparison of patients in clinical trials, it is very useful to have a clinical definition that allows identification of patients before they develop positive blood cultures and resistant hypotension. Bacteraemia signifies positive blood cultures; the term septicaemia is imprecise and unhelpful. A definition of 'sepsis syndrome' that

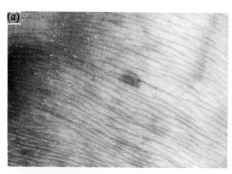
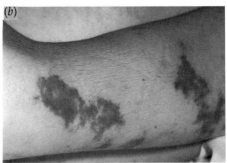

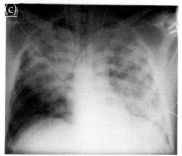

Symptoms and signs

Fever, rigors or hypothermia

Altered mental state

Evidence of pre-existing sepsis (e.g. cough or disturbance of micturition) and/or risk factors for bacteraemia (see text)

Tachycardia, tachypnoea, hypotension

Hyperventilation

Cutaneous manifestations:

Petechial or pupuric rash (particularly in septicaemia with *Neisseria meningitidis*)

Early shock: peripheral vasodilatation with warm skin

Late shock: peripheral vasoconstriction with cold, cyanotic, mottled skin

Laboratory abnormalities

Neutrophilia with 'left shift'

Thrombocytopenia

Disseminated intravascular coagulation (thrombocytopenia, prolonged prothrombin and partial thromboplastin times, reduced plasma fibrinogen and raised fibrin degradation products)

Raised urea and creatinine

Raised serum lactate

Abnormal liver function test

Positive blood cultures

Fig. 6.4. Clinical features of septic shock. (*a*, *b*) Skin changes associated with meningococcaemia. Patients with meningococcaemia may develop a skin rash that is initially maculopapular (*a*) but which then rapidly progresses to become purpuric (*b*), sometimes with frank gangrene affecting the extremities. (These photographs are not of the same patient). Patients in whom meningococcaemia is suspected should be treated with antibiotics promptly as the nature of the rash is an unreliable physical sign.

(*c*) Adult respiratory distress syndrome. This is characterised by increased alveolar capillary permeabilty and pulmonary oedema without left atrial hypertension. Clinically patients may have evidence of ventilation–perfusion mismatch, with a widened alveolar-arterial oxygen gradient and reduced lung compliance.

Table 6.9 *Definition of sepsis syndrome*

Hypothermia (<35.6 °C) or fever (>38.3 °C)
Tachycardia (>90 beats/min)
Tachypnoea (>20 respirations/min)
A presumed site of infection
and
Evidence of dysfunction of at least one organ
(altered mental state, arterial hypoxaemia (PO$_2$<10 kPa),
elevated plasma lactate or oliguria (<30 ml/h)

has been clinically tested and which has achieved widespread acceptance is shown in Table 6.9.

Septic shock is a hetergeneous condition; reported mortality varies between 20% and 80%, depending on the definition employed and the study population. Many factors influence the prognosis in patients with bacteraemia. These include the severity of underlying predisposing disease, the use of appropriate antibiotics, the nature of the pathogen involved and the magnitude of bacteraemia, the age of the patient, and the site of initial infection. Polymicrobial bacteraemia, the development of complications such as renal failure and a respiratory rather than abdominal or urinary focus of infection all indicate a worse prognosis.

Clinical features of septic shock

Risk factors for septic shock

Although there are illnesses caused by specific bacterial species, such as *Neisseria meningitidis*, that may develop rapidly in previously healthy young adults, septic shock is usually seen as a complication of underlying illness or in patients with impaired immune function. Therefore, septic shock as a presenting feature of, for example, urinary tract infection in a previously healthy young adult would be a rare event. The risk factors that predispose to the development of septic shock are generally those which indicate a worse prognosis in established disease. The presence of any severe underlying illness, including established infections such as abdominal abscess secondary to surgery, trauma or diverticulitis, or non-infectious conditions, such as diabetic ketoacidosis, that may impair host immunity and epithelial integrity is highly significant. Particular risks include trauma, malignancy and recent manipulations or surgery, including non-medical interventions such as attempted abortion or intravenous drug use. Patients at either of the extremes of age are at increased risk as are intravenous drug abusers and those with indwelling foreign bodies, in particular intravenous medical devices such as central venous cannulae.

Immunodeficiency may be overt and predictable, as in patients with HIV infection, those taking immunosuppressive drugs following organ transplantation or patients with haematological malignancy whose immune function is damaged both by their disease and by chemotherapeutic drugs. Alternatively, the immune system may be compromised in more subtle ways: for example, patients with alcoholism or cirrhosis, diabetes mellitus and renal failure are all at increased risk of developing septic shock. Patients who have undergone splenectomy are at increased risk of bacteraemia caused by encapsulated bacteria such as *Streptococcus pneumoniae*.

Organisms responsible for septic shock

Organisms causing septic shock are usually endogenous – most often translocated from the patient's gut or skin. Enterobacteriaceae, in particular *Escherichia coli*, but also *Klebsiella*, *Proteus* and *Enterobacter* spp., are responsible for the majority of infections, but since the mid-1980s there has been a rapid rise in the number of episodes caused by Gram-positive cocci, specifically *Staphylococcus aureus*, *Staphylococcus epidermidis* and *Streptococcus pneumoniae*. This reflects, in part, the emergence of antibiotic resistance, and also changes in the practice of medicine, with the much more frequent use of invasive monitoring and therapeutic techniques. These provide a portal of entry and a site for colonisation by organisms such as *Staphylococcus epidermidis*. Many patients with *Streptococcus pneumoniae* pneumonia are bacteraemic, although only some develop systemic features of septic shock.

Septic shock caused by *Pseudomonas aeruginosa* is associated with a higher case-fatality rate than that with other Gram-negative bacilli, not least because of its association with neutropenia and its resistance to many commonly used antibiotics. Anaerobic infections, particularly *Bacteroides fragilis*, also carry a high mortality, often in association with malignancy or localised abdominal abscess formation.

The risk factors discussed above determine to a large extent which organisms are likely to be isolated. Antibiotic regimens for patients with haematological malignancies undergoing chemotherapy with indwelling central lines need to take account of the likelihood of Gram-positive bacteraemia, whilst for patients with abdominal sepsis, it is important to include cover against gut-derived anaerobes.

Diagnosis and conventional management

Most patients will require intensive investigation aimed at elucidating both the cause and the severity of shock. Imaging will include chest X-ray, and ultrasound and CT scanning will often be required to exclude local collections of pus. Microbiological tests may include culture of urine, pus, sputum or cerebrospinal fluid. Blood cultures should be sent as soon as the diagnosis is suspected. A number of technological advances, including automated monitoring and antibiotic removal resins, have recently been introduced to improve the sensitivity and speed of blood culture, but this remains heavily dependent on the volume of blood cultured. At least three venepunctures should be performed in the assessment period and at least 10 and preferably 20 ml of blood should be cultured at each venepuncture.

Patients with fever and shock may not always have septic shock. It is important to consider other possibilities, including purulent bacterial pericardial effusion, peritonitis, severe pneumonia with hypoxaemia, mediastinitis (for example after oesophageal surgery or variceal sclerotherapy), anaphylaxis induced by antibiotics and toxic shock syndrome (p. 178).

Conventional management of septic shock depends on adequate doses of appropriate antibiotics, the removal of any local collection of pus and, most importantly, full supportive therapy, usually given in the context of the intensive care unit. Patients require detailed haemodynamic monitoring, which in turn may direct appropriate therapy with fluids, oxygen and vasopressors. Careful clinical trials have established that steroids do not improve prognosis in septic shock.

Progression

Patients in early shock have peripheral vasodilatation with decreased systemic vascular resistance and increased cardiac output. Those who enter the later phase of 'cold shock', with peripheral vasoconstriction, increased systemic vascular resistance and reduced cardiac output have a poor prognosis. Adult respiratory distress syndrome (ARDS) may complicate septic shock in up to 40% of patients and is associated with a very high mortality. ARDS is characterised by increased alveolar capillary permeability and pulmonary oedema without left atrial hypertension. Clinically, patients may have evidence of ventilation–perfusion mismatch, with a widened alveolar-arterial oxygen gradient and reduced lung compliance. Most patients with septic shock develop some degree of renal failure, usually the result of acute tubular necrosis secondary to hypotension.

Mortality increases with the number of systems involved and if four or more organ systems fail, mortality approaches 100%. In terminal stages, patients become progressively acidotic, with resistant hypotension refractory to treatment with fluids and inotropic drugs.

Pathogenesis of septic shock

Despite advances in biology since the mid-1980s, the pathogenesis of this condition remains incompletely understood. The development of septic shock represents a cascade, initiated by the release of bacterial components such as endotoxin into the circulation, mediated to a large extent by endogenous, host-derived inflammatory markers and culminating in severe endothelial cell damage, haemodynamic derangement and, often, death (Fig. 6.5). Capillary leakage secondary to endothelial cell damage and abnormalities of vascular tone lead to peripheral vasodilatation and maldistribution of blood flow, causing relative hypovolaemia and hypotension.

Structure of endotoxin

Much experimental work has concentrated on the role of Gram-negative endotoxin, as a large proportion of clinically significant sepsis involves Gram-negative bacilli. The Gram-negative cell wall (Fig. 6.2) consists of inner and outer cell membranes enclosing the periplasmic space. The endotoxic properties of the cell wall result from the presence,

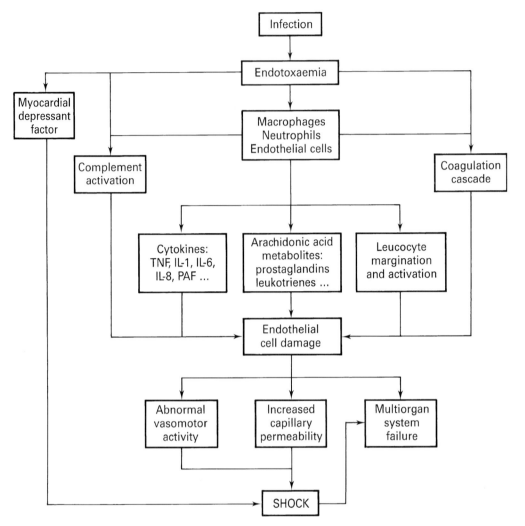

Fig. 6.5. A schematic representation of the pathophysiological cascade that leads from bacteraemia to the clinical syndrome of septic shock.

in the outer cell membrane, of bacterial LPS. LPS comprises three distinct regions: lipid A, core antigen and the outermost region, the O-specific side chain (Fig. 6.6). This last region consists of a series of repeating oligosaccharide units, the precise configuration of which is specific for a particular bacterial strain and confers serotypic specificity (the 'O' antigen). The core antigen, which is broadly similar for all the pathogenic Enterobacteriaceae is a branched oligosaccharide structure that links the O-specific side chain to lipid A. Lipid A consists of a phosphorylated glucosamine sequence linked by β-1′, 6-glycosidic bonds. The amino group of the glucosamine is generally substituted by D-3-hydroxy fatty acids, and the hydroxyl groups are esterified with long-chain saturated fatty acids.

LPS forms a physical barrier to attack by components of the humoral immune system

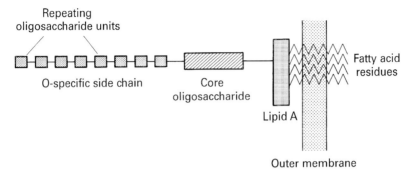

Fig. 6.6. The structure of enterobacterial LPS. Most of the pathological effects of LPS are caused by lipid A, and antibodies against lipid A can protect animals from the effects of bacteraemia.

but is also a potent activator of complement. Purified lipid A binds directly to C1q and can activate the classical pathway of complement activation *in vitro*, but this is probably of little significance *in vivo* for intact bacteria because the O-specific side chain prevents this interaction. The carbohydrate side chain is a powerful activator of the alternative pathway of complement activation, which may paradoxically protect bacteria from complement-mediated lysis: C3b is fixed mainly at the ends of the O-specific side chains, sterically preventing fixation close to the cell wall. As a consequence, the membrane attack complex (comprising the complement components that form a pore in cell membranes) is assembled at a distance from the cell membrane and is unable to insert into it. This situation may not apply to disrupted bacteria, and the activation of complement by LPS with the formation of anaphylatoxins, in particular C5a, which in turn stimulate the release of other cytokines, is one mechanism by which endotoxin can trigger the septic shock cascade.

Effects of endotoxin

LPS has numerous biological effects, most of which are attributable to the lipid A moiety. Once in the circulation, LPS stimulates cells including macrophages and endothelial cells to produce a large number of inflammatory mediators, in particular TNF, IL-1, IL-6 and IL-8, PAF and arachidonic acid metabolites such as leukotrienes, thromboxane A_2 and prostaglandins. IL-1 and IL-6 activate T cells, resulting in the production of γ-IFN, IL-2, IL-4 and GM-CSF. Complement and coagulation cascades are activated both directly and secondary to endothelial cell damage.

Receptors for endotoxin

It has recently been shown that LPS binds to a plasma LPS-binding protein forming high-affinity complexes that in turn bind to CD14, a cell surface protein present on mono-nuclear phagocytes and neutrophils. Binding of the complex of LPS and LPS-binding protein to CD14 on leucocytes *in vitro* induces TNF secretion. Monoclonal antibodies against CD14 can inhibit cell activation by LPS, and transgenic mice that express human CD14 on their leucocytes are hypersensitive to the effects of LPS. These data strongly suggest that CD14 is a major receptor for LPS, although it is probably not the only one.

Mediators of septic shock

Since many of the cytokines mentioned can stimulate the release of other cytokines and, in some cases, of themselves, and since many have synergistic or inhibitory actions, it is difficult to ascribe definite roles to any one inflammatory mediator. However, it is accepted that TNF and IL-1 play a major role in the pathogenesis of septic shock. TNF and IL-1 are both produced predominantly by mononuclear phagocytes and share most of their effects on the vascular endothelium, some of which are discussed below. It has been demonstrated that TNF levels are elevated in many patients with sepsis, and many of the stimuli that cause septic shock, such as LPS, directly stimulate TNF release from mononuclear phagocytes. Injection of LPS into animals or human volunteers results in a rise in serum levels of TNF and duplicates many of the clinical features of septic shock, including hypotension, neutrophilia and increased capillary permeability. Antibodies against TNF can protect mice against injected LPS and mice that lack the p 55 TNF receptor (TNFR-1) are also resistant to some of the effects of LPS.

However, there is also much contradictory evidence concerning the role of TNF as the central mediator of septic shock. For example, some patients with sepsis do not have elevated TNF levels in serum, and antibodies to LPS that can protect mice from LPS challenge do so without lowering the rise in TNF observed. It is likely that TNF acts locally, that serum levels do not represent its true activity and that other inflammatory mediators are also important. TNF is produced as a host defence, and interfering with its action may be harmful as well as beneficial. Therefore, mice treated with antisera to TNF or which lack TNFR-1 have increased susceptibility to infection with *Listeria monocytogenes*.

Endothelial cell changes in septic shock

The pathological consequences responsible for the clinical features of septic shock include severe endothelial cell damage, with increased capillary permeability, maldistribution of blood flow and intravascular coagulation. These changes in turn contribute to the development of multiorgan system failure. The vascular endothelium is the primary target organ in septic shock, and many of the inflammatory mediators described above have direct effects on endothelial cells. Many of these effects have recently been delineated *in vitro* in endothelial cell cultures using recombinant cytokines. It is clear that endothelial cells do not act as passive targets in the inflammatory processes operating in septic shock. In addition to morphological changes, cytokines activate a number of endothelial cell responses, including the expression of leucocyte adhesion molecules, the secretion of soluble inflammatory mediators, changes in the regulation of coagulation and alterations in vascular tone. Endothelial cells thus contribute actively to the accumulation of inflammatory infiltrates and the development of intravascular coagulation.

Morphological changes in endothelial cells

TNF and IL-1 cause alterations in endothelial cell cytoskeletal structure. Cells that normally form confluent single layers in tissue culture become misshapen and overlap extensively. Other cytokines, such as γ-IFN, synergise with TNF to produce other morphological changes. These changes, observed *in vitro*, may increase vascular permeability and promote leucocyte transmigration at sites of vascular inflammation *in vivo*.

Leucocyte adhesion molecule expression on endothelial cells

Endothelial cell expression of a number of leucocyte adhesion molecules, including ELAM-1 (E-selectin), P-selectin and VCAM-1, is induced by cytokines during the development of localised inflammatory responses (see also Chapter 5, p. 00). Expression of P-selectin (CD62) is induced within minutes by inflammatory mediators such as histamine and thrombin. ELAM-1 is expressed in response to TNF and IL-1, and surface expression peaks at 4 to 6 hours. Both P-selectin and ELAM-1 act as adhesion molecules for neutrophils. Together with the related leucocyte adhesion molecule-1 (LAM-1 or L-selectin) they make up the selectin family of transmembrane proteins.

VCAM-1 is also induced by TNF and IL-1. VCAM-1 is a member of the immunoglobulin supergene family. Expression peaks at 24 hours, much later than for P-selectin and ELAM-1. The ligand for VCAM-1 is the very late activation antigen VLA-4, a member of the integrin family that is expressed on lymphocytes and mononuclear phagocytes. ICAM-1 and ICAM-2 are also members of the immunoglobulin supergene family and both are expressed constitutively by endothelial cells. ICAM-1 expression is upregulated by TNF, IL-1 and γ-IFN, reaching a plateau at about 24 hours. Both are ligands for LFA-1, a member of the CD11/CD18 family of integrins that are broadly distributed on leucocytes.

The extent to which expression of these leucocyte adhesion molecules contributes to leucocyte margination and transmigration *in vivo* during septic shock remains to be fully established. It has been shown that injection of live *Escherichia coli* or LPS alone induces widespread *de novo* expression of ELAM-1 throughout the vascular tree of primates, and endothelial cell ELAM-1 expression is upregulated at sites of inflammation in human subjects. However, clinical studies examining this phenomenon in patients with septic shock remain to be published.

Endothelial cell secretion of soluble inflammatory mediators

Cytokines stimulate endothelial cells to produce soluble inflammatory mediators, such as IL-8 and monocyte chemotactic protein-1 (MCP-1). These cytokines, which are produced in response to TNF, IL-1 and, in the case of MCP-1, γ-IFN, attract and activate neutrophils and monocytes, respectively. Endothelial cells also produce IL-6, which is a potent stimulator of B cell proliferation and differentiation. Following margination of leucocytes, mediated by any of the processes described above, microvascular injury can result from the release of reactive oxygen intermediates and proteases from the adherent cells.

Endothelial cells as regulators of coagulation

The endothelial cell surface is normally anticoagulant, as a result of constitutive expression of molecules such as thrombomodulin and heparan and secretion of protein S. Exposure to TNF or IL-1 induces expression of tissue factor, which binds factor VIIa and initiates the extrinsic clotting pathway, as well as downregulating expression of thrombomodulin. TNF and IL-1 also increase endothelial cell synthesis of plasminogen activator inhibitor: the endothelial surface loses its anticoagulant nature and becomes prothrombotic. Experimental studies in primates have demonstrated that septic shock induces endothelial cell tissue factor expression confined to endothelial cells of the splenic vasculature, emphasising the complexity and heterogeneity of these interactions *in vivo*.

Regulation of vascular tone by endothelial cells

Endothelial cells themselves can modulate vascular tone by the release of vasoactive substances, including the arachidonic acid metabolite prostacyclin and endothelium-derived relaxant factor, of which the principal component is nitric oxide. Both of these are produced in response to inflammatory mediators such as thrombin and histamine and cause local vasodilatation.

Circulating myocardial depressant factors

Although capillary leakage secondary to endothelial cell damage and abnormalities of vascular tone leading to peripheral vasodilatation and maldistribution of blood flow are important causes of hypovolaemia and hypotension in patients with septic shock, there is also evidence for a circulating myocardial depressant factor. In patients with hyperdynamic shock, who have decreased systemic vascular resistance and normal or increased cardiac output, haemodynamic monitoring has shown that myocardial function is abnormal; typically, the ejection fraction is reduced and there is biventricular dilatation that develops 24–48 hours after the onset of sepsis and is reversible on recovery. This is not secondary to reduced coronary blood flow, which has been shown to be normal or increased in this situation. Serum from patients with septic shock reduces the extent and velocity of myocyte shortening in rat neonatal cardiac myocytes *in vitro*. The degree of this effect correlates with the clinical status of the patient. This circulating myocardial depressant factor has not been identified. It may be TNF itself, although other candidates such as leukotrienes have been suggested.

Abnormalities in peripheral oxygen uptake

Many patients with septic shock have a decrease in the arteriovenous oxygen difference, suggesting decreased peripheral oxygen use. This may reflect tissue hypoperfusion as a result of vascular endothelial damage and vascular occlusion caused by inflammation and thrombosis and inappropriate vasomotor activity. Alternatively, it may represent abnormal cellular metabolism secondary to the action of inflammatory mediators themselves. In normal individuals, tissue oxygen extraction is independent of oxygen delivery, but in a proportion of severely unwell patients with sepsis, tissue oxygen extraction increases with measures that increase oxygen delivery, such as infusion of prostacyclin, which has potent vasodilator activity. The existence of this 'oxygen debt' suggests that continued tissue hypoxia caused by hypoperfusion is an important contributor to resistant hypotension and multiorgan system failure.

Resistant hypotension

Many patients with septic shock die despite receiving adequate doses of appropriate antibiotics, and it is likely that the continued development of the sepsis syndrome does not require persistent release of endotoxin. Endothelial cell and organ damage may be sufficiently severe to cause further local cytokine release. Damaged tissues may not only allow further ingress of bacteria but will also be impaired in their ability to clear organisms and inflammatory mediators from the circulation. Tissue damage may be irreversible, and the sepsis cascade may become self-perpetuating, irrespective of the nature of the original stimulus.

New therapies for septic shock

Most of the pathogenetic mechanisms described above have been delineated in animal models or tissue culture. It is easy to imagine how the changes in endothelial cell structure and function described could lead to the clinical observations of increased capillary permeability and maldistribution of blood flow. However, definite evidence of the relative importance of any of these mechanisms in the clinical context is scanty. One method to obtain such evidence would be to try new highly targeted treatment strategies aimed at disabling just one link in the putative chain of events leading to shock, such as antibodies against TNF or endotoxin. Animal studies with polyclonal and monoclonal antibodies (mAb) against LPS and TNF have shown very significant protection against the effects of injected LPS or experimentally induced sepsis, but these have not yet been translated into clinical benefits.

A mAb against endotoxin was used in a large multicentre placebo-controlled study of patients with suspected Gram-negative sepsis. There was no statistically significant survival benefit between the treatment and placebo groups as a whole. *Posthoc* analysis did show a significant benefit in patients who were subsequently shown to have Gram-negative bacteraemia and who were not in shock at entry to the study, but it would not have been possible to identify this subset of patients at the time that the mAb was administered. A broadly similar result was obtained using a human mAb to lipid A (HA-1A). There was no significant survival benefit between treatment and placebo groups, but there was increased survival in patients subsequently found to have Gram-negative bacteraemia or endotoxaemia.

Initial enthusiasm for the use of these mAbs waned when it became apparent that the reported benefits of therapy were only statistically significant in subsets of patients and not in all those suspected to have Gram-negative sepsis. In view of their cost, it is likely that these agents will not enter routine clinical use until firmer guidelines for their use can be established, such as rapid and reliable diagnostic tests to detect endotoxaemia.

Summary

Microorganisms from many different phyla may cause human infection, but in all cases the manifestations of disease result from the interaction of microbial and host factors. Although infectious diseases are less significant as causes of mortality in the developed world than they used to be, on a global scale they still represent a major problem. Similarly, as environments and medical practices change, different infections become more prevalent. Recent advances in molecular biology and immunology have revolutionised our understanding of microbial pathogenicity and host immunity, and also of the critical interface between the two. At the same time, new diagnostic methods based on molecular and immunological technology have become available.

Therapeutic advances, such as the development of new antibiotics, now occur in the context of better understanding of the microbial processes with which they interfere, and a number of new therapeutic modalities, such as monoclonal antibodies against bacterial endotoxin or host inflammatory mediators, have become available. Many questions remain to be answered before the true usefulness of these agents can be assessed. Despite advances in the understanding of the pathogenesis of conditions such as septic shock, careful clinical trials remain the essential testing ground for treatments that show promise in the laboratory.

FURTHER READING

General
Christie, A.B. (1987). *Infectious Diseases,* 4th edn. Edinburgh: Churchill Livingstone.
Gorbach, S.L., Bartlett, J. & Blacklow, N.R. (1992). *Infectious Diseases.* Philadelphia: W.B. Saunders.
Lewin, B. (1994). *Genes V.* Oxford: Oxford University Press.
Mandell, G.L., Bennett, J.E. & Dolin, R. (1994). *Principles and Practice of Infectious Diseases,* 4th edn, Edinburgh: Churchill Livingstone.

Specific topics
Feinberg, M.B. (1996). Changing the natural history of HIV disease. *Lancet,* 348, 239–246.
Jardetzky, T.S., Brown, J.H., Gorga, J.C. *et al.* (1994). Three dimensional structure of a human class II histocompatability molecule complexed with a superantigen. *Nature,* 368, 711–718.
Kaufmann, S.H.E. (1993). Immunity to intracellular bacteria. In *Fundamental Immunology,* ed. W.E. Paul, pp. 1251–1286. New York: Raven Press.
Kollef, M.H. & Schuster, D.P. (1995). The acute respiratory distress syndrome. *New England Journal of Medicine,* 332, 27–37.
Lipton, S.A. & Gendelman, H.E. (1995). Dementia associated with the acquired immunodeficiency syndrome. *New England Journal of Medicine,* 332, 935–940.
Lynn, W.A. & Cohen, J. (1995). Adjunctive therapy for septic shock: a review of experimental approaches. *Clinical Infectious Diseases,* 20, 143–158.

Pantoleo, G., Graziosi, C. & Fauci, A.S. (1993). The immunopathogenesis of human immunodeficiency virus infection. *New England Journal of Medicine,* 328, 327–335.

Parrillo, J.E. (1993). Pathogenetic mechanisms of septic shock. *New England Journal of Medicine,* 328, 1471–1477.

Perelson, A.S., Neumann, A.V., Markowitz, M. *et al.* (1996). HIV-1 dynamics *in vivo*: virion clearance rate, infected cell life-span and viral generation time. *Science,* 271, 1582–1586.

Relman, D.A. (1993). The identification of uncultured microbial pathogens. *Journal of Infectious Diseases,* 168, 1–8.

Rosen, F.S., Cooper, M.D. and Wedgwood, R.J.P. (1995). The primary immunodeficiencies. *New England Journal of Medicine,* 333, 431–440.

Schwartz, R.S. (1993). Autoimmunity and autoimmune disease. In *Fundamental Immunology,* ed, W.E. Paul, pp. 1033–1097. New York: Raven Press.

Sissons, J.G. P. (1993). Superantigens and infectious disease. *Lancet,* 341, 1627–1629.

Wain-Hobson, S. (1995). Virological mayhem. *Nature,* 373, 102.

7

Metabolic disorders: diabetes

S. ROBINSON and D. G. JOHNSTON

- Diabetes mellitus is characterised by hyperglycaemia; patients develop specific microvascular and non-specific macrovascular complications.

- Insulin-dependent diabetes is an autoimmune disorder with abnormalities of both humoral and cellular immunity. It typically affects younger people. There is an inherited predisposition and overt disease is triggered by an environmental influence such as a viral infection. Pancreatic beta cells are destroyed over a prolonged period, resulting in severe insulin deficiency which requires treatment by insulin injections.

- Diabetic ketoacidosis is a life-threatening condition where insulin deficiency and excess of stress hormones result in hyperglycaemia and hyperketonaemia with acidosis. Patients are dehydrated and have a severe deficit of body potassium. The mainstays of treatment are intravenous insulin, saline and potassium, with careful clinical and biochemical monitoring.

- Despite being typically a disorder of middle life, non-insulin-dependent diabetes has a substantial inherited component to its pathogenesis.The development of disease in some subjects depends on environmental factors such as obesity, lack of exercise and smallness at birth. It is characterised by insulin resistance as well as insulin deficiency.

- Both kinds of diabetes are associated with complications. Microvascular complications include retinopathy, nephropathy and neuropathy. Atherosclerosis affecting the coronary, cerebral and peripheral vasculature occurs more commonly in the diabetic than in the non-diabetic – the so-called macrovascular complications. Mechanisms proposed for the production of diabetic complications include free radical damage, non-enzymatic glycosylation, lipoprotein disturbances and disorders of sorbitol and myoinositol metabolism. In insulin-dependent patients, microvascular complications are prevented by good blood glucose control.

Intermediary metabolism in the normal state

Glucose metabolism

In normal subjects, after an overnight fast, glucose is produced from hepatic glycogen (25%) and gluconeogenesis (75%). Hepatic glycogen stores are 70–80 g but they become depleted over 24 hours of fasting, such that gluconeogenesis assumes greater importance. Glucose production after an overnight fast, when extrapolated to 24 hours, is approximately 160 g per day. With prolonged starvation, glucose production decreases to 40 g per day, as many tissues adapt to other fuels, such as fatty acids and ketone bodies. The kidney in addition to the liver is capable of gluconeogenesis, and its relative contribution increases with prolonged starvation. The principal gluconeogenic precursors for the liver are amino acids, predominantly alanine and glutamine derived from muscle protein, and glycerol, derived from triglyceride hydrolysis in adipose tissue. Lactate (and pyruvate) are gluconeogenic substrates, but much of the lactate is derived originally from circulating glucose. This glucose was released from the liver, underwent glycolysis in muscle and was released again into the circulation before hepatic uptake (the Cori cycle). Glycogenolysis in muscle is an additional source of lactate, which may also be taken up by the liver after its release into the circulation.

Gluconeogenesis is controlled partly by substrate availability. As circulating glycerol concentrations increase with fasting, gluconeogenesis from glycerol also rises. Concentrations of alanine and lactate fall with fasting but the contribution to gluconeogenesis from alanine increases with prolonged starvation. Although lactate concentrations also decrease, the proportion of lactate converted to glucose rises. Factors other than substrate supply must, therefore, be important.

Both glycogenolysis and gluconeogenesis are under hormonal control. Glucagon at physiological concentrations stimulates gluconeogenesis from lactate and alanine, acting through cyclic AMP. Insulin antagonises this action. The catecholamines increase gluconeogenesis and, again, the stimulatory effect is inhibited by insulin. The regulatory sites for gluconeogenesis are those sites where substrate cycles exist in the glycolytic/gluconeogenic pathway (Fig. 7.1). Substrate cycles occur in metabolism where the forward and backward reactions are catalysed by different enzymes. The first cycle is at the phosphoenolpyruvate/pyruvate/oxaloacetate site. Pyruvate kinase (producing pyruvate from phosphoenolpyruvate) is inactivated by glucagon. Phosphoenolpyruvate synthesis is increased by glucagon. The net result of glucagon action is increased flux towards glucose. The next regulatory site is at the fructose 6-phosphate/fructose 1, 6-bisphosphate cycle. The enzyme phosphofructokinase (catalysing the formation of fructose 1, 6-bisphosphate from fructose 6-phosphate) is inhibited by glucagon. The third regulatory site in gluconeogenesis is at the glucose/glucose 6-phosphate cycle. The hepatic enzymes here are glucokinase and glucose-6-phosphatase.

Cortisol has delayed effects to increase blood glucose. It increases the synthesis of the enzymes phosphoenolpyruvate carboxykinase and glucose-6-phosphatase. Cortisol increases the supply of lactate and alanine to the liver from peripheral muscle. Growth hormone at physiological concentrations increases hepatic glucose output. Both cortisol and growth hormone also decrease glucose uptake by peripheral tissues. Glycogenolysis is increased by cyclic AMP. Glucagon and the catecholamines both increase hepatic glycogen degradation by this mechanism and the actions of both are antagonised by insulin. Glycogenolysis is also regulated at the substrate level. Glucose and glucose 6-phosphate inhibit glycogenolysis; this substrate inhibition may be important in the autoregulation of hepatic glucose production. The term *autoregulation*

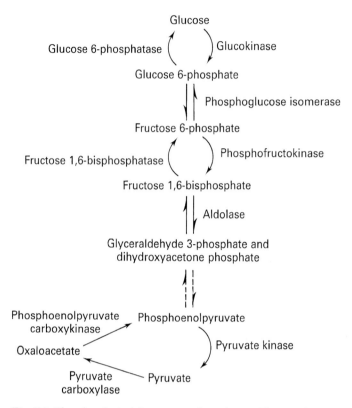

Fig. 7.1. The glycolytic/gluconeogenic pathway. The regulatory sites for hormone action are those sites where substrate cycles exist. The inhibition by glucagon of phosphofructokinase is complex. This action of glucagon is mediated through its ability to decrease the formation of fructose 2,6-bisphosphate. Fructose 2,6-bisphospate stimulates phosphofructokinase and the inhibitory effect of glucagon is mediated via inhibition of the enzyme phosphofructokinase 2, which catalyses the synthesis of fructose 2,6-bisphosphate.

refers to the ability of the liver to vary glucose production depending on the portal venous glucose level. Autoregulation does not occur if the liver has not been previously exposed to insulin.

The low levels of circulating insulin and the relatively high circulating glucagon concentrations after an overnight fast favour glycogenolysis and increased gluconeogenesis.

The blood glucose concentration after an overnight fast is usually maintained between 3 and 5 mmol/litre. Even after consuming a meal containing large amounts of carbohydrate, it rarely rises to >8.5 mmol/litre in normal subjects. In this fed state, hepatic glucose production by both gluconeogenesis and glycogenolysis is inhibited by the insulin released during and after eating. The inhibition of glucagon release by the ingested carbohydrate enhances the action of insulin. The suppression of glycogenolysis is greater than that of gluconeogenesis. The continued gluconeogenesis permits hepatic glycogen synthesis to occur during and after eating. Glucose uptake by the liver

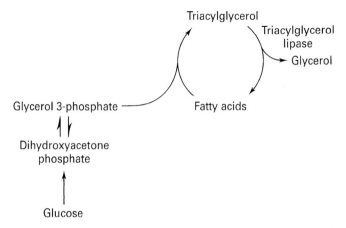

Fig. 7.2. The triacylglycerol/fatty acid cycle in adipose tissue. The glycerol released following triacylglycerol hydrolysis cannot be metabolised further in adipose tissue. The glycerol 3-phosphate necessary for triacylglycerol synthesis derives from glucose.

is enhanced, such that 20–25% of ingested glucose is converted to hepatic glycogen, mostly through the gluconeogenic pathway following glycolysis.

Ketone body metabolism

Fatty acids and ketone bodies provide alternative substrates to glucose. After an overnight fast when circulating insulin levels are low, they are metabolised by tissues such as muscle, thereby sparing glucose for metabolism by tissues or organs, such as brain, that have an obligatory requirement for glucose. Fatty acids are released from adipose tissue following triglyceride (triacylglycerol) hydrolysis (lipolysis). In adipose tissue, they may be resynthesised to triglyceride or they may be released into the circulation for metabolism elsewhere (Fig. 7.2). The glycerol released with lipolysis cannot be further utilised in adipose tissue (human adipose tissue lacks the enzyme necessary for the further metabolism of glycerol, glycerol kinase) and it too is released into the circulation. Glycerol is subsequently converted to glucose in the liver. Hormonal influences on lipolysis are exerted through triacylglycerol lipase (hormone-sensitive lipase). Triacylglycerol lipase exists in an active phosphorylated form and an inactive non-phosphorylated form. The degree of phosphorylation depends on the opposing activities of a protein kinase and a phosphatase. The protein kinase, as with many other kinases, is activated by cyclic AMP. Fatty acid esterification is also regulated, with the regulatory mediators usually having opposite effects on the lipolytic and esterification pathways. Insulin is the major inhibitory influence on fatty acid mobilisation. It does this both by an increase in esterification and by a decrease in lipolysis. The antilipolytic action is mediated in part through the effect of insulin to decrease intracellular cyclic AMP. Factors that stimulate fatty acid mobilisation include the catecholamines, adrenaline and noradrenaline, acting through β-adrenergic receptors via cyclic AMP. Stimulation of the sympathetic nervous system has similar actions. Other hormones with stimulatory effects on fatty acid release from adipose tissue include growth hormone and glucocorticoids. Glucagon is a potent lipolytic agent in certain species, but in normal humans, the lipolytic effect is small at physiological glucagon concentrations. After an overnight fast, the dominant influence leading to increased fatty acid mobilisation is the low circulating insulin concentration.

Circulating fatty acids are the major substrates for ketone body formation in the liver. Hepatic uptake of fatty acids is concentration dependent. The factors controlling fatty acid mobilisation, therefore, have a major influence on the rate of ketogenesis. Control mechanisms exist also within the liver. In the hepatocyte, fatty acids are activated to fatty acyl coenzyme A and may then be converted to triglyceride in the cytosol. The triglyceride synthesised may be stored in the hepatocyte or released into the circulation as very low density lipoprotein (VLDL). Alternatively, fatty acyl coenzyme A may be metabolised intramitochondrially by β-oxidation to acetyl coenzyme A. The metabolic fates of acetyl coenzyme A are either terminal oxidation to carbon dioxide and water in the Krebs' cycle, or conversion to acetoacetate, one of the ketone bodies. 3-Hydroxybutyrate, the other important ketone body quantitatively, is formed by the reduction of acetoacetate under the influence of the enzyme 3-hydroxybutyrate dehydrogenase.

In order to enter the Krebs' cycle, acetyl coenzyme A condenses with oxaloacetate to form citrate. In theory, ketogenesis could be regulated through variations in Krebs' cycle activity or in oxaloacetate availability. For example, alanine reduces ketosis probably through increasing oxaloacetate concentrations in the liver and through stimulation of gluconeogenesis (which requires energy as ATP produced through increased Krebs' cycle activity). Under most circumstances, however, variation in Krebs' cycle activity is not a major regulatory mechanism in ketogenesis.

Most evidence suggests that the principal regulatory site in ketone body synthesis is at the earlier stage of fatty acid transfer across the mitochondrial membrane (Fig. 7.3). This transfer is mediated by the enzyme carnitine palmitoyltransferase I (CPT I), which is situated on the outside of the inner mitrochondrial membrane. CPT I is inhibited allosterically by the metabolite malonyl coenzyme A. When hepatic synthesis of fatty acids is high, malonyl coenzyme A concentrations are also high and CPT I is inhibited. Conversely, when malonyl coenzyme A levels are low, CPT I activity is high, fatty acid transfer across the mitochondrial membrane is high and fatty acid oxidation is stimulated. The activity of CPT I is regulated by insulin and glucagon. Hepatic fatty acid synthesis and malonyl coenzyme A production are increased by insulin and decreased by glucagon. The inhibition of CPT I by insulin through increased malonyl coenzyme A, and the reverse by glucagon, are the major intrahepatic mechanisms by which insulin and glucagon control ketogenesis. During starvation in normal subjects, for example, insulin secretion is low and glucagon secretion relatively high. This results in low intrahepatic malonyl coenzyme A concentrations, increased CPT I activity, increased fatty acid transfer into mitochondria and increased ketone body synthesis.

The ketone bodies are oxidised by many tissues and organs including skeletal muscle and heart muscle, kidney, intestine and brain. 3-Hydroxybutyrate is oxidised initially to acetoacetate. The acetoacetate is converted to acetoacetyl coenzyme A under the influ-

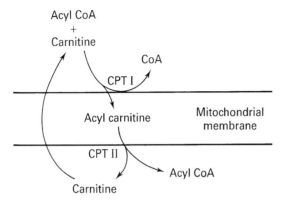

Fig. 7.3. Entry of fatty acyl CoA into mitochondria, the regulatory step in ketogenesis in the liver. CPT, carnitine palmitoyltransferase.

ence of 3-oxoacid coenzyme A transferase. Acetoacetyl coenzyme A is then converted to acetyl coenzyme A for terminal oxidation.

In the fed state, the ketone bodies are minor metabolic fuels. They assume increasing importance with fasting, such that at the end of six weeks' starvation, the brain, for example, receives 50% of its energy from ketone body metabolism.

Insulin action in normal subjects

In view of the importance of insulin in diabetes (the examplar disease), we shall consider its major metabolic actions and the mechanisms by which these actions are produced.

Mechanisms of insulin action

Insulin plays a pivotal role in the regulation of metabolism, exerting effects on carbohydrate, lipid and protein metabolism. The initial event in insulin action is its binding to the insulin receptor. This receptor is composed of two α- and two β-subunits (Fig. 7.4). Insulin binds to the α-subunits. The β-subunits lie across the cell membrane and contain tyrosine-specific protein kinase activity in the intracellular portion. Insulin binding to the α-subunits causes a conformational change in the β-subunits that activates the tyrosine kinase. Once insulin has bound, the insulin receptor complex is internalised by endocytosis and insulin dissociates from the receptor. Some receptors are degraded, whereas others pass to the Golgi apparatus; the internalised receptors join newly synthesised ones and they recycle to the cell membrane. When insulin levels are persistently raised (as happens, for example, when glucose tolerance is impaired, see below), receptor turnover and internalisation are increased, resulting in a reduced receptor number (downregulation). As more receptors become occupied, the affinity for insulin of adjacent unoccupied receptors decreases (negative co-operativity). Downregulation and negative co-operativity both serve to decrease insulin effects during sustained hyperinsulinaemia.

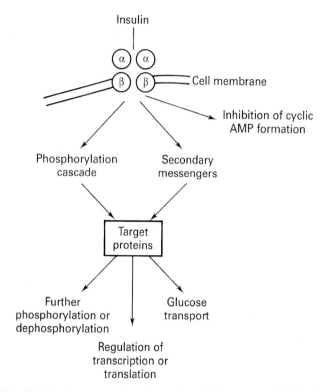

Fig. 7.4. Mechanisms of insulin action. Following insulin binding to its receptor, actions occur through the phosphorylation cascade, via secondary messengers or through inhibition of cyclic AMP production.

The multiple effects of insulin are exerted through a variety of mechanisms. Cyclic AMP is the secondary messenger mediating the actions of β-adrenergic agonists and glucagon. Insulin antagonises these actions by inhibiting the rise in cyclic AMP.

Other actions of insulin occur by different mechanisms. Insulin binding to its receptor with activation of the tyrosine kinase activity is associated with phosphorylation of the β-subunit itself (autophosphorylation). Mutations of the relevant portions of the β-subunit result in insulin resistance. Many post-receptor binding events in insulin action involve the phosphorylation and dephosphorylation of other proteins. These phosphorylation/dephosphorylation processes are mediated by serine or threonine kinases, with insulin receptor autophosphorylation as the initiating event. Still other consequences of insulin action do not rely on receptor autophosphorylation. Secondary messengers, such as membrane-linked phosphoinositols and phospholipase C, are important in mediating these actions. Finally, insulin exerts certain effects through influences on gene transcription or mRNA translation. An example here is the inhibition of synthesis of the gluconeogenic enzyme phosphoenolpyruvate carboxykinase (PEPCK), through inhibition of PEPCK gene transcription.

Skeletal muscle is the main site of insulin-stimulated glucose disposal. Glucose transport across the muscle cell membrane can be stimulated 30-fold by insulin. This stimulation is achieved by a glucose transporter glycoprotein, which transfers glucose intracellularly down a concentration gradient. The most important transporter of glucose in muscle is the glucose transporter GLUT4. GLUT4 proteins are situated intracellularly in microsomes. Following insulin binding, intracellular transporters are 'recruited' to the cell membrane. In addition to increasing the number of GLUT4 proteins in the muscle cell membrane, insulin increases the intrinsic activity of the GLUT4 transporter through mechanisms that are uncertain. Physical exercise and training increase insulin sensitivity through increased activity and synthesis of GLUT4 transporters. There may also be an increase in insulin receptor binding and an increase in other post-receptor binding events.

Insulin actions on intermediary metabolism

Insulin decreases blood glucose through both a decrease in hepatic glucose output and and increase in glucose uptake by peripheral tissues, particularly muscle. It also increases hepatic glucose uptake after food. The actions on hepatic glucose metabolism are more sensitive and occur, therefore, at lower insulin concentrations than the actions enhancing glucose uptake by muscle. The actions on the liver result from inhibition of glycogenolysis and gluconeogenesis, and stimulation of glycogen synthesis. The net effect on carbohydrate metabolism is anabolic, increasing the storage of carbohydrates.

Insulin has similar anabolic effects on lipid metabolism. It decreases lipolysis in adipose tissue. Triglyceride synthesis in adipose tissue is enhanced through an increase in glucose uptake (providing the glycerol 3-phosphate necessary); there may also be an increase in endogenous synthesis of fatty acids. Fatty acid delivery to adipose tissue from the bloodstream is increased by insulin, primarily from hydrolysis of circulating VLDL or chylomicrons, catalysed by lipoprotein lipase, the activity of which is increased by insulin. In the liver, insulin has actions that enhance fatty acid synthesis and the production of VLDL. It is evident that following ingestion of a meal containing carbohydrate and lipid, the insulin released favours the storage of excess fuel as triglyceride in adipose tissue.

Before insulin became available for the treatment of severely insulin-deficient diabetic patients, failure of growth and muscle wasting were frequently observed. These observations illustrate the important anabolic effects of insulin on protein metabolism. Insulin decreases muscle protein catabolism and decreases the release of amino acids from muscle. It also increases muscle amino acid uptake and protein synthesis. The net effect in the circulation is a decrease in amino acid concentrations, particularly the branched-chain amino acids. There are similar anabolic effects on liver protein metabolism, with increased amino acid uptake and protein synthesis, and decreased proteolysis.

DIABETES MELLITUS

A brief history of diabetes

The earliest description of clinical diabetes comes from the Ebers papyrus of Egypt in 1500 BC. It was well known to the Hindu physicians Charuka and Susruta, in 100 BC.

They referred to 'honey urine' and had insight into the pathogenesis of the disorder, in that they described it as having 'passed from one generation to another in the seed', and they also outlined the importance of 'injudicious diet'. The name diabetes, meaning to flow through a syphon, was applied in the second century A D by the Greek Aretaeus. In the seventeenth century, Thomas Willis described the sweetness of urine and in 1784 Matthew Dobson isolated sugar as the cause of the sweetness. Also in the seventeenth century, the pancreatic origin of diabetes was suggested by Brunner, and in 1869 Minkowski and von Mering showed that pancreatectomy in dogs reproduced the clinical features. In the same year, Langerhans described the islets that now carry his name. In 1894, Laguesse postulated that these islets were the source of internal secretions. In the nineteenth century also, Claude Bernard demonstrated a role for the autonomic nervous system in glucose homeostasis when he discovered that glycosuria resulted from puncture of the cerebral medulla in animals. In the years following, the concept of a hormone was developed, as a substance released by one organ to have actions at distant sites. In 1921 to 1922, Banting and Best isolated insulin and treated the first diabetic animal (a dog). The first patient to receive insulin was a 14-year-old boy Leonard Thompson, who was dying of diabetes. In a very short space of time, insulin was manufactured and distributed worldwide. In 1945, the first oral preparation for diabetic treatment was discovered by the pharmaceutical industry (by accident – they were working on sulphonamides and noted that one of their preparations lowered the blood glucose levels in animals).

Definition of diabetes

Diabetes is characterised by hyperglycaemia. It is associated with specific microvascular complications and non-specific macrovascular disease.

Diagnostic criteria

The diagnostic criteria for diabetes were laid down by the World Health Organization in 1985. They are as outlined in Table 7.1.

Classification of diabetes

Insulin-dependent diabetes (IDDM, or type 1) and non-insulin-dependent diabetes (NIDDM, or type 2) account for the great majority of patients. Diabetes, mostly NIDDM, affects 2.5% of the population of the UK.

   IDDM affects mostly young people, is associated with the development of ketoacidosis and is characterised by absolute deficiency of insulin (it is often unmeasurable in the circulation when patients first present with ketoacidosis) (Table 7.2). NIDDM usually occurs after the age of 40 years, is associated with insulin resistance and only relative insulin deficiency, and the patients do not usually become ketoacidotic. Patients with NIDDM are frequently obese. Other types of diabetes include *malnutrition-related diabetes*

Table 7.1. *World Health Organization (1985) diagnostic criteria for diabetes (75 g glucose in an oral glucose tolerance test)*

	Whole blood glucose[a]		Plasma glucose[a]	
	Venous	Capillary	Venous	Capillary
Diabetes				
Fasting	≥6.7	≥6.7	≥7.8	≥7.8
2 hour	≥10.0	≥11.1	≥11.1	≥12.2
Impaired glucose tolerance				
Fasting	<6.7	<6.7	<7.8	<7.8
2 hour	6.7–9.9	7.8–11.0	7.8–11.0	8.9–12.1

Note:
Diabetes may be diagnosed without a glucose tolerance test if classical symptoms are present and a random plasma venous glucose is ≥11.1 mmol/litre (or equivalent), or if the patient is asymptomatic and random glucose levels exceed this limit on two or more occasions.
[a] Glucose as mmol/litre.

Table 7.2. *Comparison of IDDM, NIDDM and impaired glucose tolerance (IGT)*

	IDDM	NIDDM	IGT
Prevalence (%)	0.2	2.0	Unknown
Age of onset	Usually young	Usually >40 years	Usually >40 years
Geography	Predominantly Caucasian	Prevalence greatest in non-Caucasians (e.g. Indian)	As NIDDM
Genetic factors	HLA linkage, other genetic sites	High concordance in monozygotic twins, genetic defect rarely known	Uncertain
Metabolic defect	Insulinopenia	Insulin resistance and insulin secretion deficit	Insulin resistance
Precipitants	Possibly viral infection	Obesity, exercise lack	Obesity, exercise lack
Complications	Not at diagnosis	May be at diagnosis	As NIDDM
Microvascular	Yes	Yes	No
Macrovascular	Yes	Yes	Yes
Ketoacidosis	Prone	Rarely occurs	Does not occur
HONK-C	Does not occur	Occasionally occurs	Does not occur

Note:
HONK-C, hyperosmolar non-ketotic coma.
Some NIDDM patients are insulin treated for symptoms or in an attempt to reduce the frequency of diabetic complications.

Table 7.3. *Genetic syndromes and diabetes*

Syndrome	Inheritance[a]	Chromosome[b]	Diabetes type
Ataxia telangiectasia	AR	11q	NIDDM
Friedreich's ataxia	AR	9q	IDDM
Huntington's disease	AD	4p	NIDDM
Myotonic dystrophy	AD	19q	IGT[c]
DIDMOAD[d] syndrome	AR	–	IDDM
Leprechaunism	AR	19p	IR[e]
Mendenhall syndrome	AR	–	IR[e]
Werner syndrome	AR	–	NIDDM
Haemochromatosis	AR	6p	NIDDM
APG 1[f]	AR	–	IDDM
Prader–Willi syndrome	AD	15q del	NIDDM
Growth hormone deficiency	AD	20p	NIDDM
Laron dwarfism	AR	5p	NIDDM
Klinefelter's syndrome	XLR	47XXY	IGT[c] NIDDM
Turner's syndrome	XLR	45XO	IGT[c] NIDDM

Notes:
[a] Inheritance: AR, autosomal recessive; AD, autosomal dominant; XLR, X-linked recessive.
[b] Chromosome nomenclature: p, long arm of chromosome; q, short arm of chromosome; del, deletion. The proinsulin gene is on chromosome 11 (p 15.1–15.5); the insulin receptor gene is on chromosome 19 (p 13.2–13.3).
[c] Impaired glucose tolerance.
[d] DIDMOAD, or Wolfram syndrome, comprises diabetes insipidus, diabetes mellitus, optic atrophy and nerve deafness.
[e] Extreme insulin resistance.
[f] Autoimmune polyglandular syndrome.

(which may be associated with pancreatic fibrosis and calcification), *secondary diabetes* (secondary to disease of the pancreas such as chronic pancreatitis, disease of other endocrine glands, e.g. acromegaly or Cushing's syndrome, or drug treatment, e.g. with thiazide diuretics), *insulin receptor abnormalities* (such as mutations of the insulin receptor or conditions with circulating antibodies to the receptor), *gestational diabetes* (diabetes that comes on during pregnancy and which often disappears once pregnancy is complete) and certain *rare genetic syndromes*.

Diabetes may be associated with many genetic disorders (Table 7.3). The contribution of these to the prevalence of diabetes overall is low, but the scientific importance of these disorders lies in the insight they provide into the great variety of mechanisms by which a raised blood glucose may develop. The range of mechanisms is apparent in the range of biochemical pathology; from insulinopenia in Wolfram or DIDMOAD syndrome to extreme insulin resistance in Mendenhall syndrome; from autoimmune IDDM in one of the forms of autoimmune polyglandular syndrome (Schmidt's syndrome) to a more mysterious pancreatic beta cell destruction in Friedreich's ataxia.

Table 7.3 also lists, where known, the chromosomal loci for the genes responsible for the disorders; clearly the genes responsible are not on the same chromosome. This sug-

Table 7.4. *Age-adjusted incidence of IDDM (0–14 years)*

	Incidence[a]
Finland	34.9
Sardinia (Italy)	32.4
Sweden	25.7
Aberdeen (UK)	24.0
Oxford (UK)	15.8
Pavia (Italy)	8.2
Wielkopolska (Poland)	5.0
Israel	5.9
Karachi (Pakistan)	0.7
Oran (Algeria)	5.7
Mauritius	1.3
Jefferson County (USA)	10.2
Montevideo (Uruguay)	8.2
Paraguay	0.8

Note:
[a] Incidence figures are per 100 000 of population.

gests that different genetic mechanisms underlie the diabetes in each disorder. A further inference is that diabetes can arise as a result of dysfunction in one or more genes at several possible chromosomal sites.

Patients with a strong family history of diabetes are referred to as having *potential diabetes*. *Impaired glucose tolerance* (IGT) is the term applied to those patients with glucose values during a glucose tolerance test intermediate between normal and diabetic (Table 7.1). These patients suffer the macrovascular disease but are not affected by the specific microvascular complications of diabetes. They are also at increased risk of impaired glucose tolerance worsening to diabetes (2–5% per year in Caucasian populations).

Insulin-dependent diabetes mellitus

Introduction

The incidence of IDDM in different countries is shown in Table 7.4. Examination of this table illustrates that IDDM is predominantly a Caucasian disorder most frequently encountered in Northern Europe, particularly Scandinavia. It is less common in the Southern hemisphere. There is some evidence to suggest that IDDM has increased in frequency since the 1950s. It has increased fourfold, for example, in Finland. The incidence of IDDM is highest between 10 and 14 years. It affects males and females equally, with a slightly earlier age of onset in girls (by 1–2 years). There is a seasonal variation, with a higher incidence in winter than in summer. This seasonal variation is observed in both northern and southern hemispheres, i.e. winter presentations are more likely in both. This has been taken as evidence for a possible viral aetiology or precipitant. Other environmental agents that have been implicated as aetiological factors from epidemi-ological studies include the nitrosamine compounds that are present in high concentra-tion in certain smoked food preparations. The incidence of IDDM is increased in Icelandic boys under the age of 15 years who had been born nine months after a period of traditionally high intake of smoked mutton. Smoked mutton is rich in nitrosamine compounds. These compounds are toxic to the pancreatic beta cell in experimental animals, such as mice and Chinese hamsters. There is no evidence for these compounds having an aetiological influence in other countries.

Other nutritional factors have been proposed. Foreign proteins in the diet have been implicated in susceptible individuals. The incidence of IDDM is inversely related to the prevalence of breast-feeding (in some but not in all the studies that have examined the relationship). Cows' milk has, therefore, been proposed as an aetiological factor. Antibodies to bovine serum albumin are observed more commonly in recently diag-nosed diabetics than in controls. These antibodies cross-react with a pancreatic beta cell peptide called p 69. This peptide is not normally presented on the beta cell surface, but if it were in certain circumstances (e.g. during intercurrent infection) the antibodies to bovine serum albumin would be capable of inducing cell damage. Although this is an attractive idea, a relationship between cows' milk usage in infancy and the subsequent risk of developing diabetes has not been demonstrated consistently.

A clinical syndrome that includes diabetic ketoacidosis has been observed in subjects who ingested (deliberately or by accident) the rat poison vacor. This rodenticide has been developed for the control of warfarin-resistant rat populations. The diabetes that follows is severely insulin deficient and extensive necrosis of pancreatic beta cells has been observed in those patients who died. Vacor has structural similarities to the experimental beta cell toxins streptozotocin and alloxan, and it may induce selective beta cell damage in the same way. Streptozotocin, for example, induces severe insulin deficiency when given in high dosage to adult rats. It causes beta cell necrosis in association with depletion of nicotinamide adenine dinucleotide (NAD) and ATP content. Administration of nicoti-namide prevents the development of beta cell destruction, suggesting that NAD defi-ciency is of primary importance. Nicotinamide has a similar protective effect with vacor.

The *pathology* of the pancreas in IDDM is characterised by atrophy of the islets. Our knowledge of the pathology comes from studying those patients unfortunate enough to die of their diabetes. When patients first present with IDDM, many of the islets are small with abundant fibrous stroma. The architecture of these islets is disrupted. In normal islets, the beta cells are located at the centre and the other pancreatic islet cell types are around the periphery. In IDDM islets, the cell content is predominantly alpha and delta types, and a high proportion of the alpha cells is scattered throughout the exocrine tissue, outside the islets. There are very few beta cells in these atrophic islets. Some of the islets remaining are hypertrophic and the beta cells are degranulated. The total number of beta cells in the pancreas is markedly decreased (to less than 10% of normal). The content of the other cells in pancreatic islets (the alpha cells and delta cells) is normal. Lymphocytic infiltration (so-called insulitis) is observed in the majority of patients, particularly in the younger ones. Some attempt is seen at regeneration with endocrine differentiation of ductal epithelium.

The role of viruses in the pathogenesis of IDDM

Some but not all studies have demonstrated higher titres of antibodies to *Coxsackie B viruses* in patients presenting with IDDM than are observed in the normal population. The high prevalence of asymptomatic infection with these picornaviruses in the otherwise normal population makes interpretation of the antibody data difficult. Coxsackie B4 virus is capable of infecting animal islets in culture. When injected into susceptible strains of mice, diabetes ensues. In several patients who died during their initial episode of diabetic ketoacidosis, the Coxsackie B4 virus has been isolated. Injection of a pancreatic extract from these patients into susceptible mice has been associated with beta cell necrosis and the development of diabetes. Although the case is strong for these isolated patients, the role of Coxsackie B4 in the pathogenesis of IDDM remains uncertain for the majority. For example, it would not be surprising if the non-specific stress of the infection led to the presentation with diabetes in subjects already on the way to developing the disorder.

The *mumps* virus is associated with the development of diabetes in occasional patients, often after a long delay (3–4 years). Occasional children with mumps parotitis develop circulating islet cell antibodies. Pancreatitis without diabetes is more common. Although the mumps virus can infect islets in culture, those epidemiological studies that have investigated patients with newly diagnosed IDDM have failed to show any relationship with recent mumps infection. An association with *rubella* infection is tenuous. Of patients with congenital rubella, 20% or more develop diabetes 5–20 years later. Patients who are *HLA-DR3* are more likely to develop diabetes after congenital rubella infection, while the *HLD-DR4* allele appears to be protective (p. 111). As with mumps, however, there is no evidence for rubella infection as a causative agent in the great majority of patients with IDDM.

Other viruses that have been implicated, but for which there is also no strong evidence for a role as major aetiological agents, include cytomegalovirus and the viruses causing measles, poliomyelitis, influenza, tick-borne encephalitis and hepatitis. Certain viral infections are associated with diabetes in animals, including foot and mouth disease in cattle, Coxsackie B4, encephalomyocarditis and reovirus infections in mice, and Venezuelan encephalitis in hamsters. A role for retroviruses has been proposed in the development of diabetes in the non-obese diabetic (NOD) mouse, with retrovirus particles observed frequently in the pancreatic beta cells of diabetic animals.

Viruses may, in theory, induce beta cell damage through a variety of mechanisms:

- they may damage by direct infection causing beta cell death
- incorporation of viral proteins into the beta cell membrane may induce an immune reaction targeted against the beta cell
- an autoimmune reaction may be induced through the viral genome, altering the expression of pancreatic beta cell genes and resulting in an altered beta cell-specific antigen
- a portion of viral antigen may exhibit molecular mimicry with a beta cell antigen, such that an immune response against the virus cross-reacts with normal beta cell components

- virus-induced cell damage may lead to exposure to the immune system of host intracellular antigens that are normally hidden
- the virus infection may alter the function directly of the cells of the immune system; for example with cytomegalovirus infection, which seems to be immunosuppressive in certain circumstances

Despite the possibilities, the evidence that viruses are important in the pathogenesis of human IDDM is incomplete and inconclusive. The reverse may even be the case, i.e. viruses may be protective. In animal models of IDDM (the NOD mouse and the BB rat), infection with the virus (the lymphocytic choriomeningitis (LCM) virus) protects the animals against diabetes. Our understanding of this is incomplete but it is thought that the LCM virus infection in some way modifies the host's immune response.

The genetic predisposition to IDDM

Evidence for a genetic basis for IDDM derives from population studies, studies in identical twins and family studies.

From *population* studies, there is evidence of an association between IDDM and certain HLA types. In particular, the class II molecules HLA-DR3 and HLA-DR4 are associated with IDDM, and people who are *DR3 DR4* positive have the greatest relative risk. *HLA-DR2* is protective for IDDM, irrespective of the other HLA status. Population studies have emphasised also the importance of non-genetic factors. For example, the incidence of IDDM in Asian children who migrated to Britain has increased from 3 per 100 000 per year in the years 1979 to 1981 to an incidence of 12 per 100 000 per year in 1988 to 1990.

Studies in *identical twins* have demonstrated a 30–50% concordance for diabetes. For non-identical twins, concordance rates have been similar to the rates observed for non-twin siblings. These data suggest strongly that there is a genetic predisposition to IDDM. The fact that the concordance rate is not 100% illustrates the importance of additional, non-genetic factors. Twin studies have also demonstrated that the genetic influence decreases as the age of the index twin at diagnosis increases. For example, in one study when the index twin was diagnosed under the age of 15 years, the risk of the other developing IDDM was 42%. The risk was only 13% if the index twin was >15 years at diagnosis.

Family studies have demonstrated an important influence of the *HLA-DR* region. If one family member had IDDM and the sibling was *HLA-DR* identical, the risk of developing diabetes in the sibling was increased 90-fold over that observed in the population at large. For *HLA-DR* non-identical siblings, there was no increased risk of diabetes developing. More recently, family studies have been utilised to define in more detail the genetic component. Before dealing with this, it is useful to examine data obtained from an animal model of inherited IDDM, the NOD mouse.

The *NOD mouse* develops diabetes at approximately 150 days of life (80% of females, 20% of males). The diabetes is insulin dependent and is preceded by insulitis, which is similar to that reported in human IDDM at presentation. Studies of the genetic basis of

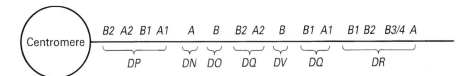

Fig. 7.5. Diagrammatic representation of the HLA class II region on the short arm of chromosome 6. The *DR*, *DQ* and *DP* genes are subdivided into *A* and *B* loci. The class II molecules consist of α- and β-chains, encoded by the respective *A* and *B* genes (see Fig. 4.2, p. 98).

IDDM in the NOD mouse have naturally focused on the MHC regions (see Chapter 3, p. 109). Class II MHC molecules (Fig. 7.5) play a similar role in the mouse to class II molecules in humans. These molecules are important in the presentation of antigen to T cells and they may be important in the development of autoimmune disorders (discussed below and p. 110). Early observations suggested that expression of a class II gene encoding a mouse protein, the IE protein, might be important in IDDM. The IE protein gene is not expressed in the NOD mouse and *IE* gene transfer to the NOD mouse prevented the development of insulitis. The class II IE molecule cannot, however, be the sole determinant of IDDM in mice, as other mouse strains do not express *IE* but do not develop IDDM.

Attention focused, therefore, on other MHC class II molecules. One of these, the IA protein, in common with other class II molecules, has a role in antigen presentation. It was observed that the amino acid that occurred at position 57 of the IA β-chain was of major importance. If this amino acid is aspartate, diabetes does not develop in the mouse. If the amino acid is other than aspartate (such as serine, valine or alanine), then diabetes is likely to occur. This observation in the NOD mouse led to study of the equivalent HLA region in humans.

The *HLA-DQβ* region is the equivalent in humans of the MHC *IA* region in the mouse. It has been observed that the presence of aspartate at position 57 in the *HLA-DQβ* gene product is protective, and that non-aspartate amino acids are associated with increased risk. Between populations, the prevalence of non-aspartate at position 57 in *HLA-DQβ* is directly proportional to the prevalence of IDDM. For example, the Norwegian population with a high prevalence of IDDM has a high frequency of non-aspartate at position 57, whereas in China there is a low IDDM prevalence and a low frequency. This genetic factor is, however, not universally associated with risk of IDDM. It is not associated with IDDM, for example, in the Japanese population. Furthermore within populations, the relationship may not be consistent. Other HLA regions have been studied. The presence of arginine in position 52 of the HLA-DQα chain is associated with disease susceptibility, but again the role of this genetic factor is limited.

Alternative approaches are, therefore, being adopted to clarify the importance of existing information in large numbers of subjects and to discover other genetic influences. The development of technologies for genome-wide searching is permitting the investigation of much of the human genome, without the requirement for prior knowledge or suspicion of a candidate gene. The recognition of microsatellite marker loci, the

construction of high-resolution human genetic linkage maps and the application of flu-orescence-based automated DNA fragment-sizing technology (p. 44) are facilitating the genome-wide exclusion mapping. For example, in a large study using sib-pairs of patients with IDDM, 20 different chromosome regions showing evidence of linkage with IDDM have been identified. Two of these had previously been suspected. The first, termed IDDM 1, is in the HLA region, as would be anticipated from previous work. The second, IDDM 2, is in the region of the insulin gene itself (some previous work had also suggested this). The remaining 18 were previously unrecognised. The specific genes involved have not yet been located, although this is likely in the next few years. IDDM, therefore, represents a disorder with multiple genetic factors contributing to its develop-ment. In individual patients, the relative importance of specific genetic influences may vary.

The autoimmune process leading to islet beta cell destruction

There is evidence for abnormalities of both humoral and cell-mediated immunity in IDDM. Mechanisms of autoimmunity are discussed in Chapter 4. *Humoral abnormalities* are present, as evidenced by circulating antibodies against islet cell cytoplasmic anti-gens. These are observed in 70–80% of patients with IDDM at presentation (and in only 0.1–3.0% of the normal population). These islet cell antibodies disappear and are usually not detectable 12 months after diagnosis. Their importance in the pathogenesis of IDDM is uncertain. They are observed in experimental diabetes caused by toxic agents (e.g. vacor poisoning, streptozotocin) and in that caused by viruses. They are likely, therefore, to be secondary phenomena, although they play some role in cell damage. When injected into experimental animals, the antibodies do not cause diabetes. Although they are of IgG class and do, therefore, cross the placenta, there is no evidence for transplacental transmission of diabetes from mother to fetus.

The potential antigens mediating the response have been intensively studied. A 64kDa antigen was identified in beta cells. Antibodies to this antigen appear early in the development of diabetes in animal models such as the NOD mouse. The antigen has now been further characterised. The full 64kDa antigen is associated with two antibody specificities. One is directed against a 50kDa fragment of the full antigen and this reacts also against the enzyme glutamic acid decarboxylase (GAD). GAD is now known to be present in two forms with different molecular size, GAD 65 and GAD 67. Antibodies in the NOD mouse arise initially against the carboxy-terminal region of GAD 65 and then spread to other antigens. The role of these GAD antibodies in the islet dysfunction of human IDDM is currently being investigated. The other antibody specificity in the 64kDa antigen is towards 37kDa and 40kDa fragments that do not contain GAD activ-ity. An antibody directed against insulin itself has also been detected in IDDM.

IDDM also is associated with disordered *cell-mediated immunity*. Transfer of spleen cells from the NOD mouse can induce diabetes in otherwise normal mice. Lymphocytes isolated from the serum of patients with IDDM have caused insulitis in susceptible mice (nude mice, which are T-cell deficient). These and other data suggest an important role for cell-mediated immune pancreatic damage.

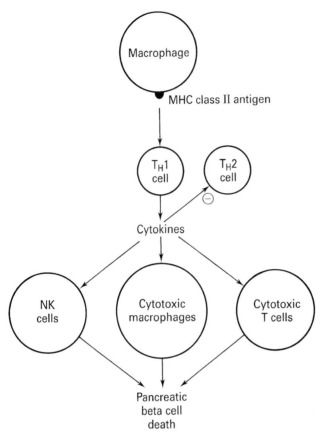

Fig. 7.6. Cellular immune process leading to death of pancreatic beta cells. An antigen-presenting macrophage is shown activating a CD4$^+$ T$_H$ cell (T$_H$1). The activated T$_H$1 cell releases cytokines that inhibit T$_H$2 cells and stimulate cytotoxic T cells, macrophages and NK cells to induce pancreatic beta cell destruction.

In order for any cell-mediated immune response to occur, antigen must be taken up by macrophages, dendritic cells or B cells. These are referred to collectively as APCs. These APCs present to T cells the processed antigen together with MHC class I or MHC class II molecules (see p. 97). The binding of the T cell to the antigen–MHC complex results in its activation. Once activated, T cells secrete cytokines and are referred to as T$_H$ cells. The majority of T$_H$ cells are CD4$^+$. T$_H$1 cells are involved classically in cell-mediated immunity; their cytokines activate endothelial cells to recruit circulating white blood cells into the tissues and they activate macrophages to destroy antigen-bearing cells. They also activate cytotoxic T cells to kill cells bearing the appropriate antigen-MHC complex. In addition, NK cells, which kill independently of MHC status, are activated. T$_H$2 cells, by contrast, stimulate B cells to make antibodies. T$_H$1 and T$_H$2 cells are mutually inhibitory. This inhibition is mediated in part through their different cytokine profiles.

The disorder of cell-mediated immunity in IDDM is considered to be an inappropriate activation of autoreactive T$_H$1 cells (Fig. 7.6). T$_H$1 cell cytokines are capable of causing

(*a*) Non-aspartate 57   (*b*) Aspartate 57

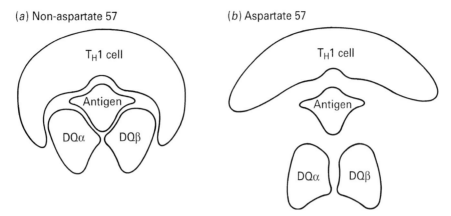

Fig. 7.7. Proposed mechanism by which HLA status may influence the efficiency of antigen presentation to T_H1 cells in the development of IDDM. (*a*) When the HLA-DQβ molecule has an amino acid other than aspartate in position 57, the presentation of antigen to T_H1 cell is efficient. (*b*) When aspartate is present in position 57, the T_H1 cell–antigen–class II complex fits together less efficiently.

beta cell toxicity *in vitro*. Antibodies to these cytokines can prevent the development of diabetes in mouse models, such as the NOD mouse. By contrast, T_H2 cell cytokine products may be protective. The concept has arisen of excessive T_H1 cell activation and decreased T_H2 cell cytokine production, together with activation of macrophages, cytotoxic T cells and NK cells. In addition to cytokine production, the activated T_H1 cells induce beta cell damage via reactive oxygen metabolites (see p. 141), via nitric oxide (NO•), through cytotoxic T cells and through NK cells. Changes in the vascular endothelium may also be important by permitting the entry of lymphocytes and macrophages to the islets.

Synthesis of autoimmune, genetic and environmental factors in the pathogenesis of IDDM

Although the mechanisms of production of IDDM remain uncertain, it is possible to speculate on a sequence of events leading to the production of diabetes. An environmental insult, such as a viral infection or chemical toxin, may lead to immunological change in susceptible individuals. The genetic susceptibility may lie in the HLA-associated efficiency of antigen presentation (Fig. 7.7). This leads to increased presentation of a normal or modified antigen (or alternatively decreased antigen presentation with impaired development of immune tolerance at some critical period). The beginning of the disease process may antedate the appearance of clinical diabetes by many years. Activated T cells have been detected in subjects at risk of IDDM up to four years before they became diabetic. Islet cell and GAD antibodies have been demonstrated in one patient 12 years before the development of diabetes. Typically, islet cell antibodies have been present for five years. Progression to diabetes is more likely if the islet cell anti-

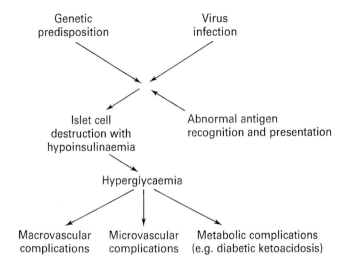

Symptoms
    Polyuria and polydipsia resulting from osmotic diuresis
    Weight loss owing to fat and protein catabolism with dehydration
    It is unusual to have symptoms owing to complications of IDDM at presentation

Signs
    There may be signs of ketoacidosis such as rapid, shallow respiration and dehydration
    There may be signs of weight loss or cutaneous candidiasis
    Glycosuria and ketones on urine dipstick testing

Complications
    Microvascular such as retinopathy, nephropathy and neuropathy
    Macrovascular such as ischaemic heart disease, cerebrovascular disease and
    peripheral vascular disease
    Metabolic complications such as ketoacidosis

Fig. 7.8. IDDM from molecular defect to complications. A virus infection may interact with a certain genetic predisposition to lead to islet cell destruction and hypoinsulinaemia. This in turn leads to hyperglycaemia and eventually the complications of diabetes.

bodies are present in high titre and if antibodies to insulin are also present. The environmental trigger must, therefore, precede the diabetes by several years. The worst outcome is cell-mediated immune damage, with T_H1 dominance over T_H2 cells and the associated cytokine changes in the pancreas. The complexity of the problem is illustrated, however, by the fact that not everyone at risk progresses to diabetes. Co-twins with activated T cells and with positive islet cell antibodies may never develop the disorder and we do not understand what dictates the outcome.

A summary of the possible pathogenetic mechanisms and clinical features of IDDM is shown in Fig. 7.8.

Diabetic ketoacidosis

Intermediary metabolism in diabetic ketoacidosis

Diabetic ketoacidosis is the first presentation of IDDM in 20–30% of patients. In one large European study of 3250 patients with established IDDM, diabetic ketoacidosis had occurred in the previous 12 months in 8.6%. The mortality from ketoacidosis is 2–5% in developed countries, 6–24% in the developing world. In the developed world, the mortality is higher in older subjects (20% in those >65 years of age) and lower in the younger age groups (2%). Ketoacidosis is precipitated by a number of factors, including infections, non-compliance with medical advice and myocardial infarction, but in 25% of patients the precipitant is unknown.

When patients without known IDDM first present in diabetic ketoacidosis, there is frequently no measurable circulating insulin. Circulating insulin is usually measurable in ketoacidotic subjects already taking insulin therapy. Mean values of 10 mU/litre have been reported, which are similar to overnight fasting levels in non-diabetic subjects. This suggests that factors other than simple insulin deficiency are important.

Insulin withdrawal in established IDDM provokes diabetic ketoacidosis, although it may take several days to develop depending on residual endogenous insulin secretion (Figs. 7.9 and 7.10). During insulin withdrawal, hepatic glucose production increases twofold over several hours. Peripheral glucose utilisation shows little change. In consequence, circulating glucose concentrations increase. The increased glucose production reflects the absence of insulin, together with a relative excess of glucagon. In established ketoacidosis, circulating glucagon concentrations are in fact increased four- to fivefold. In consequence, both glycogenolysis and gluconeogenesis are stimulated. The delivery of the gluconeogenic precursors alanine and glutamine from muscle and glycerol from adipose tissue is also increased. Insulin withdrawal is also associated with increased lipolysis and increased ketone body production by the liver. In ketoacidosis, ketone body levels are increased to a variable extent, typically to 10 mmol/litre or more. Loss of the inhibitory effect of insulin on ketogenesis, together with the glucagon excess, are the dominant factors stimulating ketogenesis. Insulin has a minor role in stimulating ketone body metabolism by peripheral tissues, which is also lost during insulin deficiency.

In patients with established diabetic ketoacidosis, stress hormone concentrations other than those of glucagon are also elevated. These include cortisol, growth hormone and the catecholamines. Sympathetic nervous system activity is increased. The catecholamines, adrenaline and noradrenaline, are increased six- to tenfold in the circulation and they stimulate both glycogenolysis and gluconeogenesis. Adrenaline also decreases glucose uptake by muscle. In addition to their effects on glucose metabolism, the catecholamines have potent lipolytic actions exerted through β-adrenergic receptors. Noradrenaline also has a direct ketogenic action at the liver, although this is probably of minor importance. Activation of the sympathetic nervous system is likely to be a major component of the stress response, although it is difficult to quantify. Cortisol secretion rates are elevated two- to fourfold in diabetic ketoacidosis. Cortisol excess causes hyperglycaemia and ketosis in insulin deficient subjects. It increases hepatic gluconeogenesis through increased synthesis of several gluconeogenic enzymes, most notably phospho-

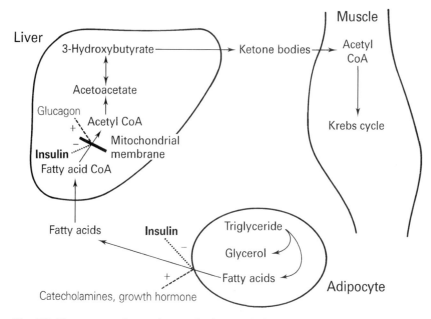

Fig. 7.9. Hormone action on ketone body metabolism. The interaction of liver, muscle and adipocyte metabolism is demonstrated. Insulin deficiency causes increased lipolysis and ketogenesis. This is aggravated by increased catecholamines, growth hormone and glucagon: − indicates inhibitory hormone actions, + indicates stimulatory actions.

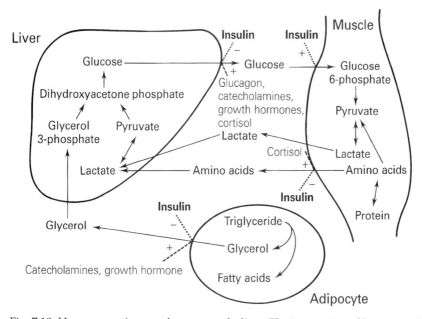

Fig. 7.10. Hormone action on glucose metabolism. The interaction of liver, muscle and adipocyte metabolism is demonstrated. Insulin deficiency causes increased lipolysis and glycerol delivery to the liver. Proteolysis (protein breakdown) is increased in muscle because of insulin deficiency. Hypoinsulinaemia also leads to increased hepatic glucose output and decreased muscle uptake of glucose. This is aggravated by increased catecholamines, cortisol, growth hormone and glucagon: − indicates inhibitory hormone actions, + indicates stimulatory actions.

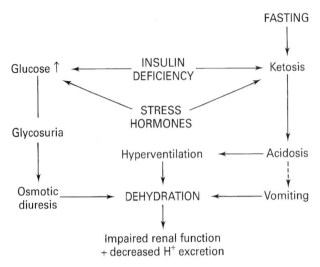

Fig. 7.11. Schematic representation of the events leading to the progression of diabetic ketoacidosis.

enolpyruvate carboxykinase. It also increases the delivery of gluconeogenic precursors from peripheral tissues to the liver, particularly amino acids such as alanine. Peripheral glucose uptake is inhibited by cortisol in a variety of tissues. In insulin deficiency, cortisol excess increases fatty acid mobilisation from adipose tissue. Growth hormone is elevated in ketoacidosis, although the elevation is not universal. Growth hormone has actions that increase hepatic glucose production and it decreases glucose uptake by muscle and adipose tissue. In insulin deficiency, growth hormone also increases lipolysis and induces a secondary increase in ketogenesis.

Therefore, the combination of insulin deficiency and stress hormone excess combine to induce hyperglycaemia and hyperketonaemia. If the precipitating illness is associated with a major stress hormone response (e.g. myocardial infarction), the onset of diabetic ketoacidosis may be very rapid.

Clinical features of diabetic ketoacidosis

The major clinical features of diabetic ketoacidosis are as follows (Fig. 7.11):

- polyuria and polydipsia
- weight loss
- vomiting, abdominal discomfort and other gastrointestinal symptoms
- clouding of consciousness and coma
- dehydration
- tachycardia and hypotension
- rapid shallow breathing (Kussmaul breathing).

The pathogenesis of these symptoms may be deduced using knowledge of the biochemical abnormalities. Insulin deficiency combined with stress hormone excess are associated with increased hepatic glucose production and decreased utilisation of glucose by tissues such as muscle. In consequence, blood glucose concentrations rise above the renal threshold. An osmotic diuresis develops, drawing fluid and electrolytes from the body. This accounts for much of the acute weight loss. At presentation with ketoacidosis, a quarter of the total body water may have been lost. The fluid lost has a tonicity of half normal (0.45%) saline. Half the fluid is lost from the intracellular and half from the extracellular compartments. Despite the excess of water lost over sodium, the plasma sodium level is often normal or low. This reflects the osmotic effect of glucose to draw water from the intracellular to the extracellular compartment. Water loss is increased by hyperventilation. Insulin has effects that retain sodium, while glucagon has natriuretic actions; the hormonal state of insulin deficiency and glucagon excess exaggerates the water and sodium loss. Stimulation of the renin–aldosterone system also leads to sodium conservation. As the intravascular volume decreases, renal perfusion declines and renal loss of glucose decreases, resulting in a further increase in blood glucose.

The weight loss that occurs as ketoacidosis develops reflects more than just this loss of fluid. There is loss also of muscle bulk and adipose tissue. The muscle loss reflects increased proteolysis as a consequence of insulin deficiency and cortisol excess. The loss of adipose tissue results from increased lipolysis caused by the insulin deficiency and stress hormone excess.

The major ketone bodies that are synthesised in excess are 3-hydroxybutyric acid and acetoacetic acid. Their accumulation produces a metabolic acidosis, which stimulates the respiratory centre (Kussmaul breathing). The coma in ketoacidosis does not seem to be attributable to the acidosis alone. Cerebral hypoxia may be a factor in some patients, with cerebral hypoperfusion secondary to intravascular volume depletion. The cause of the abdominal discomfort is also uncertain, although it may result from pancreatitis in some patients. Gastric stasis, possibly secondary to electrolyte disturbances, is common in ketoacidosis and may be the cause of vomiting.

Principles of treatment of ketoacidosis

A scheme for the immediate management of diabetic ketoacidosis is provided in the next section. Only certain aspects are described in more detail here.

The treatment of ketoacidosis requires the administration of insulin, fluid and electrolytes. Insulin therapy in the low doses conventionally used acts predominantly to inhibit hepatic glucose production. Higher doses would have a greater effect on peripheral glucose disposal. The movement of glucose into cells peripherally is also associated with the intracellular movement of potassium. This might compound the problem of hypokalaemia during therapy.

It is important to avoid hypoglycaemia in the later stages of therapy. Once the blood glucose concentration has declined to 12–14 mmol/litre, intravenous dextrose should be given as a 5% or 10% solution to maintain circulating glucose levels at this value.

Fluid is usually replaced as normal (0.9%) saline, despite the fact that there has been an excess of water lost over sodium as the ketoacidosis developed. Normal saline is required for two reasons. First, as blood glucose declines with insulin therapy and improved renal perfusion, plasma osmolality decreases. This causes water to move from the extracellular to the intracellular compartments. This movement of water intracellularly could lead to vascular collapse. The use of 0.9% saline prevents this happening. Second, the increase in intracellular water may cause cerebral oedema to occur during therapy. This rare but serious complication of treatment occurs in children and young adults and is associated with a rapid decline in plasma osmolality during treatment. The use of normal as opposed to half-normal saline may diminish the frequency of cerebral oedema, as may avoidance of a rapid decrease in blood glucose. The aim is for blood glucose concentrations to decline during treatment by 4–5 mmol/litre per hour.

Severe hypernatraemia during therapy should be avoided as it has undesirable effects on cerebral function. If the plasma sodium starts at >150–155 mmol/litre, or if it rises to this level during treatment, half-normal saline should generally be substituted.

Total body potassium is decreased in established ketoacidosis. A net loss of potassium occurs from cells as a consequence of insulin deficiency and impaired cellular glucose uptake (insulin normally stimulates potassium uptake). As acidosis develops, potassium is displaced from within cells by hydrogen ions. The extracellular potassium is subsequently lost in the urine, and the loss is exaggerated by the osmotic diuresis. The higher the blood glucose levels, the greater the potassium loss. Other causes of potassium deficiency include reduced intake, vomiting and sometimes diarrhoea. Secondary hyperaldosteronism may contribute as intravascular volume declines. Finally, insulin has actions to decrease renal potassium excretion and insulin deficiency may result in excessive renal potassium loss through this mechanism. Insulin therapy and improvement in the acidosis cause potassium ions to move intracellularly and potassium must be administered intravenously during therapy with the aim of keeping plasma potassium levels in the normal range.

As 3-hydroxybutyric acid and acetoacetic acid accumulate, the metabolic acidosis stimulates the respiratory centre and carbon dioxide is excreted in larger amounts. The carbon dioxide is formed following reaction of the hydrogen ions with bicarbonate, producing carbonic acid, which then dissociates to carbon dioxide and water. This respiratory compensation limits the fall in pH at the expense of bicarbonate. Considerable controversy exists as to the role of sodium bicarbonate administration in the therapy of ketoacidosis. With insulin treatment, excessive ketone body synthesis diminishes and the metabolism of 3-hydroxybutryic acid and acetoacetic acid results in the generation of one molecule of bicarbonate for each molecule of acid metabolised. Bicarbonate is repleted in this way. In favour of bicarbonate administration intravenously is the fact that profound acidosis has a negative inotropic effect on the heart. It may also predispose to cardiac arrhythmias, peripheral vasodilatation and respiratory depression. Against bicarbonate therapy is the potential to aggravate hypokalaemia through increased potassium movement into cells. It may also shift the oxyhaemoglobin dissociation curve to the left causing tissue anoxia, it may produce a paradoxical increase in acidosis in the central nervous system and it may induce cerebral hypoxia, through mechanisms that are uncertain. Most data suggest that sodium bicarbonate administration either has no effect, or may even delay the restoration of ketone body levels and pH to normal. It seems sensible, therefore, to reserve bicarbonate treatment for those patients with severe acidosis and cardiovascular collapse.

Scheme for the immediate management of diabetic ketoacidosis

Water and sodium

The water deficit is typically 100 ml/kg and the sodium deficit 8 mmol/kg. The fluid should be replaced as normal saline (0.9%, or 0.154 mol/litre). A typical regimen would be:

> 500 ml over 15 minutes
> 500 ml over 20 minutes×2
> 500 ml over 30 minutes×2
> 500 ml over 60 minutes×2
> 500 ml over 120 minutes (continue at this rate until fluid replete clinically).

In the elderly, central venous pressure should be assessed. When blood glucose is <12–14 mmol/litre, change to 5% glucose (it may be necessary to continue with sodium chloride concurrently).

Potassium

The potassium deficit is typically 4 mmol/kg. The potassium should be measured at outset and then 4 hourly (more frequently if abnormal). If potassium is >6 mmol/litre, no potassium is given but its level should be rechecked frequently. At potassium levels below 6 mmol/kg, the following regimens of potassium chloride treatment should be followed:

> 5–6 mmol/litre give 10 mmol/hour
> 4–5 mmol/litre give 20 mmol/hour
> 3–4 mmol/litre give 25 mmol/hour
> <3 mmol/litre give 30–40 mmol/hour.

An ECG monitor throughout therapy is a useful guide to plasma potassium. Hyperkalaemia causes peaked T waves and widening of the QRS complex. Hypokalaemia induces the appearance of a U wave and ST segment depression.

Insulin

Insulin is given as soluble (regular) insulin intravenously (e.g. Actrapid). The glucose levels are measured hourly, using a reagent strip (e.g. Glucostix) and the hourly rate of intravenous insulin infusion is altered accordingly. For the following glucose levels:

> <4.0 mmol/litre give   0.5 units/hour   (do not stop)
> 4.0–7.0 mmol/litre give   1.0 units/hour

7.1–10.0 mmol/litre give   2.0 units/hour
10.1–15.0 mmol/litre give   3.0 units/hour
15.1–20.0 mmol/litre give   4.0 units/hour
>20.0 mmol/litre give   6.0 units/hour

Bicarbonate

If the pH is less than 6.9, bicarbonate therapy should be considered (500 ml of 2.6% sodium bicarbonate (125 mmol) plus an additional 20 mmol of potassium, over 1 hour).

Other measures

Other measures that may be instituted are:

- nasogastric tube: ketoacidosis causes gastric dilatation and may lead to inhalation of gastric contents in patients with an impaired conscious level
- ECG monitor: electrolyte changes especially potassium can precipitate arrhythmias
- central venous pressure monitoring especially in elderly patients: to avoid causing cardiac failure
- antibiotics: after taking samples for culturing from all appropriate sites, give a broad-spectrum antibiotic
- catheterisation: the patient may be semi-conscious and fluid balance assessment is important
- heparin: especially in the elderly or in hyperosmolar coma when thrombosis is common, intravenous heparin should be considered. It is wise to give other patients heparin subcutaneously

Non-insulin-dependent diabetes mellitus

Introduction

NIDDM is much more *prevalent* than IDDM. It affects from 0 to 35% depending on the population (Table 7.5). Within the UK, the prevalence also varies, being much higher in ethnic minority groups, such as the Asian population (Indian subcontinent). It is a disorder of middle and late life (there is a rare subgroup of patients with diabetes that is non-insulin dependent but which presents often in the teenage years, termed maturity-onset diabetes of the young, or MODY (see p.233)). In the more common form of NIDDM, the age of presentation varies somewhat between ethnic groups, with an earlier presentation observed in the Asian compared with the Caucasian population.

The *pathology* of the pancreas in NIDDM is quite different from IDDM. The extensive beta cell destruction is not observed. Total beta cell mass is diminished but this is highly variable. On average, the beta cell mass is 60% of that observed in the non-diabetic pancreas. The lymphocytic infiltration of IDDM is also absent. Amyloid tissue, which is

Table 7.5. *The prevalence of NIDDM in different populations*

Country	Ethnic group	Age group (years)	Prevalence (%)
Japan	Japanese	20+	1.0
India	Rural	15+	1.2
	Urban		2.0
New Zealand	Caucasoid	20+	2.8
	Polynesian		7.5
Cook Islands	Polynesian (rural)	20+	2.4
	Polynesian (urban)		5.7
South Africa	African	20+	3.6
	Malay		6.6
	Indian		10.4
Fiji	Melanesian	20+	6.9
	Indian		14.8
Nauru	Micronesian	15+	34.4
USA	Pima Indian	15+	35.0

present in the non-diabetic pancreas with increasing age, is observed to a greater extent in NIDDM. A major component of this amyloid substance is the peptide amylin. Amylin is distributed within the islets in close proximity to the beta cells and appears to distort the beta cell membrane. The role (if any) of the amyloid tissue in the pathogenesis of NIDDM is uncertain at present.

Insulin resistance or reduced insulin secretion?

Both insulin resistance and insulin deficiency are observed in patients with NIDDM. The relative importance of each as a primary deficit is disputed.

Insulin deficiency

Insulin deficiency is observed in all patients with established NIDDM. Even when circulating insulin concentrations appear to be normal or even elevated above those observed in the non-diabetic state, the levels are lower than would be observed in a non-diabetic in whom the blood glucose was elevated to the diabetic values. In order to establish whether insulin deficiency or resistance is the primary defect in NIDDM, several groups have investigated subjects predisposed to NIDDM, but before the disorder appears. Such at-risk populations include first-degree relatives of patients with NIDDM, unaffected co-twins of diabetics, women with gestational diabetes in a previous pregnancy and young unaffected members of populations in which the prevalence of diabetes is particularly high. These studies have demonstrated that circulating insulin levels in response to glucose are frequently elevated early in the development of NIDDM. This hyperinsulinaemia is, however, by no means universal. It is observed, for example, in predisposed subjects with family origins in the Indian subcontinent but not in Japanese subjects at risk. As diabetes progresses and hyperglycaemia develops, insulin deficiency is universal.

Defective processing of proinsulin to insulin has been proposed as a possible primary defect. Proinsulin is converted to insulin within the beta cell granule (Fig. 7.12) under the influence of two enzymes, PC2 and PC3 (PC3 is also confusingly referred to as PC1). The intermediate split forms of proinsulin are observed in the circulation in small quantities in non-diabetic subjects (the 64, 65-split form is present in very low concentrations). Rare inherited defects of proinsulin processing have been described that result in hugely elevated proinsulin concentrations and diabetes in affected individuals. In the majority of subjects predisposed to NIDDM, concentrations of proinsulin, and of the 32, 33-split proinsulin, are present in moderately increased amounts. The primacy of processing defects in the bulk of patients with NIDDM is, however, disputed.

Insulin resistance

Insulin resistance, like insulin deficiency, is universal in established NIDDM. The term refers to the fact that there is a subnormal response to endogenous or exogenous insulin. This resistance to insulin action extends to many of insulin's actions on glucose metabolism. There is resistance to the stimulation of glucose uptake by muscle and liver, and resistance also to the action of insulin to suppress hepatic glucose production. The muscle defect is primarily in the non-oxidative pathway of glucose metabolism, i.e. in glycogen synthesis. The resistance extends to adipose tissue metabolism, with a reduced ability to suppress lipolysis. This results in an increase in circulating non-eserified fatty acid concentrations (NEFA), which reduces further the sensitivity to insulin (an increase in NEFA decreases insulin-stimulated muscle glucose uptake and metabolism (the Randle or glucose/fatty acid cycle) and increased NEFA delivery to the liver increases hepatic gluconeogenesis). The cause of the insulin resistance is unknown in the majority of subjects. In rare patients, there is a structural abnormality of the insulin receptor or of one of the proteins involved in insulin action intracellularly (e.g. insulin receptor substrate 1). For the remainder, it is likely that the insulin resistance reflects an abnormality or abnormalities early in the intracellular pathways of insulin action (a so-called post-receptor defect), in view of the universality of the metabolic defect. Occasional patients have circulating antibodies to the insulin receptor that diminish insulin action (e.g. some patients with acanthosis nigricans). For the great majority, however, the cause(s) remains unknown.

Irrespective of the cause, insulin resistance is associated with adverse effects on health. This applies even when glucose tolerance is only mildly impaired but not in the diabetic range. Notable amongst the adverse effects is the predisposition to vascular disease affecting large blood vessels, and the association with hypertension.

Insulin resistance is also associated with dyslipidaemia (raised triglyceride and decreased high-density lipoprotein cholesterol – the mechanism is described on p. 236). This dyslipidaemia is observed in insulin-resistant subjects even in the absence of dia-

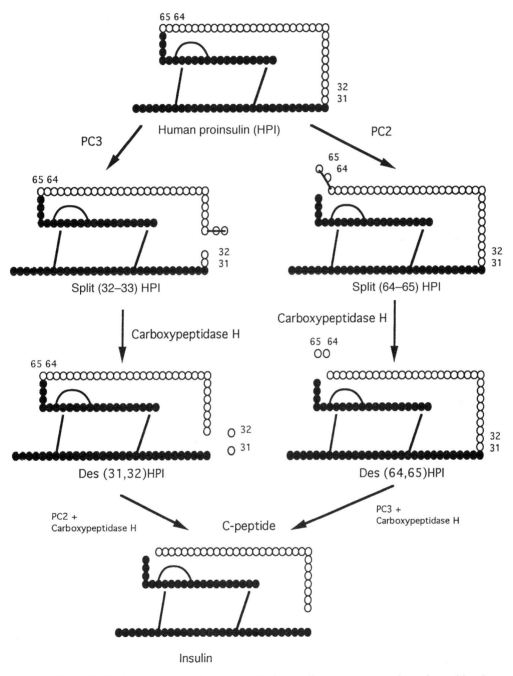

Fig. 7.12. Proinsulin within the pancreatic beta cell secretory granule is cleaved by the endopeptidases PC2 and PC3, producing 32, 33- and 65, 66-split proinsulins, respectively. This is followed by cleavage of amino acid residues by carboxypeptidase H, to form the desdiamino peptides. This series of reactions then occurs on the contralateral side to yield mature insulin and C-peptide.

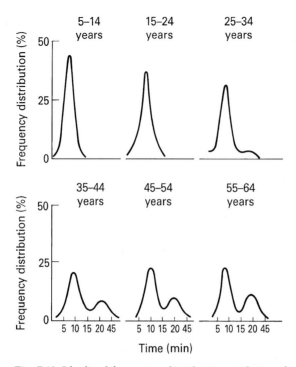

Fig. 7.13. Idealised frequency distribution with time for plasma glucose levels (mmol/litre) by age, 2 hours following an oral glucose load (100 g), in a population with a high prevalence of NIDDM (Pima Indians). Note that the plasma glucose scale is not arithmetic.

betes, although glucose tolerance is frequently impaired, by World Health Organization criteria. This combination of impaired glucose tolerance, insulin resistance, hypertension and dyslipidaemia is referred to as syndrome X (or Reaven's syndrome). Although a formal link between the lipid disturbance and the vascular disease in NIDDM and in syndrome X has not been established, a causal relationship seems likely.

Evidence for the genetic predisposition to NIDDM

Evidence for a genetic basis for NIDDM derives from population, from twin and from family studies.

Population studies

In those populations that have a high prevalence of NIDDM, fasting and 2 hour post-glucose circulating glucose concentrations demonstrate a bimodal distribution (Fig. 7.13). Such populations include the Pima Indians in North America and the Nauruan Islanders in Micronesia. In younger subjects, the blood glucose distribution is Gaussian, but in older subjects a second hyperglycaemic subgroup appears that becomes larger as the age of the population studied increases. In some populations with a high prevalence of NIDDM, the proportion of hyperglycaemic subjects increases to 30–50% once the age exceeds 50–60 years. These population data are compatible with a single dominant gene with expression increasing with age.

Twin studies

Evidence from twin studies suggests a strong genetic component. The concordance rate for NIDDM approached 100% in one large UK study. This twin study has been criticised in its design in view of the possibility of ascertainment bias, in that the twins were identified because one twin was known to be diabetic. Twin pairs where both were diabetic would be more likely to come to the attention of the investigators than discordant twin pairs. Although this criticism is valid, other studies in which ascertainment was solely on the basis of being twins (as opposed to one twin having diabetes) have confirmed the high concordance, although the rates have been somewhat lower.

Family studies

Family studies have investigated the frequency of NIDDM in first-degree relatives of patients with the disorder. From several different centres, the frequency of diabetes is approximately 30–40% in siblings. The lifetime risk for offspring is similar. Where both parents have diabetes, the risk of diabetes in the offspring is greater still. These data are also compatible with a genetic component, although the shared environment within a family may of course contribute.

Interpretation of studies

Other problems exist in the interpretation of these studies. First, it is not known if the disorder is one disease or several. Considerable phenotypic differences exist, for example in the degree of insulin resistance between ethnic groups. As already mentioned, the Asian population in the UK is markedly insulin resistant while the Japanese population in the USA appears more insulin deficient. The genetic basis may differ, therefore, in different populations or subpopulations.

Second, NIDDM is a disorder that does not develop until middle age or later. It is impossible to be certain of the disease status of the children. In other words, if glucose tolerance is normal at the time of study, NIDDM may still develop in later life. Attribution of disease status for linkage studies in families is, therefore, difficult. Third, NIDDM is associated with excess mortality, most notably from vascular disease. It may not be possible, therefore, to study siblings and parents. Fourth, the disorder is underdiagnosed and the disease status of unavailable relatives must, therefore, be uncertain. Fifth, family members with impaired glucose tolerance are difficult to ascribe. A proportion will progress to frank NIDDM but some will not. Finally, environmental factors certainly influence the expression of the disease, as discussed below.

The genetic defect underlying the NIDDM has been defined in only a small proportion of patients (less than 5%). In MODY, abnormalities of the gene for glucokinase have been observed in approximately 40–50% of families. The genetic changes in glucokinase have resulted in the predicted alterations in enzyme activity. Glucokinase in the pancreatic beta cell is, or forms part of, the 'glucose sensor' involved in the release of insulin. Glucokinase abnormalities are associated with insulin deficiency in the affected families. The majority of patients with NIDDM, however, do not have any known abnormality of the gene for glucokinase. Other genetic abnormalities have been described but they do not explain diabetes in the great majority of patients. Genes that have been studied include those coding for the insulin receptor, the insulin receptor substrate 1, the glucose transporters, particularly GLUT 4, which transports glucose across the muscle cell membrane, hexokinases, enzymes involved in glycogen synthesis and enzymes involved in insulin synthesis and proinsulin processing. Maternal transmission of NIDDM predominates over paternal transmission and this has led to a search for possible abnormalities in mitochondrial DNA (mitochondrial DNA is transmitted only from the mother). Mutations in mitochondrial DNA have been reported in certain patients with diabetes and deafness but not in the majority of adult NIDDM. Most genetic studies in NIDDM have, however, been limited to relatively small numbers of heterogenous subjects and no genetic abnormality has been definitively excluded.

The role of the environment in NIDDM

Environmental factors exert a major influence on NIDDM. The importance of *obesity* is illustrated by studies in the Nauru population. Diabetes was virtually unknown at the turn of the century. The Nauruans acquired great wealth from sales of fertiliser originating as guano (the excreta of cormorants, which nested there in great abundance). As a consequence of this increase in wealth, food intake increased and the prevalence of obesity rose to very high levels. Diabetes prevalence increased over this period such that 50% of the population over the age of 50 years is affected. Other population data have reinforced the importance of environmental factors, notably obesity. Asian Indians who have migrated to the cities have a higher prevalence of obesity compared with the rural population. The prevalence of diabetes has increased correspondingly. Within any population, cross-sectional studies have not always shown a strong association between obesity and NIDDM. In longitudinal studies, however, obesity is a strong predictor of the development of NIDDM. It should be remembered in all obesity studies that while environmental influences are strong, obesity itself may have a genetic component to its pathogenesis.

Exercise protects against NIDDM. This has been demonstrated in most but not all populations. As with obesity, the importance of exercise is supported by longitudinal studies. Women who have been athletes in youth are less likely to develop diabetes later in life than the general female population. The mechanism by which this protection occurs is uncertain, although exercise is known to increase insulin sensitivity.

The importance of the *intrauterine environment* has received attention in recent years. This emphasis has arisen from the observation in certain populations (e.g. rural Hertfordshire, UK) that NIDDM and impaired glucose tolerance were more frequent in subjects with a low birth weight and a low body weight at 12 months of age. The risk is additive with obesity, i.e. those with low birth weight and obesity in later life are most likely of all to develop NIDDM. The mechanism of this intrauterine influence is uncertain, although nutrient deficiency (particularly of amino acids) has been observed in animals to cause glucose intolerance, decreased pancreatic beta cell reserve and insulin resistance in later life. Further studies are required on this potential mechanism.

Possible advantage of the diabetic predisposition

When any condition is very common, the possibility exists that the predisposition to develop it may have held an evolutionary advantage. This applies even though the condition itself is disadvantageous, providing it does not develop until after the reproductive years. NIDDM affects up to 50% of the older members of certain populations and, as we have observed, it is a disorder of affluence and food abundance. The possibility has been raised that the predisposition to NIDDM is energy conserving, related in some way to insulin resistance. The terms 'thrifty genotype' and 'thrifty phenotype' have been applied, depending on whether it was thought to have a genetic or environmental (intrauterine) origin. Evidence recently has suggested that there may indeed be some advantage. In subjects predisposed to NIDDM, resting energy expenditure is normal but the energy lost in the digestion and assimilation of food (post-prandial thermogenesis) is reduced. This may have been advantageous during periods of food scarcity in our evolutionary past. The biochemical mechanisms underlying the decrease in post-prandial thermogenesis are unknown.

Pathogenesis of the metabolic disturbances observed in NIDDM

Much confusion has existed regarding the relative roles of insulin deficiency and insulin resistance. Patients with impaired glucose tolerance frequently demonstrate resistance to insulin-stimulated muscle glucose uptake of a similar degree to that observed in overt NIDDM. Fasting insulin levels are frequently raised at this stage. The plasma insulin response to an oral glucose load is higher than normal in impaired glucose tolerance, similar to normal in many patients with NIDDM and mild hyperglycaemia, and lower than normal in NIDDM when blood glucose concentrations are markedly elevated. NIDDM may be considered, therefore, to develop when insulin-resistant subjects are not capable of secreting sufficient insulin to compensate for their defect of insulin action.

Insulin resistance in adipose tissue may have a primary role in the metabolic disturbances of NIDDM. Adipose tissue lipolysis is normally very sensitive to insulin. Resistance to insulin's anti-lipolytic action results in elevated NEFA concentrations. The greater the increase in NEFA, the greater the degree of hyperglycaemia. The increase in plasma NEFA decreases muscle glucose uptake further, through operation of the glucose/fatty acid cycle (see p. 205). Increased hepatic NEFA oxidation leads to increased gluconeogenesis and, therefore, a rise in hepatic glucose output. The resultant increase in fasting glucose concentrations compounds the problem in two ways. First, it leads to a further decrease in insulin secretory capacity. This deleterious effect, or 'glucotoxicity', on insulin secretion is well recognised although poorly understood. Second, 'glucotoxicity' exists also for insulin action, in that a rise in fasting glucose levels inhibits subsequent insulin-mediated glucose uptake. The mechanisms of this toxic effect of glucose on insulin sensitivity are unknown, but the changes are reversible, with insulin sensitivity improving if blood glucose levels can be induced to fall.

The increase in fasting NEFA concentrations has additional effects on lipoprotein metabolism. VLDL triglyceride secretion by the liver is increased in NIDDM. This is driven by the high NEFA substrate supply (in the presence of adequate insulin for this process). In consequence, circulating triglyceride concentrations are elevated. The elevation is exaggerated by deficient activity of lipoprotein lipase. This enzyme is present on the endothelial cell surface where it hydrolyses triglyceride-rich lipoproteins such as VLDL and chylomicrons (see Table 8.4, p. 260). Levels of high-density lipoprotein cholesterol (HDL cholesterol) vary inversely with those of triglyceride-rich lipoproteins, particularly VLDL. This combination of high triglyceride and low HDL cholesterol, together with insulin resistance, has particular importance in the development of macrovascular disease in diabetes.

A summary of the pathogenetic mechanisms and clinical features of NIDDM is shown in Fig. 7.14.

Complications of diabetes

Patients with diabetes are prone to develop both micro- and macrovascular complications. The microvascular complications are specific to diabetes, whereas macrovascular disease occurs also in the non-diabetic but is more common in diabetic subjects (both IDDM and NIDDM).

Microvascular complications: early histological and functional changes

The earliest microvascular histological lesion is thickening of the basement membrane. This is observed in the capillaries in many tissues. Basement membrane contains several proteins, but the bulk of the basement membrane material is type IV collagen. It functions to provide stability to the cell and it acts as a permeability barrier. The permeability function results in part from the negative electrical charge of the membrane. Much of this charge is attributable to heparan sulphate, a large proteoglycan. Additional sulphate groups also contribute to the negative charge. In diabetes, the basement membrane thickening reflects an increase in type IV collagen content. Heparan sulphate content is decreased, as is the overall extent of membrane sulphation. In the kidney, in addition to basement membrane thickening there is an increase in mesangial material, which is similar in composition to the basement membrane.

Diabetic *microangiopathy* is associated with abnormal microvascular (arteriolar and capillary) function in many tissues. Early in diabetes, microvascular pressure and flow are increased. The resultant increase in capillary pressure is thought to damage the endothelium, leading to thickening and sclerosis of the capillary wall. Eventually, the normal autoregulatory mechanisms are lost and vasodilation is limited. This leads to the

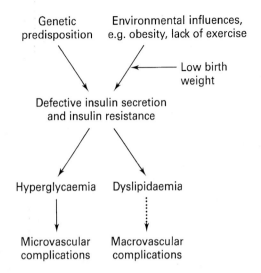

Symptoms
    Polyuria and polydipsia caused by osmotic diuresis
    The patient is often overweight
    May be no symptoms in NIDDM until major complications have occurred
    (e.g. visual disturbance owing to retinopathy)

Signs
    Signs of complications such as retinopathy or ischaemic heart disease may be
    found at presentation, as the patient may have had diabetes several years
    before diagnosis
    Glycosuria but typically no ketones on dipstick testing

Complications
    Microvascular such as retinopathy, nephropathy and neuropathy
    Macrovascular such as ischaemic heart disease, cerebrovascular disease and
    peripheral vascular disease
    Metabolic complications such as hyperosmolar non-ketotic coma

Fig. 7.14. NIDDM, from molecular defects to complications. The genetic predisposition
to NIDDM interacts with precipitants such as obesity and low birth weight. The nature
of the genetic prediposition is unknown in most patients. There is defective insulin
secretion and insulin resistance although the primary deficit is unknown. These cause
hyperglycaemia and dyslipidaemia which lead to microvascular and macrovascular
complications.

development of ischaemia in tissues such as the foot, even when the large blood vessels
remain patent.

Retinopathy

Diabetic retinopathy is the leading cause of blindness in the working population.
Background retinopathy is the term that describes microaneurysms, small haemorrhages
and exudates. This is observed in the majority of patients with long-standing diabetes
(80% show these changes at 20 years). *Maculopathy* is used to describe oedema or other
diabetic lesions occurring around the macula. Pathology in the macular region is partic-

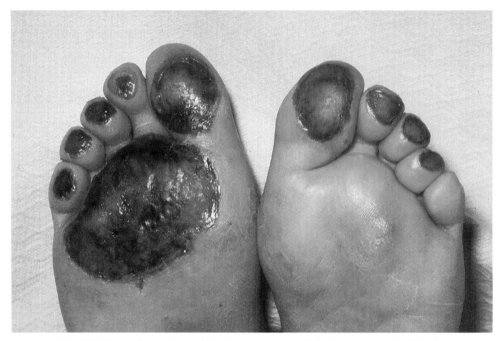

Fig. 7.15. Feet of a patient with chronic sensory diabetic neuropathy. The patient on holiday walked on hot sand, unaware of the damage sustained to the soles of the feet. (Picture courtesy of Dr R. S. Elkeles).

ularly dangerous for vision. *Pre-proliferative retinopathy* describes a situation with multiple cotton-wool spots, which represent areas of ischaemic or infarcted retina. The term *intraretinal microvascular abnormalities* refers to the shunting of blood away from such ischaemic areas. *Proliferative retinopathy* develops adjacent to areas of retinal ischaemia. New blood vessels appear in the retina (neovascularisation) and extend into the vitreous space. These new vessels are prone to bleed into the retina and vitreous space, causing blindness. Vitreous haemorrhage eventually leads to fibrosis, and as the fibrotic area contracts, the retina may become detached.

Nephropathy

Diabetic nephropathy develops in 30% of patients with IDDM of more than 15 years' duration. It is common also in NIDDM. It accounts for 35% of all patients on chronic renal dialysis. The earliest abnormality is an increase in glomerular filtration rate, at which time there is renal hypertrophy. Microalbuminuria, defined as a urinary albumin excretion rate of 20–200 µg/minute, occurs at this stage and reflects an increase in capillary permeability. Basement membrane thickening and some mesangial expansion are evident on histology. Microalbuminuria predicts later overt nephropathy, when renal impairment occurs in association with more pronounced proteinuria, which is detectable on stix testing. In both diabetic and non-diabetic subjects, nephropathy is associated also with excess mortality from cardiovascular disease, together with insulin resistance, hypertension, hypertriglyceridaemia and a low HDL cholesterol level. Once overt renal impairment develops, the risk of death from vascular disease is increased 100-fold, at least in IDDM.

Neuropathy

Diabetic neuropathy affects the peripheral nervous system and the autonomic nervous system. It increases with increasing duration of diabetes, such that 50–60% of patients are affected after 25 years. The most common clinical form is a *chronic sensory neuropathy*, with paraesthesiae or numbness in a glove and stocking distribution (Fig. 7.15). This is associated rarely with neuroarthropathy of the lower limb (a Charcot joint). *Diabetic amyotrophy* usually presents as sudden onset of pain in one thigh, with quadriceps wasting and frequently loss of body weight. This is an unusual example of *acute painful neuropathy*, which is associated with sudden onset of pain in the legs and feet. These painful neuropathies usually improve with diabetic control. Other forms of neuropathy include *diffuse motor neuropathy* with generalised muscle wasting and weakness, *pressure neuropathies*, such as carpal tunnel syndrome, and *focal vascular neuropathies*, such as isolated cranial nerve palsies. *Autonomic neuropathy* causes postural hypotension, impotence, loss of awareness of hypoglycaemia, abnormal sweating, gastric stasis, diarrhoea or occasionally constipation, and urinary retention. It is also associated with an increased frequency of sudden death.

Macrovascular complications

Macrovascular disease in diabetes increases by two- to fourfold the risk of death from cardiovascular disease. Amputation rates are five times greater than in the non-diabetic population.

The macrovascular disease results from atherosclerosis. *Atherosis* refers to the accumulation of lipid deposits in the arterial intima and *sclerosis* refers to thickening of the arterial wall resulting from accumulation of collagen in the intima and media. There is also an increase in the tone of arterial smooth muscle cells. The histology is similar to that observed in non-diabetic atherosclerosis (see Chapter 8) although some differences in protein characteristics have been reported, perhaps as a result of glycosylation. The typical lesion is the atheromatous plaque. This starts as a fatty streak, becomes a fibrous plaque and eventually more complex lesions develop. The initiating event is the uptake of low-density lipoproteins (LDL) into the arterial intima. Plaques occur most frequently at positions of focal mechanical stress, such as arterial bifurcations, which are especially vulnerable to damage.

Other diabetic complications

Certain complications of diabetes are less easily classified as micro- or macrovascular in origin. Examples include skin changes, such as necrobiosis lipoidica, and limited joint mobility.

Biochemical mechanisms of diabetic complications

Numerous biochemical mechanisms have been proposed to explain the pathogenesis of diabetic complications. It is likely that several mechanisms interact to cause functional change and structural abnormalities. Some of the likely mechanisms are outlined below, with emphasis on their interactions.

Free radical damage

A free radical is a molecule or atom with an unpaired electron. In biological systems, damage is frequently attributed to reactive oxygen metabolites, some radicals ($O_2^{\bullet-}$, OH•) and others not (HO_2^-, H_2O_2) (the dot signifies an unpaired electron). Lipids are vulnerable to attack, resulting, for example, in the peroxidation of polyunsaturated lipids in the cell membrane. Oxidative damage to proteins results frequently in their aggregation or in an alteration in their three-dimensional structure. Auto-oxidation of monosaccharides produces reactive oxygen metabolites that can then cause tissue damage. The reactive oxygen metabolites produce cell damage directly and they stimulate coagulation on endothelial cells.

Natural defences exist against such reactive oxygen species. These include the metalloprotein enzyme superoxide dismutase, which normally keeps intracellular concentrations of the very reactive $O_2^{\bullet-}$ low, by its conversion to hydrogen peroxide:

$$O_2^{\bullet-}+O_2^{\bullet-} \xrightarrow{2H^+} H_2O_2+O_2$$

The hydrogen peroxide so produced is less reactive but crosses biological membranes readily and is, therefore, potentially damaging. It is itself removed by reduction to water under the influence of the enzyme catalase:

$$2H_2O_2 \rightarrow 2H_2O+O_2$$

More importantly, hydrogen peroxide is removed by its reaction with reduced glutathione (G–SH) under the influence of peroxidase, producing oxidised glutathione (G–S–S–G):

$$H_2O_2+2G\text{–}SH \rightarrow 2H_2O+G\text{–}S\text{–}S\text{–}G$$

Oxidised glutathione is converted back to G–SH by an NADPH-dependent enzyme, glutathione reductase. Reactive oxygen species are also removed by the dietary antioxidants vitamins C and E.

Free radical production is increased in diabetes. The mechanisms are uncertain, but protein glycosylation may be involved (see below). An increase in sorbitol production may cause depletion of NADPH (see below), preventing the re-formation of reduced glutathione. Finally, superoxide dismutase activity is decreased in diabetes, preventing removal of $O_2^{\bullet-}$.

Non-enzymatic glycosylation

Glucose reacts with proteins non-enzymatically to form irreversible complexes, called advanced glycosylation end-products (AGE). The degree of glycosylation is increased by exposure to higher glucose levels. The glycosylation of haemoglobin (e.g. haemoglobin A1c) is utilised as a guide to recent diabetic control (the previous six weeks). Glycosylation of other proteins has been demonstrated in numerous tissues, including arteries and the kidneys. It has been postulated that AGE cause damage through free radical formation. AGE receptors exist on monocytes and macrophages; receptor binding increases the local synthesis of matrix proteins, cytokines and growth factors. AGE also decrease the binding of heparan sulphate to proteins and in the basement membrane: the loss of negative charge leads to increased vessel permeability. AGE quench endothelial-derived nitric oxide production leading to a loss of its vasodilatory actions. Nitric oxide also has actions to inhibit platelet aggregation and it inhibits cellular proliferation; both of these actions may be diminished. Glycosylation of collagen leads to trapping of lipid-containing lipoproteins, such as LDL, in the arterial wall. Glycosylation of LDL itself leads to increased LDL uptake by macrophages, as outlined below.

Pharmacological agents exist that inhibit AGE formation. One such agent is amino-guanidine. In animal models, aminoguanidine has beneficial effects on diabetic retinopathy and neuropathy and it prevents proteinuria in animal models of diabetic kidney disease. Long-term trials of beneficial versus adverse effects are necessary before a role for inhibitors of AGE formation can be established in human diabetes.

Lipoprotein modifications

In the arterial wall, free radical attack leads to oxidation of LDL. Insulin resistance is associated with small dense LDL, which are more prone to oxidation. Irrespective of the mechanism, oxidation of LDL stimulates their uptake by macrophages and their athero-genic potential (see p. 239). Glycosylation also stimulates uptake, as discussed previously. In the arterial intima, these lipid-laden macrophages are referred to as 'foam cells'. Oxidised LDL damages the endothelial cell wall and platelets aggregate on the endothelial cell surface. The resultant thrombus may be incorporated into a plaque. The oxidised LDL are immunogenic and high levels of autoantibodies to oxidised LDL have been observed in NIDDM. Oxidised LDL impairs nitric oxide synthesis, thereby contributing further to the deficiency of endothelial-derived vasodilation.

Sorbitol and myoinositol metabolism

Sorbitol is formed from glucose in a concentration-dependent fashion by a reaction catalysed by the enzyme aldose reductase, the so-called polyol pathway.

$$Glucose + NADPH \rightarrow Sorbitol + NADP^+$$

Aldose reductase is present in high quantities in Schwann cells and in certain other cells in peripheral nerves, the lens, cornea and retina, and in the renal glomeruli. The accumulation of sorbitol has been proposed as a mechanism for production of diabetic complications. Sorbitol in large amounts inside cells leads to cellular swelling through osmosis. Cell swelling has been observed histologically in some patients with diabetic neuropathy.

Another mechanism implicating sorbitol in diabetic complications is through depletion of myoinositol. Myoinositol is a monosaccharide from which are synthesised the secondary messengers phosphoinositides. Phosphoinositides lead to activation of protein kinase C, deficiency of which leads to decreased sodium/potassium ATPase activity and the accumulation of sodium intracellularly.

Inhibition of aldose reductase activity prevents the accumulation of sorbitol and prevents or inhibits some of the secondary changes outlined above. In experimental animals, aldose reductase inhibitors have had beneficial effects on diabetic complications, including improvements in nerve conduction velocity and a reduction in proteinuria. Results in humans have been variable and there are on-going trials to establish if benefit accrues.

Other mechanisms

Numerous other mechanisms have been proposed to explain diabetic complications. Diabetes is associated with an increase in circulating levels of procoagulant factors and a decrease in fibrinolytic factor concentrations, particularly in patients with albuminuria. Insulin resistance is associated with coronary artery disease, hypertension and excessive central body fat. The lipoprotein profile is changed, with a high proportion of small dense LDL, a decrease in HDL and an increase in circulating triglyceride levels (see p. 259). Increased oxidative damage to DNA may accelerate ageing and exaggerated oxidative DNA damage has been demonstrated in diabetic mononuclear cells. In IDDM, macrovascular disease is not associated with the dyslipidaemia observed in NIDDM. Instead, although LDL cholesterol concentrations are frequently normal, vascular disease is most severe in patients with the highest LDL cholesterol levels. There is also an association in IDDM between vascular disease and circulating levels of fibrinogen.

Relationship of diabetic complications to diabetic control

Treatment that decreases the degree of chronic hyperglycaemia delays the onset and slows the progression of complications in IDDM. The most compelling evidence to support this has arisen from a large study involving 29 centres in the USA and Canada, the Diabetes Control and Complications Trial (DCCT). In this study, 1441 patients with IDDM were followed for three to nine years. Some patients received very intensive therapy and monitoring, while others received conventional management and insulin treatment. When the study was terminated, the mean±S.D. haemoglobin A1c level was 7.23±0.96% in the intensive therapy group and 9.11±1.31% in the conventionally treated patients. Over the years of study, the risk of development of retinopathy, and the risk of established mild retinopathy progressing to vision-threatening retinopathy, were

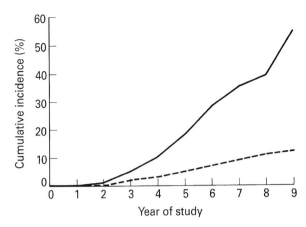

Fig. 7.16. The progression of retinopathy in the Diabetes Control and Complications Trial. The cumulative incidence of a sustained change from baseline in the progression of retinopathy in patients with IDDM receiving conventional (continuous line) or intensive (interrupted line) therapy.

reduced by 70–80% in the intensive therapy group (Fig. 7.16). Protection was also observed against nephropathy. Intensive treatment reduced the appearance of neuropathy by 69% and also prevented or retarded the progression of established neuropathy. Although intensive treatment had disadvantages also, notably a threefold increase in the frequency of severe hypoglycaemic attacks, this study demonstrated clearly for IDDM the association between poor diabetic control and complications. Equivalent data are not yet available for NIDDM, although major studies are in progress. There is little evidence currently to suggest that improvement in diabetic control limits the development or progression of macrovascular disease, although studies in progress may clarify any relationship.

Summary

IDDM and NIDDM are both characterised by hyperglycaemia but have different causes.

IDDM is caused by an autoimmune destruction of pancreatic beta cells, which usually affects young people. It has an inherited component to its pathogenesis and the disease is triggered by an environmental event such as infection with Coxsackie B virus. Treatment with insulin is required to prevent the development of ketoacidosis. Ketoacidosis develops when absolute or relative insulin deficiency, together with a stress hormone response, lead to hyperglycaemia and overproduction of the ketone bodies 3-hydroxybutyric acid and acetoacetic acid. It is a medical emergency, requiring treatment with insulin, saline and potassium, together with careful monitoring.

NIDDM also has an inherited basis, although environmental influences such as obesity, exercise and smallness at birth appear contributory. The insulin deficiency in NIDDM is typically less severe than in IDDM and all patients are insulin resistant. The insulin resistance is associated with lipid disturbances, notably a low circulating HDL cholesterol and elevated triglyceride, which may be important in the large vessel disease observed in NIDDM. This macrovascular disease is, however, also seen in IDDM, which does not show the same lipid profile, and other mechanisms may operate.

Microvascular disease causes retinopathy, neuropathy and nephropathy and is observed in both IDDM and NIDDM. The biochemical mechanisms are unknown, although evidence exists for several disturbances, including free radical damage, non-enzymatic glycosylation, lipoprotein modifications and disorders of sorbitol and myoinositol metabolism. In IDDM, the microvascular complications are prevented, or their progression delayed, by intensive control of blood glucose concentrations over several years.

FURTHER READING

Cohen, R.D., Lewis, B., Alberti, K.G.M.M. & Denman, A.M. (1990). *The Metabolic and Molecular Basis of Acquired Disease*, Vol. 1 and 2. London: Baillière Tindall. Good discussions of diabetes and metabolism.

Crofford, O.B. (1995). Diabetes control and complications. *Annual Review of Medicine*, 46, 267–269. This is a clear review of the Diabetes Control and Complications Trial and its results.

Davies, J.L., Kawaguchi, Y., Bennett, S.T. *et al.* (1994). A genome-wide search for human type 1 diabetes susceptibility genes. *Nature*, 371, 103–136. This highly technical paper gives an idea of how molecular geneticists are trying to define the genetic abnormalities.

Leslie, R.D.G. (ed.) (1993). *Causes of Diabetes. Genetic and Environmental Factors*. Chichester: Wiley. An excellent collection of review chapters on the pathogenesis of diabetes.

Newsholme, E.A., & Leech, A.R. (1983). *Biochemistry for the Medical Sciences*. Chichester: Wiley. Somewhat dated but still the best overview of human metabolism available.

Pickup, J. & Williams, G. (1995). *Textbook of Diabetes*. Oxford: Blackwell. A clearly presented description of all aspects of diabetes, particularly useful for the diabetic complications.

Rabinovitch, A. (1994). Immunoregulatory and cytokine imbalances in the pathogenesis of IDDM; therapeutic intervention by immuno-stimulation. *Diabetes*, 43, 613–621. A lucid review of the immune mechanisms in IDDM.

Reaven, G.M. (1995). The fourth musketeer – from Alexander Dumas to Claude Bernard. *Diabetologia*, 38, 3–13. This is a concise review of the pathogenesis of the metabolic disturbances in NIDDM.

8

Cardiovascular disease: atherosclerosis

A. GAW, G. M. LINDSAY and J. SHEPHERD

- Atherosclerosis is a multistage process that progresses from endothelial injury through fatty streaks to fibrolipid plaques.

- Plaques can lead to major clinical disease by haemorrhaging into an atheromatous plaque, rupturing, ulcerating or forming a surface for thrombosis. Plaque regression can also occur.

- The molecular mechanisms are complex, involving cells and cytokines. Oxidised LDL may be crucially involved.

- Clinical sequelae are coronary heart disease, peripheral vascular disease and cerebrovascular disease.

- The major modifiable risk factors are smoking, hypertension and dyslipidaemia.

Definition and terminology

Atherosclerosis is a pathological process that is defined as a focal, inflammatory fibro-proliferative response to multiple forms of endothelial injury. The response to injury hypothesis for the development of atherosclerosis was formally proposed by Ross and his colleagues in the 1970s and has been refined and developed since. There are other hypotheses that try to explain the complex pathogenesis of the atherosclerotic plaque but none has been so widely accepted as that of a normal repair process gone awry – where the healing process becomes the disease itself. The term atherosclerosis describes the pathological appearance of the lesions, encompassing as they do the soft gruel-like plaque contents (*athere*: porridge, Greek) and the fibrotic encasement of this material (*skleros*: hard, Greek). The term *arteriosclerosis* should never be used interchangeably with atherosclerosis, although it is often used as a synonym. The process of atherosclerosis may also be misleadingly applied to a number of vascular pathologies that resemble it in some of its features. For example, smooth muscle cell proliferation is a feature of atherosclerosis but it is also seen in the reactive smooth muscle cell hypertrophy of arteries in the hypertensive subject. The latter is not atherosclerosis, nor is the stenosis that occurs in patients post-angioplasty, which is again a simple response to arterial injury that falls short of full atherosclerosis.

Table 8.1. *The functions of the vascular endothelium*

Formation of a non-thrombogenic and non-adherent surface
Formation of a semi-permeable barrier
Synthesis and release of chemical regulators of vascular tone
Synthesis and release of growth factors, cytokines
Maintenance of the collagenous basement membrane
Modification of lipoproteins as they traverse the endothelium into the artery wall

Pathogenesis of atherosclerosis

Endothelial injury is thought to be the primary event in the pathogenesis of the athero-sclerotic plaque, but it is clear that gross changes, such as loss of endothelial cells with exposure of underlying matrix, do not necessarily occur at the sites of early lesions. Injury is a term that extends in meaning from cellular damage to more subtle effects such as loss of function. The arterial endothelium serves several key functions; these are listed in Table 8.1. When endothelial cells are injured by exposure to mechanical trauma or other injurious agents, such as viruses or toxins, one way that they manifest their dysfunction is to become sticky. Elegant scanning electron microscopy studies have revealed that injured endothelium allows the adherence of monocyte/macrophages and T cells (Fig. 8.1).

Endothelial 'injury' by modified lipoproteins

The principal form of injury thought to initiate atherogenesis is increasingly hypo-thesised to be mediated by lipoproteins. However, the main problem with the acceptance of this hypothesis has been that native lipoproteins are unable to induce atherogenic changes *in vitro*. Although lipoproteins certainly do enter the subendothelial space of arteries, they are neither phagocytosed by macrophages there, nor does their presence initiate any form of immune/inflammatory reaction.

A major breakthrough was made when it was recognised that when lipoproteins are chemically modified by oxidation their atherogenic potential is switched on. In this state, they are actively ingested by macrophages. These cells possess cell-surface scavenger receptors and may even have a specific receptor for oxidised low density lipoprotein (oxLDL). Unlike lipoprotein uptake mediated via the LDL receptor, uptake via these scavenger receptors is not downregulated as the cell acquires sufficient lipids for its metabolic and synthetic needs. Instead, the ingestion of oxLDL goes on unchecked to the point where the macrophage is overladen by lipids and, because of its vacuolated appearance, is referred to as a foam cell (Fig. 8.2). The oxLDL is also chemotactic for monocytes and induces their transmigration across the arterial endothelium from the circulation into the subendothelial space. Perhaps attracted by the entrapped oxLDL, these cells invade the subendothelial space by squeezing between endothelial cells. This event has even been photographed in both hypercholesterolaemic non-human primate aortae and in human coronary arteries (Fig. 8.1 and 8.2). It is then that macrophages begin their terminal path towards foam cells by phagocytosing the modified lipoproteins.

The importance of oxLDL in atherogenesis was emphasised when the drug probucol was studied. This drug is a potent antioxidant and when it was fed to hyperlipidaemic rabbits fewer atherosclerotic lesions were observed to develop. This and similar observations have prompted a renewed interest in the use of antioxidants as preventive measures for coronary heart disease (CHD). Natural antioxidants include vitamins C and E and beta-carotene all of which are found in high quantities in the so-called 'Mediterranean diet', which is reputed to be antiatherogenic. However, more recent clinical studies using antioxidant strategies to prevent atherosclerosis have been disappointing; therefore, while oxidised lipoproteins offer a plausible mechanism for the initiation and progression of atherogenesis, this explanation remains an hypothesis.

Natural history of atherogenesis

All infants have focal thickening of the coronary artery intima as a result of smooth muscle cell proliferation. Although this is an important hallmark of the developing atherosclerotic plaque, it is not unique to this condition as it is considered to be a simple adaptive response. The first lesions that may be recognised as truly atherosclerotic are called fatty streaks (Fig. 8.2). These are small lesions that on gross inspection are hardly raised and are caused by focal collections of foam cells within the intima. Necropsy studies reveal the presence of atherosclerotic plaques ranging in size from the fatty streak to larger plaques. This has been taken as evidence, albeit circumstantial, that there may be progression from one type of lesion to the other. The fatty streak lesion may be the precursor of larger atherosclerotic plaques, but they are also viewed by most workers in the field as entirely reversible phenomena. Such a belief comes from necropsy studies of infants from societies around the world where atherosclerosis as a cause of death is relatively rare. These infants, although unlikely to have died from CHD if they had lived to maturity, have many fatty streaks in their arteries.

Progression of the fatty streak to a larger more complex lesion is thought to occur through two key processes. First, the foam cells engorged with lipid begin to die and break down in the centre of the fatty streak. Releasing their cytoplasmic contents leads to the presence of extracellular lipids and the release of many chemical mediators of the inflammatory response. Smooth muscle cell migration and proliferation is the second process involved in the progression of the fatty streak. Smooth muscle cells push into the lipid-rich plaque, where they divide and begin to elaborate a connective tissue matrix composed of elastic fibre proteins, collagen and proteoglycans. The increase in cell numbers and the laying down of a collagenous matrix both serve to increase the bulk of the plaque, which now protrudes into the artery lumen and is referred to as a raised fibrolipid or advanced plaque. Such plaques are difficult to age, but necropsy studies suggest that they take 10–15 years to develop. It is also believed that new fatty streaks are continually forming throughout adult life.

Human   Nonhuman primates

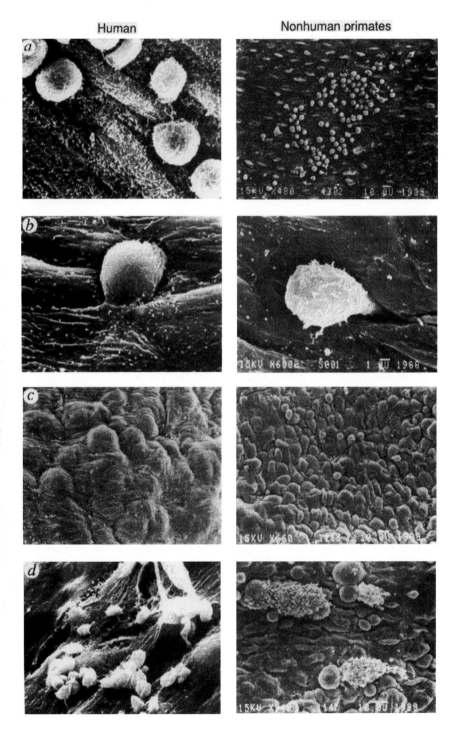

Fig. 8.1. Scanning electron micrographs taken of the aorta from hypercholesterolaemic non-human primates (right panels) versus coronary arteries obtained from human hearts with advanced atherosclerosis removed for transplant purposes (left panels).

Molecular control of atherogenesis

A complex mixture of growth factors and cytokines interact to co-ordinate cellular recruitment, migration and proliferation within the developing atherosclerotic lesion. The main players in this complex biochemical scenario are listed in Table 8.2. From a wealth of *in vitro* studies, it seems clear that none of these factors is capable of inducing atherogenesis alone. On the contrary, a complex cascade of autocrine and paracrine effects of these regulatory molecules appears to be necessary for the initiation and development of the plaque. Continued and intensive study of these growth factors and cytokines has been stimulated by the hope that the key to the control of human atherogenesis lies in the regulation of these factors, perhaps by pharmacological means.

Cellular control of atherogenesis

Macrophages have several normal functions. Principal among these is to act as scavenger cells clearing up potentially toxic materials. This coupled with their role as pro-

Fig 8.1 (*cont.*)

(*a*) (*Right*) Numerous adherent leucocytes are clustered on the surface of the endothelium in this monkey artery in an area suggesting that there are localised cell surface changes in that site. Increased monocyte and T cell adherence precedes their entry into the artery wall. (*Left*) At a somewhat higher magnification, leucocytes from a human coronary artery are similarly attached to the surface of the endothelium. Most of the cells are rounded, although a few of them appear to be in the process of spreading on the surface of the endothelium.

(*b*) (*Right*) A leucocyte that has begun to penetrate between the surface endothelial cells has extended a cytoplasmic process that appears to protrude between the endothelial cells as it enters into the subendothelial space of the monkey aorta. (*Left*) A similar process of leucocyte chemotaxis appears to be taking place in a human carotid artery; the leucocyte appears to be burrowing beneath one of the lining endothelial cells.

(*c*) (*Right*) A surface of a fatty streak taken from a hyperlipidaemic monkey. The lobular appearance of the surface of the lesion results from the large number of accumulated underlying lipid-filled macrophages, or foam cells. Monocytes and lymphocytes can be seen to continue to adhere to the surface of the lesion. In this way, their continual entry will lead to further lesion expansion. (*Left*) A similar lobulation of a fatty streak from a human coronary artery. The underlying foam cells with their lipid droplets can be seen through the stretched, thinnned endothelium. The processes in the human appear to be virtually identical to those observed in the non-human primate.

(*d*) (*Right*) Three mural platelet thrombi on the surface of an intermediate lesion of atherosclerosis in a non-human primate. When sectioned transversely and examined by light microscopy, some of these can be shown to be located on the surface of exposed macrophages, others at sites of endothelial cell separation. (*Left*) Adherent platelets are present on the surface of an atherosclerotic lesion from a human coronary artery. In this case, they are associated with an area of endothelial separation and exposure of the underlying connective tissue. In both cases, adherent, aggregated platelets undergo shape changes and characteristically release the numerous growth factors and other molecules in their granules. (Reprinted with permission from *Nature* (1993) 362, 801–809. Copyright (1993) Macmillan Magazines Limited.)

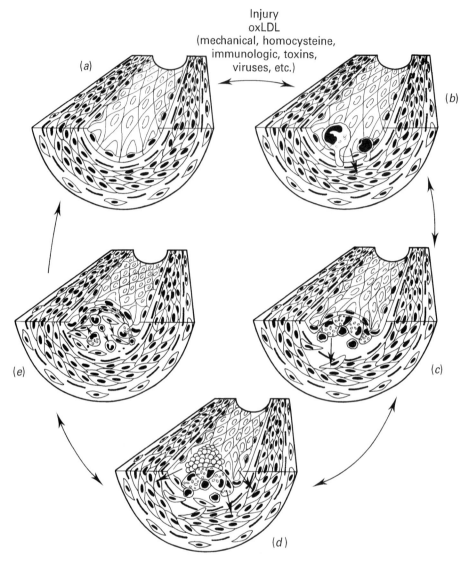

Fig. 8.2. Pathogenesis of atherosclerosis. (*a*) Cross-section diagram showing the normal architecture of coronary artery. (*b*) As a result of endothelial injury, monocyte/ macrophages adhere to the endothelial surface and begin to invade the subendothelial space. (*c*) By ingesting lipoproteins, these cells become lipid-filled foam cells and as they accumulate at the lesion site they bulge under the endothelial surface creating the physical appearance of the fatty streak. (*d*) As the lesion increases in size, smooth muscle cells proliferate and migrate into the subendothelial space and platelet mural thrombi may form on the surface. The lesion may now be called an intermediate atheromatous plaque. (*e*) Progression of these processes by continual release of regulatory molecules that stimulate and recruit other cells to the site and the laying down of fibrous tissue leads to the development of an advanced plaque. Note that this entire process (*a–e*) is by no means a one-way system and reversal of each of the steps is now thought to be clinically possible. (Taken with permission from *Nature* (1993) 362, 801–809. Copyright (1993) Macmillan Magazines Limited.)

Table 8.2. *Molecules involved in the development of the atherosclerotic plaque*

Chemical regulator	Source
Platelet-derived growth factor	E, M, P
Basic epidermal growth factor	E, M. S
Heparin-binding epidermal growth factor-like growth factor	M, S
Insulin-like growth factor 1	M, S, P
IL-1	E, M, S, L
TNF-α	E, M, S, L
TGF-β	M, S, L, P
Colony-stimulating factors	E, M, S, L
Monocyte chemoattractant protein-1	E, M, S,
oxLDL	E, M, S,
γ-IFN	M, L
IL-2	M
Nitric oxide	E
Vascular endothelial growth factor	M, S

Note:
E, endothelium; M, macrophage; S, smooth muscle cell; L, lymphocyte; P, platelet.
Source: Data taken from Ross, R. (1993). The pathogenesis of atherosclerosis: a perspective for the 1990s. *Nature,* 362, 801–809.

ducers of many of the growth factors and cytokines outlined in Table 8.2 makes the macrophage one of the most important cell types in the developing atherosclerotic plaque. It should also be noted that macrophages as well as being attracted to oxLDL can also be their source. These cells have the capacity to oxidise lipoproteins and thereby create one of the many interconnecting vicious circles that contribute to the development of atherosclerosis.

The presence of lymphocytes in the atherosclerotic plaque lends weight to the hypothesis that atherogenesis is at least in part an immunological phenomenon. This is seen most strikingly in the atherogenesis associated with the rejection of a transplanted heart, where there is clearly material present perceived by the body's immune system as foreign. More commonly, however, what could the foreign antigen be that stimulates the involvement of the immune system in the atherosclerotic plaque? To answer this we must re-examine the role of oxLDL, which may be even more important than originally thought. Autoantibodies to oxLDL have been detected in human blood, and this may account for the intrusion of lymphocytes into the plaque, which contains this potentially antigenic lipoprotein.

Plaque rupture and thrombosis

The dangers of the plaque lie in both its size and its tendency to fissure and ulcerate. The final pathway to a major clinical event such as an acute myocardial infarction is not clear, but haemorrhage into an atheromatous plaque, rupture or fissuring of a plaque, or thrombosis on the surface of a plaque are mechanisms that are likely to be involved (Fig. 8.3).

In studies by Davies and his colleagues, the role of the atheromatous plaque and thrombus formation were clarified in patients with crescendo angina and acute myocardial infarction. Thrombus formation was seen as a rapidly changing, dynamic process and of major importance in both conditions. In fatal cases of myocardial infarction, post-mortem studies have shown that coronary thrombi, in nearly all cases, are related to the fissuring of the atheromatous plaque. The factors that determine whether a thrombus does occur within the lumen are partially local, including the size and geometry of the intimal tear, whether lipid is extruded into the lumen itself, the degree of stenosis and blood flow rate at the site. Systemic factors such as the thrombotic or thrombolytic potential at the time will also play a part. Not all plaque fissuring will result in these dire consequences; the plaque may restabilise and heal over, but, at a cost: the healed plaque will now be larger than before.

Regression of the atherosclerotic plaque

The concept of therapeutic intervention producing reversal or regression of atherosclerotic lesions originated in the 1940s. Post-mortem examinations on individuals who had suffered great weight losses prior to their death revealed that the extent of plaque development in the aorta and coronary arteries was much less than expected. In response to these findings, many studies have been conducted to confirm and evaluate these observations.

Recently, the results from randomised, controlled clinical studies using different treatments for lowering cholesterol have been reported. In the Familial Atherosclerosis Treatment Study, middle-aged men who had moderately elevated LDL, a family history of CHD and angiographic evidence of CHD had reduced frequency of progression of coronary lesions and increased frequency of regression and reduced incidence of CHD events if prescribed lipid-lowering therapy (Fig. 8.4).

In the Lifestyle Heart Trial, the objective was to determine if lifestyle changes in diet, exercise, smoking and stress could affect coronary atherosclerosis. Patients with angiographically documented CHD were assigned to an experimental group or to a usual care control group. The patients in the experimental group were prescribed a regimen that included a low-fat vegetarian diet, smoking cessation, stress management training, moderate aerobic exercise and group support. After only a year, patients in the experimental group showed significant overall regression of coronary atherosclerosis in contrast to the control group, who, having made less comprehensive lifestyle changes, showed significant overall progression of coronary atherosclerosis.

The most convincing evidence of all for the benefits of cholesterol-lowering therapy comes from the 4S study, which is the first major secondary prevention trial using an HMG (hydroxymethylglutaryl) CoA reductase inhibitor or statin. In this study almost 4500 men and women with CHD were given either simvastatin or a placebo over a five year period. Those that received the lipid-lowering drug were 30% less likely to die from any cause and 42% less likely to die from CHD (Fig. 8.5).

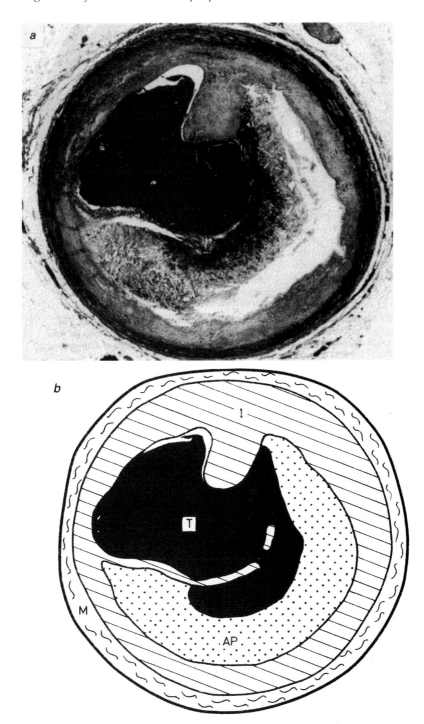

Fig. 8.3. (*a*) Histological cross-section of a major atheromatous plaque rupture. (*b*) Diagram to show the component parts. The plaque (AP) has a large defect in the fibrous cap, through which a dumb-bell-shaped mass of thrombus has formed (T), part being within the plaque and part virtually occluding the lumen (L). (Reprinted with permission from *British Heart Journal* (1985), 53, 363–373. Published by BMJ Publishing group.)

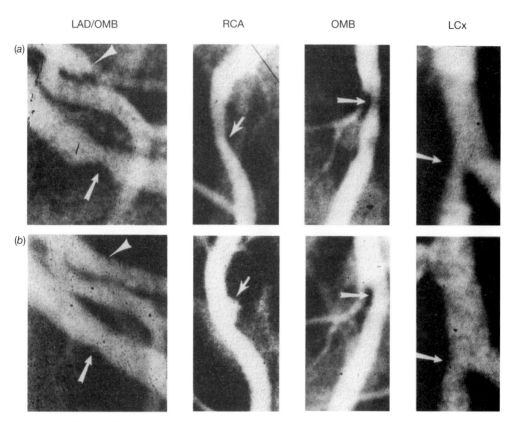

Fig. 8.4. Examples of regression in patients treated with intensive lipid-lowering therapy. (*a*) Images obtained from coronary angiography at baseline; (*b*) images obtained from the same patients after 2.5 years' therapy. LAD, left anterior descending artery: OMB, obtuse marginal branch; RCA, right coronary artery; LCx, left circumflex artery. Stenosis caused by the lesions in these vessels decreased as follows: LAD, from 100 to 28%; OMB, from 39 to 18%; RCA, from 48 to 30%; OMB from 69 to 37% and LCx, from 44 to 30%. (Reprinted by permission of the *New England Journal of Medicine* (323, 1289–1298, 1990.)

Clinical significance of atherosclerosis

Atherosclerosis is the single most important disease process in the industrialised world, where approximately 50% of all deaths are caused by atherosclerosis-related conditions. These include CHD, peripheral vascular disease and cerebrovascular disease. CHD is the single most important disease resulting from atherosclerosis and is the leading cause of death in the UK and the developed world (see Chapter 9). In 1989, CHD accounted for 26% of the annual all-cause mortality in England and Wales and the annual cost of this disease to the health service was estimated at approximately £500 million.

Clinical manifestations of atherosclerosis

Atherosclerosis is a pathological process that can occur in many different arteries. The most common clinical manifestations are seen when the coronary arteries are involved.

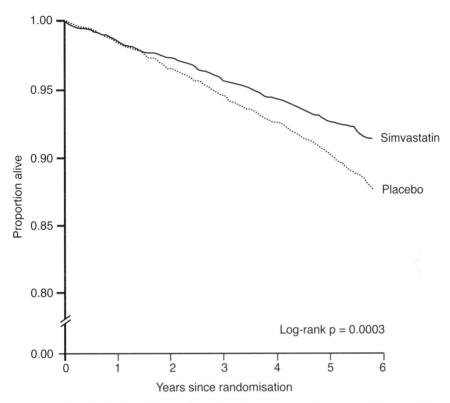

Fig. 8.5. Kaplan–Meier curves for all-cause mortality. In the 4S study, 4444 patients with CHD were randomised to receive either the lipid-lowering drug simvastatin or a placebo. The death rates in the two groups diverged after the first 18 months of therapy and then progressively separated. By the end of the study, 5 years later, the investigators could claim a very highly significant improvement in both all-cause and CHD mortality. (Redrawn with permission from Scandinavian Simvastatin Survival Study Group (1994). Randomised trial of cholesterol lowering in 4444 patients with coronary heart disease: the Scandinavian Simvastatin Survival Study (4S). *Lancet* 344; 1383–1389. Copyright by the Lancet Ltd 1994.)

With narrowing of the coronary artery lumen, the area of the myocardium supplied by that artery becomes ischaemic. This myocardial ischaemia presents as angina pectoris: retrosternal chest pain radiating up into the throat and jaws and down the arm and relieved by rest and nitrate therapy. If the coronary artery narrowing progresses to complete occlusion, the areas of myocardium supplied by the artery will become infarcted. Now the patient will complain of crushing central chest pain of longer duration that is unrelieved by rest or nitrate therapy. In many patients, an acute myocardial infarction is the very first presentation of underlying atherosclerosis and it should be noted that approximately half of all such patients die as a result.

Atherosclerosis can also affect the peripheral arteries, resulting in leg muscle ischaemia, called *intermittent claudication*. The patient will usually complain of calf muscle cramps when walking that are relieved by rest. The severity of this condition can vary from mild inconvenience to the very severe, when there is pain even at rest. Patients with peripheral vascular disease may also complain of cold extremities, poor skin and ulceration or even gangrene, all of which are the result of atherosclerotic narrowing of the peripheral arteries and reduced blood flow to the lower limbs.

The aorta is frequently affected by atherosclerosis, and although there is no occlusion of blood flow through this the largest of our arteries, there can be serious clinical consequences. The atherosclerotic lesions weaken the aortic wall and can contribute to the development of aneurysms particularly in the abdominal aorta. Rupture of an aortic aneurysm will result in sudden death.

When the cerebral arteries are affected by atherosclerosis, the patient may suffer a spectrum of effects ranging from mild neurological disturbances, such as reversible memory loss, through transient ischaemic attacks (TIAs) to a fatal cerebrovascular accident. The precise clinical presentation of cerebrovascular disease depends on the area of the central nervous system deprived of blood.

Risk factors for atherogenesis

A search for the origins, cause and the subsequent methods of prevention of CHD has proceeded from early epidemiological studies of populations to prospective cohort studies, where a population sample is identified, clinically assessed and then monitored for a number of years for signs of disease. One of the first major prospective studies to monitor and document incidence of CHD was started in the small community of Framingham in the USA.

The Framingham study began in the 1940s and was designed to generate information that would help in the early detection and prevention of heart disease. The study started with under 800 male and female volunteers in 1948 and has subsequently grown into a major prospective trial. Follow-up of the recruits, and in some cases their children, is still underway today and data from the study have given investigators valuable information about the relationship between various risk factors and CHD. It is also notable because it is one of the few large epidemiological studies of CHD that has included women.

The aetiology of atherosclerosis has been the subject of intense study since the 1940s and many contributory or risk factors have been identified. While a multitude of factors have been potentially associated with CHD, the number of well-documented risk factors is of the order of 20. However, in practice, attention focuses more commonly on the factors shown in Table 8.3, and greatest emphasis is placed on the three principal and modifiable risk factors: cigarette smoking, hypertension and dyslipidaemia.

These risk factors have been identified repeatedly throughout the literature and are now well accepted. Their modification on a population basis, particularly by dietary means, is advocated by several agencies including the British Government and the World Health Organization. That changes can be made at all, and in a relatively short time, is clear when we examine the worldwide trends in age-adjusted death rates for CHD in man between the years 1970 and 1985. The USA leads this field, having achieved an almost 50% reduction in deaths from CHD in this period, while countries such as Romania and Poland have shown marked increases of more than 70%. Scotland, in the

Table 8.3. *Major risk factors for CHD*

	Risk factors
Modifiable factors	Tobacco smoking
	Dyslipidaemia
	Hypertension
	Obesity
	Physical inactivity
Non-modifiable factors	Family history of CHD
	Diabetes mellitus
	Male gender
	Age

same 15 year period, has shown a fall of approximately 10% but remains near the top of the international league table of male CHD mortality.

Cigarette smoking

Smoking represents the most extensively documented cause of disease ever investigated in the history of biomedical research (United States Department of Health and Human Services).

There are an estimated 115 000 deaths in the UK and 3 million worldwide attributed to smoking each year. Furthermore, it has been estimated that 25% of deaths from CHD below the age of 65 and 50% of deaths in middle-aged women are accounted for by smoking. In addition to these deaths, there are a spectrum of vascular diseases, lung cancer and chronic respiratory diseases causing death and disability associated with smoking.

In many industrialised countries, the percentage of smokers is following a downward trend, e.g. in Scotland between 1986 and 1990 the number of smokers in the 12–24 age group fell from 30 to 27% while those in the 25–65 age group fell from 40 to 38%. However, in many developing countries adult cigarette consumption is both higher and increasing.

The pathophysiological mechanisms responsible for the adverse effects of smoking are by no means clear. Cigarette smoke contains a mixture of about 4000 chemicals, and the two that have received most attention are nicotine and carbon monoxide. Putative mechanisms are alterations in oxygen transport in the blood caused by the greater affinity of carbon monoxide for haemoglobin over that of oxygen; vasoconstriction and injury to the vascular wall by carbon monoxide and nicotine; and increased thrombotic tendency caused by carbon monoxide and nicotine, thereby increasing the risk of thrombosis over an atheromatous plaque. Platelet function is altered in smokers, with significantly increased aggregability even after smoking a single cigarette.

Smoking also has a number of potentially adverse effects on the plasma lipoproteins. LDL from smokers is more easily oxidised and, therefore, may be more atherogenic.

Concentrations of plasma HDL, which is thought to be an antiatherogenic lipoprotein, are generally lower in smokers than in non-smokers.

Evidence to support the view that smoking is causally associated with atherogenesis and its main clinical consequence, CHD, comes from studies examining the impact of stopping smoking on the risks of CHD mortality. Doll and Peto found that CHD deaths among male ex-smokers aged 35–55 years who had been non-smoking for less than five years amounted to approximately half the number that would have been expected had this group continued to smoke.

However, not all studies have supported the notion that the risk of CHD from smoking is completely reversible. Evidence from the British Regional Heart Study shows that both current and ex-smokers had a risk of a major CHD event more than twice that of men who had never smoked cigarettes, and even men who gave up smoking more than 20 years before were still at increased risk.

Nonetheless, all the evidence points in the same direction, i.e. smoking is closely linked to the risk of developing atherosclerosis and stopping smoking decreases that risk. These facts have already been understood by many smokers. A report from the Health Education Authority on surveys of smoking habits has shown that the majority of smokers would like to stop smoking and that each year a large proportion of smokers attempt to do so. Smoking cessation rates after one year using a number of different approaches range from 20% to 40%.

Hypertension

There is strong evidence to suggest that high blood pressure is a risk factor for CHD mortality. The earliest of these is the Framingham study, which monitored adults over a period of 24 years. Both diastolic and systolic blood pressures were measured repeatedly during the study. The major finding was that recruits who were hypertensive at the outset suffered considerably higher rates of CHD, and the rate of CHD increased as the level of blood pressure increased. Therefore, the higher the pressure the greater the risk. There appeared to be no evidence of any threshold pressure below which CHD rates ceased to decline.

The evidence from this study and others suggests that high blood pressure is a precursor of CHD, although there are doubts if this relationship is causal. These doubts arise from the results of randomised controlled trials that have set out to examine the effects on CHD mortality when mild to moderate hypertension is treated. The incidence of fatal and non-fatal myocardial infarctions indicates that, at best, the benefit is small. Analysis of the results of these and other trials of antihypertensive therapy showed that there was an overall reduction in risk of CHD of only 12% (confidence interval 0–20%) while there was a highly significant 43% reduction in the risk of stroke.

The results of the intervention trials are disappointing in terms of reduction in risk of CHD, considering the strong relationship between elevated blood pressure and CHD risk. Several theories have been postulated in order to explain these observations. One possibility is that the relationship is not causal and the two variables are only associated through an intermediary or confounding factor as yet to be identified.

Alternatively, the relationship may indeed be causal but the risk from elevated blood pressure might be irreversible. Another view is that there were deficiencies in the design of the trials.

The incidence and prevalence of hypertension in the UK is difficult to assess because of the lack of comprehensive data. However, 30% of the population have a diastolic blood pressure in the range 90–110 mmHg and 5% exceed 110 mmHg. A random assessment of clinical records in the north London area revealed that 47% of those aged 30–65 had no blood pressure reading recorded in their notes; many patients were inappropriately treated after only one reading, and even more patients had no record of a follow-up measurement. The 'rule of halves' still seems to apply in general practice, with only half of those with hypertension detected, of those half are treated, and of those treated, only half have their hypertension adequately controlled.

The mechanism by which hypertension acts as a risk factor for the development of atherosclerosis is unknown. It has been postulated, however, that increased blood pressure results in increased shear stresses on the arterial wall. This in turn will cause endothelial injury, which as we have seen above is thought to be the primary lesion in the development of the atheromatous plaque. Evidence to support this is the fact that atheromatous lesions tend to occur at sites within the arterial tree, where pressures are highest and where blood flow is most turbulent.

Increased blood pressure may also affect the transport of lipoproteins across the endothelial barrier into the subendothelial space, by increasing influx and decreasing efflux.

In animal studies, lower levels of oxygen have been demonstrated in the artery wall of hypertensive animals when compared with normals. This relative intramural hypoxia may lead to the development of oxyradicals, resulting in a more favourable environment for the modification of lipoproteins trapped in the subendothelial spaces and increasing their atherogenic potential.

Dyslipidaemia

The putative role of hyperlipidaemia in the development of atherosclerosis goes back almost 150 years to the work of Vogel. It was he who first noted the presence of cholesterol in atheromatous plaques, but it was not until the early years of the twentieth century that the association between dietary cholesterol and atherosclerotic lesions was confirmed experimentally. In 1913, the pioneering Russian scientist Anitschkow fed egg yolk to rabbits and observed the development of lesions in their aortae, identical to the atherosclerotic lesions in humans. As this work progressed, Anitschkow became convinced, only two years later, that 'there can be no atheroma without cholesterol'.

Because cholesterol, along with the other main plasma lipid, triglyceride, are insoluble in the aqueous environment of the plasma, they are transported in the bloodstream as lipoprotein complexes. There are four main plasma lipoprotein classes (Table 8.4). In the interpretation and understanding of CHD risk, the two lipoproteins LDL and HDL play key roles. The total cholesterol in the plasma is approximately distributed as follows: 60–70% transported as LDL and 20–30% as HDL. The significance of the relative amounts of these lipoproteins lies in the attributed protective property of HDL and the

Table 8.4. *The plasma lipoproteins*

Lipoprotein	Main apolipoproteins	Function
Chylomicrons	B_{48}, A-I, C-II, E	Largest liproprotein; synthesised by the gut after a fatty meal; main carrier of dietary lipid
Very low density lipoprotein (VLDL)	B_{100}, C-II, E	Synthesised in liver; main carrier of endogenously produced triglyceride
Low density lipoprotein (LDL)	B_{100}	Generated from VLDL in the circulation; main carrier of cholesterol
High density lipoprotein (HDL)	A-I, A-II	Smallest but most abundant; protective function; returns cholesterol to the liver from the peripheral tissues for excretion

atherogenic potential of LDL. Although the exact mechanism for these effects has not been fully elucidated, there is a lot of evidence to indicate that HDL is a protective factor for atherogenesis independently of other risk factors and that the correlation between total cholesterol and CHD is almost entirely owing to the concentration of LDL in the plasma.

Evidence to support the view that cholesterol is causally linked to the development and progression of atherosclerosis and CHD mortality has come from major intervention trials: two of the earliest and largest were the Lipid Research Clinics Coronary Primary Prevention Trial and the Helsinki Heart Study. The former study enrolled approximately 4000 moderately hypercholesterolaemic men with no evidence of heart disease and randomly assigned half to a lipid-lowering diet and therapy (cholestyramine) and half to a diet plus placebo. At the end of the trial, the combination of diet and cholestyramine was successful in lowering average cholesterol level by 8.5% more than that achieved in the placebo group and the prevalence of CHD was 19% lower in the treated group compared with the placebo group. The Helsinki Heart Study was also a placebo-controlled trial of similar numbers of asymptomatic men with moderate hypercholesterolaemia but used the drug gemfibrozil in place of cholestyramine. After five years of treatment, there was a marked decrease in the plasma concentrations of LDL and an increase in HDL in the treatment group, with a corresponding reduction in relative risk of CHD of 34%.

Since these studies, many other similar studies have been published. When the results of 20 trials of cholesterol lowering were pooled, a 10% reduction in blood cholesterol was associated with a 20–30% reduction in CHD. Recently published joint intervention guidelines by the European Societies of Cardiology and Hypertension and the European

Atherosclerosis Society present management strategies depending on the level of plasma total cholesterol and the presence of other risk factors for CHD.

Multiple risk factors

Much of the empirical evidence in the previous sections focused on the individual effects of the three main risk factors; however, it has become increasingly evident that CHD mortality cannot be explained solely on this basis. Analysis of the data taking into account the effects on CHD mortality when more than one risk factor is involved revealed that the risk factors interacted synergistically, i.e. in a multiplicative rather than additive manner to increase markedly the risk of CHD.

The USA Multiple Risk Factor Intervention Trial shows that in males, five-year CHD death rates per 1000 were 17.4 when the individual was a smoker, had diastolic blood pressure of greater than 90 mmHg and cholesterol levels greater than 6.5 mmol/litre. In contrast, when an individual was a non-smoker, had a diastolic blood pressure less than 90 mmHg and a cholesterol level of less than 6.5 mmol/litre then the rate was much lower, at 2.4.

Treatment of atherosclerosis

The weight of risk factors in the development of atherosclerosis may be reduced by a spectrum of activities, ranging from simple behavioural changes to an individual's life-style to direct medical and surgical management.

Smoking cessation is arguably the single most important action resulting in reduced atherosclerotic risk. This will also have other beneficial effects for an individual's health but it should not necessarily be viewed as a simple exercise. Most smokers find breaking the habits of a lifetime extremely difficult and need encouragement, support, counselling and medical aids, such as nicotine replacements.

Dietary control of obesity and/or dyslipidaemia and the instigation of a regular, moderate exercise programme are also positive actions that bring not only reduced atherosclerotic risk but also many other potential health benefits.

Medical management of dyslipidaemia and hypertension may be readily achieved with the prudent use of one or more of the many effective lipid-lowering or antihypertensive drugs now available.

The medical and surgical management of the atherosclerotic lesion itself rather than its clinical sequelae is relatively new. Surgical intervention by means of bypass grafting or angioplasty stenosed vessels provides welcome symptomatic relief for our patients but in itself does nothing to correct the underlying disease process, which will continue unabated. Such a dramatic and expensive intervention should always be accompanied by a careful atherosclerotic risk profile assessment and the correction of the major risk factors. This will only be possible with the co-operation of the patient, which in turn will depend on providing him or her with the facts.

As yet, there is no way to obtain complete dissolution of atheromatous plaques, but animal and human angiographic studies have demonstrated that powerful lipid-lowering drug therapy can halt the progression of such lesions and in many instances result in their regression, with an improved clinical outcome for the patient (Fig. 8.4). These observations place lipid-lowering drug treatments on a new therapeutic level. Previously, they were regarded as merely preventive measures to reduce the overall atherosclerotic risk of an individual; now they may be viewed as active antiatherosclerotic treatments.

Summary

Atherosclerosis is the most important underlying disease process in the industrialised world. It can be most usefully described as a focal, inflammatory fibro-proliferative response to multiple forms of endothelial injury. This endothelial injury is thought to take a number of different forms but may include the presence of modified (oxidised) lipoproteins. The processes involved in the progression of the atheromatous lesion are thought to be reversible and this concept has been the principal driving force behind many studies and new patterns of clinical practice, all aiming to prevent the sequelae of atherosclerosis, namely CHD, peripheral vascular disease and cerebrovascular disease. The major modifiable risk factors that contribute to the development of atherosclerosis are smoking, hypertension and dyslipidaemia. Numerous strategies have been employed in the last 20 years to correct these risk factors, and we are now in a position to provide our patients with sound advice and management based on accumulated research that will allow them to reduce the progression of their atherosclerotic process significantly and, in many instances, even to reverse it.

FURTHER READING

Braunwald, E. (ed.) (1988). *Heart Disease. A Textbook of Cardiovascular Medicine*. Philadelphia, PA: W.B. Saunders.

Gaw, A., Packard, C.J. & Shepherd, J. (1994). Lipids and atherosclerosis. In *Haemostasis and Thrombosis*, 3rd edn, ch. 50 ed. A.L. Bloom, C.D. Forbes, D.P. Thomas & E.G.D. Tuddenham, pp. 1153–1168. Edinburgh: Churchill Livingstone.

Gaw, A., Cowan, R.A., O'Reilly, D., St J. Stewart, M.J. & Shepherd, J. (1995). *Clinical Biochemistry, An Illustrated Colour Text*. Edinburgh: Churchill Livingstone.

Lindsay, G.M. and Gaw, A. (eds.) (1997). *Coronary Heart Disease Prevention – A Handbook for the Healthcare Team*. New York: Churchill Livingstone.

Ross, R. (1993). The pathogenesis of atherosclerosis: a perspective for the 1990s. *Nature*, 362, 801–809.

Shepherd, J. (ed.) (1987). *Lipoprotein metabolism, Ballière's Clinical Endocrinology and Metabolism*. London: Ballière Tindall.

Swales, J.D. (ed.) (1994). *Textbook of Hypertension 1994*. Oxford: Blackwell Scientific.

9

Cardiovascular disease: heart failure

A. M. HEAGERTY

- Heart failure is a clinical disorder brought about by a variety of conditions. The spectrum of signs and symptoms observed depends on the severity of the damage inflicted on the heart and, to an extent, the duration of the problem.

- There is a loss of cardiac muscle in most forms of heart failure. The residual cells undergo hypertrophy as a compensatory mechanism.

- Neurohumoral stimulation occurs systemically to support the circulation by promoting the retention of salt and water and maintaining an adequate blood pressure. These processes are potentially deleterious to the heart if the organ is exposed to them on a prolonged basis to excess.

- The condition is characterised by changes in the populations of cell surface receptors on myocytes and their functional activity. Inside the cells, the genes for alternative contractile protein isoforms are re-expressed.

- The appreciation that compensatory neurohumoral mechanisms can be deleterious to the heart has led to novel therapeutic strategies that not only improve symptoms but also, for the first time, prolong survival.

Introduction

Unlike other specific diseases described elsewhere in this book, the term heart failure embraces a number of clinical presentations and as such can be brought about by a variety of disorders. In its broadest context, Poole-Wilson has defined heart failure as a clinical syndrome caused by an abnormality of the heart and recognised by a character-istic pattern of haemodynamic, renal, neural and hormonal responses. It is caused by anything that can embarrass the pump function of the heart: if there is global myocar-dial dysfunction both the return of venous blood to the right side of the heart is reduced and the expulsion of oxygenated blood to the systemic circulation is impaired. Therefore, the constellation of symptoms that is observed depends on how much of the heart is involved and how severely it is damaged. These will be discussed briefly below. As a public health issue, heart failure is of major importance, with incidence figures acceler-ating rapidly: in the UK in 1988 around 50 000 deaths were ascribed to heart failure. The incidence rises sharply with age and it is more common in men than in women in all ages under 65 years. In 1990, heart failure was the most common cause of hospitalisation in

Table 9.1. *Causes of heart failure*

		Affected chamber		
	Examples	LV	RV	Both
Ventricular contractile dysfunction	Coronary heart disease	+++		
	Infections of myocardiun			+++
	Cardiomyopathy			+++
Increased resistance to contraction and cardiac output	Hypertension	+++		
	Aortic valve stenosis	+++		
	Coarctation of the aorta	+++		
	Pulmonary hypertension		+++	
	Pulmonary valve stenosis		+++	
Cardiac dysrhythmias	Atrial fibrillation			+++
Increased tissue needs	Anaemia			+++
	Thyrotoxicosis			+++
Inadequate cardiac filling	Constrictive pericarditis		+++	

Americans over 65 years. Before the introduction of newer therapeutic agents, the mortality over 5 years was 50%.

Haemodynamics and symptoms

It is the role of the right side of the heart to collect blood from the veins and expel it to the lungs for reoxygenation, the left side collects the resulting saturated blood and expels it into the arterial side of the circulation to perfuse the tissues. If heart failure is regarded as a failure to maintain an adequate cardiac output to the lungs, tissues or both, the consequences and resulting symptoms can be predicted. Therefore, despite the many causes of the condition (Table 9.1), the syndromes recognised as heart failure can be defined in terms of the circulatory consequences; at their most succinct these focus on salt and water retention and peripheral vasoconstriction. The cause can be regarded at its simplest as backward or forward failure. Inadequate clearance of venous blood can be characterised as **backward failure** and reduced expulsion into the pulmonary artery or aorta is **forward failure**. Of course, the two are not mutually exclusive, and in general both occur together, although one may appear to dominate when it comes to the clinical syndrome. If there is left ventricular dysfunction, which is the most common cause of heart failure, a rise in left atrial pressure leads to transudation of fluid into the lungs via backward failure. The consequent symptoms may range from mild dyspnoea to the severe breathlessness seen in overt pulmonary oedema (Table 9.2). The attendant poor forward movement of blood leads to reduced tissue perfusion and fatigue. Right ventricular dysfunction causes backward failure, manifesting as venous engorgement with transudation of fluid into the extracellular spaces. The patient presents with oedema around the ankles if ambulant, and around the sacrum if immobile. The transudation can be widespread, extending to the arms in severe cases and into serous cavities, presenting

Table 9.2. *New York Heart Association classification of heart failure*

Class	Characteristics
Class I: minimal	Patients with cardiac disease without limitation of physical activity; ordinary physical activity does not cause undue dyspnoea or fatigue
Class II: mild	Patients with cardiac disease resulting in slight limitation of physical activity; comfortable at rest; ordinary physical activity results in dyspnoea or fatigue
Class III: moderate	Patients with cardiac disease resulting in marked limitation of physical activity; comfortable at rest; less than ordinary physical activity causes dyspnoea or fatigue
Class IV	Patients with cardiac disease resulting in inability to carry on any physical activity without discomfort; symptoms of heart failure may be present even at rest; if any physical activity is undertaken, discomfort is increased

as ascites for example. Many tissues become swollen: the liver may enlarge in consequence and there may be malabsorption from a congested bowel causing weight loss: so-called cardiac cachexia.

The immediate circulatory response to a fall in cardiac output is the retention of salt and water and vasoconstriction in order to expand the blood volume compartment and hence preload, thereby restoring output to normal. This is brought about by a complex interaction of neuro-hormonal responses, including activation of the sympathetic nervous system as well as the renin–angiotensin cascade. (Figs. 9.1 and 9.2). In the short term, such as in haemorrhage, this may suffice; in chronic heart failure, these processes may ultimately become deleterious to long-term survival by inflicting further damage on the heart. Put at its simplest, these compensatory mechanisms will demand more work from an already compromised myocardium, thereby raising the real risk of cell death and a further fall in cardiac output. This is controlled by a number of cellular mechanisms: activation of the renin–angiotensin and sympathetic nervous systems will lead to increased cellular receptor activation with the consequent mobilisation of intra-cellular second messengers such as inositol 1,4,5-trisphosphate (stimulated by angiotensin II) and cyclic AMP (by noradrenaline). Both these messengers facilitate the entry of calcium into cardiac myocytes. The cardiac response is inotropic and chronotropic, and cardiac output should be enhanced. However, there is the inevitable danger of calcium overload and this can worsen diastolic relaxation problems in heart failure and predispose to transient depolarisation and sinister arrhythmias. Furthermore, although sympathetic nervous system activation may hasten calcium filling of intracellular stores, overloading may accelerate the rate of cell death in heart failure.

Myocardial function in heart failure

It has been established that contractile function in the failing heart is depressed and that relaxation is also abnormal. In many forms of heart failure, there is a loss of normal

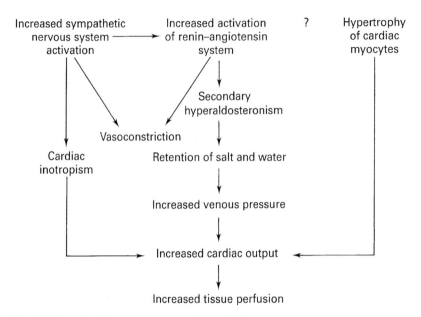

Fig. 9.1. The circulatory response to heart failure.

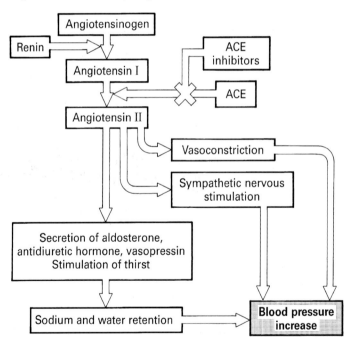

Fig. 9.2. A diagram of the renin-angiotensin cascade. The initial stimulus to renin release is low pressure in the renal glomerular afferent arterioles. The sympathetic nervous system, acting via renal nerves, and circulating cardiolamines, acting via adrenergic receptors, are also involved in the modulation of renin release. Renin cleaves a polypeptide substrate angiotensinogen in the plasma to produce a decapeptide angiotensin I, which is enzymatically attacked by the converting enzyme (ACE) to produce the octapeptide angiotensin II.

cardiac myocytes. This morphological change is not the sole cause of myocardial dysfunction; as indicated above, there are abnormalities of calcium influx and intracellular storage in cells. Disturbances of relaxation have been reported for several animal models, and in humans they are associated with the pathophysiology of cardiac diseases such as ischaemic heart disease and idiopathic dilated as well as hypertrophic cardiomyopathy. In the failing human myocardium as well as in the hypertrophied ferret ventricle, prolonged relaxation correlates with intracellular calcium metabolism. This includes dissociation from troponin C and extracellular calcium extrusion, but it is dominated by ATP-dependent calcium uptake by the sarcoplasmic reticulum. Recently, a reduction in mRNA for sarcoplasmic reticulum calcium-ATPase has been reported in specimens of human ventricle in heart failure. This ATPase belongs to a multigene family, with a single isoform, similar to that from slow skeletal muscle, expressed in ventricular and atrial myocardium. Reduced diastolic relaxation embarrasses ventricular filling and hence cardiac function. The changes in sarcoplasmic reticulum handling of calcium may also be responsible for the altered contractility through poor activation of myofibrillar proteins during systole. In short, there is a fundamental abnormality of calcium metabolism in cardiac myocytes in heart failure, which is of functional importance.

Myocardial hypertrophy and heart failure

It has been recognised for some time that hypertension is associated with left ventricular hypertrophy and that one of the consequences of long-standing uncontrolled hypertension is heart failure. This is the result of the increased load, requiring a greater force of contraction and, ultimately, the myocardial response to stretch falls off the Starling curve (Fig. 9.3). In addition, severe heart failure has been associated with the genetically determined condition of hypertrophic obstructive cardiomyopathy (HOCM) (Figs. 9.4 and 9.5). However, more recently it has become clear that there is hypertrophy of viable myocytes in a failing ventricle, although it is important to note that the cells of the hypertrophied failing heart are not normal. In consequence, there has been a great deal of interest in the molecular and cellular processes that control hypertrophy. The reasons are clear: when the heart is exposed to abnormal loads, such as in hypertension or because of loss of functional tissue in myocardial infarction, the viable cells are overloaded. Hypertrophy adds new sarcoplasmic reticula and improves myocardial metabolism. Therefore, in the short term, hypertrophy will be beneficial in heart failure. But if overload is sustained, the phenomenon may be less beneficial. This is because of the disturbance between energy production and expenditure. Hypertrophy induces capillary rarefaction and changes in oxygen diffusion, and the result can be areas of relative underperfusion in the heart and a further reduction in coronary reserve. Also hypertrophy increases the cell volume occupied by myofibrils, which increases the number of ATP-consuming fibres supplied by mitochondria, thereby worsening any energy deficit. Inevitably the response to this will be a depression in contractility.

The adult myocardial cell is terminally differentiated. Therefore, cardiac growth during hypertrophy is mainly through an increase in protein content per cell with little

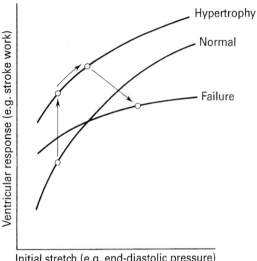

Initial stretch (e.g. end-diastolic pressure)

Fig. 9.3. The Starling mechanism in heart failure. The Starling Curves demonstrate the hypothetical relationship between a ventricular response, as represented by stroke work, and the initial stretch of myocardial muscle fibres, as represented by end-diastolic pressure. The 'normal' curve demonstrates a predicted increased ventricular response with increased end-diastolic pressure. A larger response is seen when the whole ventricle undergoes hypertrophy. Myocardial dysfunction and consequent heart failure produces a flattening of the curve so that a higher filling pressure is needed to produce stretch. This results in a poor ventricular response.

or no change in muscle cell number. In cardiac overload, after pre-initial hypertrophy there is thinning again when the end-stage of heart failure is reached. Cell death stimulates fibroblast proliferation and the replacement of myocytes with connective tissue. This is non-contractile and, in consequence, increased energy needs are placed upon the hypertrophied myocytes that surround these areas of myocardium. Ultimately such cells fail and necrose.

The principal features of myocardial hypertrophy are an increase in contractile protein content, the induction of various contractile protein isoforms and the expression of embryonic markers. An upregulation of contractile protein genes such as that for myosin light chain-2 causes an accumulation of this protein in individual cells. In addition, hypertrophy is associated with the expression of fetal forms of contractile proteins, such as β-myosin heavy chain. This controls myosin ATPase activity and muscle-shortening velocity. The expression of the V_1 (α) myosin heavy chain leads to high myosin ATPase activity and rapid shortening velocity: the expression of the V_3 isoform leads to slow shortening velocity and low myosin ATPase activity. In overload, the V_3 fetal isoform is preferred. By reducing the rate of cross-bridge cycling, contractility is reduced, but coincidentally the tension generated during systole is increased and this process enhances cardiac output in heart failure. Also the V_3 isoform is mechanically more efficient and, therefore, energy sparing, with obvious advantages in heart failure. Fetal isoforms of actin and tropomyosin are also re-expressed in response to failure and

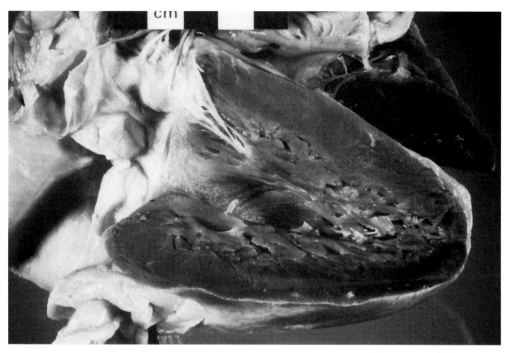

Fig. 9.4. A post-mortem specimen demonstrating severe left ventricular hypertrophy associated with hypertrophic obstructive cardiomyopathy.

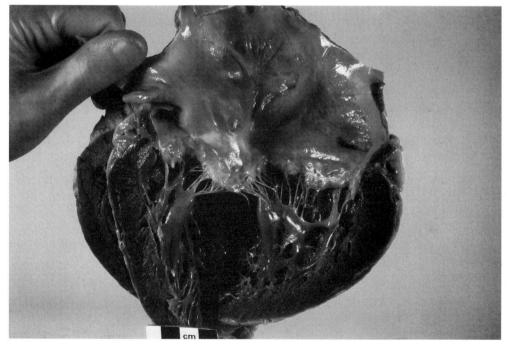

Fig. 9.5. A post-mortem specimen demonstrating severe left ventricular dilatation compatible with end-stage heart failure from a patient with congestive cardiomyopathy.

hypertrophy, although there are regional variations in expression in the myocardium. Finally, changes in isoform expression are observed for lactate dehydrogenase, creatinine kinase and the sarcolemmal pump proteins.

There is also evidence of an upregulation in non-contractile protein genes, such as atrial natriuretic factor. Downregulated after birth, this gene is re-expressed in the ventricle during hypertrophy. There is little information at present concerning the transcriptional regulation of these gene isoforms. It is clear that there are also changes in proteins synthesised in the myocardium as a result of alternative splicing, in which exons of a gene are reassembled in different configurations.

Obviously, as well as changes in contractile protein genes, there is an upregulation in the signals that promote an increase in cell size. In recent years, there has been great interest in these processes. Progress to understanding them has been rapid but is not complete yet. The main stimulus for hypertrophy appears to be an increase in load upon myocytes; how this is perceived is not clear but it may involve an as yet unidentified stretch receptor in the plasma membrane. However, in addition to this, considerable attention has been given to the possibility of sympathetic nervous system hormones, as well as angiotensin II (present in high concentrations in heart failure), being able to produce hypertrophy independent of their pressor effects. Much of the evidence for such mechanisms comes from studies of cells grown in culture, which when exposed to α_1-adrenoceptor agonists, angiotensin II or, more recently, endothelin I appear to synthesise proteins and either proliferate or undergo hypertrophy. The *in vivo* evidence for such mechanisms being important is more difficult to establish. Belief in paracrine contributions to hypertrophy from angiotensin II has been given further impetus by the discovery of the genes coding for the components of the renin–angiotensin cascade in the myocardium and the discovery that angiotensin II can be generated in the heart by a non-specific chymase.

The exact intracellular signalling systems that are activated in producing hypertrophy are also not fully understood. Studies of rat myocardium obtained within minutes after the induction of hypertension have demonstrated increased breakdown of phosphoinositide lipids and the increased expression of early response genes such as c-*myc*, c-*fos* and c-*jun*. Such proto-oncogenes encode a variety of growth factors and their receptors as well as transcriptional regulators. These genes are characterised by their rapid and transient induction, which usually does not require the synthesis of new or additional proteins. It is of interest that pressure overload in the intact heart activates a pattern of early growth-response genes that is similar to that seen in cultured cells activated by α_1-adrenoceptor agonists. Much remains to be discovered to give a complete picture of how hypertrophy is brought about. In this context, it is of interest that there is a genetically determined cardiac disorder often (although not invariably) characterised by gross left ventricular hypertrophy. This is hypertrophic obstructive cardiomyopathy, and some patients may present with severe heart failure. It is defined as enlargement of the myocardium for which no cause, such as high blood pressure or valvular heart disease, is present. This familial disorder is now known to be caused by at least four genes located on chromosomes 14, 1, 15 and 11. The phenotypic expression of other genetic familial diseases in the heart can resemble this disorder but the genes are found elsewhere; for example, in Friedrich's ataxia, which is associated with a cardiomyopathy, the genetic abnormality is located on chromosome 9. In hypertrophic obstructive cardiomyopathy, the disease is often asymmetrical and can affect different regions of the left ventricle, indeed any segment of the left ventricle free wall can be involved or the whole of the heart may be affected. Furthermore, the phenotype can alter in one particular individual with time. Whilst hypertrophy may present initially, it can give way to regression, replacement of myocytes with fibrosis, dilatation and failure. Nevertheless, the typical feature of this disorder is severe asymmetrical left ventricular hypertrophy with the production of a small interventricular cavity. By far the most important feature of this disorder is that it is associated with a high risk of sudden death from cardiac dysrhythmias, although more detailed analyses of family pedigrees indicate that not all patients are at equal risk of this complication and, indeed, in some individuals who carry the gene there appears to be little or no risk. The disorder is inherited as an autosomal dominant Mendelian trait. Put at its simplest, it would appear that there are mis-sense mutations in the β-cardiac myosin heavy chain gene and that these are a major cause of the problem. A point mutation in this gene was reported that resulted in the substitution of a single amino acid residue in the myosin polypeptide. This initial abnormality was found in all affected members of a large family pedigree. Subsequently, numerous different mis-sense mutations have been identified and 11 are single nucleotide substitutions resulting in single amino acid residue changes in the globular head or head/rod junction region of the myosin heavy chain. This cannot be the whole story because now that more families with this disorder have been identified, it is clear that defects in the β-cardiac myosin heavy chain gene account for less than half of all cases. Therefore, the search for other chromosomal abnormalities has been on-going and so far a further three genetic locations have been identified, which suggests that there are also mutations in cardiac troponin-t and α-tropomyosin. In consequence, our knowledge of this condition would indicate that the contractile apparatus of the myocardial smooth muscle cells is defective as a result of genetic abnormalities that breed true in families with this particular condition, but there is no unifying amino acid substitution that explains all hypertrophic obstructive cardiomyopathies.

The most often documented finding in this disorder of the smooth muscle contractile apparatus is hypertrophy of the left ventricle. Progression of this over a number of years has been documented in more than 70% of children with the condition, but most remain without symptoms. However, such progression has not been noted in adults and, in fact, regression may occur, as indicated above. The hearts of such patients that come to postmortem show diffuse scarring and thinning, presumed to be caused by inadequate perfusion of the rapidly enlarging heart muscle by capillaries. The natural history of the disorder in terms of clinical outcome varies: some patients remain asymptomatic, whereas others have severe heart failure or die suddenly as a result of terminal dysrhythmias. At present, it is difficult to predict family members at risk of complications.

In relation to the myocardial abnormalities in heart failure, it is worth also noting that the protein dystrophin has been linked to cardiomyopathies. X chromosome-linked cardiomyopathy presents in young males as a rapidly progressive primary heart failure and in carrier females as a later onset disease with slower progression. Linkage in two pedigrees has been established at the Duchenne muscular dystrophy (DMD) locus at Xp21; the gene encodes for a form of a protein dystrophin that is deficient in patients with Duchenne muscular dystrophy. Western blotting studies in patients with X-linked cardiomyopathy and Xp21 defects demonstrate abnormalities in myocardial dystrophin but not in skeletal dystrophin. This suggests that the dystrophin itself is abnormal and such an hypothesis is currently under intense investigation. Knock-out mice deficient of dystrophin demonstrate muscle fibres prone to sarcolemmal rupture during contraction and this has been interpreted as evidence that it acts to reinforce the muscle during activity. The fact that cardiac failure is seen in a large number of patients with Duchenne muscular dystrophy would support this view. A milder form of muscular disorder is seen in Becker's muscular dystrophy. Here the heart is less frequently involved, but there are mutations in the dystrophin gene. A recent report in such patients who had cardiomyopathies found two individuals with genetic defects around exon 1 in the absence of skeletal muscle abnormalities. Two others had deletions of exon 47 and had more typical features. Therefore, it is possible that part of the dystrophin gene controls expression in cardiac muscle only.

There are other cardiomyopathies that are seen clustered in families and associated with heart failure. The so-called dilated cardiomyopathy is such an example and although the gene(s) responsible are as yet unknown, it appears to be inherited in 20% of cases.

Changes in myocardial function in heart failure

Disturbances in cardiac rhythm

One of the most sinister prognostic developments in heart failure is cardiac dysrhythmias. These may be generated in a number of ways: first ischaemic cardiac myocytes are prone to spontaneous contractile activity and may initiate ectopic beats. Second, hypertrophy itself is known to be associated with both simple and complex ventricular arrhythmias. One of the features often seen in hypertrophy is a lengthening of the cardiac action potential. It has been suggested that at least in part this may be the result of the expression of abnormal isoforms of contractile proteins (mentioned above) or ion channels: changes in the latter would alter the slow inward calcium current that maintains depolarisation during the cardiac action potential. This is an area of intense research activity at present.

Changes in cardiac relaxation

Recently it has been shown that patients with heart failure show abnormalities in cardiac relaxation during diastole. One explanation is provided by the changes in calcium transport in sarcomeres noted above, although again this is not entirely clear, and whilst impaired relaxation would follow as a consequence of these alterations, other mechanisms may contribute. These include the increased diastolic stiffness documented in heart failure as a result of the replacement of dead myocytes by collagen and later changes in extracellular matrix effected by hypertrophied myocardial cells, which have a survival advantage by maintaining mechanical efficiency by reducing dilatation and diminishing wall tension.

Changes in myocardial and vascular receptors in heart failure

As described already, the haemodynamic consequences of the pump failing are designed to maintain blood pressure and tissue perfusion. This is achieved by increasing the hormonal output of the autonomic nervous system and the renin–angiotensin cascade, which amongst other actions will bring about vasoconstriction. But in addition, there is a dense adrenergic innervation in the heart designed to stimulate contractility and heart rate. Therefore, only in relatively advanced heart failure are symptoms and/or depressed cardiac output observed at rest. In heart failure, circulating adrenaline is increased two- to threefold and noradrenaline even more so. The reason appears to be to make available sufficient sympathomimetic hormones to bind to adrenoceptors outside synaptic clefts. In cardiac myocytes, intracellular signals are stimulated by two different internal systems: adenylate cyclase and the phosphoinositide pathway. The adenylate cyclase system couples β_1- and β_2-adrenoceptors linked via the G-protein G_s. In the human myocardium, both receptors are present and in heart failure 40% are of the β_2 type. Functionally, there is increased production of cyclic AMP. The α_1-adrenoceptors couple to phospholipase C and effect the breakdown of phosphoinositide lipids and the release of sarcomerically stored calcium, causing an inotropic effect. Proportionally α-adrenoceptors are present in lower density than the β-adrenoceptors. Two further points should be made: first the phosphoinositide lipid signalling system can lead to increased proto-oncogene expression and cell growth, which may explain the pressure-independent trophic effects of catecholamines described earlier. Second, the adenylate cyclase and phosphoinositide systems may participate in cross-talk. That is, in models with both α- and β-adrenoceptors, β-stimulation may upregulate α_1-adrenoceptor mRNA expression.

An increase in cyclic AMP brings about enhanced contractility by activating protein kinase A and ultimately increasing the phosphorylation of target structures, such as calcium channels, which provoke increased calcium influx. In heart failure, the β_1-adrenoceptor downregulates by decreasing in density. The β_2-adrenoceptor, however, does not alter in density but does uncouple from downstream signals, thereby decreasing the functional response. It should be emphasised that the G protein–cyclic AMP system is the rapid mechanism for managing cardiac performance, and β-adrenoceptor stimulation produces powerful inotropism in seconds. Therefore, overstimulation can be dangerous in the failing heart because it produces an anoxic debt and disturbances in cardiac rhythm by ischaemic cells. Therefore, it is predictably downregulated in heart failure, leading to attenuation in systolic tension. The reduced number of functionally available β_1-adrenoceptors in the heart inevitably leads to a change in the relative ratios of adrenoceptors now present, given that the β_2-adrenoceptors are largely unchanged and α_1-adrenoceptors are if anything slightly increased. This may have therapeutic implications for the development of pharmacological tools in this disease.

Downregulation of β_1-adrenoceptors can be ascribed to decreased gene expression; the increase in α_1-adrenoceptors may be the result of enhanced gene expression brought about by increased β-adrenoceptor stimulation. Uncoupling β_2-adrenoceptors may involve increased activity of inhibitory G proteins (G_i) and enhanced receptor phosphorylation. However, in the human failing ventricle, increased β-adrenoceptor kinase mRNA expression but no phosphorylation of either β_1- or β_2-adrenoceptors is reported. The net result of the changes is that myocytes undergo changes to reduce responsiveness to an already stimulated autonomic nervous system. The difficulty is that only about half of the pathways into the cell appear to be modifiable and, therefore, the cell is still susceptible to potentially significant sympathetic provocation. Certainly it is likely that this provides one of the explanations for the excess prevalence of cardiac dysrhythmias and sudden death in heart failure. Finally, it is worthwhile reinforcing the unique nature of these processes in as much as other receptor populations in the failing heart such as those for dihydropyridines, ouabain and histamine are not changed.

Treatment strategies

Until recently, the management for heart failure was largely symptomatic: obviously if a patient presented with a reversible cause for heart failure, such as disturbance of rhythm, prompt attention to its management is mandatory. But the vast majority develop the condition because of the destruction of an adequate circulation to the heart or the loss of healthy myocytes through primary muscle disease. In this context, the usual clinical course is an inexorable decline in effort tolerance, and death within five years of presentation. Therefore, the natural history of heart failure may be divided into three phases: myocardial insult, the activation of compensatory mechanisms and the development of symptoms resulting from inadequate or deleterious effects of the compensatory processes. The neurohumoral responses to a failing heart have been detailed already: the important point to stress is that a stage is often reached when potentially helpful reflexes in the acute situation also can increase the workload of the failing heart by increasing the resistance against which the heart contracts, ultimately leading to deleterious consequences themselves. The appreciation of this fact led workers to try and break the vicious circle in heart failure. Initially, it was demonstrated that the use of a systemic arterial vasodilator called hydralazine could not only improve the symptoms of heart failure but also improve survival. The rationale for treating patients with this agent, which acts as a potassium channel opener in smooth muscle, was to reduce the peripheral vascular resistance (afterload) against which the heart has to work. A similar approach is also useful in which venodilatation is produced and this reduces the preload on the heart, but the patients develop tolerance after a few months. However, armed with the knowledge gained from these studies, the next step was to attempt to block specifically the neurohumoral mechanisms initiated by myocardial injury. Therefore, a number of trials have been conducted into the use of β-adrenoceptor antagonists to reduce further the sympathetic drive to the heart. Considerable caution has to be exercised in the use of these agents because if employed at too high a dose the drugs may worsen heart failure. However, at low doses they appear to be beneficial in small trials and a large-scale study is currently on-going. However, in this context, the most significant recent advance in the pharmacological management of heart failure is the use of angiotensin-converting enzyme (ACE) inhibitor drugs. These drugs interfere with the renin–angiotensin cascade, which is stimulated in heart failure, and reduce the production of angiotensin II. This is only the second class of agent to alter prognosis and improve survival in heart failure. The reason for its success is not completely clear but may in part be a result of its ability to reduce the overproduction of angiotensin II, which is deleterious to the heart. Other strategies have been less successful: these have included the development of phosphodiesterase inhibitors and the use of antiarrhythmic drugs. In some respects, it is conceivable that the former agents might not have been very useful in as much as they were designed to stimulate contraction in residual myocardium by mimicking the action of β-adrenoceptor stimulation. An excess mortality in patients given those drugs has been noted or a failure to demonstrate superiority when compared with placebo. Antiarrhythmic drugs are being used because in many patients it is believed that death is caused by a terminal dysrhythmia. However, again, some agents have been associated with excess mortality in heart failure and trials have been abandoned. The outcome of studies with other drug classes is awaited.

Gene therapy

Clearly the definitive management of established heart failure would entail replacing the damaged heart. In this respect, one approach is human heart transplantation, but this approach is limited by the availability of donor organs and the later problems of rejection and accelerated atherogenesis seen in the coronary arteries in the transplanted heart. In order to circumvent these problems, synthetic pumps are being developed that can be used either as ventricular assist devices as a bridge to transplantation or as longer-term substitutes for the heart provided that the problems of thrombosis on the surfaces of the pump can be overcome. Another area of promise is to use latissimus dorsi muscle flaps wrapped around the heart and programmed electrically to contract in synchrony by implanted electrodes (cardiomyoplasty). However, in the long term, the major therapy for heart failure will reside in correction of the genes that are abnormally expressed either in inherited forms of heart failure or after myocardial injury has been sustained. Through gene therapy, it should be possible to stimulate intracellular repair mechanisms available to myocytes. In this regard, it should be noted that the muscle cells in the adult human heart are terminally differentiated and the major challenge is to restore the capacity of surviving cells to divide and replace injured tissue. This area of cardiovascular medicine is in its infancy. One of the major problems is an effective gene delivery system. Currently, genes are either being presented in liposomes or via inactivated, not replicating viral vectors (see p. 90). The challenge is to achieve the introduction of sufficient functional genetic material in enough cells to effect a therapeutic result. In the field of post-angioplasty re-stenosis injury, limited success is being claimed with a variety of genes attached to adenoviral vectors. In heart failure, the challenge has yet to be met with any substantial outcome.

Summary

Unlike many of the other exemplar diseases explored elsewhere in this book, heart failure belongs to a discipline where molecular and cellular biology are only now beginning to reveal clues to the mechanisms which underlie its causes. Furthermore there is more than one cause of heart failure and indeed more than one type of the disorder. Some genetically determined disorders of cardiac muscle lead to heart failure and these are mentioned. The physiological and humoral changes to the circulation effected by failure are well recognised and some of the molecular causes of these are clearly understood and described. Where therapeutics have logically interfered with the process they have been described. Major advances have been made in our understanding of heart failure but much remains to be discovered.

FURTHER READING

McKenna, W.J., Beiras, A.C. & Lado, M.P. (eds.) (1994). The cardiomyopathies. *British Heart Journal*, 72 (suppl.).

Poole-Wilson, P. (1993). Relation of pathophysiologic mechanisms to outcome in heart failure. *Journal of the American College of Cardiologists*, 22 (suppl. A), 22A–29A.

Simpson, P.C. (1989). Proto-oncogenes and cardiac hypertrophy. *Annual Review of Physiology*, 51, 189–202.

Smith, W. (1985). Epidemiology of congestive heart failure. *American Journal of Cardiology*, 55, 3A–8A.

10

Neurodegenerative disorders: Alzheimer's disease

P. G. INCE

- Alzheimer's disease is a cortical dementia and a key protein involved is microtubule-associated protein tau, which undergoes excess phosphorylation of its amino acids and truncation of the carboxy-terminal segment. The dysmetabolism of tau interferes with normal neuronal function.

- A second major protein dysmetabolism that characterises the disease is amyloid precursor protein, which aggregates forming senile plaques. These are associated with localised loss of synaptic connections in the adjacent cerebral cortex.

- The major clinical features of Alzheimer's disease do not reflect changes in a single neurotransmitter system. Multiple factors, both environmental and genetic, are responsible for the disorder. Genes involved have been located on chromosomes 1, 14, 19 and 21. The other major risk factor is age.

- The disease is a primary progressive dementing syndrome. Treatment is a challenge for social medicine. Neurotransmitter replacement therapy has had limited success.

- The distant goal in Alzheimer's disease remains to find agents that will stop or even reverse the underlying neurodegenerative processes.

Introduction

The challenge of taking a mechanistic approach to any disease entity is made all the more difficult when the knowledge at cellular and molecular levels is incomplete. This is particularly relevant in the case of neurological disorders. The information available to us from anatomy and physiology studies is abundant, but the newer technology has yet to complement this basic knowledge. Nevertheless, advances are being made: for example, the genes responsible for Alzheimer's disease are being identified, although their functional roles are not clear. Neurodegenerative disorders of middle and later life represent a major and continuing challenge at the levels of care, health service delivery and also basic pathophysiological mechanisms. This chapter and Chapter 11 will focus on the two most common neurodegenerative disorders: Alzheimer's disease and Parkinson's disease. Clinically, these are regarded as very distinct disorders, the former characterised by progressive cognitive failure and the latter by a progressive and characteristic movement disorder. However, a huge biomedical research effort in recent years has uncovered many areas of similarity between all the neurodegenerative disorders of later life, and findings in one disorder have been applied and found relevant to many others.

Several key themes underlie the, presently incomplete, understanding of these disorders and are highlighted in the basic sciences sections. A brief model of all such disorders can, however, be proposed: these are abnormalities in which the selective vulnerability of certain parts of the central nervous system (CNS) is the key determinant of the clinical features. Therefore, it is necessary to review briefly the organisation of the CNS by anatomical region, neurotransmitter systems and function. The selective degeneration of a part of the CNS is associated with abnormal metabolism (dysmetabolism) of the neuronal cytoskeleton, and an account of the normal neuronal cytoskeleton and the alterations in disease is given. This cyotoskeletal derangement is fundamental both to the death and loss of neurones and to impaired function of the remaining neurones. In addition to cytoskeletal abnormalities, there are other molecular pathological events, which are discussed.

The causes of these processes remain enigmatic, although recent research has illuminated many factors that may initiate or sustain the progressive cycle of neuronal degeneration. Since these factors remain speculative, the selection of particular aetiological or risk factors for consideration is based upon current theories, with a focus on those we believe will prove to be important for therapy or lifestyle modification in the future. For all the neurodegenerative diseases, there are a small group of patients with clear autosomal inheritance from whom genetic analysis has yielded major insights. Amongst the great majority of patients with sporadic (non-inherited) disease, there are likely to be important contributions to disease development from both inherited susceptibility factors and environmental factors. Some examples of both types of risk factor (genetic and environmental) are discussed.

The disorders are associated with characteristic clinical and pathological profiles. These typical features are described, together with the neurochemical abnormalities of specific neurotransmitter systems that underlie them. Based on the description of the pathophysiology, pathology and clinical features, the role of existing therapies and the potential to develop new ones are discussed.

The consideration of clinical care and therapy involves several aspects: first, the possibility of arresting or even reversing the disease process, although as yet there are no established therapies with this mode of action for any of these disorders; second, the possibility of supplementing or replacing defective neurotransmitter systems, a spectacularly successful strategy in Parkinson's disease but not yet fully developed for Alzheimer's disease; third, and most important at present, the general care and support required both in hospitals and the community to care for the large and increasing numbers of elderly people who are mentally or physically incapacitated (and often both).

Dementias

Alzheimer's disease is one of the most important and frequent causes of dementia in later life. It was originally described in patients under the age of 65 years (pre-senile) but

Table 10.1. *Important causes of dementia*

Origin	Examples	
Degenerative disorders	Alzheimer's disease:	Presenile onset, senile onset
	Lewy body disorders:	Parkinson's disease, dementia with Lewy bodies
	Lobar atrophies:	Frontal lobe dementia, Pick's disease, amyotrophic lateral sclerosis with dementia, corticobasal degeneration
	Huntington's disease	
	Progressive supranuclear palsy	
Vascular disease	'Multi-infarct' dementia	
	Bingswanger's (subcortical) disease	
	Lacunar state	
	Cerebral amyloid angiopathy	
	Vasculitis	
Acute cerebral insult	Post-head injury	
	Dementia pugilistica	
	Carbon monoxide poisoning	
	Cerebral anoxia	
Toxic causes	Alcohol	
	Organic solvents	
	Heavy metals	
Infective transmissible origin	AIDS-dementia complex	
	Creutzfeldt–Jacob disease	
	Neurosyphilis	
	Post-infectious syndromes:	Herpes simplex encephalitis, subacute sclerosing panencephalitis
Endocrine/metabolic origin	Vitamin deficiency:	B_{12}, folate
	Hypothyroidism	
Other	Tumours:	Primary or secondary
	Chronic subdural haematoma	
	Normal pressure hydrocephalus	

it is now clear that the same disease process produces dementia in older patients. This 'senile' group represents the most common cause of dementia in the elderly. The diagnosis is made clinically while the patient is alive largely by excluding other causes of dementia. Patients who are thus assigned a diagnosis of Alzheimer's disease and who come to autopsy have an 80% chance that the diagnosis will be confirmed pathologically. The rest will have other diseases to account for dementia. Alzheimer's disease is a clinicopathological diagnosis because there is no confirmatory diagnostic test available for use in living patients as yet.

The frequency of Alzheimer's disease as a cause of dementia compared with the other diseases that cause dementia (Table 10.1) is also not known with certainty. In hospital autopsy series, it is 50%, but these data are biased by the pattern of referral of patients for autopsy (e.g. unusual and atypical cases may be overrepresented). Data from epidemiologically representative cohorts of all dementia sufferers are not yet available, and the figure of 50% probably represents a minimum proportion of all dementia patients. However, the frequency of dementia in the population is roughly 5% for 65 year olds, rising to 15–20% in those over 85 years. Therefore, the disease is very common in a group of patients who have an increased prevalence of many other conditions, especially arteriosclerosis. As a result, the proportion of patients with mixed Alzheimer's disease and cerebrovascular disease is likely to be high, and other mixed pathologies may not be uncommon.

In the UK, it is estimated that approximately 500 000 people suffer from Alzheimer's disease of varying severity. Of these, approximately 15 000–20 000 are patients below the age of 65 years.

Normal physiology

Cerebral anatomy

Alzheimer's disease is regarded as a cortical dementia because the main changes affect cortical regions. The functional anatomy of the cerebral cortex is beyond the scope of this chapter, but several aspects are relevant. The cortex has a complex of local neuronal circuits and projecting circuits. In the former, the neurones involved have short axons that synapse locally and are often inhibitory in their effect (using the neurotransmitter gamma-aminobutyric acid (GABA)). The latter involves axons that leave the local area of the cortex and project to many other parts of the brain (mainly these are excitatory and use the neurotransmitter glutamate). Therefore, there is a massive amount of cortical interaction between the various regions. In addition to these intercortical connections, there are projection circuits, both afferent and efferent, connecting the cortex to subcortical structures in the cerebral hemispheres (e.g. basal ganglia) and also the mid-brain, brainstem and spinal cord. Some of these afferent projections into the cortex come from localised groups of neurones which use specific neurotransmitters that are not utilised in any local neuronal circuits.

The brain region of especial importance in Alzheimer's disease is the medial temporal lobe. This region includes the hippocampal formation, the entorhinal cortex and the transentorhinal cortex. These are phylogenetically ancient brain regions that are present in all mammalian species. In humans, they serve a major function in processing new memories but they also have many other functions. The synaptic circuit in this region is shown in Fig. 10.1. The entorhinal region receives axons from virtually all other cortical regions, especially the 'association' cortical regions (i.e. those brain areas especially developed in humans and excluding primary motor and sensory areas). Therefore, a tiny brain region integrates this widespread afferent activity and projects via the excitatory perforant pathway into the hippocampus. Further integrated circuits in the hippocampus result in an efferent axonal output in the fimbria/fornix that projects forwards into a region known as the basal fore-brain, a region including diverse small neuronal nuclei.

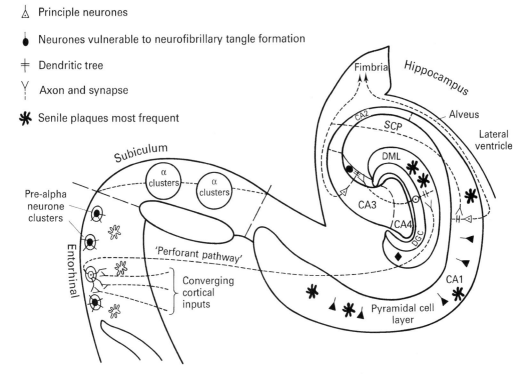

Fig. 10.1. Medical temporal lobe: hippocampus and entorhinal cortex. The pre-alpha neurone clusters of the entorhinal cortex receive afferent inputs from all association cortex regions. These are integrated into output to the hippocampus via the 'perforant pathway'. This projects to dendrites of the dentate granule cells (DGC) in the dentate molecular layer (DML). Sequential synapses of excitatory neurones relay the activity to the fimbria (which is continuous with the fornix) via pyramidal neurones in the CA3 sector. CA3 axons send the Schaffer collateral pathway (SCP) to the CA1 sector, which also projects into the fimbria. The subiculum is also a major source of efferent fimbrial axons. In Alzheimer's disease, the most vulnerable neurones are the pre-alpha, the CA1 and subicular neurones. Degeneration of these cells markedly impairs the function of the hippocampal formation, which is crucial to the formation of new memories. Senile plaque formation is also most frequent in the entorhinal cortex, CA1 sector and the DML.

Finally the division of cortical regions phylogenetically is important in relation to the progression of the disease. The hippocampus and entorhinal regions are an archicortical region, the 'oldest' category. Next are the various areas of 'limbic' cortex (e.g. cingulate gyrus) and finally the bulk of the cerebral cortex, known as isocortex. Whilst the acquisition of memory is mainly an archicortical phenomenon, most higher cognitive function, including long-term memory, is isocortical in nature.

Neuronal cytoskeleton

All cells rely on systems of filamentous structural proteins that act as a dynamic scaffold for cellular function. These cellular systems are especially important in the CNS where neurones need to maintain synaptic activity in axon terminals that may be up to 1000 mm from the neuronal cell body (e.g. motor neurones). All cell types share three classes of cytoskeletal elements (Table 10.2). Two of these – microtubules and microfilaments – are common to all cells. The third class of intermediate filament includes proteins that are relatively specific for each major tissue class. In neurones, this structural element is composed of neurofilaments that occur in three isoforms classified as low-, middle- and heavy-chain neurofilament proteins.

Microtubules are very important in the axon where they play a key role in facilitating fast axonal transport of mitochondria, house-keeping proteins and enzymes, and neurotransmitter substrates to the synaptic compartment. They are similarly crucial for retrograde axonal transport, which may include the delivery of growth factors to the cell body and nucleus.

Pathophysiology of dementias

Cytoskeletal dysmetabolism

The key protein involved in the neuronal dysfunction in Alzheimer's disease is the 'microtubule-associated protein' (MAP) tau (Table 10.2). This is one of a family of MAPs whose function is to facilitate and stabilise the polymerisation of dimeric tubulin into microtubules. The molecule is illustrated diagrammatically in Fig. 10.2. This protein undergoes a number of changes in Alzheimer's disease, which includes excess phosphorylation of amino acids that are not normally phosphorylated and truncation of the carboxy-terminal segment. These changes result from enzyme action but the protein kinases (phosphorylation) and peptidases (truncation) involved have not yet been isolated. The resulting abnormal tau has unusual properties. It loses its ability to function as a MAP and begins to self-aggregate forming fibrillary structures with a β-pleated amyloid configuration known as 'paired helical filaments' (PHF). These PHF are the predominant constituent of the characteristic neuronal inclusion body of Alzheimer's disease: the *neurofibrillary tangle*. This dysmetabolism of tau interferes with normal neuronal function and seems to be a key factor in the degeneration, death and loss of neurones that occurs on a massive scale throughout the cortex in Alzheimer's disease. However, it is important to appreciate that the PHF that are demonstrable by conventional neuropathological methods (Fig. 10.3) are the 'tip of the iceberg' of all the PHF present in the brain in Alzheimer's disease. The majority of PHF is present in the axodendritic compartment of neurones, where it has a maximum likelihood of disturbing neuronal function.

This degeneration is associated with the induction of cellular repair mechanisms. In particular, there is upregulation of the production of a cell stress (heat-shock) protein called *ubiquitin*. This 76 amino acid residue peptide is used to tag abnormal proteins to enter them into proteolytic pathways that result in their degradation. This is achieved by covalent bonding of ubiquitin to the abnormal protein, in this case PHF. The presence of ubiquitin in neurofibrillary tangles has become an important tool in diagnostic neuropathology. The next chapter on Parkinson's disease describes the 'ubiquitination' of the

Table 10.2. *Neuronal cytoskeleton and inclusion bodies in neurodegenerative diseases*

Cytoskeletal protein	Inclusion body	Ultrastructure/ immunocytochemistry	Disorder
Microtubules			
Tubulin	None known		
MAP tau	Neurofibrillary tangle	Paired helical filament or ribbon, 8–20 μm diameter; ubiquitin, tau	Alzheimer's disease
MAP tau	Neurofibrillary tangle	Straight filaments, 10 μm diameter; ubiquitin, tau	PSP
MAP tau	Ballooned neurones	Straight filaments, 10 μm diameter; ubiquitin, tau	Pick's disease, CBD
MAP tau	'Pick' bodies	Straight filaments, 10 μm diameter; ubiquitin, tau	Pick's disease
MAP tau	Astrocytic immunoreactivity	Ubiquitin, tau	PSP, CBD
MAP tau	Granulovacuolar degeneration	Ubiquitin, tau	Non-specific
Intermediate filaments			
Neurofilaments	Lewy bodies	Ubiquitin, αB crystallin	Parkinson's disease, Lewy body dementia
Unknown			
Type 1	Motor neurone disease type inclusions	Ubiquitin	Motor neurone disease
Type 2	Glial cell inclusions	Ubiquitin	Multiple system atrophy

Note:
MAP, microtubule-associated protein; PSP, progressive supranuclear palsy; CBD, corticobasal degeneration.

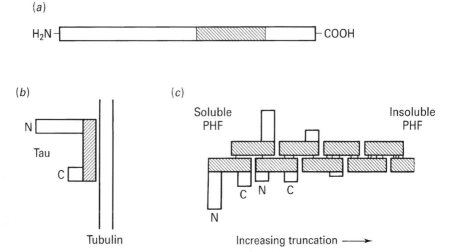

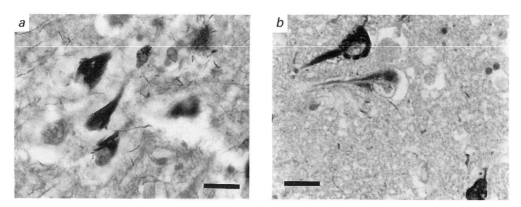

Fig. 10.2. Tau and paired helical filament (PHF) formation. (*a*) Normal tau: the shaded segment forms the PHF–tau and includes the tubulin-binding domains. (*b*) Normal binding of tau to tubulin. (*c*) Self-aggregation and truncation occurring in Alzheimer's disease to form insoluble PHF.

Fig. 10.3. Neurofibrillary tangles: (*a*) Three 'flame-shaped' tangles in pyramidal cells of the hippocampus. The intracellular lesion occupies much of the cytoplasm of the cell soma extending around the nucleus and into the apical dendrite. (Palmgren silver impregnation.) (*b*) Three pyramidal neurones stained for PHF–tau. The morphology of the lesions is similar but the intensity of staining varies. These variations may indicate differences in the cellular metabolsm of the tau protein in the tangle (Immunocytochemistry for tau.) (Scale bars: 20 μm.)

characteristic neuronal inclusion body in that disorder. This pathway appears to be common to all the neurodegenerative diseases and is important in neuropathological diagnosis and possibly in formulating potential therapeutic strategies aimed at preventing or alleviating the cytoskeletel changes that occur in these diseases.

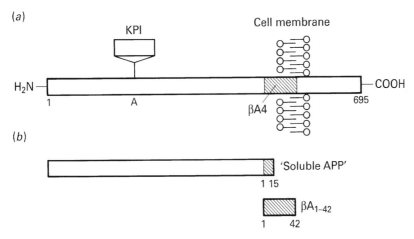

Fig. 10.4. Amyloid precursor protein (APP) and βA4. (*a*) Schematic structure of the full-length membrane-inserted APP molecule. Some isoforms include the Kunitz protease inhibitor sequence (KPI). (*b*) Proteolytic cleavage results in the formation of at least two peptides, shown schematically here. 'Soluble APP' is cleaved at βA4 $_{15-16}$. Production of the larger form – secreted APP – occurs by cleavage within the βA4 sequence. Therefore, this fragment could not give rise to βA4 amyloidosis. Production of the βA4 peptide probably occurs in the cellular endosomal/lysosomal compartment and results in some normal constitutive secretion.

Amyloid precursor protein and the amyloid β protein

The second major protein dysmetabolism that characterises Alzheimer's disease concerns a transmembrane protein called amyloid precursor protein (APP) (Fig. 10.4). This protein exists in several isoforms of varying molecular weights and is present in tissues throughout the body. The normal function of this protein is unclear but it may act in nerve cells as a trophic factor or as a cell surface receptor. Expression of the protein in the brain is rapidly upregulated by insults such as axonal damage in head injury, and it may also have a role in relation to the formation and maintenance of synapses between neurones. The discovery of this protein came about through studies of a small peptide – βA4 protein – which is now known to be a cleavage product of the larger APP molecule. This small peptide contains most of the membrane-spanning region of the APP molecule and is highly lipophilic. In Alzheimer's disease, βA4 fragments aggregate in the cerebral grey matter into an amyloid (β-pleated) fibrillar material that forms an important part of the 'senile plaque'. This pathological structure together with the neurofibrillary tangle constitute the pathognomonic lesions of Alzheimer's disease.

The molecular processing of APP has been very intensively investigated, but the processes by which the βA4 fragment is generated remain controversial. It is now clear that βA4 is a normal cleavage product of APP; probably via a proteolytic pathway involving membrane endocytosis, since this part of the molecule is normally embedded in the cell membrane and the cleavage sites are, therefore, not readily accessible to cytosolic proteases.

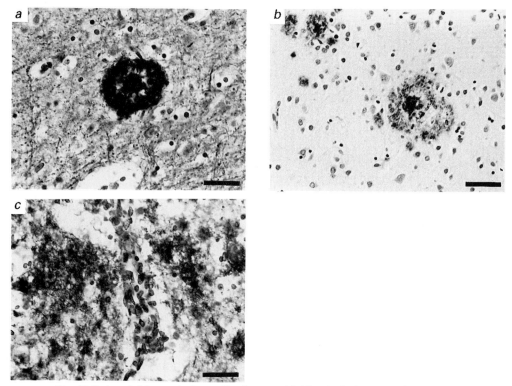

Fig. 10.5. Amyloid protein in senile plaques. (*a*) Classical plaque in the cerebral cortex. The central core and the outer halo of amyloid protein are densely stained. Glial nuclei in the background also stain, together with fine granular and fibrillary staining of the neuropil. (Methenamine silver impregnation.) (*b*) A similar plaque stained for the βA4 peptide. The amyloid halo is less intensely reactive than the core. The background shows a nuclear counterstain (haematoxylin) demonstrating glia and small neurones in the cortex. (Immunocytochemistry for βA4.) (*c*) A diffuse amyloid plaque adjacent to a cortical blood vessel. Plaques with this morphology are frequently not associated with abnormal neuritic processes. (Methenamine silver impregnation.) (Scale bars: 50μm.)

There is similar uncertainty about the processes and conditions that result in the abnormal accumulation of βA4 peptide as amyloid fibrils in the extracellular compartment of the cerebral cortex. It has been demonstrated that the βA4 peptide can be toxic to neurones in tissue culture but it is not clear if this toxicity is an important factor in the loss of neurones in the brain in Alzheimer's disease.

Senile or neuritic plaque

The senile plaque is a key component of the pathological process in Alzheimer's disease (Fig. 10.5). Unlike the neurofibrillary tangle, it is a complex structure involving extracellular amyloid deposition and cellular elements, including neuronal processes, astrocytes and cerebral macrophages (microglia). The senile plaque consists of amyloid aggregation, often with a dense core of amyloid, surrounded and permeated by abnormal den-

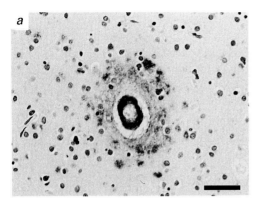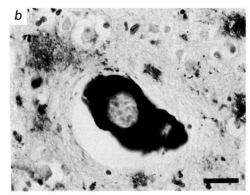

Fig. 10.6. Cerebral amyloid angiopathy in the brain of a patient with Alzheimer's disease. (*a*) The cortical capillary wall is replaced by thickened proteinaceous material in this silver impregnation. Small flecks of diffuse amyloid deposition are present in the surrounding cortical neuropil. (Methenamine silver impregnation.) (Scale bar: 30 μm.) (*b*) A similar cortical vessel stained for βA4 peptide. There is a halo of diffuse βA4 peptide deposition surrounding the vessel. Not all of this may be aggregated as amyloid and it is not detected by the silver impregnation method in (*a*) above. (Immunocytochemistry for βA4.) (Scale bar: 50 μm.)

dritic and axonal processes of neurones, which are distorted and distended and contain the other Alzheimer-related protein PHF. The other cellular elements (astrocytes and microglia) are incorporated with the lesion. This type of senile plaque is usually associated with localised loss of synaptic connections in the adjacent cerebral cortex.

The significance of these lesions is unclear because there is no animal model in which their evolution can be studied. It is likely that the structure arises from both degeneration (axonal processes that are unable to sustain form and function because of PHF accumulation) and attempts at regeneration (additional APP may be synthesised as part of the processes of re-establishing synaptic contacts). Therefore, particularly if the βA4 fragment is toxic, the processes occurring within a senile plaque may be self-sustaining once established. It is likely that senile plaques evolve until the neuronal component has completely degenerated, leaving the so-called 'end-stage' plaque, which only comprises the amyloid core.

Cerebral amyloid angiopathy

Cerebral amyloid angiopathy (CAA) is a process that commonly but not exclusively occurs in Alzheimer's disease. It involves the deposition of the βA4 peptide in and around the blood vessels of the cerebral cortex and the meninges (leptomeninges: the pia-arachnoid membranes) (Fig. 10.6). This vascular amyloidosis is very seldom present in white matter or deep grey matter structures in the brain. It causes vascular thickening and can be a cause of spontaneous haemorrhage into the cortex or meninges. However, it is not associated with abnormalities of the axodendritic processes of the cortical neuropil even when the amyloid spreads out into the neuropil from an adjacent vessel. The amyloid is formed from a $\beta A4_{1-40}$ fragment of APP and is, therefore, subtly different from the amyloid of the senile plaque. For example, this $\beta A4_{1-40}$ fragment may be less toxic than plaque amyloid ($\beta A4_{1-42}$). There is uncertainty about the origin of this amyloid component and it is not invariably present in Alzheimer's disease. Both cerebral amyloid angiopathy in the absence of Alzheimer's disease and the converse occur, although the frequency whereby both processes co-exist suggests common pathogenetic factors.

ALZHEIMER'S DISEASE

Neuropathology

The characteristic lesions of Alzheimer's disease (the senile plaque and the neurofibrillary tangle) are present in varying amounts and in different brain regions in Alzheimer's disease. There is evidence that the amount of senile plaque and neurofibrillary tangle formation is related to the severity of the disease and its duration. However, such data are always derived from cross-sectional studies (examining a single individual's brain only once) and some caution is necessary in making longitudinal assumptions about the way the disease progresses. This problem of interpretation will remain until an animal model of the disease is developed.

In a typical severely affected patient who comes to autopsy, there is a characteristic distribution of pathological changes. They are most severe in the region of the medial temporal lobe, especially the hippocampus and adjacent cortex (entorhinal cortex) (Fig. 10.7). Even within these areas, there is selective sparing of some neuronal groups, whilst others appear to represent the neurones that first manifest the changes of Alzheimer's disease and are the first to be destroyed. The disease also widely affects the neocortex, especially the limbic areas (e.g. cingulate gyrus) and the temporal and parietal lobes. The frontal lobe is often less, but significantly, affected and the occipital lobe shows most sparing. Throughout all of these areas, both senile plaques and neurofibrillary tangles are numerous. In addition, degeneration occurs in a number of 'subcortical' neuronal groups, some of which may be very important in the functional aspects of the disease. In most cases, the nucleus basalis of Meynert in the basal fore-brain shows neuronal loss with neurofibrillary tangle formation. This is a nucleus composed of large cholinergic neurones that send axons projecting to the whole of the cortex and which give rise to all the neurotransmission relying on acetylcholine in the cortex. The locus coeruleus, a noradrenergic nucleus with similar widespread cortical and subcortical projections, and the brainstem raphé nucleus, a similar serotonergic nucleus, are also regularly involved by the disease.

Although the senile plaque and the neurofibrillary tangle are the most conspicuous lesions present in the brain, especially using traditional staining methods, they may not be the best indicators of neuronal dysfunction. It has been shown that loss of synapses is a major part of the pathology of Alzheimer's disease and quantification suggests that at least 50% of cortical synapses are lost from the neocortex. In addition to this loss of synapses, it may be that the function of surviving pre-synaptic terminals is affected by the cytoskeletal abnormalities present within axons and dendrites. This probably occurs in many neurones in which neurofibrillary tangle formation in the neuronal perikaryon

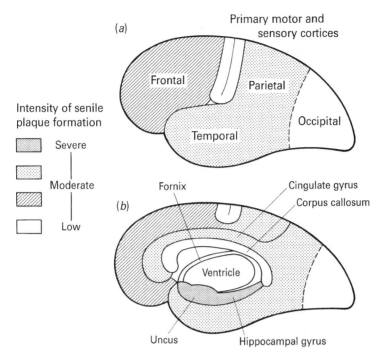

Fig. 10.7. Relative severity of cortical Alzheimer-type pathological changes. (*a*) Lateral view; (*b*) medial view. The medial temporal lobe areas (uncus, hippocampal gyrus and hippocampus) are most severely affected. Frontal lobe involvement is variable and may be equal to or more severe than temporal or parietal lobe involvement. Individual patients may show other variations from the stereotypical pattern.

is not yet developed, and the extent of brain dysfunction will be underestimated from quantification of the neurofibrillary tangles alone. Biochemical methods for detecting abnormal tau in homogenised brain tissue show greatest abundance of tau in white matter and suggest that much of the cytoskeletal abnormality in the brain in Alzheimer's disease is not revealed by routine neuropathological methods. It is possible to demonstrate by histopathology a diffuse element of abnormal neuronal processes, which have been called 'neuropil threads', in the cortex, which may be a morphological marker of this phenomenon.

Correlations have been made between the severity of dementia, as measured by a variety of clinical and neuropsychological scoring methods, and various neuropathological indices. In general, the severity of dementia correlates least well with counts of cortical senile plaque density and correlates best with biochemical estimates of abnormal tau or quantification of synapses. Counts of neurofibrillary tangle densities show correlations with severity of dementia that are intermediate between these other indices.

Finally, a great variety of subgroups of patients with Alzheimer's disease have been described in relation to pathological features. The most frequent of these groups comprises demented individuals with high neocortical senile plaque densities and marked involvement of the medial temporal lobe but who have few or absent neocortical neurofibrillary tangles. Since it is most likely that neuronal changes are primarily responsible for the cerebral dysfunction of Alzheimer's disease, it is still unclear what causes dementia in these patients. It is possible that the phenomenon of abnormal axonal tau metabolism and cytoskeletal dysfunction described above predominates in this group, but in the absence of widespread neurofibrillary tangle formation. The factors that cause some patients to present in this way rather than with the classical pattern of involvement are entirely unknown.

Neurochemistry

In contrast to Parkinson's disease, the major clinical features of Alzheimer's disease do not reflect changes in a single neurotransmitter system. Rather they reflect more global involvement of both cortical and subcortical neuronal populations that utilise a variety of neurotransmitters. Therefore, the involvement of the locus coeruleus and the raphé nuclei in the brainstem is associated with reduced noradrenergic and serotonergic input to the cortex. Many of the cortical neurones involved, and especially the hippocampal and entorhinal circuits, are excitatory and use the excitatory amino acid glutamate (or a related compound) as neurotransmitter. In general, all attempts based on neurotransmitter phenotype to identify specific subgroups of cortical neurones that are either especially vulnerable or resistant to degeneration in Alzheimer's disease have been unsuccessful.

However, neurochemical studies have revealed some features of potential therapeutic significance. This is particularly true of the cholinergic system in Alzheimer's disease since degeneration of the nucleus basalis of Meynert is a consistent and early feature. The specific functional effects of such loss are not known in humans but animal studies suggest a profound influence on memory acquisition, retrieval of memories and procedural skills in relation to memory. The potential role of a cholinergic replacement strategy as a pharmacological therapy in Alzheimer's disease remains controversial and is discussed further below. The neurochemical pathology associated with this degeneration includes features both of loss of afferent axons and of local cortical degeneration. Thus, in the cerebral cortex there is a loss of the enzyme choline acetyltransferase, which is involved in neurotransmitter synthesis and is a marker of presynaptic terminals on afferent axons. The loss of this component correlates with the numerical density of surviving neurones in the nucleus basalis of Meynert. The population of post-synaptic cholinergic neurotransmitter receptors is usually maintained but not increased in Alzheimer's disease. Normally, the post-synaptic response to a loss of pre-synaptic input (deafferentation) is to upregulate receptor numbers. The absence of such upregulation in Alzheimer's disease may reflect the severity of local cortical degeneration and the loss of the nerve cells and processes that normally express these receptors. Thus, the relative inefficacy of neurotransmitter replacement in Alzheimer's disease compared with Parkinson's disease probably reflects the extent of diffuse degeneration in the target regions of the particular neurotransmitter projection systems (i.e. extensive cortical degeneration in Alzheimer's disease versus slight basal ganglia degeneration in Parkinson's disease). Similarly, neurotransmitter replacement within a single system may show little clinical benefit when multiple neurotransmitter systems are abnormal.

Aetiology

Most patients with Alzheimer's disease appear to have a sporadic disease. A small proportion of patients clearly have a familial inherited disease showing an autosomal dominant mode of inheritance (p. 79). It is apparent that multiple factors, both environmental and genetic, can produce Alzheimer's disease. The families with inherited forms of the disease have been of immense value in characterising key molecular events that give rise to the disease, and the various genetic abnormalities that have been described are presented in the first section below. However, even among families with autosomal dominant disease, the clinical presentation within individual patients is in middle or later life. Therefore, these genetic factors clearly operate in such a way that other factors associated with ageing are necessary prior to the development of disease. Clearly, while the role of environmental factors is of major importance, it is more controversial. None of the environmental risk factors currently proposed can be unequivocally demonstrated to cause the disease. Indeed, the only risk factor that undoubtedly operates is ageing. The best model of the development of sporadic Alzheimer's disease involves an interaction between incompletely characterised genetic and environmental factors in the ageing brain.

Genetics

Familial Alzheimer's disease can be divided into those with early and late onset. In general, early onset disease is regarded as having an age of onset below 65 years. Among these early onset cases, there is considerable heterogeneity in the gene mutations that have been described. The chromosomal locations that have been assigned to the various familial forms of Alzheimer's disease are shown in Table 10.3.

Early onset familial disease

Chromosome 21

Interest in the role of genes located on chromosome 21 in relation to Alzheimer's disease stems from the observation that virtually all patients with Down's syndrome (trisomy 21 or chromosome 21 translocation) develop intellectual decline and the neuropathological features of Alzheimer's disease. Clinically, Alzheimer's disease develops in early middle age in Down's syndrome and by the age of 60 years is almost universally present. Interest in chromosome 21 increased when it was found that a small proportion of patients with familial early onset Alzheimer's disease could be linked to this chromosome by restriction fragment length polymorphism techniques. The region of the chromosome that includes the mutant gene was further defined and found to include the gene that encodes for APP. Eventually this gene was sequenced in these families and the presence of a variety of specific single or double amino acid substitutions has been found to correlate with affected members. Therefore, it is clear that minor changes in the amino acid composition of this protein will cause amyloid accumulation and the clinical

Table 10.3. *Chromosomal location and gene products associated with genetically determined Alzheimer's disease*

	Protein	Onset	Comments
Chromosome			
21	APP	Early	Point mutations
14	Presenilin 1	Early	Point mutations
1	Presenilin 2	Early	Point mutations
19	Apolipoprotein E, alleles 2, 3 and 4	Late	Risk factor
Other genetic factors			
Trisomy 21	APP (?)	Early	Down's syndrome related disease

Note:
APP, amyloid precursor protein.

development of Alzheimer's disease. An important point to remember is that all forms of inherited Alzheimer's disease, including the trisomy 21 and the APP gene mutation families, involve the development of a disease that is characterised by both senile plaque and neurofibrillary tangle formation. Therefore, the interlinked cascades whereby APP and tau dysmetabolism both develop can be initiated by structural protein changes in APP. Many APP gene mutations have been described and there is some remarkable clinical and phenotypic diversity. Thus, one mutation (the 'Dutch' amyloid mutation) is associated with a syndrome of cerebral amyloid angiopathy and cerebral haemorrhage with minimal Alzheimer-type changes. These differences in phenotype are very important for molecular geneticists and protein chemists who are attempting to understand the normal processing and function of APP and the way in which these diverse mutations initiate disease.

In Down's syndrome, it is believed that abnormal APP metabolism arises through a 'gene dosage' effect, whereby the presence of three APP alleles is associated with overproduction of APP. Theoretically, this excess of APP might result in an increased proportion that is processed by the pathway that initiates amyloid formation and the Alzheimer's disease process. Neuropathologically, this theory seems plausible because the first abnormal feature in the Down's syndrome brain is the accumulation of amyloid plaques composed of βA4 fragments in which no neuritic component is present (diffuse plaques). These can be present in teenage Down's syndrome individuals decades prior to the development of Alzheimer's disease. However, this model should not be interpreted as applying to all forms of Alzheimer's disease and it is by no means certain that cerebral βA4 amyloidosis is the primary event in most patients with Alzheimer's disease.

Chromosome 14

Familial cases that map to a specific region of chromosome 14 comprise the largest group of early onset familial Alzheimer's disease patients. The specific gene S182 has been identified recently and will undoubtedly provide major new insights into the disease process. Phenotypically these cases are associated with onset around age 45 to 55 years and pathologically there is early and intense senile plaque formation and neurofibrillary degeneration. The functional effect is to initiate the cascade of biochemical changes which lead to all the manifestations of Alzheimer's disease that are seen in sporadic cases.

Other chromosomes

A small number of early onset familial occurrences appear not to map either to the chromosome 21 or to the chromosome 14 loci. The chromosomal location of the gene abnormalities in these cases has also been determined recently and linked to a gene, STM2 or E5-1 on chromosome 1. Both appear to be causative through autosomal dominant missense mutations.

Late onset familial disease

Chromosome 19

A very significant finding in late onset familial Alzheimer's disease concerns the role of the protein known as apolipoprotein E (ApoE). This is known to be a major component of the vascular metabolism of lipids and cholesterol and has been very well characterised in that system. Genetically, it is encoded by multiple alleles that produce specific isoforms, the most frequent of which are $\varepsilon 2$, $\varepsilon 3$ and $\varepsilon 4$. Recent genetic studies in familial late onset Alzheimer's disease have shown that the disease is dependent on the expression of the $\varepsilon 4$ allele. Since all individuals have two alleles, a number of homozygous and heterozygous combinations are possible and Table 10.4 compares the frequency of these combinations in normal elderly people, those with late onset familial Alzheimer's disease and in sporadic cases of Alzheimer's disease. It is clear from this table that it is quite possible to develop Alzheimer's disease in the absence of the $\varepsilon 4$ allele and, therefore, this allele is not a cause of the disease (*cf.* APP gene mutations) but an important risk factor both in familial and sporadic cases. In addition to affecting the age of onset (younger in $\varepsilon 4$ carriers, older in $\varepsilon 2$ carriers), these ApoE alleles may also affect the rate of disease progression. These are recent findings and the metabolic events associated with these different ApoE alleles are not well defined in the brain. ApoE is known to be expressed in the brain, may be synthesised in astrocytes and is present within neurones. It has been proposed that the $\varepsilon 4$ protein may preferentially interact with APP or the $\beta A4$ peptide and stimulate amyloid formation. However, no difference in the total amount of amyloid or senile plaques has been demonstrated between the different allelotypes. Other workers have emphasised a possible role for the $\varepsilon 2$ allele since this is under-

Table 10.4. *Apolipoprotein E allele frequencies in familial and sporadic Alzheimer's disease*

Patient group	allele frequency[a]		
	$\epsilon2$	$\epsilon3$	$\epsilon4$
Normal controls	0.08	0.77	0.15
Spouse controls	0.08	0.78	0.15
Familial late onset disease	0.05	0.55	0.4
Sporadic late onset disease	0.02	0.48	0.5
Early onset familial disease with mutations affecting chromosome 14 and the APP gene	0.08	0.72	0.19

represented in Alzheimer's disease. It is proposed that the $\varepsilon2$ allele confers protection against the disease, possibly by interacting with tau protein and stabilising and reducing cytoskeletal dysfunction. These various interpretations are further confounded by 'cohort effects' resulting from the impact of ApoE allelotype on other diseases. For example, the ApoE isoform from $\varepsilon4$ is associated with an increased risk of vascular disease, including coronary artery disease and cerebrovascular disease. Both of these conditions are associated with significant premature death in the population and will affect the probability of surviving into the age range when Alzheimer's disease is prevalent. For this reason, the frequency of allelotypes in normal young people and normal elderly people need to be taken into consideration when interpreting the impact of ApoE in Alzheimer's disease. A further problem concerns the differing frequencies of ApoE alleles between different racial groups.

To conclude, despite these reservations, ApoE is undoubtedly a major risk factor for late onset disease. While it is not the basis for genetic testing, either for confirmation or exclusion of the risk of developing Alzheimer's disease, studies defining the mechanisms by which these various alleles interact with the abnormal brain metabolism that causes Alzheimer's disease will significantly advance understanding of the disease process.

Sporadic Alzheimer's disease: risk factors

Most cases of Alzheimer's disease, roughly 90% of patients with late onset disease, are not associated with any discernable familial pattern of inheritance. Genetic susceptibilities almost certainly have a major role in determining which individuals will develop the sporadic disease, and one such factor, the ApoE allelotype, has been characterised. These cases must inevitably have other contributing aetiological factors and there has been much interest in determining these. As yet the only proven risk factor is age. Certain 'environmental' factors (e.g. head injury, aluminium) are also strong candidates for a role in the pathogenesis of Alzheimer's disease.

Age

It is clear that the risk of developing Alzheimer's disease increases markedly with age. Therefore, while the prevalence of the disease in 60 year olds in the UK is 2%, this rises to around 20% of people in their eighties, at a rate of roughly 5% per decade. The reasons for this increasing prevalence are not entirely certain. Some of the biological features of Alzheimer's disease also vary with age. It seems that the burden of the neuropathological lesions of Alzheimer's disease in the brain is much higher on average in younger patients than in older patients. Similarly, neurochemical observations show a convergence in the oldest age groups between neurotransmitter levels in Alzheimer's disease and those in normal individuals. These observations may reflect a degree of normal age-related brain atrophy and diminished 'functional reserve' in the ageing brain. Perhaps in a younger brain, with greater initial functional reserve, the disease process must be more advanced before clinical effects are manifested. A related concept has been proposed concerning brain function and cognitive reserve, which may also affect susceptibility. This is the concept of 'use it or lose it'. It is possible that intellectual activity may, through unknown feedback mechanisms, possibly involving neurotrophic factors reduce the extent of age-related brain atrophy and retard the onset of Alzheimer's disease. This is extremely difficult to study in patients. Attempts have been made to correlate age of onset with 'years of schooling' as a marker of intelligence and intellectual development. Even where such studies do show an effect on age of onset, it is not clear to what extent years of schooling actually correlates with pre-morbid intellectual interest and activity in later life.

A final issue concerning age is the possibility that among the 'oldest old' (i.e. patient above 90 years), there may be a levelling off or even a reduction in the prevalence of Alzheimer's disease. If this were so, it would indicate that the disease is not an inevitable consequence of ageing and is contrary to the concept that if people lived long enough all would develop Alzheimer's disease. If a group of patients can be defined who were 'immune' to the disease, their study would be invaluable in identifying susceptibility factors and environmental influences. Such data would greatly assist in directing research into preventitive strategies.

Head injury

Epidemiological studies have repeatedly shown that amongst patients suffering from Alzheimer's disease there is more likely to be a history of significant head injury compared with controls. This does not mean that all such patients have a disease precipitated by a head injury nor, conversely, that a severe head injury will inevitably be associated with subsequent development of the disease. Because of these epidemiological links, attempts have been made to understand the molecular events that may be involved. Bearing in mind the linked cascades of tau and APP dysmetabolism that contribute to Alzheimer's disease, several interesting observations have been made.

First, APP is known to be a protein that is upregulated during neuronal injury (a cell stress or heat-shock protein). Many head injuries associated with coma involve a pathological condition known as 'diffuse axonal injury'. This implies a widespread traumatic disruption of axons in various parts of the white matter of the cerebral hemispheres and brainstem. This damage ranges from complete axonal shearing through to minor stretching and disruption of axon segments and is caused by the movement and deformation of the brain during sudden angular acceleration. It is now clear that one of the earliest pathologically demonstrable features of diffuse axonal injury is increased synthesis and axonal transport of APP. Therefore, it is possible that in susceptible individuals this massive acute rise in APP synthesis results in an excess of APP being metabolised in a way that triggers the amyloidosis pathway. That this may be so is supported by the finding of extracellular diffuse βA4 protein deposits in the brain following head injury. These deposits can begin to accumulate within the first 24 hours of the injury.

Second, it has long been recognised that the cerebral disorder associated with boxing – 'punch drunk syndrome' or dementia pugilistica – is associated with widespread neuronal degeneration and the formation of neurofibrillary tangles. Modern methods of characterising the biochemical constituents of these tangles show that they are composed of abnormal tau protein and are indistinguishable from the type of tangles seen in Alzheimer's disease. Therefore, head trauma can induce altered metabolism of both APP and tau, resulting in changes similar to those seen in Alzheimer's disease.

Aluminium

A major controversy has raged over the possible role of environmental exposure to aluminium in the pathogenesis of Alzheimer's disease. A range of evidence including epidemiology, reports of experimental neurotoxicity, elemental analysis of senile plaques and neurofibrillary tangles, clinical trials of aluminium chelators and studies of aluminium exposure in chronic renal failure have all been cited as evidence. Whilst the extent of these data is considerable, as yet all constitute circumstantial evidence only. Of particular importance are studies of the human brain showing that aluminium can enter the brain using the iron transport pathways and is carried by transferrin. The distribution of transferrin receptors in the brain closely mirrors the regions susceptible to Alzheimer-type degeneration. This whole field is too extensive to be adequately discussed here. It is the personal view of the author that aluminium remains a likely factor to contribute to sustaining the pathogenetic cascade that results in Alzheimer's disease. Whether this applies to the majority of patients, only a small minority, or none at all remains to be determined.

Other factors

A particularly interesting finding from recent epidemiology in Alzheimer's disease is that smoking tobacco products may retard the disease process. Similar data have been reported for Parkinson's disease. A possible biological explanation for this may be the effect of nicotine on the nicotinic subclass of acetylcholine receptor in the cerebral cortex. There is increasing evidence that receptor activation is linked to the activity of nerve growth factor and possibly other neurotrophic factors. This is an area of great potential therapeutic importance since selective nicotinic agonists are already in development.

Clinical aspects: presentation and diagnosis

Dementia can be defined as a clinical syndrome of impairment of multiple domains of cognitive function in a patient with normal alertness and conscious level. Thus, confusional states are regarded as distinct from dementia. The dementia syndrome may be progressive (e.g. in neurodegenerative disease) or static (e.g. following head injury or an encephalitis).

Alzheimer's disease is a primary progressive dementing syndrome, the vast majority of patients presenting in later life (60 years and older) (Fig. 10.8). The prevalence of the disease is higher in women, although the incidence of new cases is equal in men and women. This probably reflects the greater numbers of women than men in these older age groups. However, the possibility that gender is itself a susceptibility factor is a developing area of research interest. The initial manifestations include impaired short-term memory and reduced ability to acquire new memories. Difficulty in abstract thought and disorientation in time and place are also important primary symptoms. Particular problems include language difficulty (word finding and comprehension) and visuospatial dysfunction. The disease process is characterised by inexorabe progression, which may result in an end stage of vegetative existence. Seizure activity may also characterise very advanced stages of the disease. These latter stages are associated with severe physical incapacitation and a cachetic state equivalent to that of malignant neoplastic diseases. Many patients die of intercurrent illnesses, especially pneumonia, but a substantial proportion die through this terminal physical incapacitation. Several stages of disease progression can be defined, and are summarised in Table 10.5. These are important because of the likelihood of increasing dependency that accompanies transition from one stage to another, which has major implications for clinical care and the management of patients. The memory changes in Alzheimer's disease usually involve both early impairment of memory acquisition and a retrograde loss of existing memories. Because of this, patients will gradually fail to recognise and acknowledge people and events in their lives in a retrograde fashion. Therefore, they may forget where they have recently moved to live and may begin to wander. In many patients, such wandering may not be as purposeless as is often perceived but may represent attempts to return to a neighbourhood or house that was previously familiar to the patient. Similarly, close relatives may find that the patient no longer recognises them and loss of memory can thus excise familiarity with the patient's offspring and eventually their spouse, a situation that is extremely upsetting to these relatives. The neurochemical and neuropathological basis for this memory disorder is one of the few areas in Alzheimer's disease where a relatively simple mechanism can be proposed. The early involvement of the hippocampus and medial temporal cortex affects an area of the brain with a key role in the acquisition of new memories. The subsequent and progressive degeneration of the nucleus basalis and the frontotemporal neocortex is presumably responsible for the failure to recall, process or even retain established long-term memories.

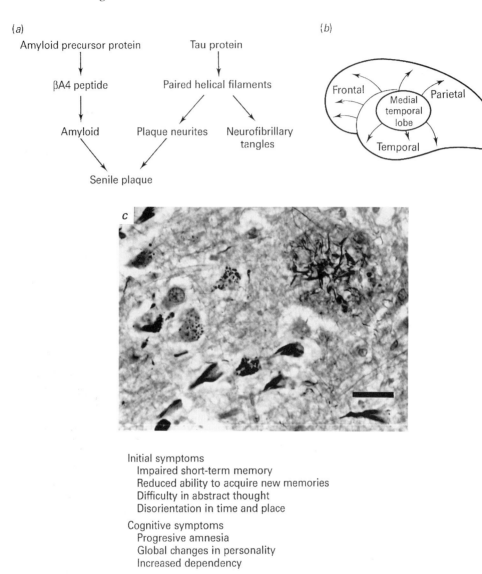

(a)

Amyloid precursor protein → βA4 peptide → Amyloid

Tau protein → Paired helical filaments → Plaque neurites / Neurofibrillary tangles

Senile plaque

(b)

Frontal — Medial temporal lobe — Parietal — Temporal

(c)

Initial symptoms
    Impaired short-term memory
    Reduced ability to acquire new memories
    Difficulty in abstract thought
    Disorientation in time and place

Cognitive symptoms
    Progresive amnesia
    Global changes in personality
    Increased dependency

Non-cognitive symptoms
    Depression
    Hallucination
    Aggression and agitation

Fig. 10.8. Alzheimer's disease: neural changes and the resulting clinical featurers. (*a*) Converging protein cascades leading to senile plaques, plaque neurites and neurofibrillary tangles. (*b*) The probable spread of pathology from the medial temporal lobe. (*c*) Neurofibrillary tangles, granulovacuolar degeneration, and a senile plaque in the pyramidal cell layer of the hippocampus. The plaques appear as dark 'flame-shaped' structures within individual neurones. Granulovacuolar degeneration is the dot-like appearance within other neurones. The senile plaque is stained to show the network of abnormal neuronal processes (dystrophic neurites) which permeate its structure. The amyloid component of the plaque is shown in Fig, 10.5. (Palmgren silver impregnation.) (Scale bar: 30 μm.)

Table 10.5. *Functional assessment staging (FAST) in Alzheimer's disease*

Stage[a]	Characteristics	Clinical diagnosis
1	No objective or subjective functional decrement	Normal adult
2	No objective deficit; subjective deficit in word finding, or naming; recalling location of objects, recalling appointments	Normal aged adult
3	Deficits noted in demanding occupational or social settings	Compatible with incipient AD
4	Deficits in performance of more complex tasks of daily life	Mild AD
5	Deficits in choosing proper attire, and patients requires assistance for independent community functioning	Moderate AD
6a	Requires physical assistance to dress	Moderately severe AD
6b	Requires assistance to bathe properly	Moderately severe AD
6c	Requires assistance with use of toilet	Moderately severe AD
6d	Urinary incontinence	Moderately severe AD
6e	Faecal incontinence	Moderately severe AD
7a	Speech limited to about six words of vocabulary	Severe AD
7b	Intelligible vocabulary limited to one or two words	Severe AD
7c	Ambulatory ability lost	Severe AD
7d	Ability to sit up lost	Severe AD
7e	Abilty to smile lost	Severe AD
7f	Ability to hold head up lost	Severe AD

Note:
[a] The FAST score is the highest ordinally enumerated score.
Source: Adapted from: Reisberg, B. (1986). *Geriatrics* 41, 30–46.

   Coupled with memory loss, there is an increasing inability to function normally in activities of daily life. This may affect the ability to do tasks such as shopping, cooking, housework or household administration, and a change in the role of the patient in a household may be a presenting feature. In addition, there may be an increasing disinhibition or the development of abnormal behaviours including aggressiveness and wandering. A significant proportion of patients have an element of depression, especially early in the disease, which further impairs their ability to function normally. All of these symptoms create major emotional problems for the close relatives and carers who have to cope with a patient with Alzheimer's disease. Because the disease is prevalent in the elderly, there is the possibility that their spouse may themselves be frail, demented or have died. Frequently, patients will progress to a stage where family carers are no longer able to cope and the patient must be admitted to residential accommodation with an appropriate level of general and nursing care. Additional psychiatric features are not uncommon in Alzheimer's disease (non-cognitive and behavioural symptoms). These include visual and auditory hallucinations, delusions and misidentification syndromes. The significance of these symptoms in the diagnosis of Alzheimer's disease resides in the recognition that their occurrence is consistent with the diagnosis. Occasionally, they may be solitary presenting features of the disease. From the point of view of the underlying brain disease, it is not yet clear which neurochemical and neuropathological features constitute the 'substrate' of these clinical manifestations. For some, such as depression, there is a possible correlation with degeneration of brainstem monoaminergic nuclei. For most, the complexity of brain interconnections and function responsible for such symptoms is virtually unknown. When considered alongside the widespread involvement of brain areas by the disease process, it is likely that they result from complex neurochemical imbalances in multiple neurotransmitter systems.

A further feature of Alzheimer's disease is the very marked clinical heterogeneity between individual patients. For both early and late onset cases, the rate of disease progression can be extremely rapid (e.g. two to three years between diagnosis and death) or protracted (15 years or more). Some patients have a very passive illness, characterised by ready compliance with carers and little interest in physical activity, whereas others may be aggressive or show restlessness or wandering. The presence of hallucinations and the other psychiatric features is equally variable. The biological correlates of these variations in clinical features are not yet established and they, therefore, remain unpredictable from patient to patient.

Criteria for diagnosis, clinical ratings and investigations

The most widely used criteria for the diagnosis of dementia are those of the American Psychiatric Association Diagnostic and Statistical Manual (DSM IV). Criteria for the specific diagnosis of Alzheimer's disease have been published in the USA (NINCDS-ADCDA) and in Europe (MRC working party). The American criteria are most frequently used and divide patients into three categories: definite, probable and possible. Only two of these (probable and possible) can be made in life because the definite category requires histopathological verification at autopsy.

An even greater plethora of clinical rating scales have been used to assess the extent of intellectual impairment in Alzheimer's disease (Table 10.6). These involve tests or observations regarding both cognitive function and function in daily activities. They include simple measures (MMSE, Blessed score), which can easily be applied in a routine clinical setting, through to highly specialised examinations (CAMDEX, CANTAB), which are only appropriate in research studies.

In relation to investigation, all patients should receive some form of dementia rating to assess the severity of cognitive deficit. Other investigations are based upon the exclusion of treatable conditions (see Table 10.1) or the demonstration of brain diseases other than Alzheimer's disease that may be responsible for the dementia.

Management and therapy

Despite the abundant insights into the pathogenesis of Alzheimer's disease, the 'cause' remains obscure. Of course there is not a single cause and as a result a whole range of therapeutic interventions may have a role to play. Unfortunately, as yet there are no interventions available that will reverse or even slow down the progression of the disease. Similarly, there are no preventative strategies that have been demonstrated to reduce the

Table 10.6. *Clinical ratings scales used in dementia assessments[a]*

Ratings scale	Scoring system	Comments
Global staging scales		
		Provide an overall clinical impression and an overall estimate of clinically meaningful change in longitudinal course and treatment studies
Global Deterioration Scale (GDS)	7 stages	Stage 4 and higher indicate dementia
Clinical Dementia Rating (CDR)	0, 0.5, 1, 2, 3	Score of at least 1 indicates dementia
Cognitive evaluations		Document and characterise the primary cognitive symptoms including memory dysfunction
Blessed Dementia Scale (BLS-D)	0 to 28	Low scores show *least* impairment
Blessed Information/Memory/Concentration Test (IMCT)	0 to 27	Low scores show *most* impairment
Mini-mental State Examination (MMSE)	0 to 30	Low scores show *most* impairment
Mattis Dementia Rating Scale (DRS)	0 to 144	Low scores show *most* impairment
Activities of Daily Living (ADL)		Rate daily activities necessary for personal self-maintenance and independence
Katz ADL scale	3-point rating of six activities	1, independent; 2, requires assistance; 3, totally dependent
FAST score	see Table 10.5	
Behavioural symptoms		Characterise non-cognitive symptoms commonly observed including depression, delusion, hallucinations and aggression
Geriatric Depression Scale	30-point questionnaire	Either self or observer rated
Computer test batteries		For use especially in research settings
Cambridge Neuropsychological Test Automated Battery (CANTAB)		Based on 'touch screen' use; the tests used are based on animal neuropsychology

Note:
[a] Only the most frequently encountered clinical scales are listed. For a more complete list see Kluger, A., Reisberg, B. & Ferris, S. H. (1994). In *Dementia*, A. Burns & R. Levy, pp. 355–370. London: Chapman & Hall.

Table 10.7. *Therapeutic strategies in Alzheimer's disease*

	Molecular mechanism	Therapy
Neuroprotection: general		
Inflammation	Possible role of cytokines and their receptors in sustaining degeneration	Anti-inflammatory agents
Oxidative stress	Possible role of oxygen-free radical-mediated damage to neurones and glia	Anti-oxidants, e.g. vitamin E, lazaroids
Excitotoxicity	Possible role of abnormal intracellular calcium homeostasis as a result of inappropriate activation of glutamate receptors and calcium channels	Anti-glutamatergic therapy
Neuroprotection: specific		
Beta-amyloidosis	If β-amyloid is toxic and causes degeneration (note that β-amyloid may not be toxic but merely a marker for the disease process)	Drugs to: (i) inhibit proteolysis of APP to form the $\beta A4_{1-24}$ peptide (ii) inhibit $\beta A4_{1-42}$ fibrillisation into amyloid (iii) enhance reabsorption of β-amyloid
Neurofibrillary tangles	If neurofibrillary tangle formation is toxic to neurones or results in a lack of normal tau available to stabilise the cytoskeleton	Drugs to prevent the abnormal metabolism of tau into PHF tau, e.g. phosphorylation of key sites
Neurotransmitter replacement		
Cholinergic	Especially the nicotinic subclass of receptors	Drugs to modulate neuro-transmitters: (i) increased synthesis or release (ii) decreased breakdown, e.g. anticholinesterase (tacrine)
Monoaminergic	Dopamine, serotonin, noradrenaline	(iii) synthetic agonists, antagonists, reuptake inhibitors

risk of developing the disease. However, the biology of Alzheimer's disease as it is so far understood does signpost a variety of theoretical therapies, which are summarised in Table 10.7.

Although it is currently impractical to treat Alzheimer's disease in order to halt disease progression, it is quite possible to manipulate neurotransmitter function pharmacologically to give symptomatic treatment. The neurotransmitter defect that has attracted most interest in Alzheimer's disease is the loss of cortical cholinergic input. It will be recalled that this results from degeneration of the cholinergic projection neurones of the nucleus basalis of Meynert. Neurotransmitter replacement can be achieved by several theoretical routes: increased intrinsic synthesis, extrinsic neurotransmitter replacement, synthetic neurotransmitter agonists, decreased neurotransmitter breakdown and finally reduced neurotransmitter reuptake. The most popular strategy in Alzheimer's disease has been to reduce the breakdown of acetylcholine in the synaptic cleft using an acetylcholinesterase inhibitor. The most widely known drug of this type that has been tested is 9-amino- 1, 2, 3, 4-tetrahydroacridine (THA, tacrine). Clinical trials have reported very varied success in treating cognitive symptoms of the disease with tacrine. It seems that no more than 30% of patients show clinical improvement, which is usually modest and not long sustained. Therapy may be complicated by side effects, including systemic cholinergic symptoms and liver toxicity. However, these can be managed in most patients. Since no other effective therapies are available, this treatment is now licenced for use in Alzheimer's disease in the USA and France, but not in the UK.

The other major pharmacological strategy in Alzheimer's disease is the use of psychotropic agents to control non-cognitive and behavioural symptoms if these cause problems in the general life of the patient. A particular example is the subgroup in whom aggressive behaviour is frequent and disruptive. The most commonly used drugs include the phenothiazine major tranquillisers and drugs such as haloperidol. The phenothiazines, in particular, interact with dopaminergic neurotransmission and may cause extrapyramidal (parkinsonian) side effects. In modern psychogeriatric practice, such drugs are used only with care and monitoring to ensure that the side effects are minimised. The role of other drugs with known activity in the brain (e.g. selective serotonin reuptake inhibitors) has not been established but they may be of use in the treatment of other psychological features, such as depression.

The distant goal of therapy in Alzheimer's disease remains to find agents that will stop or even reverse the underlying neurodegenerative processes.

It is very important to acknowledge the extent to which the management of Alzheimer's disease on a practical level at present is concerned with social medicine as much as with therapeutics. Once the diagnosis has been made, there remains the responsibility to assist in maximising the care and assistance given to patients, with their carers matched appropriately to need as the disease progresses. This requires a multidisciplinary approach in which geriatricians, psychogeriatricians and general practitioners work with many professional and lay groups to optimise care and minimise stress and suffering. The involvement of general physicians and surgeons to treat intercurrent illness must be seriously considered. Such illness may cause deterioration of mental function that is reversible, but a diagnosis of co-existent Alzheimer's disease often causes reluctance to consider such treatments. The correct clinical decision can only be made by careful evaluation of the underlying severity of the dementing syndrome.

Summary

All the major neurodegenerative disorders are conditions of later life, even when they are genetically determined as autosomal dominant diseases. Therefore, ageing is a constant requirement for the development of these conditions and is the single most important risk factor.

All these disorders result in neuronal degeneration that is characterised by dysfunction of the cytoskeleton. This frequently manifests itself as specific inclusion bodies whose major constituent proteins are presumed to be the primary molecular target in the disorder. However neuronal death and dysfunction are not necessarily caused by these lesions *per se*. They may simply be markers of aberrant processing that depletes the neurone of sufficient normal cytoskeletal elements to function adequately.

All of the neurodegenerative disorders show some degree of selective vulnerability in that specific neuronal systems, nuclei or regions are affected to varying degrees. Some parts of the brain are usually unaffected, except at very late stages. The determinants of the differing patterns of selective vulnerability in each of the disorders are not yet understood and are likely to be a direct consequence of the particular pathogenetic factors operating.

REFERENCES

Burns, A. and Levy, R. (1993). *Dementia*. London: Chapman & Hall.

Davidson, F.G. (1995). *Alzheimer's. A Practical Guide for Carers to Help you Through the Day*. London: Piatkus.

Davies, D.C. (ed.) (1988). *Current Problems in Neurology, 11: Alzheimer's Disease*. London: Libbey.

Wilcock, G.K. (ed.) (1993). *The Management of Alzheimer's Disease*. Petersfield, UK: Wrightson Biomedical.

Wurtman, R.J., Corkin, S., Growdon, J.H. and Ritta-Walker, E. (eds.) *Advances in Neurology*, Vol. 51, *Alzheimer's Disease*, pp. 1–78. New York: Raven Press.

11

Neurodegenerative disorders: Parkinson's disease

D. J. BURN

- Animal models of Parkinson's disease have indicated that there is a significant increase in tonic neuronal activity in the globus pallidus and the subthalamic nucleus. The net effect is to produce increased inhibitory output to the ventrolateral thalamus. The Lewy inclusion body is always present.

- The main neurochemical feature of Parkinson's disease is a decrease in brain dopamine concentration resulting from degeneration of central dopaminergic neurones.

- Recent studies have suggested that Parkinson's disease is caused by a combination of environmental and genetic factors, although simple Mendelian genetics will not account for most cases. A number of genes probably each make small contributions to an individual's susceptibility.

- Clinical features usually begin unilaterally in an arm or leg with slowness and poverty of movement. Many patients have a rest tremor. Therapy focuses upon restoring dopamine levels in the central nervous system. Life expectancy is now near normal.

Introduction

Originally described as 'the shaking palsy' by James Parkinson in 1817, Parkinson's disease is one of the most common neurodegenerative diseases encountered by the neurologist. The identification of a profound deficiency of the neurotransmitter dopamine in the basal ganglia of patients with Parkinson's disease in the early 1960s led to the development of replacement therapy and the transformation of patients' lives. Although problems may occur in the long term with drug treatment of these patients, no other neurodegenerative disorder can, to date, be treated as effectively.

Based upon a tetrad of bradykinesia, resting tremor, rigidity and postural instability, the clinical diagnosis of Parkinson's disease would seem to be straightforward. In recent years, however, it has become clear that the clinicopathological correlation may not be as accurate as assumed previously. Several large series have yielded remarkably consistent figures suggesting that an ante-mortem diagnosis of Parkinson's disease is correct in only 70 to 80% of patients. Such error rates are more than of academic interest, since they may seriously affect conclusions that are drawn from epidemiological and therapeutic studies. Like Alzheimer's disease (Chapter 10), the ultimate diagnosis of Parkinson's disease is a pathological one, since ancillary ante-mortem tests are of limited help.

In this chapter, the anatomy of the basal ganglia will first be briefly reviewed, since dysfunction of these areas of the brain and their allied nuclei play a fundamental role in the pathogenesis of parkinsonian symptomatology. Next, the characteristic neuronal inclusion of Parkinson's disease, the Lewy body, will be considered including its relationship to normal ageing and the so-called subclinical disease state. Neurotransmitter defects, especially that of dopamine, will conclude the basic science section.

The clinical section will then deal with the epidemiology of Parkinson's disease, potential pathogenetic factors, the clinical diagnosis of the condition and its management, including both current and possible future strategies.

Physiology

The anatomy of the basal ganglia

The chief nuclei of the basal ganglia are the striatum (sometimes referred to as the neostriatum) and the pallidum, or globus pallidus. The striatum is subdivided into both dorsal and ventral compartments. The former comprises caudate and putamen, while the ventral striatum is composed of the ventral continuation of the caudate and putamen, the nucleus accumbens septi and parts of the olfactory tubercle. The globus pallidus is composed of internal and external segments and the ventral pallidum. The amygdala is also part of the basal ganglia but will not be considered any further here.

Two other nuclei, the substantia nigra, located in the mid-brain, and the subthalamic nucleus, in the diencephalon, are closely allied to the basal ganglia in functional terms (see Fig. 11.1). The substantia nigra is itself subdivided into the dopamine-rich pars compacta and the dopamine-poor pars reticulata. The latter, histologically and functionally, is closely related to the globus pallidus, internal segment; together both constitute the main output nuclear complex of the basal ganglia.

The internal architecture of the striatum is complex, and in the mammalian fore-brain is a mosaic of two interdigitating, neurochemically distinct compartments. These two compartments, the 'patch' (or 'striosomes') and 'matrix', have distinct afferent and efferent connections and, thus, appear to be functionally distinct. There is, for instance, a topographic arrangement of corticostriatal afferents, with cortical inputs to the patch compartment originating from the deep layer V and layer VI of the cortex, while those to the matrix arise from superficial layer V and the supragranular layers. The patch and matrix compartments may be linked by somatostatin-positive interneurones.

A number of peptide neurotransmitters co-localise with GABA in striatal efferent neurones. The arrangement of these neurones into discrete pathways and their relationship with the globus pallidus (both internal and external segments) and subthalamic nucleus are of central importance in current theories of basal ganglia function and pathophysiology. While there is good evidence for the existence of several basal ganglia–thalamo-cortical circuits, each with different functions, only the so-called 'motor circuit' will be

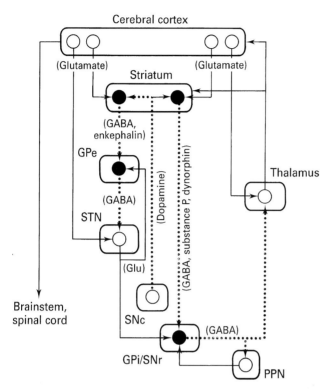

Fig. 11.1. Simplified diagram showing the relationship between the striatum and the pallidum. GPi and GPe, globus pallidus pars interna and externa, respectively; PPN, pedunculopontine nucleus; SNc, substantia nigra, pars compacta, SNr, substantia nigra, pars reticulata; STN, subthalamic nucleus. Inhibitory pathways are dotted; excitatory pathways are continuous.

considered further, since this is of direct relevance to the pathogenesis of Parkinson's disease.

The main pathways involved in the 'motor circuit' are shown in Fig. 11.1. In primates, the basal ganglia motor pathways are focused principally on the putamen and its connections. This part of the neostriatum receives topographic projections from the primary motor cortex and from at least two pre-motor areas. The putamen also receives topographic projections from the primary somatosensory cortex and from the somatosensory association cortex. The terminal fields of these projections occupy the bulk of the putamen, the nerve endings converging upon medium-sized, densely spiny neurones.

As Fig. 11.1 illustrates, there are two distinct groups of striatopallidal efferents. One group, whose cell bodies are preferentially located in the striatal patches, projects directly to the internal globus pallidus and substantia nigra, pars reticulata complex. This is often referred to as the 'direct ' pathway. The terminal fields of these striatopallidal neurones stain heavily for substance P, dynorphin and GABA. The other group of striatal efferent neurones, which originate in both the striatal patches and the matrix, project to the external globus pallidus, which, in turn, projects via the subthalamic nucleus to the internal globus pallidus and substantia nigra, pars reticulata. This pathway is known as the 'indirect' pathway. The terminal fields of these striatopallidal neurones stain heavily for enkephalin, as well as for GABA. The internal globus pallidus and substantia nigra, pars reticulata project, in turn, to ventral thalamic nuclei. The motor circuit is closed by means of thalamocortical projections to the supplementary motor area.

The dense dopaminergic projection from the substantia nigra, pars compacta to the neostriatum is of crucial importance in the control of movement. The effect of this projection upon striatal neurones depends upon the post-synaptic dopamine receptor subgroup. Within striatal patches, dopamine receptors are mainly D_1 in type, and dopamine exerts an excitatory effect upon the striatopallidal efferents. By contrast, in the matrix, dopamine receptors are largely D_2, and dopamine inhibits these striatal efferents.

Figure 11.1 does not show the striatonigral pathway. This inhibitory projection contains not only GABA, but also enkephalin, dynorphin and substance P. A close anatomical relationship between enkephalinergic striatonigral terminals and dopaminergic neurones in the substantia nigra has been demonstrated.

Animal models of Parkinson's disease have indicated that there is a significant increase in tonic neuronal activity in both pallidal segments as well as in the subthalamic nucleus. This occurs through the divalent action of the nigrostriatal dopaminergic projection to the putamen. Loss of the inhibitory dopaminergic projection feeding into the indirect pathway leads to increased activity of the inhibitory neurones projecting to the globus pallidus external segment. Inhibitory output to the subthalamic nucleus is, therefore, reduced, leading to a relative overactivity of excitatory projections from this nucleus to the globus pallidus internal segment. The loss of excitatory nigrostriatal dopaminergic input to the directly projecting striopallidal neurones reduces what would otherwise be an inhibitory influence upon the output nuclear complex of the basal ganglia (see Fig. 11.1). In Parkinson's disease, there is, therefore, an overactivity in the indirect pathway and a reduction in activity of the direct pathway feeding into the globus pallidus external segment (as well as the substantia nigra, pars reticulata). The net effect is to produce increased inhibitory output to the ventrolateral thalamus, leading to excessive inhibition of thalamocortical neurones. One theory of the pathogenesis of bradykinesia, which is core to the diagnosis of Parkinson's disease, is that reduced tonic activity in these thalamocortical projections lessens the responsivity of the pre-central motor fields that are engaged by the motor circuit.

The Lewy body

The Lewy body is a hyaline eosinophilic neuronal inclusion body that is always present in Parkinson's disease. These inclusions were first described at the beginning of the twentieth century by Friederich H. Lewy. The Lewy body is not, however, pathognomonic for Parkinson's disease and may occur in a number of other disorders (see Table 11.1). These other conditions are mostly familial, occur at a young age and are associated with other pathological lesions. Furthermore, while Lewy bodies are always present in

Table 11.1. *Conditions in which Lewy bodies may found*

Parkinson's disease
Asymptomatic (pre-clinical) Parkinson's disease
Lewy body dementia
Subacute sclerosing panencephalitis
Autosomal dominant olivopontocerebellar atrophy
Joseph disease
Hallervorden–Spatz disease
Ataxia telangiectasia
Familial motor neurone disease
Neuroaxonal dystrophy

Parkinson's disease, they are not invariably present in these other disorders: they are reported in only 10–15% of patients with Hallervorden–Spatz disease, for example.

Classical Lewy bodies occur in monoaminergic and cholinergic neurones of the brainstem, diencephalon, basal fore-brain, cerebral cortex and autonomic ganglia. In the brainstem and basal fore-brain (brainstem-type Lewy bodies), the Lewy bodies are usually round and 5–25 μm in diameter, with a spherical dense hyaline core surrounded by a pale-staining halo. Ultrastructurally, the body is formed from aggregated filament, 8–10 nm in diameter, arranged in a radially orientated or haphazard formation. The dense osmiophilic core is composed of granular and vesicular material.

Cortical Lewy bodies are generally smaller, with no distinct core and are located in the small to medium-sized pyramidal neurones of deeper cortical layers. The amygdala, insular cortex, cingulate gyrus and frontotemporal neocortex are sites where cortical Lewy bodies are found in greatest numbers. The application of immunohistochemical techniques such as anti-ubiquitin immunohistochemistry has made the detection of these inclusions far easier than was possible using conventional staining methods. Further phenotypes of Lewy body are located in the sympathetic ganglia (serpiginous in shape), basal fore-brain and certain brainstem nuclei, such as the dorsal motor nucleus of the vagus (non-spherical, not confined to the neuronal perikarya). It is currently believed that variations in the morphology of the Lewy bodies relate to developmental stage and location. The typical neuropathology of Parkinson's disease and the associated distribution of the Lewy bodies will be described below but, suffice it to say, the distribution is relatively restricted to monominergic neurones, raising the possibility of an intrinsic vulnerability of these neurones to Lewy body formation.

The ultrastructural similarity of the Lewy body filaments and neurofilaments led to the investigation of the cytoskeletal composition of Lewy bodies, using immunohistochemical methods from 1983 onwards. So far, 26 antigenic determinants have been detected in Lewy bodies and these may be divided into four groups (Table 11.2).

Group 1 antigenic determinants are postulated to be structural elements of the Lewy body fibril. Neurofilaments are composed of three subunits, with molecular masses of about 70 kDa (neurofilament-light, NF-L), 150 kDa (neurofilament-medium, NF-M) and 200 kDa (neurofilament-heavy, NF-H), which form polymers. There is a differential

Table 11.2. *The division of some of the molecular components of Lewy bodies into four antigenic groups*

Antigenic group	Functional status	Molecular components
1	Structural elements of the Lewy body fibril	Neurofilaments (NF-L, NF-M, NF-H), gelsolin-related amyloid protein[a]
2	Proteins implicated in cellular response to fibrils	Ubiquitin, ubiquitin carboxy-terminal hydroxylase, ingestin,[b] α2-macroglobulin, αB-crystallin, complement
3	Enzymes of phosphorylation dephosphorylation system	Calcium–calmodulin-dependent kinase II
4	Passively diffusing cytosolic proteins	TH, high-molecular-weight MAPs, calbindin, tubulin

Notes:
TH, tyrosine hydroxylase; MAP, microtubule-associated proteins; NF-(L,M,H), light, medium and heavy molecular subunits of neurofilaments, respectively.
[a] Single or limited studies, so classification should be interpreted with caution.
[b] Ingestin is also known as multicatalytic proteinase.

distribution of these epitopes within the Lewy body. For example, monoclonal antibodies directed against carboxy-termini of NF-M and NF-H label Lewy bodies with a peripheral accentuation, while antibodies directed against NF-L, and those directed against the amino-termini of NF subunits, label Lewy bodies diffusely. The reason for the differential distribution of these epitopes is at present uncertain. Both heavily and minimally phosphorylated epitopes of NF-H are found within Lewy bodies. Although there has been some debate, it is generally agreed that there is a lack of tau immunoreactivity in Lewy bodies. One study has suggested that antibodies to gelsolin-related amyloid may label both cortical and brainstem Lewy bodies; this protein would thus represent a major structural component of the inclusions.

Group 2 proteins are involved in non-lysosomal ATP-dependent protein degradation (see Table 11.2 for individual proteins). They are evenly distributed throughout the Lewy body, implying the uniform presence of proteolytic activity. Ubiquitin is one of the group 2 proteins and is a small protein of 76 amino acid residues that is found universally in plants and animals. It is synthesised in response to a range of cellular insults and becomes linked to abnormal proteins or proteins undergoing rapid turnover. It is, at present, unclear whether the presence of ubiquitin in Lewy bodies is indicative of saturation of the ubiquitin-dependent protein degradation pathway, leading to fibril accumulation, or whether it is related to ineffective proteolysis owing to abnormalities in the substrate protein or the degradative pathway. One possible explanation is that, because of post-translational modification in the phosphorylation of the structural elements of the Lewy body, resistance to the effects of ubiquitin and ingestin is conferred upon these elements. Although αB-crystallin is only found in around 10% of Lewy bodies, it is almost never detected in neurofibrillary tangles, suggesting a specific role in Lewy body pathogenesis for this heat-shock promoter.

Enzymes of the phosphorylation/dephosphorylation system constitute group 3 proteins. Again their presence leads to a constant theme underpinning the formation of Lewy bodies: that there is faulty phosphorylation or dephosphorylation of structural proteins as a key event. This is, therefore, a common feature to the possible aetiopathogenesis of both Alzheimer's disease (Chapter 10) and Parkinson's disease. Either hyperphosphorylation or phosphorylation at abnormal sites in neurofilaments and other structural epitopes could conceivably confer resistance to phosphatases and proteases, leading to accumulation of these proteins.

Group 4 proteins (Table 11.2) are likely to be passively acquired components of the Lewy body, diffusing in from the surrounding cytosol, and are not clearly involved in fibrillogenesis.

To summarise, the constitution of Lewy bodies is becoming clearer by the use of immunohistochemistry. The processes by which these constituents aggregate and are modified to form the inclusions is, however, far less certain. It seems that the self-assembly and aggregation of protein, possibly accelerated by altered phosphorylation (post-translational processing), are key events. Insoluble Lewy body neurofilaments may undergo degradation by proteolysis. Until an experimental model becomes available to study Lewy body formation, such schemes will, however, remain purely speculative.

PARKINSON'S DISEASE

Neuropathology

The distribution of Lewy bodies and their predilection for monoaminergic neurones is discussed above. In Parkinson's disease, the involvement of pigmented brainstem nuclei is characteristic, particularly in the substantia nigra and locus coeruleus. Macroscopically, the brain of a patient with Parkinson's disease may show depigmentation of these nuclei, with few other changes evident. Microscopically, the power of the Lewy body as an indicator of Parkinson's disease is such that disease is excluded if they are absent in two unilateral 7 μm nigral sections, 330 pigmented nigral neurones or 150 pigmented neurones in the locus coeruleus. The neuropathological accompaniments of the Lewy bodies are neuronal loss and slight-to-moderate gliosis. Neuronal loss is also observed in the dorsal motor nucleus of the vagus, with variable involvement of the nucleus basalis of Meynert and other subcortical nuclei. The occurrence of cortical-type Lewy bodies in Parkinson's disease is currently being debated, with some claiming that with anti-ubiquitin immunocytochemistry Lewy bodies are *always* seen, while others have reported the absence of such cortical inclusion bodies in some patients, despite careful searching.

The process involving the substantia nigra is not homogenous, and it is the ventrolateral tier of the pars compacta part of this nucleus that bears the brunt of neuronal loss. Specifically, it is the melanised (pigmented) neurones of the ventrolateral tier that are targeted, with a 60–70% loss being typical, compared with a loss of only 25% non-pigmented neurones. This suggests that the non-melanised cells are more resistant to neuronal damage, a phenomenon perhaps in part mediated by the presence of higher concentrations of the calcium-binding protein calbindin in these neurones. Although an attractive hypothesis, neither the presence of melanin nor the lack of calbindin can satisfactorily explain the neuronal susceptibility in Parkinson's disease, since the nucleus basalis of Meynert (which is affected by Lewy body formation and cell loss) contains calbindin and is devoid of melanin.

Neurones from the ventrolateral tier of the substantia nigra, pars compacta project preferentially to the putamen. As explained above, the putamen is important in the control of movement through so-called motor loops feeding back to the ventral thalamus. Unlike several other forms of parkinsonism, the striatum is spared in Parkinson's disease, and transynaptic degeneration does not seem to occur.

Incidental Lewy body disease and pre-clinical Parkinson's disease

Incidental Lewy body disease comprises patients coming to post-mortem who in life had no evidence of parkinsonism, but in whom Lewy bodies are found on examination of the substantia nigra and/or locus coeruleus. Such patients are, on balance, felt to represent pre-clinical incidents of Parkinson's disease, though some have suggested that incidental Lewy bodies are a feature of normal ageing. This seems unlikely from pathological studies, where the microarchitecture of the substantia nigra has been studied in controls of varying age and in Parkinson's disease patients. When the pars compacta of the caudal substantia nigra is divided into ventral and dorsal tiers, a linear fallout of pigmented neurones with advancing age has been observed in control brains, preferentially affecting the dorsal tier. In patients with Parkinson's disease, an exponential loss of pigmented neurones has been found when loss is plotted against clinical disease duration, with a pattern of nigral regional loss opposite to that of normal ageing (i.e. affecting the ventrolateral tier most and the dorsal tier least). In cases of incidental Lewy body disease, cell loss has been found to be confined to the ventrolateral tier of the substantia nigra, congruent with the ventrolateral selectivity of symptomatic Parkinson's disease. On the basis of these findings, it seems probable that incidental Lewy body disease represents a pre-symptomatic phase of Parkinson's disease.

How extensive is incidental Lewy body disease? In a number of pathological series, incidental Lewy body-positive patients comprised those where the inclusions were found in the substantia nigra and/or the locus coeruleus. There were some important differences in case ascertainment between the different series. For instance, in the majority, causes of death were a wide range of neuropsychiatric and systemic diseases. Some, however, excluded any patient coming to post-mortem with a history of overt dementia, to avoid inadvertent inclusion of cortical (or diffuse) Lewy body disease (see below). Notwithstanding methodological differences, with increasing age there is a general rise in the prevalence of incidental Lewy body disease; this reaches a maximum of 14.4% in the 80- to 89-year-old group. Estimates of the overall prevalence of Lewy bodies in the population over age 60 are approximately 10%, whereas the frequency of Parkinson's disease in the living population over the age of 40 is only between 0.35 and 0.40%. It has been calculated that, at any given date, perhaps no more than 1 in 15 patients with nigral Lewy bodies over the age of 40 will have clinically identifiable Parkinson's disease.

If incidental Lewy body cases truly represent pre-clinical Parkinson's disease, the frequency of such cases suggests an iceberg effect, where only the tip of those suffering from Parkinson's disease may be being identified *in vivo*. This clearly has major implications for any ante-mortem study examining genetic and environmental influences upon the condition, where significant underascertainment may be leading to erroneous conclusions.

Neurochemistry

The main neurochemical feature of Parkinson's disease is the decrease in brain dopamine concentrations as a result of degeneration of central dopaminergic neurones. This is of such over-riding importance and severity that efforts to replenish the brain's dopamine content therapeutically have met with considerable success. The nigrostriatal dopaminergic projections are particularly vulnerable, with the mesocortical and mesolimbic dopaminergic projections being less severely affected. Furthermore, not all dopaminergic systems appear to degenerate, with sparing , for instance, of the descending neurones to the lumbar spinal cord.

The striatal dopamine deficiency that results from the loss of the nigrostriatal projections is uneven, because the degeneration of the substantia nigra is also uneven. The posterior putamen is particularly severely affected, since this receives input from the ventrolateral substantia nigra. There is great reserve within the nigrostriatal neurotransmitter system, with parkinsonian signs only appearing when striatal dopamine levels fall to 70–80% of normal. Some of this reserve may derive from increased presynaptic dopamine turnover (as reflected by an increased homovanillic acid/dopamine ratio), as well as from post-synaptic dopamine receptor hypersensitivity. The massive dopamine deficiency in the nigrostriatal system plays a major role in the genesis of the bradykinesia, tremor and rigidity of Parkinson's disease. Such symptoms may be reproduced to a remarkable degree in monkeys exposed to the toxin 1-methyl-4-phenyl-1,2,3,6-tetrahydropyridine (MPTP). This toxin is thought to destroy selectively the nigrostriatal dopaminergic neurones, leaving other classical neurotransmitter systems unaffected.

In addition to the dopaminergic loss, a number of other neurotransmitter systems may be affected in Parkinson's disease, but to a lesser degree. These systems include the noradrenergic system (especially the coeruleo–corticolimbic projections), serotoninergic system (selected raphé nuclei) and the cholinergic system (especially projections to the neocortex from the nucleus basalis of Meynert and pedunculopontine nucleus). The functional consequences of such losses are uncertain but they may be implicated in the cognitive changes that can accompany the disorder, as well as the loss of smooth and subtle modulation of motor programmes. It should be mentioned that while subcorticocortical cholinergic deficiency is common to both Alzheimer's and Parkinson's disease, the deficiency in the former is inevitable, early and severe, while in Parkinson's disease, the deficiency is very variable and may be extremely mild.

Epidemiology

It will be apparent from the above that there are a number of additional pitfalls inherent in any study of the epidemiology of Parkinson's disease over and above potential failings that may accompany any epidemiological study. Specifically, these are completeness of ascertainment and diagnostic accuracy. Nevertheless, such studies provide a useful framework to aid identification of potential pathogenetic factors, and until a simple, cost-effective and accurate means of identifying Parkinson's disease (be it clinical or subclinical) in everyone within a given population exists, they are still of fundamental importance.

Parkinson's disease is more common with increasing age, although it can occur, albeit rarely, in individuals before the third decade. Parkinson's disease is probably less common in non-Caucasians, especially Chinese and Africans; most studies have found a higher prevalence in men than in women, although there are several notable exceptions.

The incidence of Parkinson's disease in Rochester, Minnesota, where a relatively stable population was assessed over a 35-year period, showed that rates varied within a narrow range of 16 to 21 new cases per 100 000 population per year, with no general trend towards an increase or decrease in rates. This gave an age-adjusted figure (to 1960 US population) of 17.9 per 100 000 per year. The corresponding incidence rates for Carlisle, England over a four-year observation period were 12.1 (uncorrected) and 9.4 (age-adjusted).

The prevalence of Parkinson's disease in Aberdeen was determined to be 164.2 per 100 000 of the population, using a survey of multiple public health records and personal examination of patients to verify diagnosis. A door-to-door survey of persons in Copiah County, Mississippi, however, yielded a figure of 347 per 100 000. Such differences may, of course, be real and relate to geographical or other factors, but the differences may also come from study design.

The lifetime incidence rate of a person developing Parkinson's disease in North America is of the order of 2.5%. A similar figure is probable in the UK. Analytical epidemiological results are discussed below in the context of possible environmental pathogenetic factors.

Potential pathogenetic factors

The cause of Parkinson's disease is not yet known. It is not inconceivable that there may be several different and independent causes, each producing nigral neuronal loss and Lewy body formation as the 'common end-point'. At present, it seems likely that neither purely genetic nor purely environmental factors can account for the majority of cases of Parkinson's disease, so a useful approach is the multifactorial threshold model. In this model, it is assumed that there is some underlying graded attribute that is related to the causation of Parkinson's disease. This is referred to as the individual's liability, which includes both genetic and environmental factors and which renders them more or less likely to develop the disease. The curve of liability has a normal distribution in both the general population and the relatives of probands, but the curve for relatives is shifted to the right because they have a higher mean liability. The point on the curve beyond which all individuals are affected is the threshold. In the general population, the proportion beyond this threshold represents the *population* frequency, while among relatives this proportion is the *familial* frequency. The levels of putamen dopamine and nigral cell loss (80% and 50% of normal, respectively) that must be reached before symptoms of Parkinson's disease develop could act as the threshold in a clinical study.

Genetic factors

Such is the frequency of Parkinson's disease in the population that an index case has a 15 to 20% chance of having at least one relative also affected by the condition. Although initial twin and family studies concluded that genetic factors were unlikely to play a major role in the aetiopathogenesis of Parkinson's disease, this view has recently been challenged. Functional neuroimaging studies using positron emission tomography to examine the integrity of the nigrostriatal dopaminergic projections in both affected twins and their so-called 'unaffected' co-twins have indicated a high frequency of subclinical dopaminergic abnormalities in the co-twins, raising concordance rates to as high as 45% in monozygotic twins. The numbers of twin pairs studied have, however, been too small to distinguish between genetic and environmental mechanisms.

In the most recent study of familial Parkinson's disease, the families of 20 British probands were examined; they were selected on the basis of having clinically typical Parkinson's disease and at least one affected relative. In all, 49 secondary cases were identified, clinically indistinguishable from 'sporadic' Parkinson's disease. Pedigree and segregation analysis suggested that an autosomal dominant inheritance pattern, with reduced penetrance, was the most likely to account for familial Parkinson's disease.

Furthermore, a number of families have been identified where the inheritance of pathologically proven Parkinson's disease is clearly autosomal dominant. One such kindred originated from Contursi in Southern Italy, and, intriguingly, the autosomal dominant pattern was maintained in both the family members who remained in Contursi and those members who emigrated to the USA, thereby eliminating local environmental factors. Several of the large kindreds where Mendelian genetics appear to be involved have clinically atypical Parkinson's disease: the Contursi kindred was one such example, with a relatively early age of onset, rapid course and mild or absent tremor.

It is unlikely that simple Mendelian genetics account for the vast majority of Parkinson's disease cases. If a genetic component is involved, it may come from a number of genes, each making a small contribution to an individual's susceptibility. One way in which genetic susceptibility and environmental factors could interact is through xenobiotic enzyme profiles. For example, hepatic S-oxidation of S-carboxymethyl-L-cysteine has been shown to be more likely to be slow in Parkinson's disease than in controls. A defect in the gene for the enzyme responsible, cysteine dioxygenase, could be inherited as an autosomal recessive trait, as occurs in Hallervorden–Spatz disease, which is also associated with nigral damage (as well as abnormal basal ganglia iron deposition).

Mitochondrial mechanisms have also been considered, although since the transmission of mitochondrial genes is matrilineal, a tendency towards maternal transmission would be expected; this has not been observed in any family study to date.

Environmental factors

One of the most exciting discoveries in recent years relating to the pathogenesis of Parkinson's disease was the observation that a relatively simple toxin MPTP, which is a structural analogue of meperidine, can lead to a syndrome clinically identical to Lewy body Parkinson's disease, including levodopa responsiveness. The toxin also causes selective degeneration of the substantia nigra and locus coeruleus, with eosinophilic inclusions found in primate brains in the areas where Lewy bodies are found in humans. MPTP is biotransformed to the 1-methyl-4-phenylpyridinium ion, MPP^+, by monoamine oxidase type B, located in glial cells. MPP^+ is then probably taken up by neurones via the catecholaminergic uptake system and cell death occurs via interference with NADH-linked respiration in mitochondria. Since MPTP and MPP^+ are relatively simple molecules, it has been argued that similar compounds, either naturally occurring or artificial, could lead to nigral cell damage, perhaps over a prolonged period of time or through depleting nigral reserve in a single exposure (even *in utero*?)

An association between pesticide use and Parkinson's disease has been reported, while others have noted the condition to be more common in rural areas and linked to drinking well water. Interestingly, a number of studies have found smoking to have a relatively protective influence upon an individual developing Parkinson's disease. No consistent links have been detected with previous head injury, vaccinations, exposure to anaesthetics or specific drugs, birth order, birth weight, alcohol or coffee consumption.

Overall, several possible pathogenetic environmental influences have been identified for Parkinson's disease, although these have mainly been elicited from case-control analytical epidemiological studies and do not apply to many individuals. Furthermore, no MPTP-like substance or other neurotoxin has yet been identified in the environment.

Clinical features

Table 11.3 lists the common symptoms and signs associated with Parkinson's disease. The disease typically begins unilaterally, in an arm or leg, and initial symptoms may be subtle or even misleading. Sensory symptoms, for example, are not often considered to be part of the condition and this may lead to a number of unnecessary investigations being carried out. The dragging of a leg may lead to the suspicion of a pyramidal tract disorder.

In 60% or more of patients, however, a typical 'pill-rolling' rest tremor develops at a frequency of 3–5 Hz. Slowness and poverty of movement are also early features leading to a loss of dexterity for fine tasks, such as doing up buttons, and complaints of smaller, illegible writing (micrographia). The more complex the task, the greater the impact of

Table 11.3. *Symptoms and signs occurring in Parkinson's disease*

	Symptoms and signs
Main features	Bradykinesia/akinesia (poverty of movement)
	Rest tremor (3–5 Hz)
	Postural tremor (6–8 Hz)
	Rigidity (lead-pipe±cog-wheeling)
	Reduced arm swing and shortened stride length
	Postural instability and falls
Other features	Slowness of thought and memory retrieval (bradyphrenia)
	Frank global dementia
	Depression
	Sensory symptoms, including restlessness and pain
	Constipation
	Drooling of saliva and dysphagia
	Weight loss
	Autonomic impairment, especially urogenital

the bradykinesia. The patient may have difficulty turning in bed or initiating getting out of a bath. The voice becomes softer and monotonous and the facial expression 'masked', with reduced blink frequency (facial hypomimia). The patients may feel 'stiff'; on examination, this is manifest as a 'lead-pipe' type of rigidity in the limbs, which develops superimposed 'cog-wheeling' if tremor is also present. The gait is very characteristic in Parkinson's disease, with earliest signs being a shortened stride length and reduced arm swing. As the condition progresses, postural reflexes become impaired, leading to falls in which the patient does not throw out their arms to protect themselves. It should be emphasised that early postural instability is not a typical feature of Parkinson's disease and may suggest another condition associated with parkinsonism, such as multiple system atrophy or Steele–Richardson–Olszewski syndrome. A number of other symptoms and signs may occur in Parkinson's disease and these are listed in Table 11.3.

The differential diagnosis of conditions that may feature parkinsonism is listed in Table 11.4. These will not be discussed any further here.

The diagnosis of Parkinson's disease is, therefore, relatively straightforward when the characteristic clinical features are established. In the early stages, the diagnosis may be less easy to make, and both evolution of the signs over a period of time, and the patient's response to treatment (see below) may be further clues. As mentioned above, the neurologist's clinical accuracy in making a diagnosis of Parkinson's disease ante-mortem is still only of the order of 70–80%. A number of clinical diagnostic criteria, such as those

Table 11.4. *The differential diagnosis of parkinsonism: this list is not exhaustive and does not include rare parkinsonian manifestations in uncommon diseases (e.g. prion disease)*

Idiopathic (Lewy body) Parkinson's disease
Multiple system atrophy
Steele–Richardson–Olszewski syndrome
Corticobasal–ganglionic degeneration
Dopamine receptor-blocking agent exposure
Alzheimer's disease
Hydrocephalus
Multi-infarct state
Carbon monoxide and cyanide poisoning
MPTP poisoning
Manganese poisoning
Post-encephalitic parkinsonism
Wilson's disease
Parkinsonism–dementia–ALS complex of Guam
Dementia pugilistica ('punch-drunk' syndrome)

suggested by the UK Parkinson's Disease Society Brain Bank, have been developed to aid diagnosis.

Treatment

Current strategies

After making the diagnosis of Parkinson's disease, it should always be remembered by the physician involved that the patient is being told they have a lifelong condition that in all likelihood will adversely affect their work and domestic situations to an increasing degree. It is also important to stress that life expectancy is now near to normal and that effective treatment is available. An unhurried and sympathetic approach, coupled with an early review for questions and, if the individual wishes it, contact with the Parkinson's Disease Society, should, therefore, be the norm.

Table 11.5 lists, in three rather arbitrary groups, the drugs currently used to treat Parkinson's disease. At present there is no treatment available that is truly 'neuroprotective'. The large multicentre American DATATOP study (deprenyl and tocopherol antioxidant therapy of Parkinson's disease) suggested that the use of the monoamine oxidase type B inhibitor selegiline retarded the need for levodopa treatment and prolonged time spent in employment. The rationale was that by inhibiting the monoamine oxidase enzyme the oxidative stress associated with dopamine metabolism would be reduced. Furthermore, selegiline was shown to prevent MPTP causing experimental parkinsonism in subhuman primates. Selegiline also has a modest symptomatic antiparkinsonian action, so it has proved impossible to show whether or not the perceived benefits were neuroprotective or symptomatic in nature.

Table 11.5. *Drugs used currently in the treatment of Parkinson's disease*

Group	Drugs
Group 1 (mild antiparkinsonian effects)	Amantadine (Symmetrel), Anticholinergics, e.g. orphenadrine (Disipal), benzhexol (Artane) Antidepressants, e.g. amitriptyline (Lenitizol, Saroten) Selegiline
Group 2 ('gold standard')	L-DOPA preparations (carbidopa (Sinemet), benserazide plus levadopa (Madopar))
Refinements	1. Including a dopa decarboxylase inhibitor 2. Multiple-sized tablets available (e.g. Sinemet-275, Sinemet-LSIIO) 3. Slow-release preparations (e.g. Sinemet-CR)
Group 3 (usually used in more advanced disease)	Dopamine agonists, e.g. pergolide (Ly-141B), bromocriptine (Parlodel) Apomorphine (Euporphin)

The use of selegiline is still a useful first step, since it is usually well tolerated. An anticholinergic drug may also be helpful at this stage, particularly to reduce embarrassing tremor, although such agents are best avoided in the elderly patient with memory impairment, prostatism or glaucoma.

The therapeutic hallmark of Parkinson's disease is the responsiveness of the condition to oral levodopa therapy, with over 70% patients deriving an 'excellent' response from such treatment. Oral levodopa is coupled with a peripherally acting dopa decarboxylase inhibitor (carbidopa or benserazide), which minimises levodopa-induced peripheral side effects such as nausea and postural hypotension and allows more of the administered dose of levodopa to reach the nigrostriatal neurones. After uptake, conversion of the levodopa then takes place within these surviving neurones to dopamine.

Levodopa preparations are still the 'gold standard' of antiparkinsonian drugs in terms of efficacy, but their use in the long term is associated with troublesome side effects, which broadly divide into wearing-off effects and involuntary movements. It is, therefore, best to tailor the need for levodopa introduction to the individual's disabilities and handicaps, rather than their neurological impairments, and to use the lowest possible dose. The rate of emergence of levodopa-related side effects is roughly 10% per year of use, so that by 10 years of treatment almost all patients will be affected.

Some authorities prefer initial monotherapy with directly acting dopamine agonists, such as the synthetic ergoline derivatives pergolide and bromocriptine. These agents differ in their affinities for dopamine D_1 and D_2 receptors and, in theory, retard the need for levodopa introduction. They are also associated with a much lower incidence of wearing-off effects and involuntary movements than levodopa. Unfortunately, only around 30% of patients can manage on such monotherapy, either because of lack of efficacy, or because of side effects. Dopamine agonists are, nevertheless, helpful as levodopa 'sparing' agents when long-term levodopa side effects occur, and their long half lives may improve quality of sleep as well as smooth the rapid fluctuations in motor performance that occur by day in advanced disease.

Apomorphine is a parenterally administered (by subcutaneous injection or sublingual tablet) dopamine agonist that acts rapidly and thus may reverse sudden deteriorations in motor performance. It is reserved at present for severe, difficult-to-control Parkinson's disease cases and usually requires the prophylactic use of domperidone as an antiemetic.

Future therapies

The ideal future management of Parkinson's disease would be the ability to identify preclinical cases in a cost-effective manner and to administer a neuroprotective agent of low toxicity to prevent the emergence of symptoms. A 'second-best' approach would be to treat patients in the early stages of the disease with neuroprotective and symptomatic therapies. In the more immediate future, the use of better symptomatic drug treatments and neurosurgical procedures are being actively explored.

Although the use of peripherally acting dopa decarboxylase inhibitors allows more levodopa to reach the nigrostriatal neurones, levodopa is still metabolised in the periphery to a significant extent by the ubiquitous enzyme catechol-O-methyl transferase. Trials are currently underway of inhibitors of this enzyme that appear to prolong the benefit obtained from a given levodopa dose, with few associated serious side effects.

As explained above, there appears to be an overactivity of the subthalamic nucleus and its glutamatergic output in Parkinson's disease. Both antiglutamatergic medical treatments, such as N-methyl-D-aspartate antagonists like remacemide, and stereotactic neurosurgical procedures to the subthalamic nucleus are currently undergoing trials to reduce subthalamo–pallidal output. Initial results using both strategies are encouraging.

Refined neurosurgical techniques, largely achieved using MRI-guided stereotaxis, have also meant that accurate targeting can be made to structures other than the subthalamic nucleus. Continuous electric stimulation of the ventrolateral thalamus (specifically the nucleus ventralis intermedius) has the advantage over ablation in having a lower complication rate, especially when performed bilaterally. This procedure seems to be very effective at suppressing tremor and possibly also some levodopa-induced involuntary movements.

Posteroventral pallidotomy is another 'old' operation undergoing a renaissance. Recently published evidence suggests that this method may improve not only tremor and rigidity but also akinesia, gait and speech.

Finally, neurosurgical advances have been coupled with meticulous basic science studies to implant substantia nigra neurones harvested from aborted fetuses into the caudate and/or putamen of patients with Parkinson's disease. Patients can derive considerable benefit, mainly on the side contralateral to the graft. Studies using positron emission tomography have indicated that the graft remains viable, while the non-grafted striatum contains to lose function as a result of 'native' disease. Only a small number of patients have received such fetal grafting, not least because of the practical problems, and the method remains experimental. Future strategies may include the development of tumour cell lines or animal-derived fibroblasts transfected with the gene for tyrosine hydroxylase (the rate-limiting enzymatic step in the synthesis of endogenous dopamine) for use as striatal implants.

Since the mid 1980s, a number of trophic and mitogenic factors have been identified for the central nervous system. A neurotrophic factor, in its narrow definition, is a survival factor for embryonic neurones either of the peripheral or central nervous system. Nerve growth factor and brain-derived neuronal factor are two such factors. Animal studies of neurotrophic agents have been directed at their ability to prevent or rescue lesions to nerve cells, although, to date, a specific neurotrophic factor for embryonic, let alone adult, dopaminergic neurones has not been identified. Brain-derived neuronal factor has, however, been shown to increase the number of tyrosine hydroxylase-immunoreactive cells in mid-brain cultures. If a trophic factor for dopaminergic neurones was identified, and it could be produced in sufficient quantity, the timing, mode and site of administration would be further major challenges to both basic scientists and clinicians.

Summary

Parkinson's disease is a distinct clinicopathological entity with a significant lifetime incidence. Initially, the pathological basis for the condition has been described and related to dysfunction of the basal ganglia. Despite much greater understanding of the neuroanatomy of the basal ganglia, the precise ways in which these nuclei influence control of movement in health, let alone disease, is still poorly understood. Further understanding of the Lewy body, and its unique composition, undoubtedly holds the key to answering many questions, not least why the ventrolateral substantia nigra and locus coeruleus are so specifically targeted in Parkinson's disease. Unlike Alzheimer's disease, a dominant neurochemical deficiency of dopamine in Parkinson's disease allows a rational replacement therapy to be undertaken.

Pathogenetic factors have been discussed. It now seems highly probable that a combination of environmental and genetic factors interact to cause Parkinson's disease, although the relative balance between these factors may vary from individual to individual. Emphasis has been placed both on the possible large pool of 'pre-clinical' Parkinson's disease cases, which hampers interpretation of conventional epidemiological studies, and on our limitations in accurately diagnosing the condition in life. Drug treatment is usually highly successful in the early stages of the illness, although a number of problems arise in the long term. Future strategies include improved medical and surgical treatments for advanced disease and the development of neuroprotective agents.

FURTHER READING

Alexander, G.E., Crutcher, M.D. & De Long, M.R. (1990). Basal ganglia-thalamocortical circuits: parallel substrates for motor, oculomotor, 'prefrontal' and 'limbic' functions. *Progress in Brain Research*, 85, 119–146.

Gibb, W.R.G. & Lees, A.J. (1988). The relevance of the Lewy body to the pathogenesis of idiopathic Parkinson's disease. *Journal of Neurology, Neurosurgery and Psychiatry*, 51, 745–752.

Golbe, L.I. (1990). The genetics of Parkinson's disease: a reconsideration. *Neurology*, 40 (suppl. 3), 7–14.

Marsden, C.D. & Fahn, S. (ed.) (1994). *Movement Disorders 3. Neurology*, vol. 12: Oxford: Butterworths International Medical Reviews.

Pollanen, M.S., Dickson, D.W. & Bergeron C. (1991). Pathology and biology of the Lewy body. *Journal of Neuropathology and Experimental Neurology*, 52, 183–191.

Stern, G.S. (ed.) (1990). *Parkinson's Disease*. London: Chapman & Hall.

12

Neoplasia

H. S. PANDHA AND K. SIKORA

■ In normal circumstances, there is a balance between growth-promoting and growth-restraining signal transduction elements so that cellular proliferation only occurs as appropriate. Neoplastic growth is characterised by abnormalities in the activity of critical signalling molecules so that this balance is disrupted and abnormal cell growth ensues.

■ Cancer-related genetic abnormalities include chromosomal deletion, translocation or gain of material. The consequences may include inactivation of a tumour suppressor gene or activation or amplification of an oncogene.

■ There is evidence of an increased risk of cancer amongst first-degree relatives of individuals with a similar tumour. This is also seen in colorectal cancer.

■ Colorectal cancer is clearly a disease caused by defective somatic cell genetics. Currently there is intense interest in gene therapy strategies to interfere with its spread.

The mechanisms of neoplasia

In the UK, one person in three will develop cancer during their lifetime. The term 'cancer' comprises over 200 diseases that differ in their genetic basis, aetiology, progression and final outcome to sufficient degrees to be classified as separate entities. Genetic alterations are at the very centre of tumorigenesis so that, at a cellular level, cancer can be designated a genetic disorder. The period from the mid-1980s has witnessed remarkable progress in the understanding of the pathogenesis of cancer. This knowledge, however, has yet to have a positive impact on the treatment and survival of affected individuals. In this chapter, the molecular and cellular basis of neoplasia is discussed using colorectal cancer (CRC) as the exemplary condition. This common cancer has been studied extensively and represents a truly multifactorial disease, as the detailed discussion of the relative contributions of genetic and environmental factors will demonstrate.

The clinical presentation of any cancer depends on the tissue type affected and the location but usually involves an expanding tumour mass, which causes symptoms through local invasion, local expansion or the production of biologically active molecular products such as hormones or cytokines. Each tumour type has its own natural history, which has been altered successfully only in a few 'curable' malignancies such as certain germ cell tumours, leukaemias and lymphomas.

Fundamentally, cancers represent a form of de-differentiation or, more generally, a disturbance of the normally differentiated state that is associated with loss of growth control. Genetic changes or mutations in somatic cells of the body are the main initiating events and are responsible for tumour progression. It is clear also that changes in cell chromosomes either in number or in organisation are key events in tumorigenesis and that the immune system plays a role in limiting or eliminating cancer to an extent through the recognition of novel antigens on cancer cells. There is considerable evidence that some cancers are caused by viruses either indirectly by suppression of the host immune system and impaired elimination of tumour cells, or directly by activation of oncogenes or the insertion of viral DNA into host chromosomes to augment or destroy normal gene expression.

Normally, there is a balance between growth-promoting and growth-restraining signal transduction elements so that cellular proliferation only occurs as appropriate. There is an equilibrium between stem cells capable of replication and the cellular deficit resulting from natural cell loss. In specific circumstances, this balance is capable of upregulation in favour of a controlled increase in cell number, such as during embryogenesis, wound repair or immune response and in normal tissue turnover. Neoplastic growth, in contrast, is characterised by abnormalities in the activity of critical signalling molecules so that the balance is disrupted and abnormal cell growth ensues. Proteins encoded by overexpressed or mutant proto-oncogenes and loss of tumour suppressor gene products are important to this scenario. As a result, complex effector responses are initiated, including ion transport, pinocytosis, glycolysis, changes in cytoskeletel architecture and the synthesis of DNA and RNA. Deregulation of these events creates the biological framework driving aberrant cell proliferation, loss of differentiation and the development of metastases.

Behaviour of cancer cells

A number of characteristics have been used to describe how cancer cells behave differently from their normal counterparts:

> Clonality
> anaplasia
> autonomy
> metastasis.

Clonality

Genetic markers can be used to show that the vast majority of cancers are clonal (i.e. originating from a single stem cell). In addition to this clonality, there may be numerous epigenetic events to create the environment for change from normal cell division, such as chronic inflammation or persistent stimulation of the immune system. Virtually all solid tumours and a majority of haematological malignancies display abnormalities in the chromosomal karyotype that is inherited by the population of tumour cells. These

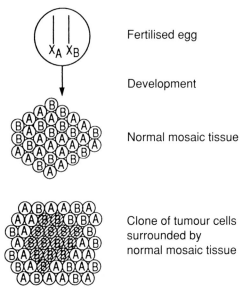

Fertilised egg

Development

Normal mosaic tissue

Clone of tumour cells
surrounded by
normal mosaic tissue

Fig. 12.1. The clonal origin of tumours. The X-linked marker G6PD can be inherited in two forms, A and B. A female who is heterozygous has a mosaic of cells, some expressing G6PD A and some G6PD B depending on which X chromosome is active in each somatic cell. A tumour arising in such a female will only express one variant of G6PD (G6PD B here) if its development is clonal, i.e. arising from a single progenitor cell. (Reproduced with permission from Bodmer, W.F. (1991). In *Cellular and molecular biology of cancer,* 2nd edn, ed. L.N. Franks and N.M. Teich, Oxford: Oxford University Press.)

abnormalities may involve the translocation, deletion or addition of part of chromosomes or of whole new chromosomes.

Studies on leukaemias occurring in patients with glucose 6-phosphate dehydrogenase (G6PD) deficiency have demonstrated the clonal nature of certain cancers. This condition is common in Africa and is inherited in two forms, A and B, easily distinguished by electrophoresis. A female who is heterozygous G6PD A/B is a mosaic of cells half of which express G6PD A while the other half express G6PD B. A tumour arising in such a female, if it is clonal, should not be a mosaic – all cells will arise from A or B. Leukaemias occurring in these individuals always arise from either A or B and this confirms clonal proliferation (Fig. 12.1). The observation of uniform karyotypic abnormalities in all cells in, for example, chronic myeloid leukemia, which has the 9 to 22 translocation, also provides strong evidence for clonality. Furthermore, since these types of translocation are never seen in normal cells, the chromosomal abnormalities may serve usefully as 'tumour markers' indicating the presence of a common malignant state in the individual; these changes should not be detectable after successful treatment and their subsequent detection may then be the first indication of disease relapse. The techniques available currently to the molecular geneticist allow clonal genetic abnormalities to be identified in non-dividing cells, including gene mutation, rearrangement, translocation, deletion and amplification (Chapter 2).

Anaplasia

Cancer cells may show some of the morphological characteristics of their normal counterparts, but the lack of normal cellular differentiation is a feature recognised readily by light microscopy. Anaplasia is a lack of normal co-ordinated cellular differentiation. The cells have large nuclei, increased nucleus to cytoplasm ratio, with more apparent chromatin and prominent nucleoli. There may be increased mitoses, giant cells containing multiple nucleoli and abnormal mitosis, reflecting failure of karyokinesis. The presence of aneuploid cells, as detected by techniques such as flow cytometry, now has diagnostic and prognostic value. The process of anaplasia may be expressed at:

1. The cellular level, with morphological derangement and/or loss of normal tissue architecture, invasiveness, destruction of normal tissue, pleomorphism and a high mitotic rate
2. The biochemical level, with inappropriate and poorly controlled secretion of growth factors, hormones or peptides such as immunoglobulins

Autonomy

The many local and distant environmental factors that control normal cellular proliferation are circumvented when the process of malignant transformation occurs. This autonomy is usually relative and requires a minimal number of supporting factors, such as platelet-derived growth factor (PDGF), epidermal growth factor (EGF) or insulin-like growth factors (IGF-I, IGF-II). In certain circumstances, clonal proliferation results in further autonomy through the production of a growth promoting factor by the tumour itself; this is termed autocrine stimulation. The first molecule identified with the potential for autocrine stimulation was transforming growth factor α (TGFα). Other mechanisms by which tumour cells show less dependence on growth factors include the expression of increased numbers of receptors, such as that for EGF on the cell surface and the activation of internal biochemical processes that normally require exposure to a growth-promoting agent for activity. For example, a protein tyrosine kinase ordinarily dependent for activity upon binding of a specific growth factor to a cell surface receptor may be permanently activated, thereby completely bypassing the need for exposure to the growth-promoting agent.

Metastasis

Dissemination of cancer occurs through the process of contiguous spread and metastasis. Cells lose their adherence and restrained position within an organised tissue, develop the capacity to invade and become capable of proliferating in unnatural locations and tissue environments. These changes in growth patterns are accompanied by biochemical changes that may promote the metastatic process. The first step probably involves the attachment to the extracellular matrix via binding to receptors on the cell membrane that bind specifically to glycoproteins such as fibronectin and laminin. The tumour then progresses from a homogeneous proliferating clone to a group of hetero-

Table 12.1. *Cytogenetic abnormalities in solid tumours and lymphoma*

Tumour	Area affected
Translocations	
Non-Hodgkin's lymphoma	t(8;14)(q24;q32)
	t(14;18)(q32;q21)
	t(11;14)(113;q32)
Alveolar rhabdomyosarcoma	t(2;13)(q37;q14)
Ewing's sarcoma	t(11;22)(q24;q12)
Chromosomal deletions	
Renal cell carcinoma	3q 13–21
Wilms' tumour	11p 13
Retinoblastoma	13q 14
Meningioma	Monosomy 22
Small cell lung cancer	3p 13–23
Neuroblastoma	1p 32–36
Colorectal carcinoma	17p, 18p

geneous subpopulations of cells, some of which have progressively accumulated the entire array of enzymes and surface molecules such as collagenases and lysosomal hydrolases required for metastasis.

The aetiology of cancer

Cancer genetics

Chromosomal analysis of human cancer cells has yielded a huge amount of information about the nature and incidence of chromosomal abnormalities in malignant cells. Certain cytogenetic abnormalities have diagnostic and prognostic significance in both haematological and solid malignancies (Table 12.1). Although there are a wide variety of cancer-related cytogenetic abnormalities, these are relatively small in number and non-randomly distributed throughout the genome. They may be caused by:

- deletion of part of a chromosome or of a whole chromosome; this may inactivate a tumour suppressor gene
- translocation; this may inactivate a tumour suppressor gene or activate an oncogene
- gain of chromosomal material; this may promote cell proliferation by amplification of an oncogene or it may interfere with normal cell development.

Chromosome aberrations may be primarily related to the formation of a specific tumour and may be the only genetic abnormality present. Secondary aberrations are not random, are rarely the only phenomenon and occur in the presence of the primary change; they may be epiphenomena (incidental event occurring as an accompaniment of a developing tumour, but not essentially or typically linked with it) or they may determine the biological behaviour of the tumour including invasion, metastasis and response to treatment. Primary aberrations would be expected to occur early in tumorigenesis, whereas secondary changes would become more frequent in the later stages.

A number of constitutional chromosomal abnormalities are associated with predisposition to cancer, and examples are shown in Table 12.1. These may be associated with numerical or structural abnormalities of chromosomes, or chromosome breakage syndromes. In some cases, the molecular pathology of the chromosome rearrangement has been delineated and a translocation or deletion has been shown to inactivate a tumour suppressor gene, as in del(11p 13) and the Wilms' tumour gene (WT1). We will discuss in detail below the condition adenomatous polyposis coli, which predisposes to colonic cancer in all individuals with a specific chromosomal deletion, 5q21, and show that for patients and families with family histories of this disease genetic analysis facilitates diagnosis and screening and makes genetic counselling a vital part of their management.

Other mechanisms by which there is a systemic inherited susceptibility to tumorigenesis include disorders characterised by genomic instability, which can be recognised by increased spontaneous chromosome breakage in cultured cells. The pattern of this breakage is specific for each disorder. Conditions predisposing to cancer in this way include xeroderma pigmentosa, in which there is extreme sensitivity to the effects of sunlight and carcinogens because of a reduced ability to repair damaged DNA, and Bloom's syndrome, in which there is a defect in a gene encoding a DNA ligase, leading to inefficient joining of nucleotides. Other examples include ataxia telangiectasia and Fanconi's anaemia. Certain carcinogens increase the risk of developing cancer, both through causing genetic mutations by interfering with chromosome organisation and by acting as tumour promoters so that the possibility of developing cancer after a cell has been initiated increases significantly. For example, there are inherited differences in the ability to metabolise drugs such as debrisoquine. In the general population, 10% are poor metabolisers in the homozygous state and this is associated with increased toxicity when the drug is administered in normal doses. Studies have shown that there is a sixfold reduced frequency of lung cancer in slow metabolisers.

The immune system may also determine susceptibility to tumour formation, through HLA and antibody formation and T cell receptors. The HLA system controls two main sets of cell surface determinants, which are involved in interactions between lymphocytes and other cells in the control of the immune response. A number of associations between HLA and virus-associated cancers such as nasopharyngeal carcinoma and Kaposi's sarcoma have been noted. In these situations, inherited differences in immune responses associated with HLA variation as well as with variation in other aspects of the immune system, such as antibody and T cell responses, may be relevant in susceptibility to virally induced human cancers.

Viral carcinogenesis

While there are many examples of viruses that are unequivocally carcinogenic in animals, evidence in humans for truly oncogenic viruses has been lacking until recently. Oncogenic viruses can be separated into broad categories based on the type of nucleic

Table 12.2. *Viruses associated with human cancers*

Viruses	Cancer(s)
RNA viruses	
Human immunodeficiency virus	Lymphoma, (?)Kaposi's sarcoma
Human T cell leukaemia virus I	T cell leukaemia, lymphomas
Human T cell leukaemia virus II	(?)Hairy cell leukaemia
DNA viruses	
Human papilloma virus	Anogenital carcinoma, skin carcinoma, laryngeal carcinoma
Herpes simplex virus-2	Cervix carcinoma
Epstein–Barr virus	Nasopharyngeal carcinoma, African Burkitt's lymphoma, immunoblastic lymphoma
Cytomegalovirus	Kaposi's sarcoma, (?)cervix carcinoma
Hepatitis B virus	Hepatoma

acid in their chromosome (Table 12.2). Most of the RNA viruses are retroviruses and they vary in the time taken to complete cellular transformation (i.e. acutely or chronically). The mechanisms underlying retroviral oncogene activation are well characterised and include the transduction of cellular proto-oncogenes, insertional mutagenesis and the transactivation of cellular genes by viral-encoded transcription factors. The DNA sequences involved in tumour induction, viral oncogenes, are identified by the prefix v, as in v-*myc*. Cellular homologues of these have the prefix c-.

Oncogenes

Proto-oncogenes are the normal cellular counterparts of a gene identified as causing a tumour; they do not have transforming potential in their native state. Proto-oncogenes are a family of genes that act in a dominant fashion to induce or maintain cell transformation. They have a role in normal cellular growth and differentiation but when mutated may function as oncogenes. Proto-oncogenes may be changed to promote cell transformation by:

- abnormal regulation of the gene, resulting in constitutive overproduction
- gene amplification leading to increased production of oncoprotein
- translocations that activate the proto-oncogene or result in fusion genes encoding a novel protein product
- point mutations that alter the function of the gene product and produce a transforming protein

The biochemical actions of proto-oncogenes may involve protein phosphorylation, with serine, threonine and tyrosine as substrates, G-protein interaction or they may act as transcription factors (Table 12.3). Protein phosphorylation can result in cell transformation by a variety of mechanisms; for example, the oncogene may encode a growth factor or the oncogene product is a normal or modified growth factor receptor such as the EGF

Table 12.3. *Proto-oncogenes and oncoproteins associated with cancer*

	Protooncogene	Oncoprotein
Growth factors and growth factor-like molecules	*sis*	B chain of PDGF
	int-2, hst	Related to fibroblast growth factors Others: EGF, TGFα, TGFβ, IGF-1, IGF-2
Growth factor receptors and receptor-like molecules	*erbB-1–4*	EGF receptor
	fms	CSF-1 receptor
	ros	Insulin receptor
	Others: *ret, msk, trk, met, kit*	
Intracellular signal transduction molecules	H-, K- and N-*ras*	Membrane-associated GTP-binding proteins
	BCR/*abl, src, syn, fgr*	Membrane-associated/cytoplasmic protein tyrosine kinases
	raf/mil, mos, cot, pim-1	Cytoplasmic protein Ser-Thr kinases
Nuclear transcription factors	*erbA*	Thyroid hormone receptor
	c-, L- and N-*myc, myb, jun, fos, scl, lyl-1*	DNA-binding proteins
Apoptosis blocking factors	*bcl-2*	Blocks c-*myc*-induced apoptosis

receptor. Other oncoproteins derive from protein tyrosine kinases genes, which are suggested to be receptors for as yet unidentified growth factors; these include Met, Ret and Trk. There is evidence that activated Raf1 may provide a link between cytoplasmic membrane-generated signals and nuclear proteins that regulate gene expression and cell division. G-proteins (guanine nucleotide-binding proteins) are involved in signal transduction. When stimulated by a receptor protein, they exchange bound GDP for GTP and the activated G-protein – GTP complex then interacts with second messenger systems such as adenylate cyclase (which generates cyclicAMP) and phospholipase C (which generates diacylglycerol, a protein kinase C activator, and inositol trisphosphate, which increases intracellular calcium levels). G-proteins possess an intrinsic GTPase activity that terminates the signal. The *ras* oncogene family (H-*ras*, K-*ras* and N-*ras* (the prefix denotes the origin of the gene, e.g. H for Harvy sarcoma virus)) each encode a 21 kDa protein, p21, which shares homology with the G-proteins but has sustained mutations that render it constitutively active by maintaining the protein in the GTP-bound activated state. In the appropriate genetic background, GTP–Ras is growth promoting and part of the cascade of somatic genetic events that lead to the development of cancer. *ras* mutations appear in nearly 30% of all tumours examined, with particularly high rates in pancreatic carcinomas (95%), thyroid tumours (60%) and adenocarcinoma of the colon (50%). *ras* is known to require other co-operating activated oncogenes such as p53 or *myc* to cause full transformation in various model systems.

A number of proto-oncogenes, such as *myc*, *fos* and *jun*, encode transcription factors and so modulate gene expression. The role of *myc* in colorectal carcinogenesis will be discussed in detail.

Tumour suppressor genes

The first indication that tumour suppressor genes may exist came from cell fusion experiments by Harris *et al*. Fusing normal cells with tumour cells leads to a loss of some or all malignant features. Over time, some cells regain their malignant potential ('revert') and this correlates with the loss of particular chromosomes or parts of chromosomes. Further evidence comes from cytogenetic studies that have shown consistent karyotypic abnormalities, particularly deletions. Analysis of restriction fragment length polymorphisms (RFLPs) has enabled the examination of regions of chromosomal loss on a smaller scale, not visible macroscopically (see Chapter 2). Using this method, it is possible to map precisely the loci that have lost heterozygosity (termed loss of heterozygosity (LOH) analysis) and hence are the likely sites for tumour suppressor genes. It is interesting to note that some loci appear to be associated with tumours of a restricted histogenetic type (e.g. 13q14 and retinoblastoma), whereas others have been associated with a wide variety of malignancies (e.g. 3p 13–23 in small cell lung cancer, ovarian adenocarcinoma and renal cell carcinoma) (Table 12.1). Some aberrations are associated with tumour progression or a more advanced stage of malignancy, and some tumours have been shown to have multiple allelic loss.

The retinoblastoma paradigm

The conceptual basis for the genetic study of tumour suppressor genes was laid by Knudson and Strong in a series of epidemiological studies of retinoblastoma, Wilms' tumour and neuroblastoma. These childhood tumours were of interest in that 10–30% of patients presented with bilateral disease. Bilateral tumours arose at an earlier age than the more common unilateral cancers and in some cases were associated with a positive family history. Knudson predicted that two rate-limiting genetic events or 'hits' were required for tumour development. Children with genetic predisposition for cancer had inherited the first hit and only one additional genetic event was needed for cancer to arise. In contrast, the sporadic cases required two 'hits', and so bilateral tumours were extremely unlikely to occur and the unilateral tumours occurring were observed to present much later. Subsequent studies have suggested that the two hits of the Knudson model could be explained by the inactivation of both alleles of a tumour suppressor gene, typically with a point mutation in the first allele followed by a gross chromosomal deletion or rearrangement affecting the second allele (Fig. 12.2).

Genetic syndromes and predisposition to cancer

There is compelling epidemiological evidence of an increased risk of cancer amongst first-degree relatives of individuals with a similar cancer. In a minority of cancer patients, genetic factors may be the primary determinant; in others, cancer may develop

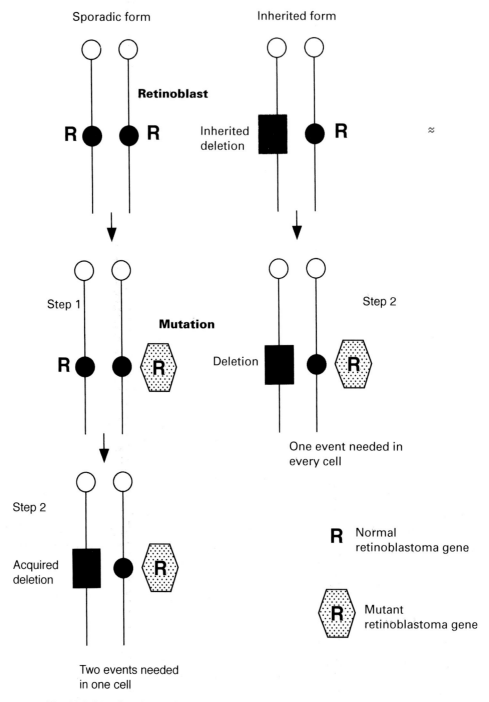

Fig. 12.2. Knudson's two hit hypothesis and retinoblastoma.

Table 12.4. *Examples of syndromes predisposing to cancer and their chromosomal location*

Name of disease	Chromosomal location
Autosomal dominant	
Familial adenomatous polyposis	5q
Tuberose sclerosis	9q, 11q
Multiple endocrine neoplasia type 1	11q
Multiple endocrine neoplasia type 2	10q
Neurofibromatosis type 1	17q
Neurofibromatosis type 2	22p
Von Hippel–Lindau disease	3
Li Fraumeni syndrome	17p
Autosomal recessive/X-linked	
Fanconi'a anaemia	1q
Ataxia telangiectasia	11q and others
Bloom's syndrome	?12
Xeroderma pigmentosa	7 types
Albinism	11q
Wiscott–Aldrich syndrome	Xp
Bruton syndrome	Xp

because an inherited factor increases susceptibility to environmental carcinogens. An increasing number of genes causing familial cancer syndromes have been mapped and several have been identified. These are usually recognised by a clinical phenotype, such as multiple colonic polyps in familial polyposis coli, or by laboratory tests, such as detection of structural chromosomal abnormalities. The syndromes may be autosomal dominant or recessive or X-linked. Recognition of clustering of common cancers in families may be put down to chance occurrences or shared environmental factors such as diet, but a genetic cause of cancer is suggested by early age at onset, multiple tumours or bilateral disease, and a pattern of familial clustering compatible with a Mendelian segregation of the cancer (Table 12.4).

At the molecular level, two forms of cancer susceptibility gene might be distinguished in this group of high-risk patients:

1. The inherited susceptibility is a mutation in genes involved directly in tumorigenesis (oncogene or tumour suppressor gene)
2. The predisposition to cancer is a secondary effect, as in DNA repair disorders discussed earlier

None of the dominant oncogenes have been implicated in inherited human cancer, but both recessive tumour suppressor genes and DNA repair defects may have an inherited predisposition. The Li–Fraumeni syndrome, for example, is a syndrome affecting young patients, inherited, paradoxically, in autosomal dominant fashion, in which there

Table 12.5. *Five-year survival for CRC according to stage of disease, using the Aster–Coller modification of Duke's staging*

Extent of tumour	Stage	Proportion of all patients presenting with CRC (%)	Five-year survival by site of cancer (%)	
			Colon	Rectum
Confined to the mucosa	A	2	82	40
Extending through muscularis mucosa but not through muscularis propria	B1	11	65	65
Extends beyond muscularis propria	B2	30	50	40
Stage B1 with regional lymph nodes involved	C1	2	40	33
Stage B2 with regional lymph nodes involved	C2	22	15	15
Distant metastases	D	33	<5	<5

is the predisposition to develop multiple tumours such as soft tissue sarcomas, leukaemias, adrenocortical, breast and brain tumours. It is now known that this syndrome results from the germ-line transmission of a mutant allele of the tumour suppressor gene p 53. This defect has subsequently been seen in a variety of adult solid tumours and is thought to be the most common genetic abnormality seen in human tumours.

Genetic disorders in which there is an increased predisposition to cancer are uncommon. It will be increasingly important to identify genetic factors that interact with environmental carcinogens as these potentially will affect most people. Furthermore, the identification of those factors causing genetic syndromes is likely to lead to novel treatments such as gene therapy, as well as earlier identification, monitoring and prevention of common cancers.

COLORECTAL CANCER

The exemplar disorder that will be discussed to illustrate the development of cancers is colorectal cancer (CRC).

CRC is the second most common malignancy in the UK and is responsible for approximately 20 000 deaths yearly. It has a peak incidence at 65 years and a lifetime incidence of 1 in 27 (both males and females). The incidence appears to be rising and therapeutic advances have made little impact on the 5-year survival since the 1960s. Table 12.5 shows expected survival for stages of the disease. It has been long postulated that factors in the environment and especially diet either promote or directly cause CRC. Dietary constituents, changes in gut flora or intraluminal pH may be important co-factors in tumour formation, but none of these have been individually substantiated by epidemiological studies. Instead, the development and application of modern techniques of molecular biology have increased our understanding at the cellular level of what is now regarded as essentially a genetic disease. An understanding of the specific and sequential genetic changes eventually responsible for malignant transformation are providing us with directions for developing new techniques for diagnosis and monitoring disease, and for the design of new therapeutic systems.

Aetiology and risk factors

CRC is a disease of the West; the highest rates are in urban areas in high socio-economic groups. Industrialised nations, particularly in North America, northern and western Europe, Australia and New Zealand, show markedly elevated incidence rates of CRC compared with those of developing countries in Asia, Africa and Latin America. Epidemiological studies have shown strong correlations between mortality from CRC and per capita consumption of calories, red meat and dietary fat and oils, as well as with elevation in serum cholesterol. Migrant groups adopt the local incidence of CRC within one generation. A number of specific factors may contribute to the development of colorectal tumours:

- bile acids
- dietary fibre
- faecal pH
- dietary calcium
- faecapentanes
- non-dietary factors

Bile acids

It is thought that diets high in fat cause an increased concentration of faecal bile acids and cholesterol metabolites in the stool. These are converted by faecal bacteria into carcinogens, cause the numbers of anaerobic bacteria and levels of bacterial enzymes in the stool to increase, and lead to activation of procarcinogens. Cholecystectomy results in high levels of bile acids in the caecum and ascending colon and may be associated with a greater frequency of right-sided colonic tumours.

Dietary fibre

The protective effect of dietary fibre has been demonstrated both in rat models and in human studies, the latter particularly in groups such as Vegans and Seventh Day Adventists, who eat no animal fat and who consequently have a high fibre intake. In rats with carcinogen-induced colon cancers, dietary supplementation with either pectin or wheat bran also produced a protective effect. Since Burkitt's observations of low rates of CRCs in Africans with high dietary fibre intake, several large studies have shown an inverse relationship between fibre intake and colon cancer incidence. This relationship has been more consistent for fruit and vegetables than for cereals. The postulated mechanisms by which dietary fibre is protective include decreased stool transit time, resulting in less exposure to potential carcinogens, lowering of faecal pH, resulting in decreased bacterial enzyme activity, and decreased concentrations of secondary bile acids through a dilutional effect.

Faecal pH

The products of the fermentation of complex carbohydrates include short-chain fatty acids and hydrogen, and this results in a lowered faecal pH. Several comparisons in humans have shown that these products are lower in individuals at risk for colon cancer compared with controls. Alkaline environments support higher concentrations of free bile acids and other potential carcinogens. In particular, one specific short-chain fatty acid, butyric acid, may affect cellular differentiation and susceptibility to carcinogenesis.

Dietary calcium

Calcium salts modulate damage to colonic epithelium by reducing the concentration of free bile acids through the formation of insoluble bile salt complexes. Individuals with colon cancer have been shown to have a lower intake of calcium. Other factors thought to be protective include dietary supplementation of selenium, vitamins A and C, flavones and indoles, although there are no good data to demonstrate their effectiveness.

Faecapentanes

Faecapentanes are potent mutagenic compounds found in human faeces as a result of microbial metabolism. There is a correlation between the level of stool faecapentanes and tumour incidence, and incidence of pre-malignant colonic polyps. Intraluminal levels of faecapentanes are reduced by increased intake of dietary fibre, vitamin C and vitamin E.

Non-dietary factors

Factors that may contribute to CRC include decreased physical activity, increased parity and occupational exposure to asbestos and organic solvents. A recent study by the American Cancer Society suggests that aspirin ingestion has a protective effect; a prospective study of 424 adults revealed that the mortality rates from colon cancer decreased with more frequent aspirin use in both men and women. This appears to correlate with studies showing the decreased rate of adenoma growth with the non-steroidal anti-inflammatory drug sulindac. Established risk factors for CRC are shown in Table 12.6.

Symptoms

The clinical presentation of CRCs depends to a large degree on the location and rate of growth of the primary tumour. Features common to any type of tumour and in all sites include anorexia, malaise and weight loss but more specifically CRC may present with pain, mucorrhoea, chronic blood loss leading to iron-deficient anaemia, and as a change

Table 12.6. *Lifetime risk of death from CRC*

Average population risk	1:50
One first-degree relative affected	1:17
One first-degree, one second-degree relative affected	1:12
One first-degree relative under 45 years affected	1:10
Two first-degree relatives affected	1:6
Three first-degree relatives affected	1:3

in bowel habit, occasionally with the classical symptoms of alternating constipation and diarrhoea. Right-sided lesions may be very insidious in nature and often present as vague abdominal pain or sometimes mimicking cholecystitis or peptic ulcer disease. Left-sided colonic lesions are more often circumferential and, therefore, may present as partial or total obstruction; they are more likely to present with blood visibly mixed in with stool or frank haematochaezia. Tenesmus and pelvic pain are usually features of advanced rectal or sigmoid tumours and indicate invasion into local tissues and/or sacral nerve roots.

Screening

The natural history of CRC suggests that it may be amenable to intervention through screening. The prognosis is related to the depth of invasion of the cancer, and since surgery cures approximately 90% of cancers limited to the mucosa and submucosa, early diagnosis could improve survival. Since CRC usually arises in adenomas, removing adenomas should prevent most cases of cancer. Population screening studies using faecal occult blood tests have shown that a higher proportion of cancers at an early stage (Dukes, A) are detected in groups offered screening compared with unscreened controls. These tests are low in cost but to date have been found to have disappointing uptake and poor yield. Despite the increased facilities to perform flexible sigmoidoscopic examination in recent years, no randomised clinical trial has yet demonstrated that screening by sigmoidoscopy improves survival in patients with CRC. The main evidence for reduced mortality from any type of screening comes from case-control studies. The three commonly used screening tests are (i) digital rectal examination; (ii) faecal occult blood test; and (iii) sigmoidoscopy.

Digital rectal examination

Digital rectal examination is of limited efficacy; most recent studies have shown that no more than 10% of CRCs are detectable by this method.

Faecal occult blood test

The faecal occult blood (FOB) test usually involves the use of the haemoccult card in which the peroxidase-like activity of haemoglobin catalyses the phenolic oxidation of guaiac-impregnated paper to an easily recognisable blue colour. Its sensitivity is estimated at 50–65% and in order to be reliable it requires at least 20 ml blood loss from the tumour per day. It is essentially a test for the haematic moiety of haemoglobin and relies on an optimum degree of haemoglobin degradation, which is most commonly achieved by blood loss from sigmoid cancers. An alternative method of detection, the 'Haemeselect' test, utilises fixed chicken erythrocytes that have been coated with an anti-human haemoglobin antibody. A positive test is observed when erythrocyte agglutination occurs in the presence of haemoglobin in a small faecal solution obtained from a smear of faecal matter. This method has a sensitivity of 94%.

False negative results occur in the presence of dietary vitamin C (which inhibits the chemical reaction), if there is insufficient bleeding from the tumour, if the blood loss is intermittent and in bleeding from right-sided colonic lesions where there has been time for degradation of haemoglobin in the faecal environment.

False positive results occur as a result of blood loss from non-malignant conditions such as haemorrhoids and sigmoid diverticulosis, and also from ingestion of fruit and vegetables with peroxidase activity, which can mimic that of haemoglobin. The number of false positive results are markedly reduced by combining the sensitive guaiac test with the immunoassay for haemoglobin.

Sigmoidoscopy

There are now a number of large multicentre studies showing the benefits of screening sigmoidoscopy; the routine use of the 65 cm flexible sigmoidoscope has been shown to detect 2.5 times the number of adenomas and carcinomas that were detected with the older more uncomfortable 25 cm rigid sigmoidoscopes. Flexible sigmoidoscopy is a sensitive method for detecting CRC distal to the splenic flexure, an area which harbours over 75% of all adenomas and 90% of all adenomas over 1 cm in size. The American Cancer Society in 1992 recommended non-selective screening of all individuals at 50 years by flexible sigmoidoscopy, to be repeated every three to five years.

Colonoscopy

Colonoscopy uses a flexible colonoscope to examine the interior of the entire colon and rectum. It can be used to obtain specimens and to remove polyps.

Colonoscopy is used mainly for follow-up of patients at substantially high risk of CRC as a result of a familial tendency or inherited syndrome, after previous colonic resection and in patients with extensive or severe inflammatory bowel disease. A possible way to maximise the effectiveness of screening programmes in CRC is the establishment of family cancer clinics, such as the unit at St Mark's Hospital in London. In these units, genetic counselling is made available, and risk estimates for relatives of patients with CRC are obtained. Of 715 patients interviewed at the unit at St Mark's Hospital in the period up to 1993, 90% accepted screening. Relatives with a lifetime risk of 1 in 10 or greater were offered screening five yearly by colonoscopy, and those for whom the risk was between 1 and 10 and 1 in 17 were offered yearly screening for faecal occult blood (Table 12.6). In addition, for women with Lynch II syndrome, additional screening for breast and pelvic tumours was offered. Of 382 high-risk patients assessed, 62 patients were found to have polyps and five patients had carcinomas. These were detected on colonoscopy; faecal occult blood testing was of poor sensitivity and was thought to be unsuitable as a tool for screening high-risk groups.

In Fig. 12.3, a clinical overview of CRC shows the sites of colon tumours and the symptoms and signs of CRC.

Mechanisms of colorectal tumorigenesis

The development of CRC results from an interplay of environmental factors on the genetic background of the individual. The risk of colorectal tumorigenesis has been related to a number of factors, which are shown in Table 12.7. Like all cancers, CRC, whether sporadic or secondary to a genetic predisposition, is a consequence of a series of poorly understood changes in the genome of the normal cells. As we will subsequently see, CRC is currently an excellent model for understanding the sequential molecular changes that occur during the development of malignancy.

The multistep process of colorectal carcinogenesis involves the formation of adenomas either from hyperplastic epithelium or from polyps, with subsequent progression to carcinoma, as suggested by Morson (Fig. 12.4). Recognition of this sequence has allowed the molecular events at each stage leading to eventual tumour formation to be studied. Almost all CRCs (98%) are adenocarcinomas, and it is likely that such carcinomas arise in a small number of pre-existing adenomatous polyps. The evidence for a sequential change from adenoma to carcinoma comes from a number of observations. Minute adenocarcinomas generally arise within adenomatous polyps and removal of polyps diminishes the incidence of cancer in those patients. Adenomas co-exist with carcinomas in over a third of patients. Foci of cancer may be detected within large dysplastic adenomas, or a residual region of adenoma can often be noted at the margins of a carcinoma specimen. A markedly increased frequency of cancer is seen in the familial polyposis syndromes, and oncogene and tumour suppressor gene abnormalities are seen in both adenomas and carcinomas (Fig. 12.5). This process of tumour initiation and progression is likely to be continuous and probably occurs over a period measured in years or decades. In particular, the study of relatively common forms of inherited CRC have been extremely useful; they have been well described and analysis of large family cohorts have been possible.

Both neoplastic and inflammatory polyps occur in the large and small intestine. Adenomatous polyps may be tubular or, less commonly, villous. Tubular adenomas are distributed evenly along the length of the colon whereas villous adenomas are usually rectal. Adenomas over 2 cm in diameter and those of villous shape are most likely to transform. Although it is not necessary to have a polyp detected before or coincidental with a cancer, this sequence occurs five times more frequently than cancer alone.

Solitary colonic polyps are found in the general population with an incidence increasing with age, from about 15% at 50–59 years to 75% over the age of 75 years.

Three stages of growth of tumours are recognised (Fig. 12.4). The preneoplastic stage consists of hyperplastic growth of colonic epithelium, leading to the formation of polyps or adenomas, which are outgrowths into the colonic lumen (Fig. 12.6). These adenomas,

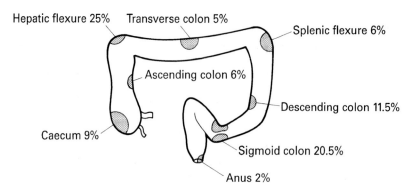

Symptoms
  Bleeding
  Altered bowel habit (constipation or diarrhoea)
  Pain
  Anorexia
  Weight loss
  Vomiting
  Tenesmus
  Awareness of an abdominal mass
Signs
  Anaemia
  Cachexia
  Abdominal distension from tumour mass, ascites or bowel obstruction
  Hepatomegaly
  Jaundice
  Rectal mass
  Pelvic mass
  Fistulae to bladder or vagina
  Stigmata of a predisposing syndrome, e.g. CHRPE in FAP
  Endocrine, metabolic or haematological paraneoplastic phenomena
Diagnosis
Determine the nature and anatomical level of lesion by:
  Barium enema

  Sigmoidoscopy/colonoscopy: examination and also allows biopsy to be taken upon visualisation

  Ultrasound scan: abdominal, pelvic or transrectal; determines the extent of local spread and screens for liver metastases

  Computer axial tomography (CAT) scan: also allows accurate tumour staging after surgery before considering chemotherapy and/or radiography
  Magnetic resonance imaging (MRI)

  Tumour markers, e.g. carcinoembryonic antigen; CA 19-9 is usually not tissue or tumour specific

Fig. 12.3. A clinical overview of CRC. The diagram shows the incidence of tumours at the various sections of the colon. (Some tumours (15%) have no clear area of occurrence.)

Table 12.7. *Groups at risk for CRC*

Risk	Associated disease
Markedly increased risk	
Familial polyposis coli and associated syndromes:	Gardener's syndrome, Turcot's syndrome, Field's syndrome, juvenile polyposis, inherited adenomatosis (Lynch type 1) Cancer family syndrome (Lynch type II) Total ulcerative colitis for >8 years
Moderately increased risk	Previous gynaecological or breast cancer Ureterosigmoidostomy Previous *Streptococcus bovis* bacteraemia Other gastrointestinal tract polyposis syndromes

which may vary greatly in size, shape and complexity, do not necessarily progress to form tumours. However, it is thought that all tumours arise from adenomas. The final stage is the formation of adenocarcinomas (Fig. 12.7), which may invade locally or metastasise into the bloodstream. The majority of CRCs arise sporadically, but between 5 and 25% of all tumours may have a specific genetic basis. A number of inherited clinical syndromes have been identified on the basis of their different clinical and pathological characteristics (Table 12.8).

Hereditary CRC

Patients with hereditary gastrointestinal polyposis syndromes have a very high incidence of colorectal malignancies.

Familial adenomatous polyposis

Familial adenomatous polyposis (FAP) was first described by Harrison Cripps in 1882. It is an autosomal dominant syndrome with high penetrance and a prevalence of approximately 1 in 8000 in the UK. FAP may account for 0.5 to 1.0% of all CRCs. The age of onset is variable and the mutation rate is thought to be up to 30%. Although it is a rare cause of colonic cancer, it provides a model of tumorigenesis and may also reveal factors that are important in the formation of sporadic tumours. A number of extracolonic manifestations are also associated and include sebaceous cysts, dentiginous cysts, desmoid tumours, black lesions of the retina and congenital hypertrophy of retinal pigment epithelium (CHRPE) (Fig. 12.3, Table 12.8). Where these extracolonic features are common, the disorder may be known as Gardner's syndrome, which is not a separate disease and is caused by the same genetic abnormality. There is also an association with extraintestinal cancers, including papillary carcinoma of the thyroid, astrocytomas, medulloblastomas and hepatoblastoma. Individuals with FAP or its variant syndromes develop up to several thousand adenomas in their large intestine, duodenum and stomach during childhood and adolescence, which then increase in number and size by

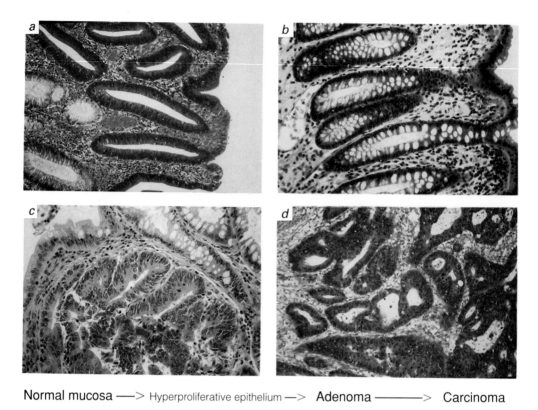

Normal mucosa ——> Hyperproliferative epithelium —> Adenoma ————> Carcinoma

Fig. 12.4. The progression of normal colorectal mucosa to carcinoma (after Morson, 1974). (*a*) Normal mucosa. (*b*) Mild dysplasia, a low-power view of darkly staining regular adenomatous glands with mild dysplasia next to non-neoplastic crypts. (*c*) severely displastic adenomatous gland, which shows complex branching, multilayering and focal cell death. (*d*) Carcinoma, moderately differentiated invasive adenocarcinoma with some complex gland formation. (Colour plates kindly provided by Dr G. Stamp, Hammersmith Hospital.)

the end of their second to fourth decades of life. The diagnosis of FAP is confirmed by finding more than 100 adenomatous polyps in the colon and rectum (Fig. 12.8). Although only a small number of the adenomas present actually progress to carcinoma, all patients eventually will develop malignant tumours if resection of the large intestine is not performed. Approximately 12% also develop carcinomas of the stomach and duodenum. Patients with FAP should be offered total colectomy with ileorectal anastomosis or pan-proctocolectomy with restorative ileoanal anastomosis if colonic polyps have already developed. Subsequent management includes lifelong assessment of the rectal stump and also endoscopic assessment every three years of the stomach and duodenum. Most carcinomas occur in patients between the ages of 30 and 50 years if proctocolectomy is not performed, and this contrasts with the expected peak incidence of non-inherited CRC of between 60 and 70 years.

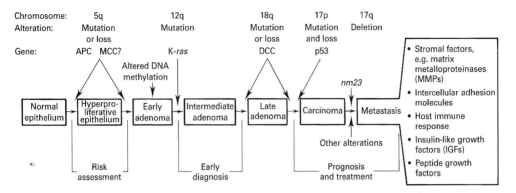

Fig. 12.5. Molecular changes during the development of CRC. The genes are the proto-oncogene K-*ras*; p 53, a tumour suppressor gene; and three genes called APC, adenomatous polyposis coli; DCC, deleted in colon cancer; and MCC, mutated in colon cancer. (After Fearon, E.R. and Vogelstein, B. (1990). A genetic model for colorectal tumorigenesis. *Cell*, 61, 759–767, with permission.)

The APC (for adenomatous polyposis coli) gene, which when mutated leads to FAP and Gardner's syndrome, was localised to chromosome 5q21 in 1986, following the report of a male patient with mental retardation who had Gardner's syndrome and a constitutional deletion of chromosome 5q. Identification at the molecular level by White, Nakamura and Vogelstein followed in 1991. Using RFLP analysis and *in situ* hybridisation of DNA from 13 families of patients with FAP, the location of the FAP gene was found to be close to a marker at 5q21–q22. The gene for FAP has been cloned and sequenced independently by two groups. It encodes a large protein product of 2843 amino acid residues that acts primarily as a tumour suppressor gene. At present germ-line mutations have been identified in affected individuals in about two-thirds of the families with FAP and Gardner's syndrome who have been studied. All inherited mutations in the APC gene identified so far appear to inactivate the gene; they include gross deletions in a minority of patients and, more often, localised mutations that cause frame-shifts or create stop codons or missense mutations in the gene product. It is of great interest that a potential mouse model of polyposis coli, the min mouse, has a germ-line mutation in the murine homologue of the APC gene.

Relatives of affected individuals should be entered on a genetic register, and those at risk of inheriting the gene offered genetic counselling and screening. Screening of at-risk relatives by annual sigmoidoscopy usually begins between 11 and 15 years of age, since the rectum is involved by adenomata at an early stage, and polyps rarely develop before the age of 11 years. If polyps are found they are biopsied to confirm that they are adenomas and to exclude carcinomas, and timing of colectomy is carefully considered. In the absence of any suspicious lesions, sigmoidoscopy is continued annually until the age of 40, when there is less than 1% risk to an individual of developing the disease. The age-specific risk of FAP in relatives with negative gastrointestinal examinations can be further modified by including the results of ophthalmoscopy to detect CHRPE. Specifically, these are discrete, darkly pigmented rounded lesions 50–200 μm in diame-

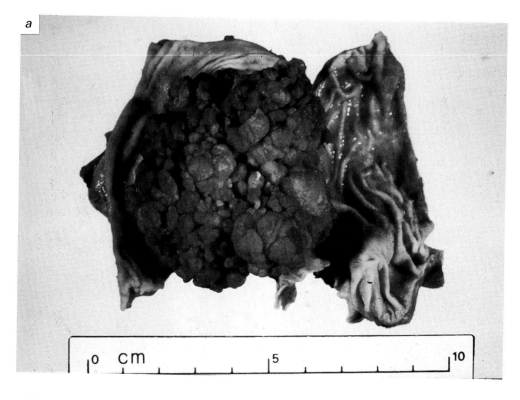

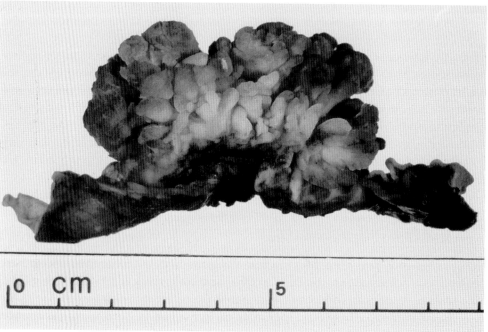

Fig. 12.6. Villous adenoma of the colon (kindly provided by Dr D. Parums, Hammersmith Hospital).

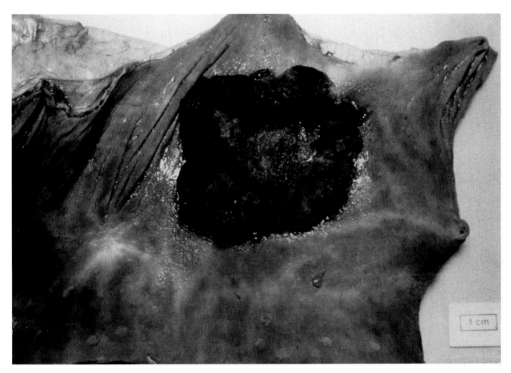

Fig. 12.7. Carcinoma of the colon (kindly provided by Dr D. Parums, Hammersmith Hospital).

ter (Fig. 12.9). Smaller solitary unilateral lesions may be seen in normal individuals, but it is rare for normal individuals to have more than three lesions. Most patients with FAP have four or more CHRPEs. These are present at birth so can be used as biological markers at that age. It has been estimated that, in families in which CHRPEs appear to be a feature of the disease, the finding of fewer than three lesions in an individual at 50% risk of inheriting FAP reduces their estimated risk to approximately 1 in 13, whereas more than three lesions conveys a very high probability that the individual is affected. Pre-natal diagnosis is available by linkage analysis or by direct mutation detection.

Hereditary non-polyposis CRC

The hereditary non-polyposis colon cancer syndrome (HNPCC) has been recognised since the 1950s in that certain families could be identified with a pre-disposition to CRC in an autosomal dominant pattern of inheritance. This became known as the Lynch or family cancer syndrome. In Lynch type I families, tumours were common under the age of 50 years, confined in two-thirds of patients to the caecum and ascending colon, and were often metachronous. In Lynch type II, in addition to all Lynch type I features there was also an added pre-disposition to gynaecological, renal and other gastrointestinal

Table 12.8. *Syndromes associated with an increased risk of gastrointestinal cancer*

Syndrome	Inheritance	Location of gene	Cancer site	Associated manifestations
Site-specific colon cancer (Lynch type I)	Autosomal dominant	?	Colon, most lesions on right side	None
Cancer family syndrome (Lynch type II)	Autosomal dominant	2p 16	Colon, other gastrointestinal sites, ovary, uterus, renal tract, pancreas, breast	None
Muir–Torre syndrome	Autosomal dominant	?	As in Lynch type II, larynx, bladder, breast	Keratocanthoma, sebaceous adenomata, basal cell carcinoma
Familial adenomatous polyposis/Gardner's syndrome	Autosomal dominant	5q21–22	>100 colorectal adenomata, colorectal, other gastro-intestinal sites, thyroid, brain	Sebaceous cysts, adontogenic jaw cysts, retinal changes (hypertrophy of retinal pigment epithelium), desmoids
Gorlin's syndrome	Autosomal dominant	9q	Skin, fibrosarcoma, jaw, nasopharyngeal, harmartomatous colonic polyps	Multiple skin basal cell carcinomas, odontogenic keratocysts of jaw, multiple skeletal abnormalities, palmar and plantar pits
Peutz–Jegher's syndrome	Autosomal dominant	?	Gastrointestinal harmartomas, gastrointestinal, ovarian, breast, testicular	Mucocutaneous pigmentations (freckling)
Juvenile polyposis	Probably autosomal dominant	?	Juvenile polyposis of gastrointestinal tract; risk of gastrointestinal cancer	Congenital heart disease, clubbing, macroencephaly, polydactyly
Turcot's syndrome	Autosomal recessive	?17p	Numerous colorectal polyps, but <100; colorectal and central nervous system	Cafe au lait spots, sebaceous cysts, pigmented spots

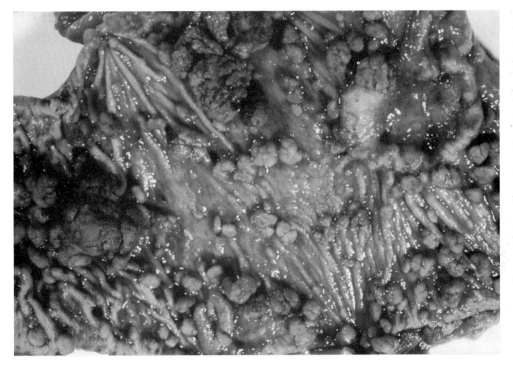

Fig. 12.8. Carcinoma of the colon arising in a patient with FAP.

cancers. They are thought to represent 5–10% of all CRCs (Table 12.8). The HNPCC syndromes are heterogeneous at the phenotypic and probably the genetic level. There are no clinical features other than a few adenomatous polyps to alert the clinician to the diagnosis of Lynch syndrome, although in the Muir–Torre syndrome, which may be a variant of the family cancer syndrome, sebaceous adenomata and keratoacanthomata may be seen on the skin. In first-degree relatives of patients with Lynch type II syndrome, there is a sevenfold increase in the incidence of CRC, markedly higher than the risk to relatives with sporadic cancer (Table 12.6). Accurate recording of family history and genetic counselling are currently the only means of identifying those at increased risk. A limited cytogenetic study suggested linkage of HNPCC to the Kidd blood group on chromosome 18q; however, no germ-line mutations or deletions in the DCC (deleted in colon cancer) gene located on chromosome 18q were found in 500 kindreds with HNPCC. In companion studies, there was evidence of germ-line genetic changes indicative of errors in DNA replication on chromosome 2p. Subsequently, independent investigations have identified the gene for HNPCC as hMSH2, a human homologue of the prokaryotic gene *mutS*, which itself is involved in the repair of DNA mismatches. A variety of mutations in this gene have been detected in affected family members.

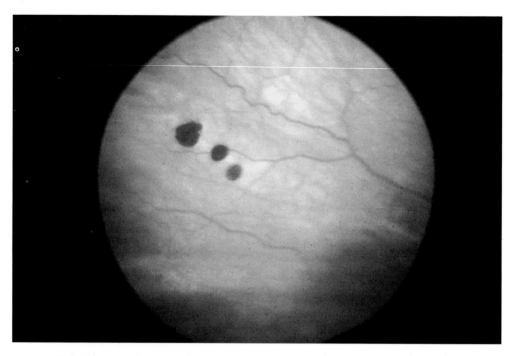

Fig. 12.9. Congenital hypertrophy of the retinal pigment epithelium (kindly provided by Mr S. Schulenberg, Hammersmith Hospital).

Non-hereditary CRC

First-degree relatives of patients with CRCs have a threefold to fivefold increase in the risk of developing the disease; this is not seen in studies of spouses, who presumably share the same diet and environment but not the genetic make-up. The risks of cancer to relatives is shown in Table 12.6. The increased risk is as a result of increased formation of adenomatous polyps; the susceptibility to this follows a pattern of dominant inheritance.

Inflammatory bowel disease and CRC

Patients with ulcerative colitis have an increased susceptibility to tumour formation although molecular studies indicate that the early events of neoplasia appear to differ in this population. The most important factors associated with the highest risk of malignancy are the extent of colitis and early age of onset. The relative risk of cancer varies also with chronicity of disease and is thought to be 0.3% after 10 years, 12–15% after 20 years, and 50% after 30 years, although some reports have included a risk of only 4.5% at 30 years. There may also be a different genetic basis for cancers arising from long-standing ulcerative colitis. A low rate of *ras* mutations and high expression of *myc* p 62/64 oncoproteins are associated features.

Table 12.9. *Somatic mutations in CRC*

Gene	Type of mutation	CRCs with alteration (%)
Tumour suppressor genes		
p 53	Point mutation, LOH	75–85
APC	Point mutation, small deletion (LOH)	>65
DCC	LOH, insertion, deletion, point mutation	70–75
Oncogenes		
K-*ras*	Point mutation	48
N-*ras*	Point mutation	<2
neu (HER2/*erb*-2)	Amplification	<5
c-myc	Amplification	<5
myb	Amplification	<5

Tumour formation may be through adenoma formation or through non-specific routes. Specific mutations have been identified at a later stage of tumorigenesis.

In Crohn's disease, the reported increased risk of occurrence of CRC has been between 4 and 20%. Average age of onset is 10 years younger than sporadic CRC, at 55 years, and there is a higher prevalence of mucinous carcinoma.

Oncogenes

The abnormal expression of a number of oncogenes have been implicated in CRC. The most important of these are *ras* and *myc* (Table 12.9).

The ras *family*

Members of the *ras* gene family have a critical role in the development of a number of cancers including CRC. As discussed earlier, *ras* proteins promote hydrolysis of GTP to GDP, acting synergistically with GTPase-activating protein. The Ras–GDP couples extracellular signals from growth factors and their receptors to second messengers and eventually leads to cellular proliferation. Mutations in *ras* may either initiate the development of adenomas, which may eventually transform into carcinomas, or promote the growth of a small adenoma with little dysplasia into a lesion with a higher malignant potential. Increased levels of the p 21 protein product of *ras* have been associated with CRC but are not specific for neoplasia.

Mutations in one of the three *ras* genes can be identified in at least 50% of CRCs and in about 45% of adenomas that either are greater than 1 cm in size or appear dysplastic. In adenomas with minimal dysplasia or that are less than 1 cm in size, there is a 10% *ras* mutation rate. Activation of *ras* in CRC is usually by point mutation and almost always involves K-*ras* at the twelfth codon. Mutations in *ras* are found in up to two-thirds of all colonic tumours; increased mutation frequency has been associated with increased malignant phenotype. In FAP, these mutations are seen in both polyps and adenomas at all stages of evolution as well as in carcinomas. Acquisition of the *ras* point mutation is a relatively early event in the adenoma–carcinoma sequence but does not appear to be the initiating event. Such mutations are seen along the entire length of the large intestine, in contrast to *myc* overexpression and chromosomal losses, which are seen mainly in distal tumours, and suggest that different genetic lesions may predominate at different sites. Mutation analysis is a potential method of screening of CRC. A recent study of stool samples from CRC patients found that K-*ras* mutations could be identified in stool samples in eight of nine patients in whom the mutations were present in the tumour. Although K-*ras* mutations are only present in 40% of CRCs, they are present at the pre-malignant stage and so facilitate the early identification of an adenoma or of a recurrent carcinoma.

The myc *oncogene*

The *myc* gene is located on chromosome 8q24 and encodes two polypeptides. Their natural function is not known but their structure suggests a role in transcriptional regulation and as co-factors for DNA polymerase. High levels of *myc* expression are seen in left-sided colonic cancer, although gene amplification is uncommon. In studies using polymorphic DNA probes linked to the APC gene on chromosome 5q, 50% of CRCs with raised *myc* expression also had deletions in the regions of the APC gene. In FAP patients, high levels of *myc* expression and *myc* mRNA are associated with two-thirds of adenomatous polyps. Increased transcription of *myc* is associated with increasing tendency towards malignant transformation.

Tumour suppressor genes

The existence of recessive genes that when altered lead to tumour formation has been suspected for many years. Evidence for them comes from large family studies of FAP patients and their relatives, studies on cell fusion and somatic hybrids, and studies of consistent chromosomal loss and loss of DNA in tumours. This work enabled candidate areas for tumour suppressor genes to be localised in the human genome. Four genes involved in CRC have been identified; two (the APC and MCC (mutated in colon cancer) genes) were identified through FAP family studies, and two (the p53 and DCC (deleted in colon cancer) genes) through the study of loss of heterozygosity in sporadic tumours (see Fig. 12.5 and Table 12.9).

The 'two hit' hypothesis leading to loss of tumour suppressor gene function in the Knudson model was described above. Testing for allele loss in both FAP and sporadic CRC has uncovered a number of regions of the genome that are consistently altered during the development of CRCs. Five tumour suppressor genes are now discussed.

The APC gene

Inactivation of the APC gene is important in the development of adenomas in patients with polyposis and sporadic CRC. Somatic mutations that inactivate the APC gene, either those localised specifically in the APC gene or LOH for chromosome 5q, can be detected in 60–65% of CRC and adenomas that are not a part of FAP. Mutations of this gene appear to be the first step in neoplasia and initiate adenoma formation. Such mutations are seen in tiny early adenomas and precede *ras* mutations. Mutation analysis of non-FAP colon cancer patients also reveals the presence of less severe inherited mutations that result in a milder phenotype and lower penetrance. This may reveal an underlying predisposition to CRC.

The MCC gene

The MCC gene lies close to the APC gene and was thought originally to be responsible for FAP. It is mutated in 15% of sporadic CRCs but is not associated with FAP. Its role in colorectal carcinogenesis is uncertain.

p53

The p 53 tumour suppressor gene is located on the short arm of chromosome 17 and encodes a 53 kDa nuclear phosphoprotein that functions as a negative regulator of cell proliferation. The p 53 protein binds specific DNA sequences and appears to be a transcription factor that may regulate the expression of particular cellular genes. Normal (wild-type) p 53 acts as a 'molecular policeman'. It blocks the growth of many transformed cells at various points in the cell cycle and arrests replication in DNA-damaged cells. Wild-type p 53 may also be involved in restricting precursor populations by mediating apoptosis, or programmed cell death, and may modulate the cytotoxicity of anticancer drugs. Experimentally, transfection of p 53 into human cancer cell lines suppresses malignant phenotype and growth. Abnormal or mutant p 53 allows the accumulation of gene mutations and chromosomal rearrangements and has been associated with virtually every sporadically occurring malignancy, including 60% of CRCs.

The DCC gene and loss of heterozygosity

Some tumour suppressor gene alterations were identified originally by the frequent loss of DNA detected by means of LOH analysis (see p. 35). Comparison of allele loss in hereditary and sporadic cancer indicated that there are common mechanisms fundamental to the development of both types of tumour. LOH events are thought to be selected for during tumorigenesis because they can inactivate tumour suppressor genes.

The most common site of loss is chromosome 17p, which is deleted in over 75% of CRCs studies; 18q is lost in 70% and 5q in 50%. A candidate tumour suppressor gene from the region of chromosome 18q affected by LOH has been identified and is termed DCC (deleted in colon cancer). The gene product has a predicted amino acid sequence similar to that of a neural cell adhesion molecule, which may explain in part some of the cellular properties of invasion, motility and metastatic behaviour seen in cells from CRCs. Levels of product were reduced to less than 5% of those in normal colonic mucosa. The introduction of normal chromosome 18 by cell fusion results in loss of tumorigenicity in certain experimental CRC lines. These observations suggest a role for DCC as a candidate tumour suppressor gene but does not prove it has a direct role in carcinogenesis. The tumour suppressor gene presumed to be the target of these allelic losses is p 53. In more than 90% of the CRCs with the 17p LOH, the remaining copy of the p 53 gene encodes a mutant p 53 protein; p 53 mutations are infrequent in CRC without 17p LOH or in adenomas. Therefore, both events – point mutation of one p 53 allele and the loss of the remaining wild-type p 53 allele by LOH – occur frequently only in later stages CRC and perhaps most often during the transition from adenoma to carcinoma.

The nm23 *gene*

The *nm23* gene is located at 17q21 and deletions of this area have been detected in CRCs. The *nm23* transcript has been found in normal colonic mucosa and increased expression has been demonstrated in polyps and in both metastatic and non-metastatic CRC. Expression of *nm23* may also have prognostic value for the development of metastatic disease.

Other genetic and cellular factors

It is likely that tumour suppressor genes and oncogenes interact with a number of other important genes and epigenetic events to bring about the further changes that will eventually lead to tumour formation. Some of these events are now described.

DNA hypomethylation

DNA methylation appears to be a controlling factor in the regulation of gene expression. A decrease in methylation of cytosine/guanine nucleotides is associated with gene activation. DNA hypomethylation may cause chromosomal instability leading to abnormalities associated with cancers. More specifically, hypomethylation can affect very small regions in DNA and may lead to abnormal transcription or inappropriate expression of genes important for neoplastic cell growth, so giving the cells a selective growth advantage. Hypomethylation may also inhibit chromosomal condensation, leading to somatic non-dysjunction. Hypomethylation of the *erbB-2* and *myc* oncogenes has been found in a significant number of polyps and adenocarcinomas compared with normal mucosal tissue. Comparison of methylation status in normal mucosa, polyps and carcinomas showed that DNA from polyps and carcinomas was similarly methylated, suggesting that a decrease in the methylation status was an early event in tumour formation.

Tumour-associated antigens

Specific tumour cell surface characteristics have been sought for some time in order to direct treatment most specifically. Carcinoembryonic antigen (CEA) is one member of a group of heavily glycosylated single-chain peptides that was originally discovered in extracts of colonic adenocarcinoma. It is not specific for colorectal malignancy, with raised levels found in 30–50% of all patients with breast carcinomas; it is also found in a number of benign conditions. Its function *in vitro* is as a cell adhesion molecule, and its altered expression may be involved in the process of liver metastasis. Serial CEA levels can detect tumour recurrence in otherwise asymptomatic patients; in two-thirds of patients an elevated CEA may be the first indicator. Pre-operative levels reflect tumour burden. Approximately 25–50% of patients with locoregional and 95% of patients with liver metastases will have raised levels. The rate of rise may be more important than absolute levels. Steele *et al.* have shown that raised levels of CEA have prognostic value for colonic carcinoma but not for rectal carcinoma. Further studies at the Mayo clinic have drawn a similar conclusion but noted that within different stages of colonic carcinoma CEA was only an independent prognostic factor for Duke's stage C patients with four or more lymph nodes involved. Immunocytochemical studies have shown the presence of CEA in normal columnar epithelial cells and goblet cells. Monoclonal antibodies have demonstrated a large number of epitopes in health and disease, and further studies of individual epitopes may increase the specificity of CEA assays. Recently, the gene for CEA has been cloned and characterised. The molecule is encoded by a member of a gene family belonging to the immunoglobulin superfamily and mapped to chromosome 19. CEA has been used as a target antigen for localisation of tumours and their metastases using radiolabelled antibodies, and as a potential target for therapy with either drug–antibody or isotope–antibody conjugates. However this approach has so far been unsuccessful. The expression of CEA is not specific.

Growth factors and growth factor receptors

Insulin-like growth factor

Insulin-like growth factors (IGFs) are polypeptides that are structurally related to insulin. IGF-I and IGF-II are important anabolic and mitogenic peptides and are thought to be significant endocrine, autocrine and paracrine factors involved both in normal cellular growth and proliferation and malignancy. IGF-I, IGF-II are potent stimulators of CRC cell proliferation *in vitro*. IGF-I is produced mainly by hepatocytes and is a basic single-chain polypeptide of 70 amino acid residues that has some homology with proinsulin. IGF-II is produced mainly during fetal life and its normal function in adults is largely unknown.

Two factors that significantly affect the extent of cellular response to IGFs include the membrane receptors for IGFs and their high-affinity binding proteins (IGFBPs), which modulate the action of IGFs at the receptor level. All three components of the IGF system play an important role in the proliferation of colonic tumours. The evidence for this includes the widespread existence of high-affinity binding sites for IGF-I in several colon cancer cell lines and in freshly resected tumours. These studies plus those showing the proliferative effect of IGF-I in several cell lines demonstrate the importance of IGF-I in growth regulation. Lambert *et al.* found that IGF-II mRNA was increased up to 800-fold in CRC compared with normal tissues; this increase in expression was observed specifically in distal and Duke's C carcinomas. The same group also detected an RFLP in 1 of 13 patients, suggesting a structural modification of one of the IGF-II alleles in the tumour compared with normal tissues.

Peptide growth factors

Like the IGFs, peptide growth factors (PGF) are potent regulators of cellular proliferation. They appear to be the paracrine mediators of epithelial–mesenchymal interaction and growth. The important PGFs include EGF and TGF-α, the fibroblast growth factors (FGFs), TGF-β, as well as a number of oncoproteins that are either single peptide growth factors or peptide growth factor receptors that are constitutively active, such as c-erbB-2 and int-2 (FGF-3). Cancer cells, including CRC, have the ability to sustain growth through autocrine and paracrine loops. This may occur through the production of certain growth factors and/or enhanced expression of their receptors. These factors may give a survival benefit to the cells once transformed. Several autocrine and paracrine loops have been demonstrated in 80% of primary and metastatic CRC. Using specific ligand-binding assays to its receptor, EGFR is shown to be normally expressed or found to have an even lower expression than in unaffected colon mucosa.

Metastasis in CRC

CRC has a high propensity to metastasise by the haematogenous, lymphatic and intraperitoneal routes. However, it is not clear whether the complex process of metastasis occurs in a number of discrete steps, as first suggested by Ziedman (multistep theory), is a truly random process (stochastic theory) with all cells having more or less equal ability to metastasise, or is a combination of both processes. Ziedman proposed that only a specialised subset of cells within tumour populations possesses all the attributes necessary for metastasis. Studies of B16 murine melanoma lines have shown that certain cells express properties that specifically provide an advantage for survival in the circulation and tissues in mice. Tumour dissemination then is achieved by cell movement and digestion of limiting factors, such as basement membranes, by proteolytic enzymes. The eventual site of arrest of tumour cells depends on their ability to escape host defence mechanisms, on their adherence to vascular endothelium by inducing endothelial retraction and on binding to glycoproteins of the basement membranes. Finally, local invasion and cell migration is facilitated by the action of local enzymes such as type IV collagenase.

A number of observations have supported the stochastic theory. The expression of metastatic behaviour by an individual cell is often influenced by local events. Although the cell populations in most CRCs are heterogeneous, cells derived from metastases are not necessarily more aggressively disseminating then parental lines. Factors that would normally limit tumour spread, such as basement membrane, are absent in the liver sinusoids and occasionally in blood vessels and lymphatics. Furthermore, proteases released as a result of the normal response to tumour antigens by leucocytes, occlusion of small capillaries by tumour emboli leading to local thrombus formation, tissue ischaemia and infarction may all lead to disruption of basement membranes and allow tumour metastasis.

Invasive factors and metastasis

Invading and disseminating cells come into contact with a variety of extracellular molecules that constitute the extracellular matrix. This is an active biological compartment that provides physical support for tissues and regulates the physiological behaviour of cells that are in contact with it; these include enzymes such as the matrix metalloproteinases (MMPs) and local growth factors. The extracellular matrix is made up of proteins with specific tasks, such as structural support (the collagens), and fibrous proteins that have adhesive properties (fibronectin and laminin). As discussed above, invasion of tumour cells into blood vessels and lymphatics is a prerequisite for metastasis. However, local penetration by the tumour may be achieved by a combination of enzymatic digestion of the extracellular matrix and enhanced cell motility. The most extensively studied enzymes thought to be involved at the level of the extracellular matrix are the MMPs and their inhibitors – the tissue inhibitors of MMPs (TIMPs).

The matrix metalloproteinases

There has recently been great interest in the inappropriate activity of the MMPs, which are tissue proteinases that may facilitate local invasion and metastasis by degrading the extracellular tissue matrix. The MMPs are a widely distributed family of enzymes that play a key role in the turnover and remodelling of the extracellular matrix. MMPs originate from stromal cells, monocytes, macrophages and polymorphonuclear lymphocytes in normal circumstances or in the presence of tumour cells or inflammation. They are tightly regulated through control of gene expression, and at a post-translational level are activated by the cleavage of a propeptide. MMPs are involved in both physiolgical processes, including embryonic development, and in tumour invasion. To date five subgroups of MMPs have been identified based on the relationship of each enzyme to bacterial zinc-containing proteinases; a further division into three subclasses is made on the basis of substrate specificity. Although basement membranes are effective barriers to tumour invasion, some tumours secrete specific enzymes that degrade these membranes or are associated with impaired membrane synthesis. These tumours have been shown to have a high propensity to metastasise. Basement membranes from CRCs have low levels of two components: laminin and type IV collagen. Recent studies have shown that the occurrence of laminin-negative tumours correlated with the frequency of metastasis (which was not the case for laminin-positive tumours) and that laminin expression may be a better prognostic indicator than histological tumour grade. Limited deposition of type IV collagen has been associated with a shorter survival, particularly with patients with Duke's C and D disease.

Increased expression of MMP-2, MMP-7 and MMP-9 has been detected in a number of sporadic CRCs; it is thought that this overexpression may reflect biological aspects of tumour behaviour related to the metastatic process rather than tumour burden. TIMP suppresses tumour invasion and metastasis in certain tumours. Paradoxically, high levels of these tissue inhibitors have been found in CRC and this has been associated with the extent of tumour invasion. This may reflect a role for TIMP as a growth enhancer in addition to its inhibitory properties.

Cell surface and metastasis

The role of intercellular adhesion molecules (ICAMs) in tumour progression has been of considerable interest in recent years, particularly as a result of studies of leucocyte behaviour during immune responses. The interaction between host and tumour cells and the extracellular matrix may be determined by one or many ICAMs and their receptor density; it does not simply consist of cells 'gluing together'. The expression of receptor molecules is associated with the expression of other developmentally important proteins affecting cell division, cell interactions, cell shape and cell movement.

A large number of adhesion systems are used by any one cell. We shall consider the role of the integrins, the cadherins and the immunoglobulin superfamilies.

Integrins

There are at least three families of integrin receptor. These include the fibronectin receptor and related receptors that bind to collagen and laminin, a receptor on platelets that binds fibronectin and fibrinogen and finally two receptors on leucocytes that play a role in the adhesion of neutrophils to endothelial cells. The integrins recognise a specific tripeptide amino acid sequence Arg–Gly–Asp (known as RGD) in the extracellular protein, which is common to a number of extracellular adhesive proteins.

Cadherins

The cadherin family of cellular adhesion receptors is important for cell-to-cell binding; a cadherin molecule on one cell will only bind an identical cadherin molecule from another cell. Four subclasses have been described (E, P, N and L), although cells express multiple classes of cadherin. Changes in cadherin expression have a direct effect on cell morphology and may contribute to the release of tumour cells from the primary site and be associated with a more aggressive phenotype.

Immunoglobulin superfamily

Expression of ICAM-1 has been correlated with depth of invasion and metastatic potential of human malignant melanomas. The tumour suppressor gene DCC is involved in colorectal tumour progression and encodes a glycoprotein that is a member of the immunoglobulin superfamily. It has been suggested that CRCs that have lost one copy of the DCC gene have a greater propensity to metastasise. CEA, discussed above, is a glycoprotein that may also have a function as a cell adhesion molecule. It has been hypothesised that CEA is released from certain CRCs, taken up by macrophages and hepatocytes and presented on the cell surface. The homophilic binding that then occurs between CEA-expressing tumour cells and hepatocytes may encourage tumour migration arrest and begin the formation of a liver metastasis.

Host immune response and metastasis

Despite many thousands of tumour cells entering the circulation each day, very few survive to become metastases. The efficiency of host effector systems such as the immune response are thought to be responsible for this. The host responses may be innate or acquired. Potential effector cells include cytotoxic T cells and natural killer cells. The former effect cell killing by binding to target cells through T cell receptor recognition of 'foreign' antigen in association with self antigens encoded by the MHC class I genes. Although T cells are frequently seen infiltrating tumours, their exact role in inhibiting metastasis is not clear. Natural killer cells are large granular lymphocytes distinct from T and B cells. They have been implicated in the eradication of disseminating tumour cells in experimental models of metastasis. Allogeneic tumour cells highly metastatic in other mice are frequently less metastatic in adult nude mice; this has been attributed to higher levels of natural killer cells in the nude mice. Despite intensive research in cytokines and the immunology of CRC, immunotherapy using interferons, interleukins and tumour-infiltrating lymphocytes has been largely disappointing, both in treating bulk tumours and in the adjuvant setting.

A summary of a possible genetic model for CRC is shown in Fig. 12.2; the interaction between the specific genetic and local tissue factors discussed may account, at least in part, for the transition from normal colonic epithelium to metastatic and/or locally invasive carcinoma.

Potential therapies based on molecular genetics

CRC is clearly a disease caused by defective somatic cell genetics. Gene therapy strategies, therefore, seem an appropriate avenue for further research.

The main problem facing the gene therapist is how to incorporate new genes into every tumour cell. If this cannot be achieved then any malignant cells that remain unaffected will emerge as a resistant clone. Presently we do not have ideal vectors. Despite this drawback, there are already over 100 protocols accepted for clinical trial in cancer patients worldwide – the majority in the USA. The ethical issues are fairly straightforward with oncology providing some of the highest possible benefit–risk ratios. There are six strategies currently under investigation:

- genetic tagging
- enhancing tumour immunogenicity
- vectoring cytokines to tumours

- inserting drug-activating genes
- suppressing oncogene expression
- replacing defective tumour suppressor genes.

Genetic tagging

There are several situations where the use of a genetic marker to tag tumour cells may help in making decisions on the optimal treatment for an individual patient. The insertion of a foreign marker gene into cells from a tumour biopsy and replacing the marked cells into the patient prior to treatment can provide a sensitive new indicator of minimal residual disease after chemotherapy. The most common marker is the gene for neomycin phosphotransferase (*neoR*), an enzyme that metabolises the aminoglycoside antibiotic G418. This gene when inserted into an appropriate retroviral vector can be stably incorporated into the host cell's genome. Originally detected by antibiotic resistance, it can now be picked up by the more sensitive PCR approach. In this way, as few as one tumour cell amongst one million normal cells can be identified. This procedure can help in the design of aggressive chemotherapy protocols.

A particularly elegant use of this strategy has been the analysis of the reasons of failure in autologous bone marrow transplantation for childhood acute myeloblastic leukemia (AML). Failure can be caused by inadequate chemotherapy or by reinfusion of viable tumour cells in the stored marrow. Reinfused marrow was labelled with *neoR* and recurrent tumour was analysed for the presence of this gene. In the majority of patients, tumour cells contain the marker, indicating a failure of the purging process. Similar studies are now in progress for neuroblastoma as well as for chronic myeloid leukemia and acute lymphoid leukemia. So far, no marking protocols for CRC have been developed.

Enhancing tumour immunogenicity

The presence of an immune response to cancer has been recognised for many years. The problem is that human tumours seem to be predominantly weakly immunogenic. If ways could be found to elicit a more powerful immune stimulus then effective immunotherapy could become a reality. Several observations from murine tumours indicate that one reason for weak immunogenicity of certain tumours is the failure to elicit a T helper cell response. These cells, in turn, release the necessary cytokines to stimulate the production of cytolytic T cells, which can destroy tumours. The expression of cytokine genes such as those for IL-2, TNF and interferon in tumour cells has been shown to bypass the need for T helper cells in mice. Similar clinical experiments are now in progress. Melanoma cells have been prepared from biopsies and infected with retrovirus containing the gene for IL-2. These cells are being used as a vaccine to elicit a more powerful immune response.

Many tumours express low amounts of the products of the MHC. These molecules are necessary for antigen presentation and their absence may help tumours evade immune scrutiny. There are now several examples of mouse model systems where tumour cells transfected with MHC class II genes can be used not only to prevent tumour spread when given as a prophylactic vaccine but also to induce remission of established leukaemias, lymphomas, carcinomas and sarcomas. Clinical experiments involving the direct intratumoral injection of foreign HLA genes are currently in progress for several tumour types including CRC.

Vectoring cytokines to tumours

Cytokines such as the interferons and interleukins have been actively explored for their tumoricidal properties. Although there is evidence of cytotoxicity, they also have profound side effects which limit the dose that can safely be administered. It is possible to insert cytokine genes into cells that can potentially home on tumours so enabling high concentrations of their protein product to be released at or in the tumour. TNF genes have been inserted into tumour-infiltrating lymphocytes from patients with melanoma and the lymphocytes given systemically. These experiments are controversial for two reasons. First, it appears from *in vitro* studies that the amount of TNF expressed from such cells was unlikely to be sufficient to cause a significant cytotoxic effect and, second, the insertion of a foreign gene limits the ability of the lymphocyte to target into tumour masses. Over 15 patients have so far been treated at the US National Cancer Institute and formal publication of the results are eagerly awaited.

Inserting drug-activating genes

The main problem with existing chemotherapy is its lack of selectivity: active drug killing any cell it comes into contact with. If drug-activating genes could be inserted that would only be expressed in cancer cells, then the administration of an appropriate prodrug could be highly selective. There are now many examples of genes preferentially expressed in tumours. In some cases, their promoters have been isolated and coupled to drug-activating enzymes. Examples include CEA in CRC (Fig. 12.10), α-fetoprotein in hepatoma, prostate-specific antigen in prostate cancer and c-*erbB-2* in breast cancer. Such promoters can be coupled to enzymes such as cytosine deaminase or thymidine kinase, so producing unique retroviral vectors that are able to infect all cells but can only be expressed in tumour cells. These suicide or Trojan horse vectors may not have absolute tumour specificity but this may not be essential; it may be possible to perform a genetic prostatectomy or mastectomy, so effectively destroying all tumour cells.

Much work is currently in progress to develop both the promoter systems, which rely on differential transcription control, and the design of the drug-activating systems. Cytosine deaminase, for example, converts the relatively non-toxic antifungal drug 5-fluorocytosine to the cytoxic 5-fluorouracil. Both drugs are already in clinical use and provide a useful system for further development. Other drug-activating systems are being explored that release even more potent toxins. An example is the enzyme linamarase, which converts amygdalin to cyanide. Clinical trials using genetically activated prodrugs are anticipated shortly in hepatoma, melanoma and pancreatic and breast cancer.

Normal cell

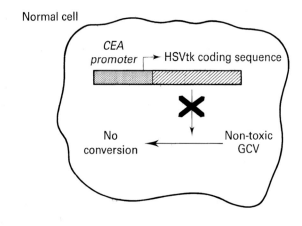

CRC cell

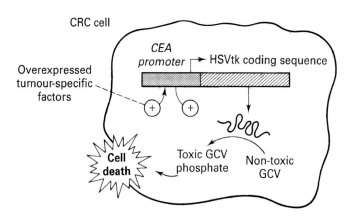

Fig. 12.10. Genetically directed enzyme prodrug therapy (GDEPT). This is a strategy where a foreign gene is delivered into both normal and tumour cells using a retrovirus. The foreign gene codes for a prodrug-activating enzyme, such as herpes simplex virus thymidine kinase (HSVtk). This enzyme can convert ganciclovir (GCV) to a toxic phosphorylated derivative. By linking tumour-specific transcription sequences upstream of the foreign gene, for example a CEA promoter, the enzyme is only produced in tumour cells. Hence when the patient is given the harmless prodrug GCV, only cancer cells can convert it to the cytoxic form, resulting in tumour-specific cytotoxicity.

Suppressing oncogene expression

The downregulation of abnormal oncogene expression has been shown to revert the malignant phenotype in a variety of *in vitro* tumour lines. It is possible to develop *in vivo* systems such as the insertion of genes encoding for complementary (antisense) mRNA to that produced by the oncogene. The antisense mRNA binds to the oncogene mRNA and prevents translation. Such antigenes specifically switch off the production of the abnormal protein product. The mutant form of the c-*ras* oncogene is an obvious target for this approach. Up to 45% of CRCs contain a mutation in the twelfth amino acid of this protein and reversion of this change in cell lines will lead to the restoration of normal growth control.

Clearly the major problem is to ensure that every single tumour cell becomes infected. Any cell that escapes will have a survival advantage and produce a clone of resistant tumour cells. For this reason, it may be that future treatment schedules will require the repetitive administration of vectors in a similar way to fractionated radiotherapy or chemotherapy.

Replacing defective tumour suppressor genes

In cell culture, malignant properties can often be reversed by the insertion of normal tumour suppressor genes, such as RB-1, wild-type p 53 and DCC. Although tumour suppressor genes were often identified in rare tumour types, abnormalities in their expression and function are abundant in common human cancers. Defects in p 53 occur in up to 60% of CRCs. As with antigene therapy, the difficulty in this approach lies in the delivery of actively expressed vectors to every single tumour cell *in vivo*. Nevertheless, clinical experiments are in progress in non-small cell lung cancer, where retroviruses that encode wild-type p 53 genes are being administered bronchoscopically. No results are as yet reported.

Summary

In this chapter, the changes that result in ungoverned cell proliferation have been discussed with emphasis on colorectal tumours. The defects in somatic cell genetics in CRC are outlined and the potential therapies based on molecular genetic manipulation are discussed.

Perhaps the biggest risk from gene manipulation *in vivo* is the possibility of insertional mutagenesis and the activation of oncogenes leading to neoplasia. Such risks are clearly important factors in the consideration of the ethical basis for gene therapy for disorders such as cystic fibrosis, haemophilia and the haemoglobinopathies. For patients with metastatic cancer, the risks are low. Such patients are often desperate for some form of treatment and are already searching for the gene therapy programmes described in the media. Therapies with even minimal potential benefit will be avidly considered. In this situation, the biggest problem is offering false hope. It is unrealistic to expect such new strategies to be effective immediately. The first patients entering trials will provide much information for little personal benefit. This must be recognised by both the investigator and patient to reduce the 'breakthrough' mentality that surrounds novel cancer treatments.

There have been remarkable advances in our understanding of the molecular biology of cancer. Interventional genetics is now poised to provide new selective tumour destruction mechanisms for patients with widespread cancer. But there are many hurdles still to overcome: how to transfer efficiently and stably genes into tumour cells *in vivo*, how to ensure safety for both patient and staff, and how best to place genetic approaches alongside more familiar therapies. We are witnessing the beginnings of molecular therapy. Fifty years ago in the late 1940s, the first alkylating agents were discovered and were about to enter clinical trial as systemic chemotherapy. None of our predecessors could have predicted the successes and disappointments that have led to the practice of modern medical oncology. We are now leaving an era of empiricism and entering an age when our knowledge of genetics and logical molecular design is likely to change radically the future face of cancer treatment.

FURTHER READING

Lemoine, N., Neoptolomus, J. & Cook, T. (eds.) (1994). *Cancer: A Molecular Approach.* Oxford: Blackwell Scientific.

Franks, L.M. & Teich, N.M. (eds.) (1993). *Introduction to the Cellular and Molecular Biology of Cancer.* Oxford: Oxford University Press.

Price, P. & Sikora, K. (eds) (1995). *The Treatment of Cancer,* 2nd edn. London: Chapman and Hall.

Devita, T., Hellman, S. & Rosenberg, S.A. (eds.) (1993). *Cancer: Principles and Practice of Oncology,* 4th edn. Philadelphia: Lippincott.

Latchman, D.S. (ed.) (1994). *From Genetics to Gene Therapy: The Molecular Pathology of Human Disease.* Oxford: Bios Scientific.

13

Toxic mechanisms: drugs

M. PIRMOHAMED, B. K. PARK and A. M. BRECKENRIDGE

- Drug toxicity is a major complication of drug therapy. It can mimic disease and it can cause death.

- There are three major types of adverse drug reaction: (i) *pharmacological*, which are an exaggeration of the known pharmacological actions of a drug; (ii) *chemical*, which are the result of the physicochemical properties or chemical reactivity of the drug or its metabolites; and (iii) *idiosyncratic*, which are bizarre reactions not predictable from the known pharmacology of the drug.

- Age, concomitant disease and certain genetically determined enzyme deficiencies act as pre-disposing factors for adverse drug reactions. With idiosyncratic reactions, pre-disposition is often caused by multiple factors with variable levels of influence acting in combination to produce the toxicity.

- Drug–drug interactions represent an important risk factor and can predispose to all types of adverse reaction by interfering with either the handling of the drug in the body or its action within the body.

- Prevention depends on the type of adverse reaction. Pharmacological adverse reactions are usually amenable to dose reduction. Prevention of the other forms of toxicity depends on the development of predictive tests and/or the development of newer chemical entities that do not have the propensity to cause the toxicity.

Drug toxicity is a major complication of modern drug therapy. The importance of adverse drug reactions can be illustrated by the fact that (i) they are a significant cause of patient morbidity, accounting for about 2% of hospital admissions; (ii) they occur in approximately 10–20% of hospital inpatients; (iii) they cause deaths in 0.1% of medical inpatients and 0.01% of surgical inpatients; (iv) they represent an unnecessary burden on already overstretched medical resources; (v) with idiosyncratic toxicity, the occurrence of the adverse reaction in a subgroup of the population may result in withdrawal of the drug at the expense of denying the majority of the population an otherwise effective treatment; and (vi) drug toxicity may take many forms, and indeed, drugs have taken over from syphilis and tuberculosis as the great simulators of disease. Therefore, the occurrence of an adverse drug reaction may interfere with the normal diagnostic process, and may lead either to unnecessary treatment and investigation or to a delay in treatment. Table 13.1 lists some of the major drug catastrophes that have occurred over the years, starting with the thalidomide disaster.

Table 13.1. *Some of the drugs which have been withdrawn as a result of adverse drug reactions*

Drug	Adverse reaction	Year
Thalidomide	Congenital malformations	1961
Clioquinol	Subacute myelo-optic neuropathy	1975
Practolol	Oculo-mucocutaneous syndrome	1977
Benoxaprofen	Hepatorenal damage	1982
Zimeldine	Guillain–Barré syndrome	1983
Perhexilene	Hepatotoxicity and neuropathy	1983
Osmosin	Gastrointestinal ulceration and perforation	1984
Nomifensine	Haemolysis and hepatotoxicity	1986
Metipranolol	Anterior uveitis	1991
Terodiline	Cardiac arrhythmias	1992
Temafloxacin	Anaphylaxis, hepatotoxicity and haemolysis	1993
Remoxipride	Aplastic anaemia	1994

Many classifications of adverse drug reactions have been proposed. For this chapter, in order to provide a mechanistic approach to drug toxicity, the adverse reactions will be divided into three broad categories:

- pharmacological: an exaggeration of the known pharmacological actions of the drug
- chemical: physicochemical properties or reactivity of the drug causes effects
- idiosyncratic: unpredictable effects.

Pharmacological drug toxicity

Pharmacological adverse drug reactions basically represent an augmentation of the known pharmacological actions of the drug and can be rationalised in terms of either the primary or the secondary pharmacological effects of the drug (and its metabolites). These reactions are usually dose dependent and can be alleviated by dose reduction. This type of drug toxicity is the most common form, accounting for about 70–80% of all adverse reactions. In general, the reactions account for a great deal of morbidity; fortunately, because they tend to be mild, they are rarely fatal.

Some examples of pharmacological adverse reactions are given in Table 13.2. Those reactions that obviously represent an exaggeration of the known therapeutic actions of the drug are classified as being the result of the primary pharmacology of the drug, while those reactions that are less obvious, being effects at sites other than the primary pharmacological site, are termed secondary pharmacological effects. For example, among the most common secondary pharmacological adverse effects seen in clinical practice is the problem of gastrointestinal toxicity in users of non-steroidal anti-inflammatory drugs (NSAIDs). This is because NSAIDs are inhibitors of cyclo-oxygenase; inhibition of this enzyme in the gut mucosa impairs mucosal ability to resist attack by gastric acid, resulting in peptic ulceration and sometimes haemorrhage. The relative risk

Table 13.2. *Examples of pharmacological adverse drug reactions*

Drug class	Drug	Adverse effect
Primary pharmacology		
Anticoagulant	Warfarin	Haemorrhage
Antihypertensive	Captopril	Hypotension
Oral hypoglycaemic	Chlorpropamide	Hypoglycaemia
Corticosteroids	Prednisolone	Cushing's syndrome
Secondary pharmacology		
Beta-blocker	Atenolol	Bronchospasm
Antiarrhythmic	Amiodarone	Thyroid dysfunction
Nucleoside analogue	Zidovudine	Bone marrow suppression
Opiate	Morphine	Respiratory depression
Tricyclic antidepressant	Imipramine	Anticholinergic side effects
Antibiotic	Ciprofloxacin	Seizures
Non-steroidal anti-inflammatory drug	Indomethacin	Gastro-intestinal bleeding

of upper gastrointestinal haemorrhage in aspirin users is about 3.3 and for users of non-aspirin NSAIDs it is 3.1. The risk of perforation is higher with NSAIDs (5.9) as is the relative risk of death (7.6). Inhibition of renal cyclo-oxygenase is thought to be responsible for the renal toxicity often witnessed with NSAIDs.

Factors predisposing to such reactions may result from pharmaceutical variation in drug formulation, pharmacokinetic or pharmacodynamic abnormalities, and drug–drug interactions.

Pharmaceutical variation

The active substance represents only a very small part of the drug, which also contains many inactive ingredients used as bulking agents and to confer certain release characteristics on the drug. Therefore, alteration in the release characteristics of the active substance may predispose to drug toxicity. In order to avoid such toxicities, particularly when changing patients from one formulation of a compound to another, for example from the brand leader to a generic drug, the two compounds must be shown to fulfil criteria laid down by the drug regulatory authorities, in that they must be bioequivalent in terms of the amount and rate of drug absorbed. A typical example was seen with the NSAID preparation Osmosin (a rate-controlled preparation of indomethacin), which caused a high rate of gastrointestinal bleeding. The characteristics of the formulation were such that very high local concentrations of indomethacin were achieved, which together with high concentrations of potassium (also present in the formulation) led to the gastrointestinal toxicity.

ABSORPTION

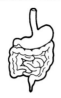

The process by which a drug passes from its site of administration to the circulation

Adverse effects may arise as a result of changes in the extent and rate of absorption, although the usual consequence is a loss of efficacy

DISTRIBUTION

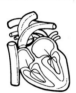

The process by which a drug passes from the circulation to the tissues

Of importance when liver blood flow is affected in heart failure for drugs such as lignocaine

Important for drugs that exhibit extensive tissue binding; for example, tetracycline binds to newly formed bone, resulting in growth retardation; chloroquine binds to melanin and can lead to retinopathy

METABOLISM

The process of conversion of lipid-soluble drugs to water-soluble compounds prior to excretion occurs mainly in the liver

Hepatic metabolism is reduced in hepatic disease and in extrahepatic diseases such as cardiac failure and hypothyroidism. It affects the elimination of lipophilic drugs, which can lead to accumulation and toxicity, particularly with drugs that have a narrow therapeutic index

EXCRETION

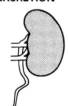

The process of elimination of drugs and their metabolites, which is predominantly performed by the kidneys

Impaired excretion and tissue accumulation is seen in renal failure, usually with hydrophilic compounds such as digoxin, lithium and aminoglycoside antibiotics

Fig. 13.1. The pharmacokinetic processes of drug absorption, distribution, metabolism and excretion.

Pharmacokinetic considerations

Pharmacokinetics is the mathematical description of the processes of drug absorption, distribution, metabolism and excretion (Fig. 13.1). In many cases, alteration of pharmacokinetic parameters for a drug leads to reduction in plasma levels and loss of efficacy. A reduction in elimination of the drug (or its metabolites) because of impairment of hepatic metabolism and/or renal excretion will lead to high plasma levels with consequent dose-dependent toxicity. Therefore, hepatic disease may be expected to affect the elimination of (lipophilic) drugs that undergo hepatic metabolism. However, in practice, because of the enormous reserve of the liver parenchyma, adverse reactions resulting

Table 13.3. *Pharmacological adverse drug reaction occurring as a result of pharmacodynamic variation*

Drug	Pharmacodynamic adverse effect	Predisposing factor
Opiates	Coma	Hepatic encephalopathy
Indomethacin	Left ventricular failure	Underlying left ventricular dysfunction
Quinidine	Torsades de pointe	Hypokalaemia
Kanamycin	Paralysis secondary to neuromuscular blockade	Myasthenia gravis/treatment with muscle relaxants

from impaired hepatic elimination only occur with severe disease and often only with drugs that have a narrow therapeutic index, such as phenytoin and theophylline. Reduction in administered dose and monitoring of plasma concentration may need to be carried out in such cases to avoid toxicity. Extrahepatic disease may also be associated with reduced hepatic metabolism. For example, cardiac failure by reducing hepatic blood flow can reduce clearance of drugs with a high extraction ratio, such as lignocaine and propranolol. Hypothyroidism is also associated with decreased hepatic metabolism. Renal failure will affect the excretion of (hydrophilic) drugs, which do not undergo hepatic metabolism, leading to accumulation and consequent toxicity. Pharmacologically active metabolites produced by hepatic metabolism may also accumulate in renal failure, leading to toxicity. In these cases, drug accumulation can be avoided by individualising dosage requirements on the basis of the patient's creatinine clearance.

Pharmacodynamic considerations

In certain patients, the effect of a drug at its site of action may be either reduced or accentuated, leading either to reduced efficacy or to toxicity, respectively. Such interindividual variability in drug response is usually a result of concomitant disease (Table 13.3). For example, in patients with underlying left ventricular dysfunction, the administration of a NSAID such as indomethacin, which causes salt and water retention, may tip the patient into overt failure.

Drug–drug interactions and pharmacological adverse drug reactions

Pharmacokinetic and pharmacodynamic interactions between drugs are common, although such reactions are of clinical significance in only a small proportion of patients. The chance of a drug–drug interaction increases with the number of drugs prescribed. It has been estimated that if five drugs are given simultaneously, there is a 75% chance of causing an adverse drug interaction. Therefore, patients on multiple drugs, for example the elderly, or those with chronic diseases who require continuous drug therapy are particularly at risk of adverse drug interactions. The clinically important drug interactions tend to involve drugs with a narrow therapeutic index, such as warfarin, phenytoin, theophylline, digoxin, lithium and cyclosporin.

Drug interactions can be classified into pharmaceutical, pharmacokinetic and pharmacodynamic interactions. Examples of clinically important interactions involving all these processes are given in Table 13.4.

Pharmacokinetic drug interactions, in general, may have two types of effect:

1. Elevation of plasma levels of the object drug by the interacting drug, resulting in dose-dependent toxicity.
2. Reduction in plasma levels of the object drug, with consequent therapeutic failure and recurrence of the disease for which the drug was originally prescribed.

Of particular importance are those interactions that involve drug metabolism and drug excretion. The role of drug metabolism is to convert lipophilic, non-polar compounds by a combination of phase I and phase II metabolic pathways into water-soluble polar compounds that can be readily excreted from the body (Fig. 13.2). Phase I reactions are mainly carried out by the cytochrome P450 enzymes, a superfamily of haemoprotein enzymes whose main location is the endoplasmic reticulum of hepatocytes. Phase II reactions are performed by a variety of enzymes, including the glucuronyl transferases N-acetyl transferase and glutathione-S-transferases. Drug metabolism, and in particular the cytochrome P450-dependent reactions, may be perturbed by other drugs that act as either inducers or inhibitors of these enzymes. Drug excretion is performed predominantly by the kidneys (Fig. 13.1). Perturbation of excretion may lead to elevation of drug levels in the plasma and, sometimes (particularly with drugs that have a narrow therapeutic index), to dose-dependent toxicity.

Pharmacodynamic drug–drug interactions are basically of two types: those that lead to an additive or synergistic effect and those that result in antagonism of drug action (Table 13.4).

The clinical importance of the different forms of pharmacokinetic and pharmacodynamic drug interaction can be illustrated by using NSAIDs as an example.

Pharmacological toxicity involving NSAIDs

Pharmacokinetic interactions of NSAIDs

Metabolism. The metabolism of warfarin is inhibited by several NSAIDs, including high-dose aspirin, azapropazone and phenylbutazone. The interaction of warfarin with phenylbutazone is particularly complex. Warfarin is administered as a racemic mixture of two enantiomers: (R)-warfarin and (S)-warfarin. Phenylbutazone inhibits the metabolism of the more potent (S)-warfarin while at the same time increasing the metabolism of (R)-warfarin. Thus, although there will be no overall change in plasma levels of the racemic mixture, a greater proportion of the drug will be the more potent (S)-warfarin, which may result in haemorrhage.

Table 13.4. *Some examples of clinically important drug interactions which lead to pharmacological adverse drug reactions*

Category	Object drug	Interacting drug	Adverse effect	Mechanism
Pharmacokinetic				
Absorption	Cyclosporin	Erythromycin	Cyclosporin toxicity	Inhibition of metabolism in gut wall (and liver)
Distribution	Phenytoin	Sodium valproate	Phenytoin toxicity	Protein-binding displacement; also inhibition
Metabolism	Terfenadine	Ketoconazole	Torsades de pointe	Enzyme inhibition
	Oral contraceptive	Phenytoin	Unwanted pregnancy	Enzyme induction
Excretion	Digoxin	Verapamil	Digoxin toxicity	Reduced renal clearance
	Lithium	Indomethacin	Lithium toxicity	Reduced excretion
Pharmacodynamic				
Synergistic	Captopril	Amiloride	Hyperkalaemia	Decreased potassium excretion
Antagonistic	Captopril	Indomethacin	Reversal of hypotensive effects	Decreased intrarenal prostaglandin production

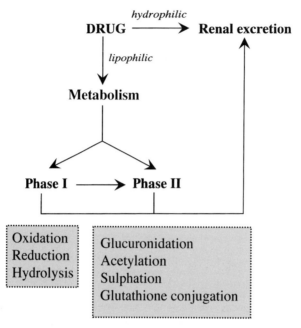

Fig. 13.2. The process of drug metabolism. The metabolic processes in the body are divided into two phases, phase I and phase II. Some drugs undergo sequential phase I and phase II metabolic biotransformations, while other drugs only undergo metabolism by either phase I or phase II.

Excretion.   Salicylates cause a 50% reduction in the renal clearance of methotrexate, which has resulted in patient deaths. The dose of methotrexate should be halved in patients requiring the concomitant administration of NSAIDs.

Pharmacodynamic interactions of NSAIDs

Synergistic.   Aspirin and the other NSAIDs all reduce platelet adhesiveness and are prone to causing gastric erosions. In addition, aspirin in high dosage and some of the other NSAIDs cause hypoprothrombinaemia. The combination of these actions together with the anticoagulant action of warfarin can greatly increase the risk of a life-threatening haemorrhage.

Antagonistic.   The antihypertensive action of drugs such as ACE inhibitors is antagonised by concomitant administration of NSAIDs; this is thought to be because NSAIDs reduce the intrarenal production of prostaglandins.

Chemical drug toxicity

Chemical drug toxicity can be rationalised in terms of either the physicochemical properties or the chemical reactivity of the drug or its metabolites. These reactions are dependent on the relative rates of accumulation and clearance of the compound. A dose–response relationship may be discernible, although this is not always the case.

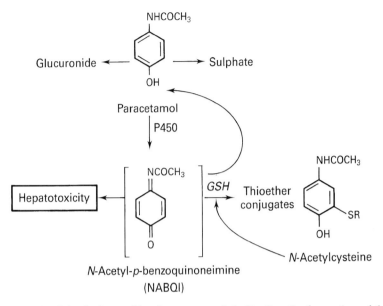

Fig. 13.3. Metabolic profile of paracetamol, indicating the formation of the reactive quinoneimine metabolite, thought to be responsible for the hepatotoxicity seen in overdose. *N*-Acetylcysteine, which is antidote of choice, acts by increasing intracellular glutathione (GSH) levels, thereby restoring the balance between activation and detoxication.

Chemical drug toxicity may occur either with therapeutic doses of the compound or with an overdose of the drug. If we consider the latter, most drug overdoses result in toxicity that is in keeping with the known primary and secondary pharmacological actions of the drug. In certain cases, however, overdosage results in chemical toxicity that does not obviously correspond to the known pharmacology of the drug. The prime example of this is paracetamol overdosage, which along with viral hepatitis is the most common cause of acute liver failure worldwide. In the UK, it causes approximately 160 deaths per year.

Drug metabolism plays an important role in the pathogenesis of paracetamol hepatotoxicity. In therapeutic doses, paracetamol undergoes sulphation and glucuronidation in the liver, with only a small proportion (5–10%) undergoing oxidative metabolism by the cytochrome P450 enzymes. The product of oxidative metabolism, *N*-acetyl-*p*-benzoquinoneimine, is chemically reactive and is normally detoxified by glutathione to form harmless metabolites (thioether conjugates) that can be excreted from the body (Fig. 13.3). After overdosage, this balance between activation and detoxication is disturbed because of saturation of sulphation and depletion of the liver glutathione stores, which leads to hepatic necrosis. The mechanism by which hepatocellular necrosis occurs is not fully understood, but it may involve modification of free sulphydryl groups, lipid peroxidation, oxidative stress and covalent binding of essential cell macromolecules. Intravenous *N*-acetylcysteine, which is the antidote of choice, acts by increasing intracellular glutathione levels, thereby restoring the balance between bioactivation and detoxication.

Although paracetamol hepatotoxicity is dose dependent, there is interindividual variation in susceptibility. For example, chronic alcoholics are more susceptible because of (i) increased bioactivation as a result of induction of particular P450 isoforms by alcohol; and (ii) a relative deficiency of intracellular glutathione consequent to the poor nutritional status. The clinical importance of this observation is that chronic alcoholics should be treated with N-acetylcysteine at lower plasma paracetamol levels than non-alcoholics. In contrast, children are less susceptible to paracetamol hepatotoxicity because of an enhanced sulphation capacity.

At therapeutic doses, the physicochemical properties of a drug can lead to cell-selective accumulation and, thus, organ-specific toxicities. The best known example of this is with perhexilene (an antianginal), which has been associated with hepatotoxicity and neuropathy. Perhexilene tends to become trapped in lysosomes because of its physicochemical properties, where it inhibits the actions of phospholipases and leads to the accumulation of phospholipids. This can lead to liver toxicity that is variable in severity and, in some cases, is indistinguishable from alcohol-induced liver injury. Subjects who have a mutant form of the P450 isoform CYP2D6 (see p. 385), an enzyme involved in the oxidation of perhexilene, have a higher risk of developing liver disease (and neuropathy) than subjects who are extensive metabolisers of CYP2D6.

Idiosyncratic adverse drug reactions

Idiosyncratic adverse drug reactions are totally aberrant effects that are not predictable from the known pharmacological actions of a drug. There is no simple dose–response relationship and factors within the affected patient may be important in the pathogenesis of the reactions. Although they only affect a minority of individuals, they are often serious, accounting for many drug-induced deaths. Such reactions are not detected by pre-clinical toxicology testing in animals and indeed cannot be reproduced in animal models.

The possible mechanisms of idiosyncratic drug reactions are:

- pharmaceutical variation
- receptor abnormality
- abnormal biological system that is only apparent in the presence of the drug
- abnormality in drug metabolism
- immunological
- drug–drug interactions
- multifactorial.

With some reactions, only one of the above mechanisms may be implicated, while for the majority of idiosyncratic reactions, a combination of mechanisms may be responsible for producing a multifactorial predisposition to toxicity.

Pharmaceutical causes

Excipients (substances added as a vehicle) in drug formulations, degradation of the active substance and contamination with toxic substances in the manufacturing process can all lead to idiosyncratic adverse drug reactions. For example, tartrazine, a colouring agent used in many drug formulations, can lead to skin rashes. A more recent example is the eosinophilia–myalgia syndrome associated with the use of L-tryptophan. This condition is characterised initially by eosinophilia, myalgia and subsequently by myositis, fasciitis, skin sclerosis and peripheral neuropathy. A contaminant introduced into the formulation as a result of a change in the manufacturing process, which has subsequently been chemically identified as a tryptophan dimer, has been suggested to be the aetiologic agent.

Receptor abnormality

A structural abnormality in a receptor not normally associated with the drug may produce an altered and bizarre response to the drug resulting in an idiosyncratic drug reaction. Malignant hyperthermia, a dominantly inherited disorder that is triggered by the administration of some general anaesthetics, represents the best example of such a mechanism. The disorder is characterised by hyperthermia, muscle rigidity, cardiac arrhythmias and rhabdomyolysis. It carries a high mortality unless treatment is instituted early in its course.

Malignant hyperthermia is thought to result from disruption in the control of intracellular free calcium. The primary defect is in the ryanodine receptor. The defect makes it more sensitive to lower concentrations of stimulators of opening of calcium channels. This results in enhanced rates of calcium release from the sarcoplasmic reticulum during anaesthesia, which in turn results in sustained muscle contraction and the glycolytic and aerobic metabolism characteristic of malignant hyperthermia. Molecular studies have identified at least three mutations in the ryanodine receptor gene, which is located on chromosome 19.

Abnormal biological system unmasked by the drug

A biochemical deficiency that may otherwise have remained asymptomatic may become unmasked by the administration of a drug, resulting in idiosyncratic toxicity that is characterised by a qualitative abnormality in the response of the target organ.

The best example of this is glucose 6-phosphate dehydrogenase deficiency, which is a sex-linked disorder affecting about 200 million people worldwide. It causes red cell haemolysis only in the presence of stress, for example infection or drugs. A large number of drugs, including primaquine and the sulphonamides, can induce red cell haemolysis in patients with a deficiency of this enzyme.

Normally, glucose 6-phosphate dehydrogenase functions to reduce NADP while oxidising glucose 6-phosphate, thus providing a source of reducing power that maintains cellular glutathione in the reduced form. In the absence of reduced glutathione, the red cell is susceptible to oxidative damage from drugs, which clinically is manifest as haemolysis, a fall in the haemoglobin concentration, fever and the formation of dark urine.

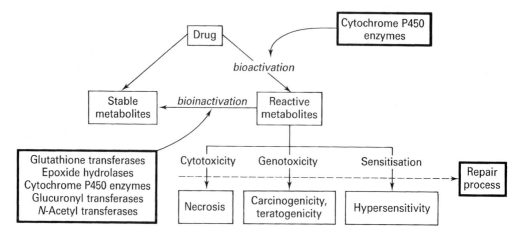

Fig. 13.4. The role of chemically reactive metabolites in causing various forms of drug toxicity. Bioactivation is dependent on the cytochrome P450 enzymes, while bioinactivation can be performed by various enzymes. In cases of inadequate bioinactivation of a chemically reactive metabolite, various repair processes may come into play and prevent the toxicity.

Abnormalities of drug metabolism

Drug metabolism can normally be considered a drug *detoxication* process (Figs. 13.2 and 13.4). In certain circumstances, however, drug metabolism, and in particular the cytochrome P450-mediated phase I metabolic pathways, can lead to the formation of toxic, chemically reactive metabolites, a process termed **bioactivation** (Fig. 13.4). Fortunately, in the majority of individuals, the formation of the chemically reactive metabolites is counter-balanced by detoxication mechanisms, a process termed **bio-inactivation** (Fig. 13.4), which leads to harmless excretion of the metabolite. It has been postulated that, in susceptible individuals, this balance between bioactivation and detoxication is disturbed either by genetic factors or by host factors such as age, enzyme induction and disease, all of which may allow the metabolite to escape detoxication.

An inadequately detoxified chemically reactive metabolite can combine with and damage cellular macromolecules, such as proteins and nucleic acids, and may cause various forms of toxicity (if repair mechanisms are overwhelmed), including teratogenicity, carcinogenicity, cellular necrosis and hypersensitivity (Fig. 13.4). The last two mechanisms are responsible for the majority of the idiosyncratic drug toxicities seen in clinical practice.

Direct (metabolite-mediated) toxicity is caused by indiscriminate covalent binding of the toxic metabolite to cellular macromolecules, which may interfere with their normal physiological function and lead to cellular necrosis. Direct toxicity rather than immune-mediated toxicity is particularly likely to occur when covalent binding involves a protein that has a critical function in the cell, for example the plasma membrane Ca^{2+}-ATPase.

Immunological effects

The mechanism by which a drug can lead to immune-mediated idiosyncratic toxicity (hereafter termed hypersensitivity reactions) is based on the hapten hypothesis. This states that most drugs (or their metabolites) are of low molecular weight (<1000 Da) and, therefore, cannot act as immunogens *per se*. They act as immunogens only when the drug (or more usually its toxic metabolite) becomes covalently bound to autologous macromolecules such as proteins. The term hapten has, therefore, been coined to describe a substance that becomes immunogenic only when it is conjugated to a macromolecular carrier. Certain drugs such as the penicillins, because of their intrinsic chemical reactivity, can form drug–protein conjugates directly. The majority of drugs, however, are not intrinsically chemically reactive and, therefore, do not react directly with proteins but require prior bioactivation to a chemically reactive intermediate by the cytochrome P450 enzymes (Fig. 13.4). The immune response to the hapten–protein conjugate may be characterised by specifically committed T lymphocytes and/or antibodies (Fig. 13.5) directed against the drug (haptenic epitopes), the carrier protein (autoantigenic determinant) or the neoantigen created by the combination of the drug and the protein (new antigenic determinant) (Fig. 13.5).

T lymphocyte activation, which is crucial in the whole process of generating an immune response against a hapten–protein conjugate, requires the antigen to be taken up and undergo intracellular catabolism in so-called antigen–presenting cells (Fig. 13.5) prior to presentation (in association with MHC molecules) of recognisable epitopes on the surface of these cells (see also Chapter 4). The antigen may contain many possible epitopes, although only a few are recognised by the immune system. The predominance of one epitope, called immunodominance, may be dictated by the expression of a particular MHC allele. This phenomenon is known as MHC restriction, and in essence what this means is that the high level of polymorphism of the MHC genes results in a subset of individuals in the population who can respond vigorously to drug-related antigens and, therefore, are more likely to develop drug hypersensitivity.

Once an immune response against a hapten–protein conjugate has been elicited, the interaction between the antigen and the immune system causes tissue damage through four general mechanisms of hypersensitivity (Fig. 13.6). Such mechanisms are not exclusive since a particular drug reaction may involve more than one type of hypersensitivity.

The distinction between direct and indirect immune-mediated idiosyncratic toxicity is primarily based on clinical criteria (Table 13.5), although laboratory tests such as the eosinophil count and the presence of autoantibodies may provide useful supplemental information.

The whole process can be illustrated with reference to the penicillins, which can induce a vast array of adverse reactions (Fig. 13.7) mediated by the four types of hypersensitivity reaction (Fig. 13.7). The most severe reaction is anaphylaxis, which is IgE-mediated. Anaphylaxis with penicillin occurs in 1 in 2000 patients and has a mortality of 1 in 500 000. Penicillin can react directly with proteins because the β-lactam ring is chemically unstable and can open spontaneously to form intermediates that combine

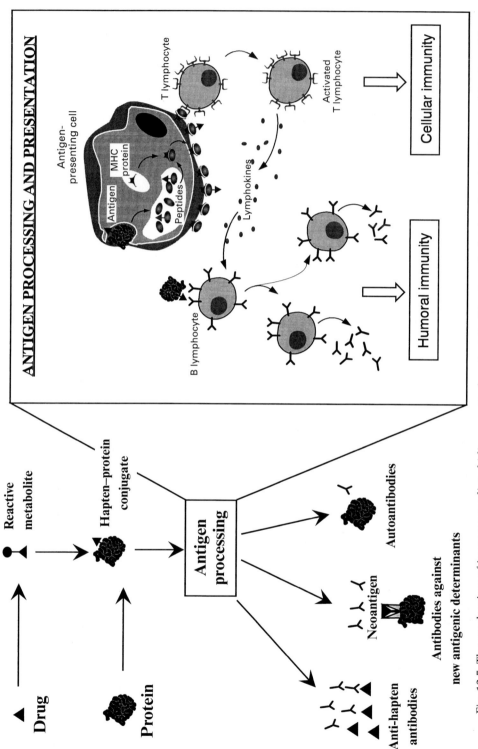

Fig. 13.5. The mechanism of immune-mediated idiosyncratic drug toxicity. The drug-derived antigen (usually a combination of drug metabolite and carrier protein) is ingested by antigen-presenting cells and processed so that the antigenic peptides are presented in combination with MHC antigens on the surface of the cells. These are recognised as being 'foreign' by T lymphocytes that become activated and undergo blast transformation. Lymphokines are secreted by these cells, which mobilise other components of the immune system, including B lymphocytes. The resulting immune response is mediated by B lymphocytes (humoral immunity), which differentiate into plasma cells and secrete antibodies, and/or T lymphocytes (cellular immunity). The response may be directed against the drug, the drug-altered antigen (neoantigen) or against the carrier protein (autoantigen).

Type I Specific IgE antibodies bind to mast cells via their F receptors. Binding of multivalent antigen to adjacent IgE induces degranulation and release of mediators, such as histamine and leukotrienes

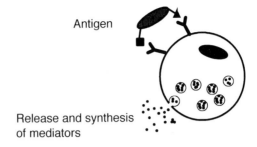

Type II Antibody (IgG, IgM) is directed against an individual's own cells. This may lead to cell destruction by killer T cells (K-cells) or complement-mediated lysis. Alternatively the cells may be removed by phagocytosis

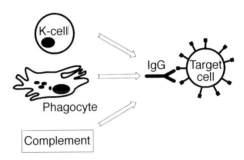

Type III Immune complexes are deposited in tissue (e.g. small blood vessels, glomerular basement membranes). Activation of complement leads to recruitment of polymorphs and a local inflammatory response

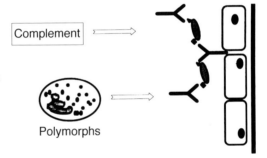

Type IV Specific T cells bind to fixed antigen. Lymphokines are released which induce an inflammatory reaction and attract and activate macrophages, which release mediators

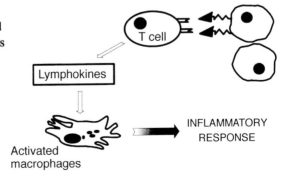

Fig. 13.6. The four types of hypersensitivity reaction.

Table 13.5. *Distinction between direct and immune-mediated idiosyncratic toxicity*

Feature	Direct toxicity	Immune-mediated toxicity
Time to adverse reaction	Variable but often rapid	2–6 weeks
Time to toxicity on rechallenge	Similar to primary exposure	Sooner than on primary exposure, often within 24–48 hours
Associated symptoms	Symptoms of organ affected	Symptoms of organ affected, plus rash, fever, adenopathy, arthralgia ('hypersensitivity manifestations')
Laboratory features		
Eosinophilia	No	Yes, in many reactions
Antibodies	No	Yes, but only demonstrated for a few reactions
Specific T cells	No	Yes, but only demonstrated for a few reactions

with proteins, forming several antigens, the most common being the penicilloyl antigen (Fig. 13.7). Antigen formation from the semi-synthetic penicillins such as amoxycillin can involve either the penicillin nucleus or the synthetic side chains.

Several factors determine the likelihood that a patient will develop an anaphylactic reaction (and other immunologic reactions) to penicillin. Such factors may also apply to hypersensitivity reactions caused by other drugs. It has been found that in patients on high doses of penicillin, there is little interindividual variability in circulating penicilloyl groups, yet less than 40% show a detectable serological response, suggesting that the ability to mount an immune response to the penicillin antigens is under genetic control. Interestingly, patients with an atopic diathesis, a condition characterised by high IgE levels, are disproportionately represented among individuals who experience anaphylactic reactions to penicillin. Furthermore, the half life of the IgE antibodies, once formed, is enormously variable, ranging from 10 days to > 1000 days. Therefore, it can be surmised that those individuals who either do not respond serologically or only respond transiently will be at the lowest risk of IgE-mediated allergy. Other risk factors include the age of the individual and the route of administration, with adulthood and parenteral drug use increasing the risk of anaphylaxis. The factors responsible for translating the serological response to tissue damage are poorly understood but relate to the ability of the mast cell to release chemical mediators, including histamine, serotonin and leukotrienes. These mediators, which are released upon cross-linking of the IgE antibodies on the mast cell surface, cause vasodilatation and increased permeability of the small blood vessels, and bronchospasm, resulting in the clinical syndrome of anaphylaxis.

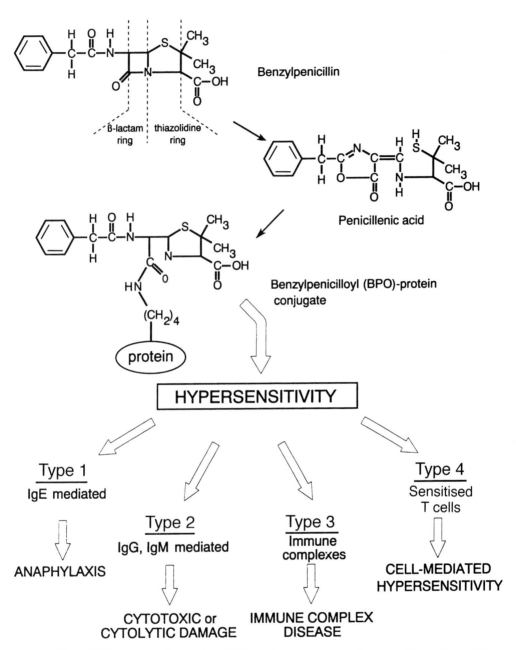

Fig. 13.7. Structure of benzylpenicillin and postulated mechanism of formation of the major antigenic determinant the benzylpenicilloyl (BPO) antigen. The penicillins have been reported to cause a wide variety of adverse reactions which are mediated by the four types of hypersensitivity reactions, as illustrated at the bottom of the figure.

Drug–drug interactions

Concomitant administration of drugs that induce the drug-metabolising enzymes, particularly the cytochrome P450 enzymes, may alter the balance between drug bioactivation and detoxication and lead to idiosyncratic toxicity. There are several examples where this seems to be important. Valproic acid-induced hepatotoxicity is more common in children on polytherapy with other enzyme-inducing anticonvulsants than in children on monotherapy. Hepatitis induced by isoniazid occurs in 1% of patients when given alone, while co-administration of rifampicin, a potent enzyme inducer, increases the incidence to 5–8%.

Conversely, inhibition of the metabolising enzymes, particularly when their major role is in the detoxication of toxic metabolites, also increases the risk of toxicity. For example, teratogenicity caused by administration of phenytoin or carbamazepine is increased several-fold with the concomitant prescription of valproic acid. This is because valproic acid is an inhibitor of the detoxication enzyme microsomal epoxide hydrolase; its administration increases fetal exposure to the drugs and, thus, covalent binding to fetal DNA of the chemically reactive epoxide metabolite formed from phenytoin or carbamazepine.

Multifactorial aetiology

The process whereby a drug can cause an idiosyncratic reaction is complex and for most drugs is akin to the situation with many polygenic diseases: a multitude of factors acting in combination may be necessary to produce the toxicity. In different patients, a different number and combination of factors may be responsible. It can be hypothesised that the frequency of a particular adverse reaction will be dependent on the number of factors which need to act together to produce the toxicity, those reactions requiring one predisposing factor being relatively more common than those reactions where four factors acting sequentially are required. This may explain the rarity of some idiosyncratic drug reactions as well as the variability in frequency of the same form of toxicity seen with different drugs.

Sites of metabolite-mediated idiosyncratic toxicity

Any organ system can be affected by idiosyncratic toxicity, either in combination or in isolation. The most commonly affected organs are the liver (Fig. 13.8), formed elements of the blood (Fig. 13.9) and the skin (Fig. 13.10), while kidneys, nervous system and lungs are less commonly affected. Comprehensive lists of drugs known to cause organ-specific toxicities are not provided in this section: for these the reader is referred to some of the texts mentioned at the end of the chapter.

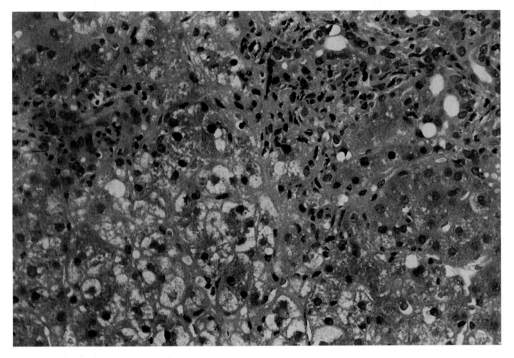

Incidence
Mild cases occurring in up to 20% of patients, e.g. with isoniazid
Severe cases rare, 0.1%

Form of toxicity
Wide ranging, most commonly hepatitis and cholestasis. Drugs can also cause
neoplasia, steatosis and granuloma

Severity
Variable ranging from 'transaminitis' to fulminant hepatic failure

Diagnosis
Clinical
Liver function tests
    transaminases elevated in hepatocellular damage
    alkaline phosphatase elevated in cholestatic hepatitis
    mixed hepatitis: mixed biochemical picture
Immunological tests including autoantibody screening
Liver biopsy

Mechanism
Variable, dependent on form of toxicity. For drug-induced hepatitis, toxicity often
results from the formation of chemically reactive metabolites, which cause toxicity
either directly or by acting as a hapten and initiating an immune response

Fig. 13.8. Drug-induced hepatotoxicity. Histology of a liver biopsy specimen taken from
a 23-year-old patient with hepatitis induced by erythromycin, showing features of
inflammation including infiltration by various types of white cells including
eosinophils. (Provided by Dr Paul Johnson, Department of Pathology, University of
Liverpool.)

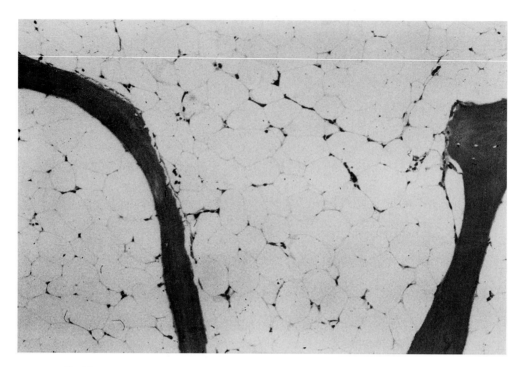

Incidence
30–60% of all cases of aplastic anaemia result from drugs
Incidence of agranulocytosis 2.6 per million inhabitants (Sweden); incidence higher with clozapine (1 in 100) and captopril (1 in 250)

Form of toxicity
Variable; effect on pluripotential stem cell leads to aplastic anaemia, while more selective destruction of platelets, red cells or white cells may lead to thrombocytopenia, haemolysis or agranulocytosis, respectively

Severity
Variable, often recovering on withdrawal of offending drug, except for aplastic anaemia, which may require specific treatment

Diagnosis
Clinical
Peripheral blood count
Coombs' test
Platelet antibodies
Bone marrow biopsy

Mechanism
Often caused by a chemically reactive metabolite that produces either direct cell damage or damage by an immune-mediated mechanism

Fig. 13.9. Drug-induced haematological toxicity. Bone marrow biopsy taken from a 85-year-old patient with aplastic anaemia induced by a NSAID, showing replacement of normal bone marrow by a fatty marrow. (Provided by Dr Paul Johnson, Department of Pathology, University of Liverpool.)

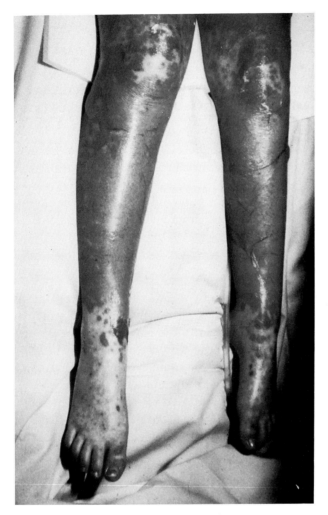

Incidence
Variable, depending on the drug; may be as common as 3% for drugs such as carbamazepine. Almost every drug in clinical practice has been reported to cause mild cutaneous eruptions.

Form of toxicity
Variable in terms of type and extent of toxicity

Severity
Variable, ranging from fixed drug eruptions to toxic epidermal necrolysis (shown here)

Diagnosis
Usually clinical
Occasional requirements for skin biopsy

Mechanism
Usually immunological, consequent to binding of drug–hapten conjugate to epidermal tissues

Fig. 13.10. Drug-induced cutaneous toxicity. Toxic epidermal necrolysis induced by carbamazepine in an 18-year-old epileptic patient.

Factors affecting drug toxicity

Age

Toxic reactions to drugs are more common at extremes of age. In the elderly, 10% of all hospital admissions may be the result of adverse drug reactions. Several factors may be responsible for this predisposition:

- drugs are used more frequently in the elderly than in any other age group
- polypharmacy is more common in the elderly, increasing the risk of adverse drug interactions
- age-related changes in physiology may lead to alterations in pharmacokinetics and pharmacodynamics of certain drugs and thus contribute to the increased incidence of toxicity
- disease is more common in the elderly, which may alter the handling of the drug and result in toxicity.

Most of the reactions that occur in the elderly as a result of these predisposing factors are of the pharmacological type. On occasions, however, some idiosyncratic drug reactions also occur more frequently in the elderly. The reasons for this are unclear, but reduced clearance of the parent drug and/or its toxic metabolites may be important.

The very young are also more susceptible to certain toxicities. For example, valproic acid-induced liver damage is most common in children under the age of 2 years, particularly if they are on polytherapy. The idiosyncratic hepatotoxicity is thought to result from direct toxicity of the reactive metabolites: the 4-ene and 2, 4-diene. The formation of these toxic metabolites is enhanced by enzyme induction, while detoxication is dependent on glutathione conjugation. It has been suggested, therefore, that susceptibility to valproic acid-induced hepatotoxicity is a result of a combination of enhanced production of toxic metabolites and a deficiency of detoxication, the latter being dependent on mitochondrial glutathione levels and glucuronidation, which may be functionally immature in the young.

Disease

Certain diseases can predispose to adverse drug reactions, usually of the pharmacological type but occasionally of a chemical and idiosyncratic nature. The effect of hepatic disease and renal disease on the elimination of lipophilic and hydrophilic compounds, respectively, has already been mentioned. Such diseases usually lead to drug accumulation, resulting in dose-dependent toxicity.

Atopic patients have a higher incidence of hypersensitivity reactions, although the reason for this is unclear; it may be a reflection of 'immune hyper-responsiveness'. Autoimmune diseases such as Sjögren's syndrome also predispose to immune-mediated idiosyncratic toxicity. Patients with AIDS have a much higher incidence of hypersensitivity reactions to drugs such as sulphonamides, clindamycin and thiacetazone than non-AIDS patients. The mechanism of this is unclear, but it may be related to altered immune responsiveness in HIV-positive patients.

Pharmacogenetics

The considerable interindividual variation seen with drug responses results from a combination of environmental factors and host genetic constitution. The field of genetic variation in drug response has been termed pharmacogenetics. Genetic variation can either affect the metabolism of the drug (altering its rate and/or route of elimination) or the response to the drug, both of which can predispose to drug toxicity. The abnormality occurs because of a mutant allele that causes either a quantitative enzyme deficiency, or more commonly, a qualitative change in gene expression (i.e. structural abnormality with altered substrate specificity). Of the genetic influences affecting drug response, glucose 6-phosphate dehydrogenase deficiency and malignant hyperthermia are two of the more important conditions; these have already been discussed. The rest of the section will concentrate on genetic polymorphisms affecting the drug-metabolising enzymes, the classic examples of which are

- the hydrolysis of succinylcholine
- the acetylator status
- drug oxidation polymorphisms.

Succinylcholine hydrolysis

Succinylcholine, a neuromuscular-blocking agent, produces paralysis of short duration because of its rapid hydrolysis to the inactive succinylmonocholine by cholinesterases present in the plasma and liver. In about 1 in 3000 individuals, succinylcholine administration causes paralysis and apnoea lasting several hours because of an atypical plasma cholinesterase that has a substrate affinity at least 100-fold less than the normal variant.

Acetylator status

The acetylation of drugs is one of the major phase II metabolic inactivation pathways. The ability to N-acetylate xenobiotics is under genetic control, the fast acetylator phenotype being inherited as autosomal dominant and the slow acetylator phenotype as autosomal recessive. Slow acetylators have a deficiency in the cytosolic enzyme N-acetyltransferase (NAT-1). The frequency of the slow acetylator phenotype varies according to the population studied: 52% of the British population are slow acetylators, while less than 10% of the Japanese population are slow acetylators. In general, slow acetylators tend to eliminate the drug more slowly and, therefore, have higher plasma levels of the parent drug and/or phase I oxidative metabolites, which can predispose to toxicity. For example, antinuclear antibodies and systemic lupus erythematosus caused by hydralazine, procainaminde or isoniazid develop more quickly in slow acetylators than in fast acetylators, because a larger proportion of the drugs undergoes oxidative metabolism. The slow acetylator phenotype has also been shown to predispose to the development of bladder cancer. Fast acetylators eliminate the drug more rapidly and have lower plasma levels after ingestion of equivalent doses than slow acetylators. This can occasionally lead to therapeutic failure, for example with isoniazid in the treatment of tuberculosis.

Drug oxidation polymorphisms

The most common pharmacogenetic polymorphism affecting phase I oxidative metabolic pathways is the debrisoquine hydroxylation polymorphism. The poor metaboliser (PM) phenotype, which is inherited as an autosomal recessive trait, is characterised by a deficiency in the metabolism of debrisoquine (a now little-used antihypertensive agent) when compared with the extensive metaboliser (EM). Patients with PM phenotype, which has a frequency of 5–10% in the Caucasian population, have a deficiency of the cytochrome P450 isoform CYP2D6. Molecular studies have identified at least four mutations responsible for the PM phenotype. Cytochrome P450 2D6 (CYP2D6) has broad substrate specificity and has been found to be involved in the metabolism of at least 20 commonly used drugs, including antidepressants, antipsychotics and anti-arrhythmics. A deficiency of this enzyme may lead to either therapeutic failure or drug toxicity. The former has been described with drugs such as codeine, which need to be metabolised to their active components by the enzyme. Three types of adverse reactions are possible in PM. First, poor metabolism of the drug will diminish first-pass metabolism, increase bioavailability and, therefore, result in an exaggerated pharmacological response, for example hypotension with debrisoquine. Second, diminished metabolism prolongs the half life of a drug and leads to accumulation, with consequent toxicity; for example, neuropathy and hepatotoxicity with perhexiline are much more common in PM. Third, the deficiency of the usual metabolic pathway can alter the route of metabolism of a drug, causing the formation of toxic metabolites, for example phenacetin.

Carcinogenicity and teratogenicity

The possibility of serious delayed toxicities, including carcinogenicity and teratogenicity, is of major concern during drug development, which necessarily involves extensive pre-clinical evaluation of the mutagenic, carcinogenic and reproductive toxicology. The assessment of such toxicities in humans is largely dependent on post-marketing surveillance and retrospective analysis of the National Cancer Registries.

It is now generally accepted that the induction of cancer in humans by chemicals, including pharmaceuticals, involves several consecutive independent steps. Drugs may cause cancer by acting either as direct genotoxins, which have as their primary biological activity the alteration of the information encoded by DNA, or as non-genotoxic carcinogens, which can act by a variety of mechanisms to promote the initial damage caused by a genotoxin.

Only a small number of pharmaceutical agents have been identified as possible carcinogens in humans. The main classes of drug are antineoplastics, immunosuppressants and hormones. Therefore, in most instances, the carcinogenic potential of these compounds is compatible with their pharmacodynamic properties. However in certain cases, for example with the analgesic phenacetin, there is no apparent relationship between their primary mode of action and the toxic manifestation. Phenacetin was withdrawn from clinical use because of an association with a higher risk of renal tumours, which are thought to arise because of bioactivation of the drug to a reactive metabolite by renal enzymes.

The phocomelia induced by the sedative thalidomide provided a milestone in the appreciation of the devastating effects drugs may have with respect to human disease. The particular mechanism involved in the selective developmental toxicity of thalidomide in the fetus has not been elucidated, although it is now appreciated that there are more than 20 mechanisms by which chemicals may induce fetal abnormalities. Drugs in use that are associated with a risk of teratogenicity include anticonvulsants, steroids and retinoids. Given the limitations of pre-clinical tests for reproductive toxicity, caution must be exercised in the use of any drug in pregnancy.

Summary

There is no doubt that toxic reactions to drugs are common. The majority of the adverse reactions will be of the pharmacological variety, i.e. an exaggeration of the normal pharmacological actions of the drug. Although these reactions account for a great deal of morbidity, fortunately they are only rarely fatal. An understanding of the mechanism of these reactions will depend on a knowledge of the pharmacology of the drug, and they should be preventable by the good clinical practice of rational prescribing. Alleviation of this form of toxicity only usually requires dose reduction, although, in some cases, the drug may have to be withdrawn completely.

A small proportion of adverse reactions are of the chemical variety, being dependent on the physicochemical properties or chemical reactivity of the drug or its metabolite. A knowledge of the mechanism of the toxicity may allow the development of preventive strategies, such as the use of specific antidotes (for example in paracetamol hepatotoxicity) or inhibition of the formation of the reactive metabolite.

The idiosyncratic reactions are bizarre, unpredictable from the known pharmacology of the drug and do not show a simple dose relationship. Although less common than the dose-dependent toxicities, in general they tend to be more severe, accounting for many fatalities. Management of such toxicity includes withdrawal of the offending drug, together with supportive and symptomatic treatment when required; treatment is dependent on the major organ system(s) affected. At present, for most of the drug-induced idiosyncratic toxicities, we have no method of prevention. Prospective prediction of susceptibility is a possibility for certain idiosyncratic reactions and may already be in clinical use, for example the caffeine–halothane contracture test for prediction of susceptibility to malignant hyperthermia. However, for many of the reactions, because of their multifactorial nature, absolute predictive tests may be neither practical nor possible. An understanding of the mechanism for the idiosyncratic toxicity may provide an alternative method of prevention by the development of new compounds incorporating structural features that prevent them from being toxic or forming toxic metabolites while at the same time ensuring that they retain their pharmacological efficacy.

FURTHER READING

General

Ammus, S. & Yunis, A.A. (1989). Drug-induced red cell dyscrasias. *Blood Reviews*, 3, 71–82.

Hughes, W.T. (1995). Postulates for the evaluation of adverse reactions to drugs. *Clinical Infectious Diseases*, 20, 179–182.

Mueller-Eckhardt, C. (1987). Drug-induced immune thrombocytopenia. *Baillière's Clinical Immunology and Allergy*, 1, 369–389.

Pessayre, D. & Larrey, D. (1988). Acute and chronic drug-induced hepatitis. *Baillière's Clinical Gastroenterology*, 2, 385–423.

Pohl, L.R., Satoh, H., Christ, D.D. & Kenna, J.G. (1988). Immunologic and metabolic basis of drug hypersensitivities. *Annual Reviews in Pharmacology*, 28, 367–387.

Uetrecht, J.P. (1992). The role of leukocyte-generated reactive metabolites in the pathogenesis of idiosyncratic drug reactions. *Drug Metabolism Reviews*, 24, 299–366.

Specific topics

Brodie, M. & Feely, J. (1991). Adverse drug interactions. In *New Drugs*, 2nd edn, ed. J. Feely, pp. 29–39. London: BMJ.

de Smet, P.A.G.M. (1991). Drugs use in non-orthodox medicine. L-Tryptophan and the eosinophilia-myalgia syndrome. In *Side Effects of Drugs Annual 15*, ed. M.N.G. Dukes & J.K. Aronson, pp. 514–531. Amsterdam: Elsevier Science.

Koopmans, P.P., van der Ven, A.J.A.M., Vree, T.B. & van der Meer, J.W.M. (1995). Pathogenesis of hypersensitivity reactions to drugs in patients with HIV-infection – allergic or toxic? *AIDS*, 9, 217–222.

Park, B.K. & Kitteringham, N.R. (1990). Drug–protein conjugation and its immunological consequences. *Drug Metabolism Reviews*, 22, 87–144.

Park, B.K., Coleman, J.W. & Kitteringham, N.R. (1987). Drug disposition and drug hypersensitivity. *Biochemical Pharmacology*, 36, 581–590.

Park, B.K., Pirmohamed, M. & Kitteringham, N.R. (1992). Idiosyncratic drug reactions: a mechanistic evaluation of risk factors. *British Journal of Clinical Pharmacology*, 34, 377–395.

Pirmohamed, M., Kitteringham, N.R. & Park, B.K. (1994). The role of active metabolites in drug toxicity. *Drug Safety*, 11, 114–144.

Pirmohamed, M. & Park, B.K. (1993). Prediction of idiosyncratic drug reactions. *Adverse Drug Reaction Bulletin*, 163, 615–618.

Rawlins, M.D. & Thompson, J.W. (1991). Mechanisms of adverse drug reactions. In *Textbook of Adverse Drug Reactions*, 4th edn, ed. D.M., Davies, pp. 18–45. Oxford: Oxford University Press.

Roujeau, J.-C. & Stern, R.S. (1994). Severe adverse cutaneous reactions to drugs. *New England Journal of Medicine*, 331, 1272–1285.

Tucker, G.T. (1994). Clinical implications of genetic polymorphism in drug metabolism. *Journal of Pharmacy and Pharmacology*, 46 (suppl. 1), 417–424.

14

Toxic mechanisms: alcohol

J. NEUBERGER

- The toxic effects of alcohol have public health implications in that alcohol contributes not only to liver and other organ damage but also to death from accidents, suicides and homicides. Within the UK alcohol is estimated to cost in excess of £2 billion annually with a cost to the National Health Service, of £100 000 000. The incidence of cirrhosis of the liver caused by alcohol in the UK is approximately 10 per 100 000. About 25 000 die each year as a consequence of alcohol.

- The main site of metabolism of ethanol is the liver: there are three pathways of ethanol metabolism: via alcohol dehydrogenase, via the mitochondrial ethanol oxidising system (MEOS) and by catalase. The alcohol dehydrogenase pathway plays a central role in the metabolism of ethanol.

- There is considerable variation in the response to alcohol. Among the factors implicated are genetic variations, which include polymorphisms in both alcohol dehydrogenase and acetaldehyde dehydrogenase, and variations in the volume of distribution of alcohol. The reasons why females are more susceptible to alcoholic liver damage than males are not clear. There are many immunological abnormalities in patients with alcoholic liver disease, including disorders of the cellular and humoral immune system; whether these are involved in the pathogenesis of liver disease or are a consequence of it remains uncertain.

- The mechanism of alcohol toxicity is poorly understood. Ethanol itself is not very toxic to liver cells but acetaldehyde forms more toxic reactive metabolites, which may result in complement activation, the generation of antigens leading to immune-mediated cell damage and direct toxic effects. The last includes alterations to the structure of liver cells and the development of lipid peroxidation.

- Clinically, alcoholic liver disease may be difficult to detect. An increasing number of serological markers has been developed. The histological spectrum of liver damage varies from fatty liver (usually reversible) to cirrhosis (irreversible) and alcoholic hepatitis, which is often fatal. The reasons for the wide spectrum of liver damage remain to be established.

Alcohol has long been associated with the development of liver damage. Despite the fact that alcohol liver disease is the major cause of liver cirrhosis in patients in the Western world, the mechanisms responsible for the liver damage remain unclear. The spectrum of liver damage induced by alcohol varies considerably, ranging from minimal changes to cirrhosis and alcoholic hepatitis. However, there exists considerable individual variation in susceptibility to the effects of alcohol in inducing liver damage. Those factors responsible for this variation are poorly defined: metabolic, immunological and genetic factors have been implicated. Treatment remains largely supportive; abstinence is the most effective form of therapy.

In this chapter alcohol will be used to describe alcoholic drinks; ethanol will be used where the specific metabolic aspects are discussed.

Epidemiology

Assessment of alcohol consumption is difficult and often unreliable. An approximate estimate of the consumption of alcohol can be obtained by dividing the amount of alcohol consumed by the population by the number of adults legally permitted to drink. Such figures make the false assumption that only legally sold alcohol is consumed and ignores individual variations in alcohol consumption. There is great variation in the pattern of consumption; for example, in the USA, 50% of the alcohol consumed is accounted for by 10% of the drinking population. Overall about one-third of the population are light drinkers, one-third are moderate to heavy drinkers and the rest are abstainers. Abstinence is more common amongst women than men and amongst older people of both sexes than amongst younger adults.

Alcohol is associated with a variety of diseases and disorders (Table 14.1) but the greatest risk is alcoholic liver disease. Death rates from cirrhosis are higher for men than women and higher for non-whites than whites. Alcohol also contributes to death by accidents, suicides and homicide. This is particularly marked in men aged below 35. Indeed, alcohol is associated not only in half of all violent deaths but also in one-third of drownings and one-quarter of homicides, boating and aviation deaths. Furthermore, nearly half of convicted jail inmates in the USA were under the influence of alcohol at the time of committing the offence and over half of those who were drinking at the time of the offence were drunk. More than half of people convicted of violent crimes were drinking at the time of the offence.

In the UK, estimates suggest that alcohol contributes to up to 40 000 deaths each year; this compares with 2000 deaths a year with cervical cancer. The financial cost in the UK of alcohol excess is estimated to be over £2000 million per year, through lost production and the medical and social services caring for the individual. The cost to the National Health Service has been estimated to be about £100 million.

In hospital, estimates in England suggest that problem drinking occurs in 15–30% of males and about half that number of women. Alcohol excess contributes to 27% of drug overdoses, 20% of head injuries, 17% of road accidents and 10% of gastrointestinal haemorrhages.

Alcohol and the liver

It has long been recognised that there is a close relationship between the amount of alcohol consumed and alcoholic liver disease. There is a broad consensus that there is a

Table 14.1. *Extrahepatic manifestations of alcohol toxicity*

System	Disease
Gastrointestinal tract	
Oesophagus	Reflux
	Oesophageal cancer
Stomach	Gastritis
	Gastric ulcer
Small intestine	Malabsorption
	Altered motor activity
Pancreas	Pancreatitis (acute and chronic)
	Carcinoma
Cardiovascular system	Congestive cardiomyopathy
	Hypertension
Central nervous system	Cerebellar degeneration
	Wernicke–Korsakoff syndrome
	Polyneuropathy
Muscle	Myopathy: acute/chronic
Haematological	Haemolysis
	Impaired cryothropoeisis
	Abnormal morphology:
	macrocytosis, triangulocytes
	Neutropenia
	Thrombocytopenia
Endocrinological/metabolic	Hypogonadism
	Hyperoestrogenaemia
	Pseudo-Cushing's syndrome
	Hypoglycaemia
	Ketoacidosis
	Gout
	Osteopenia
Pregnancy	Fetal alcohol syndrome
	Increased risk of abortion and
	still birth

'safe-limit': below 14 units (1 unit equates to 10g alcohol) a week for women and below 21 units a week for men, the risk of developing alcoholic liver disease is small. Above these limits, the risks rise proportionally. The general public has latched onto these figures and it is unusual for any reader of a broad-sheet newspaper to admit to drinking over these amounts! However, these figures must be taken with caution and levels may well be revised. A 1995 report *Sensible Drinking* from the UK Department of Health recommends a daily maximum intake of 2–3 units (women) and 3–4 units (men), a move not without opposition from the medical profession. Alcohol has many effects and some, such as the effect on cardiovascular disease, may be beneficial. It must not be forgotten that alcohol is enjoyed by many, including medical students and doctors, so that draconian restrictions may be counterproductive.

The annual mortality in the UK attributed to alcohol is about 25 000; but estimates vary between 5000 and 40 000; the annual incidence of alcoholic cirrhosis in the UK is about 10 per 100 000 and the mortality from alcoholic liver disease is about 2000 per year.

Alcohol metabolism

Absorption

Ethanol is absorbed from the gastrointestinal tract by simple diffusion, primarily in the duodenum and upper jejunum. The rate of absorption of ethanol is affected by the gastric emptying time and by the presence of the intestinal contents. Therefore, in patients with a gastroenterostomy, the rate of absorption is increased, whereas in the presence of food, absorption is reduced. Animal studies have suggested that carbohydrates, amino acids and peptides will enhance ethanol absorption. If alcohol is given in a more concentrated form (as in whisky), the rate of absorption is greater than in a weak form (as in beer or wine).

Distribution

Ethanol is relatively lipid insoluble and is, therefore, distributed throughout the body, but relatively little is found in fat.

Excretion

The average man is able to excrete about 1 g of ethanol per hour per 10 kg body weight. The rate of excretion will vary considerably. Over 90% of ethanol is oxidised and secreted as carbon dioxide and water (see below). Smaller amounts of ethanol are eliminated via urine (less than 1%) and breath (1–3%). The distribution of ethanol between blood and expired air is 2100:1.

Site of ethanol metabolism

Although ethanol is metabolised in the kidney, stomach, intestine and bone marrow cells, the main site of ethanol metabolism is the liver.
There are three main pathways for ethanol metabolism (Fig. 14.1)

> alcohol dehydrogenase (ADH)
> mitrochondrial ethanol oxidising system (MEOS)
> catalase.

The main pathway for ethanol metabolism is via the enzyme ADH, which metabolises ethanol to acetaldehyde with the production of reduced NAD (NADH) (Fig. 14.2). This takes place in the cytosol; the acetaldehyde formed diffuses into the mitochondria where it is converted by acetaldehyde dehydrogenase (ALDH) to acetate. The acetate is released into the blood and oxidised by the peripheral tissues with the production of carbon dioxide, water and fatty acids.

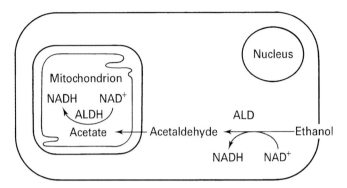

Fig. 14.1. Ethanol metabolism by alcohol dehydrogenase (ALD). ALDH, acetaldehyde dehydrogenase.

Alcohol dehydrogenase

$$C_2H_5OH + NAD^+ \longrightarrow CH_3CHO + NADH + H^+$$

MEOS

$$C_2H_5OH + NADPH + H^+ + O_2 \longrightarrow CH_3CHO + NADP^+ + 2H_2O$$

Catalase

$$C_2H_5OH + H_2O \longrightarrow CH_3CHO + 2H_2O$$

Fig. 14.2. Major routes of ethanol metabolism.

Alcohol dehydrogenase

ADH plays a central role in the metabolism of alcohol. There exists considerable polymorphism in ADH, which has been related to ethanol metabolism, alcohol dependence and alcoholic liver disease. The three classes of ADH isoenzyme are shown in Table 14.2.

Hepatic ADH activity is low in fetal life but adult levels are reached by the age of 5 years.

The pH optimum for ADH oxidation of ethanol is near 11 so that physiologically the rate of reaction is less than half the maximum, with a K_m for ethanol less than 1 mmol. Therefore, ethanol is metabolised from the blood at a constant rate until very low blood levels are achieved.

Oxidation of ethanol to acetaldehyde by ADH requires NAD^+ as a co-factor, which is reduced to NADH. Since NADH reduction exceeds its rate of re-oxidation under normal conditions, the increased ratio of NADH to NAD^+ is associated with a significant reduction in the redox state of the liver. This is thought to account for the major metabolic effects of ethanol metabolism, including inhibition of hepatic glyconeogenesis, decrease of fatty oxidation and decrease in citric acid cycle activity. This results in, amongst other consequences, raised blood lactate, ketosis, hyperuricaemia and hepatic trapping of triglycerides.

Table 14.2. *Isozymes of ADH*

Class	Locus	Peptide
I	ADH1	
	ADH2	$\beta_1, \beta_2, \beta_3$
	ADH3	$\gamma_1 \gamma_2$
II	ADH4	
III	ADH5	
IV	ADH7	
V	ADH6	

In addition to the polymorphism of ADH (discussed below), several factors may affect the activity of ADH. These include: intracellular acetaldehyde concentration, shuttle mechanisms transporting reduced equivalents into the mitochondria, and the rate of mitochondrial respiratory chain activity. The rate of ethanol elimination *in vivo* correlates with the basal metabolic rate; this suggests that the rate of mitochondrial NADH oxidation is the main rate-limiting factor in the ADH pathway. However, this cannot be the only limiting factor because in renal failure, where hepatic ADH activity is increased, blood ethanol clearance remains normal.

Other factors inhibit the rate of ethanol elimination: prolonged fasting reduces ethanol clearance. By comparison, fructose and corticosteroids enhance ethanol elimination. This may be related to the increased conversion of NADH to NAD^+. Cimetidine, a weak enzyme inhibitor that is commonly taken for digestive upsets, reduces metabolism.

Ethanol metabolism can also be inhibited by the ADH inhibitors: pyrazole and its derivatives may lead to high blood levels.

MEOS system

The MEOS system is located in the endoplasmic reticulum and requires NADPH and oxygen. The importance of the MEOS system in ethanol metabolism overall remains uncertain.

The cytochrome responsible for the MEOS system is designated P45IIE1. This has been characterised and localised to chromosome 7. The MEOS system has also been demonstrated in mucosal cells of the upper gastrointestinal tract and the colon.

Catalase

Catalase is a haemoprotein located in the perioxomes and is capable of oxidising ethanol *in vitro* in the presence of hydrogen peroxide; the physiological role remains uncertain.

Table 14.3. *Isozymes of aldehyde dehydrogenase*

Class	Isozyme	Distribution
E1	ALDH1	Cytosolic
E2	ALDH2	Mitochondrial periportal > perivenous
E3		Not involved in acetaldehyde oxidation
E4		Not involved in acetaldehyde oxidation

Acetaldehyde metabolism

Acetaldehyde is oxidised rapidly under normal circumstances. Over 90% is metabolised to acetate in the liver by the enzyme aldehyde dehydrogenase; this enzyme is NAD^+ dependent and has a very low K_m value and a high reaction rate so that under normal circumstances very little acetaldehyde is found outside the liver. Acetaldehyde dehydrogenase activity is found in the microsomes, mitochondria and cytoplasm, but the functional activity is probably entirely a mitochondrial process. There are two forms of aldehyde dehydrogenase, I and II (see below) (Table 14.3).

Oxidation of acetaldehyde to acetate results in reduction of cytosolic and mitochondrial redox status. This low redox state is associated with increases in the liver and blood lactate/pyruvate and β-hydroxybutyrate/acetoacetate ratios.

Acetaldehyde dehydrogenase may be inhibited by a number of compounds, of which disulphiram (Antabuse), a tetramethylthiouram sulphide is the most familiar. Similar reactions occur when sulphonurylureas are administered. Metronidazole and cefamandole may also inhibit aldehyde dehydrogenase, resulting in increased production of acetaldehyde and leading to the so-called sensitising reactions. Patients on these agents are at increased risk of developing alcohol flush syndrome; the 'Antabuse reaction.' The alcohol flush reaction is characterised by pulsating headaches, tachycardia and erythema of the face and upper chest. In severe cases, asthma, hypotension, angiooedema and vascular collapse can occur. These reactions occur probably as a direct consequence of acetaldehyde toxicity.

MECHANISMS OF ALCOHOL TOXICITY

As indicated above, alcohol toxicity is, in general, compatible with features of a direct or predictable toxin. However, there remains a large variation in sensitivity to alcohol toxicity: only 8–18% of people who abuse alcohol in the long term develop cirrhosis; in some patients, liver damage will not progress beyond the stage of fatty liver even in the face of continued alcohol excess; of those who drink about one bottle of spirits per day (surely a group self-selected by relative wealth and determination), only half will develop a cirrhosis in two decades.

To explain the relationship between the amount of alcohol consumed and the probability of developing severe liver damage that has been reliably demonstrated in many populations and the apparently contradictory data derived from individual studies, it is important to understand not only the direct metabolic mechanisms of ethanol toxicity but also those idiosyncratic mechanisms that account for most variation; these factors are genetic or immunological.

Genetic factors in ethanol metabolism

Metabolism of ethanol is dependent on many factors, including whether alcohol is consumed when fasting or with food, rates of gastric emptying (which may be affected by fats or hypertonic solutions), the extent of metabolism by the gastric or intestinal mucosa, the presence of drugs, the extent of chronic alcohol ingestion, age, body habitus and even the time of day. Nevertheless, when these factors are considered, a variation of less than 10% in the rate of metabolism of ethanol is seen *within* an individual. In contrast, when individuals are compared, there may be up to a threefold difference in the rates of ethanol metabolism, which cannot be explained by the above factors.

The importance of genetic factors for ethanol metabolism has been shown by studies in mono- and dizygotic twins. Nearly two-thirds of the variability in peak blood ethanol concentration and nearly half of the variability in elimination rates may be owing to genetic factors. In contrast, about 10% of the variation in peak blood ethanol concentration could be attributed to differences in alcohol intake and the effects of age, weight and degree of fat. The difference in susceptibility to develop alcoholic liver damage between males and females is largely related to volumes of distribution.

As a result of these observations, research has concentrated on the importance of the ethanol metabolising enzymes. There is increasing evidence, however, that other genetic factors are also important in determining susceptibility to alcoholic liver damage (Table 14.4). The dopamine D_2 receptor has been linked to alcohol addiction, and some of the genes associated with fibrosis, namely those for collagen type 1 (*COL1A1* and *COL1A2*), are thought to be important.

Isozymes of ADH

ADH consists of dimeric molecules with subunits of 40 kDA. Currently, seven different ADH genes have been identified with five classes of enzyme. These have been sequenced and analysis of data suggests that there are two functional groups: one with the α-, β- and γ- subunits and a second with π, ψ and σ-subunits. Furthermore, polymorphism occurs at ADH1 and ADH2 (see Table 14.2). The differences result from amino acid substitutions at two residues, which result in different co-enzyme-binding sites and affect the kinetic constants.

ADH1 and ADH2 appear with different frequencies in different racial groups. Thus, within ADH2 polymorphism occurs in the β-subunit: the β_1 form is predominant in black and white populations whereas the β_2 form is predominant in the Chinese and Japanese. The β_3 form appears in 25% of the black population. In ADH3 polymorphism, the two γ

Table 14.4. *Genes that may influence susceptibility to alcohol*

	Genes
Alcohol metabolism	For ADH For aldehyde dehydrogenase For cytochrome P450IIE2
Fibrosis	Type I collagen genes (COL1A1, COL1A2)
Immune system	HLA alleles
Addiction	Dopamine receptor gene
Other	Gene for α_1-antitrypsin, TNF polymorphism

alleles appear with equal frequencies in the white populations but the γ_1 form dominates in the Japanese, Chinese and black populations.

There is tissue distribution of the different isoenzymes. For example, in rats the class I enzyme is expressed equally in perivenous and periportal areas. In the gastrointestinal tract, different isoenzymes predominate.

Isozymes of acetaldehyde dehydrogenase

As with ADH, there are multiple molecular forms of aldehyde dehydrogenase (Table 14.3). Of these, only classes E1 and E2 are important in acetaldehyde metabolism.

Both ALDH1 and ALDH2 are tetrameric molecules with subunits of about 500 amino acid residues. Polymorphism has been identified for both isozymes.

Isozymes in relation to alcoholic liver disease

A number of studies have shown that the rate of ethanol excess and of alcoholic liver disease varies between populations and some of this has been attributed to genetic patterns of ethanol metabolism. Many of the early studies were hampered by the fact that subjects were not specifically genotyped.

Facial flushing after alcohol consumption is well recognised in the Chinese and Japanese and this has been attributed to elevated acetaldehyde levels and has been highly correlated with ALDH2 deficiency. Those who are homozygous for ALDH2*2 have the most severe flush reaction and higher acetaldehyde levels than those with other genotypes of the enzyme. These reactions occur when acetaldehyde concentrations reach between 40 and 60 mmol/litre.

Amongst the Japanese, nearly three-quarters report flushing after alcohol and the vast majority of these are ALDH2 deficient. In contrast, nearly all those who do not flush are ALDH2 active. However, this situation is not clear-cut since around 10% of Caucasians also report facial flushing following alcohol ingestion, but the ALDH2*2 isoenzyme has not been found in Caucasians.

A number of studies have shown that those who flush and are ALDH2 deficient are less likely to be heavy alcohol drinkers. However, amongst alcoholics who are ALDH2 deficient, drinking problems occur later in life.

Immunological factors in alcoholic liver disease

Although within the population there is a clear dose–response relationship in the effects of alcohol, there is considerable variation in the hepatic susceptibility to alcohol consumption. That immune reactions may be implicated in determining the rate of progression or development of alcoholic liver disease is suggested by a number of factors, including evidence of disturbance of the immune system and the clinical observation that in some patients liver damage may progress even when alcohol consumption is stopped.

HLA antigens

The importance of HLA antigens has remained confusing; part of the problem arises from the fact that distribution of HLA antigens varies between different populations. Most studies have relied on serotyping, which is unreliable for HLA assignment. It is difficult to control for many of the other factors already described that may affect susceptibility. An association between HLA-B8 and the development of alcoholic cirrhosis has been described but data are conflicting. Other studies have implicated HLA-B5, HLA-B13 and HLA-B40.

Serological abnormalities in alcoholic liver disease

Of the autoantibodies in patients with liver disease, elevation of serum IgA has been recognised for many years. IgA (mainly IgA 1 subclass) may be deposited in the kidneys, giving rise to IgA nephropathy leading to glomerulonephritis and renal failure. Monomeric IgA is also present in the hepatic sinusoids of patients with alcoholic liver disease but it does not correlate with serum levels of IgA. Other reports have emphasised the importance of elevated serum levels of IgG. The hypergammaglobulinaemia may be the result of the increased availability of gut-derived antigens as a consequence of reduced Kupffer cell function and portosystemic shunting. This is confirmed by the presence of increased titres to gut-derived antigens. An alternative explanation is that the hypergammaglobulinaemia is consequent on impaired suppressor cell function.

Non-organ-specific autoantibodies are also present in increased concentrations in patients with alcoholic liver disease. These include the smooth muscle antibodies and antinuclear antibodies, which are found usually in low titre and more commonly in women than in men. Liver-specific antibodies (both IgG and IgA) include those that react with liver membrane antigens, the liver-specific lipoprotein and the asialoglycoprotein receptor. Of greater interest has been the presence of antibodies towards alcohol-altered liver cell determinants. These antibodies, which can induce antibody-dependent cell-mediated cytotoxicity, appear to be related to neoantigens associated with acetaldehyde rather than with ethanol. Thus, acetaldehyde may act as a hapten or may induce structural alterations to other proteins leading to development of a neoantigen. Others have identified antibodies to alcoholic hyaline in patients with severe alcoholic liver disease.

Cell-mediated immunity

Delayed hypersensitivity is reduced in patients with alcoholic liver disease and reactivity is reduced to all recall antigens. Patients with alcholic hepatitis and cirrhosis have a reduced number of circulating lymphocytes; this is primarily through a reduction in T cells, with the B cell numbers being relatively well preserved. This may be a result of sequestration of T cells within the liver. Functional studies have shown that in patients with alcoholic liver disease, lymphoblast transformation is increased by ethanol or acetaldehyde. Leucocyte migration to acetaldehyde is reduced only in those patients with alcoholic hepatitis. Thus, lymphocytes from patients with alcoholic liver disease can be shown to be sensitised to antigens in normal liver, alcohol hyaline and alcohol-treated liver. It is difficult to determine whether these immune reactions are primary, or secondary to alcohol-mediated liver damage.

The reticuloendothelial system

A decreased phagocytic capacity is found in patients with alcoholic liver disease. This may be a direct consequence of ethanol acting on the cells of the reticuloendothelial system, or a blockage of capacity by circulating immune complexes. Decreased reticulo-endothelial system activity is associated with an increased susceptibility to infections, particularly bacterial.

Cytokines and inflammatory markers

Alcoholic liver disease shows features of an inflammatory response, with increased circulatory levels of inflammatory cytokines and increased tissue expression of inflammatory and adhesion molecules. In patients with alcoholic hepatitis, levels of TNF-α, IL-1 and IL-6 are increased. The first two cytokines remain elevated for several months, whereas IL-6 falls with recovery. Whether these (and other) cytokines are implicated in the generation or perpetuation of liver or extrahepatic organ damage or whether these changes represent a healing response to alcohol-induced liver damage remains uncertain.

Metabolic toxicity

Ethanol toxicity

There are a number of mechanisms by which it is suggested that alcohol toxicity can occur:

- membrane alterations
- membrane lipid peroxidation
- enzyme dysfunction
- abnormal redox state
- increased cellular oxygen requirement
- inflammation
- fibrogenesis.

Ethanol will alter membrane fluidity but the consequences of this in the pathogenesis of the disease remain uncertain.

Toxicity of acetaldehyde

Acetaldehyde metabolism results in reduction of hepatocyte redox levels, as indicated above; production of acetaldehyde from ethanol results in increased amounts of NADH. This has a number of effects on the liver and general metabolism.

Hyperlacticaemia

The enhanced $NADH/NAD^+$ ratio results in an increased ratio of lactate to pyruvate as a consequence of decreased utilisation and enhanced production of lactate within the liver. The high level of lactate contributes to the generalised acidosis and reduces renal uric acid excretion, resulting in hyperuricaemia. This may lead to gout. The effect of alcohol in causing ketosis will also promote raised uric acid levels.

Depressed lipid oxidation and enhanced lipogenesis

The increased $NADH/NAD^+$ ratio increases the concentration of α-glycerophosphate, leading to retention of triglycerides within the hepatocyte as a consequence of trapping fatty acids. Fatty acid synthesis is also enhanced by excess NADH. Because mitochondria preferentially use hydrogen equivalents from ethanol rather than those from oxidation of fatty acids, there is decreased fatty acid oxidation, which results in accumulation of fat within the liver and the development of megamitochondria.

Protein metabolism

Whilst *in vitro* ethanol will inhibit protein synthesis, the effect in humans is less clear-cut. The malnutrition seen in patients with alcoholic liver disease is largely related to poor dietary intake and to liver cell failure.

Glucose metabolism

The effect of ethanol on glucose metabolism is complex since ethanol may inhibit hepatic gluconeogenesis as a consequence of the increased $NADH/NAD^+$ ratio, when glycogen

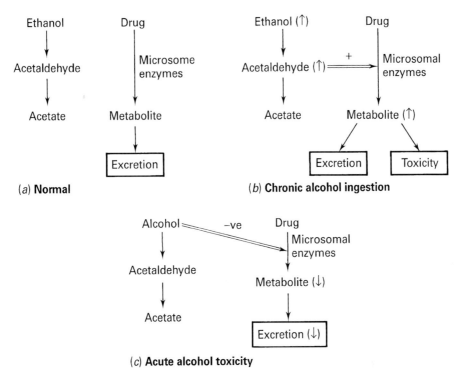

Fig. 14.3. Effect of ethanol on drug metabolism. (*a*) Normal. (*b*) Chronic alcohol ingestion.(*c*) Acute alcohol toxicity.

stores are released, or under other circumstances, gluconeogenesis is actually acceler-ated.

Hepatic hypoxia

Histologically, the main lesions caused by alcohol in the liver are detected in the cen-trilobular or perivenular zone, where the pO_2 is least. Ethanol induces an increase in hepatic portal blood flow (as indeed will any meal), but in the situation of chronic alcohol consumption there appears to be defective oxygen utilisation. Again tissue hypoxia will enhance the amount of NADH and increase the lactate/pyruvate ratio. Furthermore, since there is more ADH in those hepatocytes in the perivenular zone, it is likely that more toxic metabolites of ethanol are generated by metabolism.

Consequences of ethanol as an enzyme inducer

Ethanol is a potent enzyme inducer and particulate cytochrome P45OIIE1 is enhanced. Those compounds that are converted by this enzyme to potentially toxic intermediates are metabolised faster (Fig. 14.3). For example, paracetamol is metabolised to a toxic intermediate (NAPQI) which, if not removed by glutathione, accumulates in the liver resulting in increased toxicity (Chapter 13, p. 371). In those patients with chronic alcohol consumption, the cytochrome P450 activity is enhanced, leading to a greater generation of metabolites and a subsequent increase in toxicity of paracetamol. Other clinically important interactions include those with the oral contraceptive (potentially leading to reduced contraceptive effect) and warfarin (leading to reduced anticoagulation). In contrast, acute ingestion of alcohol may inhibit enzyme activity and so reduce toxicity of drugs such as paracetamol as less toxic metabolites are generated (Fig. 14.3).

Toxic effects of acetaldehyde adducts

Acetaldehyde may form reactive adducts with protein that may result in

- increased complement activation
- generation of neoantigens
- disruption of microtubule formation
- inhibition of enzyme activity
- increased lipid peroxidation

Acetaldehyde binds to cysteine and glutathione, resulting in reduced levels of glutathione in the hepatocyte. Since glutathione is a free radical scavenger, the radicals produced by, amongst other things, ethanol metabolism by the MEOS system may make the cell more susceptible to lipid peroxidation damage. Acetaldehyde also interferes directly or indirectly with other enzyme activities.

Ethanol metabolism and immune processes

As indicated above, patients with alcoholic liver disease have evidence of disturbance of the immune system, with abnormal immunoglobulin levels and organ-specific and non-specific autoantibodies. The extent to which these are secondary to liver and other target cell damage involved more acutely in the pathogenesis is unclear. Nonetheless, there is increasing evidence that some immune mechanisms may be involved in the mechanisms of liver damage.

Complement activation

Acetaldehyde has been shown to form adducts with plasma membranes which, *in vitro*, activate complement. This may result in organ damage.

Role of white cells

In patients with alcoholic liver damage, there is increased appearance of the three main endothelial adhesion molecules (ICAM-1, VCAM-1 and E-selectin). In alcoholic hepatitis, E-selectin is found on inflamed endothelium at the site of neutrophil infiltration and increased ICAM-1 and VCAM-1 levels are found on sinusoidal endothelium. In contrast, in cirrhosis, ICAM-1 and VCAM-1 are strongly expressed on sinusoidal endothelium. The distribution of adhesion molecules would allow the T cells and monocytes to transmigrate in alcoholic hepatitis and cirrhosis.

It is possible that these adhesion molecules are induced by TNF-α, which is secreted in increased amounts in alcoholic hepatitis and cirrhosis. It has been suggested that the increased TNF-α is produced by macrophages stimulated by endotoxin reaching the systemic circulation from ethanol-induced gut damage.

Alcohol and fibrosis

One feature of alcohol-induced liver injury is the proliferation of perisinusoidal cells, including myofibroblasts, fibroblasts and transitional cells. The most important of these are the lipocytes (Ito cells), which contain ADH and, therefore, are able to metabolise ethanol. These cells are able to secrete collagens type I, II and IV and laminin. Since these cells are located in greatest concentration in the perivenular region, damage by ethanol of these cells may explain the distribution of fibrosis. The mechanism by which ethanol induces collagen formation is unclear. This may relate to inflammation from ethanol or acetaldehyde or the associated hyperlactataemia. The increased deposition of collagen in the space of Disse results in reduced blood flow and features of portal hypertension. Thus, portal hypertension may be present before the onset of frank cirrhosis.

Lipocytes, on appropriate stimulation, are transformed into myofibroblasts and can produce collagen. *In vitro*, acetaldehyde and other aldehydes will stimulate these cells. Collagen deposition represents the results of a balance between secretion and removal. Polyunsaturated lecithin stimulates collagenase activity and can, at least *in vitro*, reduce the collagen secretion by acetaldehyde-stimulated lipocytes. Circulating tissue inhibitors such as the metalloproteinase inhibitor TIMP may prove to be reliable markers of hepatic fibrosis.

Alcohol and other conditions

It is now clear that patients with chronic viral hepatitis (resulting from infection with hepatitis virus B or C) are at greater risk of alcohol-induced liver damage. Furthermore, those patients who are heterozygous or homozygous for haemochromatosis and those with α_1-antitrypsin deficiency are also at greater risk of alcohol-induced liver damage. Whether this represents an additive effect of two different toxins on the liver or whether there is a more involved interaction remains to be determined.

Clinical aspects

History

The history in patients with possible alcohol-related liver damage is divided into two aspects: obtaining an alcohol history and looking for evidence of and the extent of target organ damage. Alcohol dependence and alcoholic liver damage do not necessarily occur together.

It is often very difficult to take an accurate drinking history since patterns of drinking will vary throughout the lifetime of the individual and it may be difficult accurately to recall patterns of drinking 10–15 years earlier. Furthermore, alcohol intake is rarely

Table 14.5. *Cage questionnaire: two or more positive answers imply a possibility of alcohol dependence*

C	Have you ever felt you should cut down on your drinking?
A	Have you felt annoyed when others have criticised your drinking?
G	Do you feel guilty about your drinking?
E	Do you ever have an eye opener (an early morning drink to steady your nerves)?

regular and the extent and frequency of binges may be difficult to determine. Traditionally, the amount of alcohol consumed is measured by units, with one unit of alcohol being approximately half a pint of beer, one pub measure of spirits or one wine glass of wine. This corresponds to about 10g alcohol. The use of units is now moderately well understood by the general public, but care must be taken against over reliance, since pub measures of spirits may vary and the strength of spirits and beer may also vary considerably. Evidence of alcohol dependency should be sought and the simple CAGE questionnaire is a useful guide to follow (Table 14.5). Symptoms of organ failure should be sought.

Clinically, the patient may show evidence of alcohol consumption, with alcohol on the breath or features of intoxication. Nutritional deficiencies are common. The features of chronic liver disease are well described and include jaundice, spider naevi, hepatosplenomegaly, ascites, leuconychia and, rarely, encephalopathy. Differentiation between alcohol intoxication, withdrawal and hepatic encephalopathy may be difficult, but withdrawal tends to be associated with stimulation and excitement. None of these clinical features is specific to alcoholic liver disease. Dupuytren's contractures (palmar fasciitis) is *not* associated with alcoholic liver disease.

Investigations

Blood tests

There are no specific tests to show alcoholic liver damage but simple screening blood tests may point to the possibility (Table 14.6). These involve measurement of changed levels of normal blood constituents and detecting substances that are indicative of deranged liver metabolism or liver cell damage.

Haematology

Ethanol is toxic to the bone marrow and this may result in a pancytopenia and macrocytosis. It must be remembered that there are many other causes of macrocytosis including folate and vitamin deficiency, hyperlipidaemia and hypothyroidism. Morphologically abnormal red cells may be seen and a finding of triangulocytes is said to be characteristic of alcoholic liver disease. Both the mean cell volume and the morphological changes slowly resolve after alcohol withdrawal.

Table 14.6. *Blood markers associated with alcoholic liver disease*

	Specificity	Usefulness
Raised mean cell volume	+	+++
Gamma-glutamyl transpeptidase	+	+++
Gamma-aminobutyric acid	++	+
Carbohydrate-deficient transferrin (CDT)	++	+
Mitochondrial aspartate aminotransferase	++	+
Acetate	++	+
Aspartate aminotransferase/alanine aminotransferase ratio	++	++

Liver enzyme levels in serum

As a result of damage to liver cells, some enzymes that are typically liver in origin are released into the bloodstream and can be measured.

Gamma-glutamyl transferase (GGT). This is the most commonly used serum biochemical marker of alcohol consumption. It is an inducible enzyme of hepatic origin and may be increased by any enzyme-inducing agent, including some drugs such as anticonvulsants. Increase may also occur as a result of biliary or hepatocellular damage, hyperlipidaemia type IV, diabetes, trauma, obesity and pregnancy. Although GGT is a marker of enzyme induction it poorly reflects the degree of liver cell damage.

Aminotransferases. Serum aspartate aminotransferase (AST) and alanine aminotransferase (ALT) are elevated in up to three-quarters of alcohol abusers but rarely exceed five times the upper limit of normal. Again, elevated transferase activities are not specific to alcohol and may occur in any type of cell damage. Some workers rely on the selective increase in the mitochondrial isoenzyme of AST, a marker of the mitochondrial damage discussed above. In contrast to many other forms of liver damage, AST is increased more than the serum ALT in alcoholic damage and this has been used to help distinguish the disease from other causes of liver damage.

Other blood tests of liver alcoholic damage

Ethanol is an enzyme inducer, as outlined above and, therefore, enhanced glucaric acid excretion may be found in those with a high alcohol intake; similarly, aminopyrine clearance may be increased. Plasma proteins may be reduced (albumin, haptoglobins and transferin), whereas acute-phase proteins such as α_2-macroglobulin and caeruloplasmin may be increased.

Serum transferrin may be increased in those drinking excessively and a carbohydrate-deficient form (CDT) has been reported to be a useful marker; current techniques are more reliable now, although this diagnostic test has not achieved widespread use. Plasma lipids may be increased and, in particular, hypertriglyceridaemia may be a feature of acute alcoholic liver disease, with the values reaching 20 mmol/litre or more.

HDL cholesterol, HDL phospholipids and apolipoprotein A_1 and A_2 are increased by ethanol.

Other investigations

Liver scan.   The technetium liver scan is now performed less rarely than before and findings in alcoholic liver disease are non-specific although in the presence of alcoholic hepatitis there may be a complete 'white-out' where there is no uptake of radioisotope by the liver. This is found only in alcoholic hepatitis and in acute Wilson's disease. The ultrasound may show an enlarged liver with a bright echo as a result of fat infiltration.

Liver biopsy.   The most useful investigation is liver biopsy, which not only helps make the diagnosis and establish the severity of alcoholic liver damage but also excludes other causes of abnormal liver tests.

Liver lesions

There are three main liver lesions in alcoholic liver disease:
- fatty liver
- alcoholic hepatitis
- fibrosis and cirrhosis.

The lesions tend to be most marked in the perivenular region. This may be a consequence of the possible hypermetabolic state of the hepatocytes in people consuming excess alcohol because of the effect of ethanol on hepatic oxygenation, or it may reflect the tissue distribution of the oxygen metabolising enzymes.

Fatty liver

Fatty liver (Fig. 14.4) is characterised by accumulation of fatty droplets within the hepatocytes; commonly, this is in a macrovesicular pattern, but when there is a microvesicular pattern it is associated with a poor prognosis. Fatty accumulation normally starts in the perivenular area, around the central vein. The hepatocytes enlarge and may compress the sinusoids. This may contribute to the portal hypertension that is seen in patients with fatty liver in the absence of fibrosis.

There are many other causes of fatty liver, including obesity, diabetes, malnutrition, inflammatory disease and toxic reactions, so the lesion is not specific for alcohol.

Clinically, the patients are well and usually asymptomatic, the condition is often detected on routine examination. In the great majority, the lesion resolves on alcohol withdrawal.

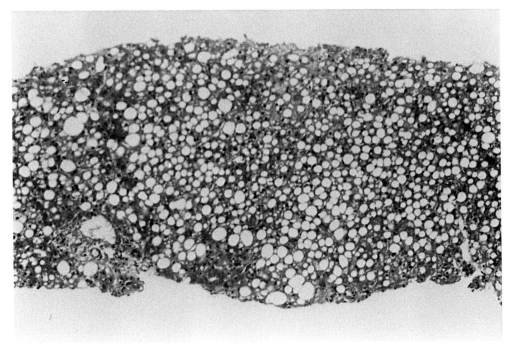

Clinical features
  May be well and asymptomatic
  Reversible on alcohol withdrawal
  There are many other causes

Fig. 14.4. Liver biopsy of a patient showing fatty liver. There is macrovesicular distribution of fat throughout the entire lobule but no evidence of cellular infiltration or disruption of the normal hepatic architecture. The fat is distributed within the droplets. (Courtesy of Dr S. Hubscher.)

Alcoholic hepatitis

Alcoholic hepatitis (Fig. 14.5) is also called sclerosing hyaline necrosis and may lead to cirrhosis. Fatty infiltration is usually present, as are ballooned hepatocytes, often containing Mallory bodies. The three features of alcoholic hepatitis are fibrosis, inflammation and parenchymal cell damage.

The inflammatory response consists predominantly of polymorphonuclear leucocytes. These inflammatory cells are found around the damaged hepatocytes.

Fibrosis is always present and is usually pericellular in distribution. Other types of fibrosis include perivenular fibrosis or sclerosis where lesions of the terminal hepatic vein (the central vein) occur. This may lead to veno-occlusive-type lesions; this is not specific for alcoholic hepatitis and may be found in cirrhosis.

Parenchymal damage is characterised by swelling of the hepatocyte cytoplasm, resulting in balloon degeneration and necrosis. The ballooned hepatocytes are believed to result from decreased endocytosis and decreased microtubular assembly as a

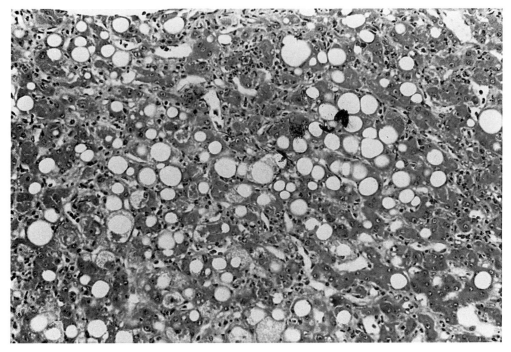

Clinical features
    Patients may be well, but are usually ill
    Jaundice
    Fever
    Right upper quadrant abdominal pain
    Abnormal blood tests (see text)

Fig. 14.5. Picture of liver biopsy showing alcoholic hepatitis. In addition to macrovesicular fat, there is infiltration of the liver parenchyma by white cells, especially polymorphs. There is evidence of ballooning of hepatocytes and Mallory's hyaline. (Courtesy of Dr S. Hubscher.)

consequence of ethanol metabolites. This leads to a switch in the production of the normal hepatocyte cytokeratin to bile duct-type cytokeratin. This is associated with cell swelling and Mallory body formation. The cell swelling compresses sinusoids. Mega-mitochondria may be seen and this may be a reflection of recent heavy alcohol consumption. It is interesting that the megamitochondria in the periportal hepatocytes are different in shape from those in the centrilobular hepatocytes. The periportal megami-tochondria are not specific to ethanol damage and may be found in steatohepatitis from any cause, whereas the focal centrilobular megamitochondria are most specific for alcoholic liver disease. Megamitochondria are associated with a poor outcome.

    Mallory bodies, or alcohol hyaline, is associated with cholestasis of any cause, but they are found frequently in patients with alcohol hepatitis and cirrhosis. These bodies appear to be aggregates of altered intermediate cytoskeletal filaments. Again, these features of alcoholic hepatitis are not specific to ethanol and may be found in chronic cholestasis and Wilson's disease. Pericellular fibrosis and fatty liver with polymorph infiltration may also be seen in obesity, diabetes, gastrointestinal bypass and following

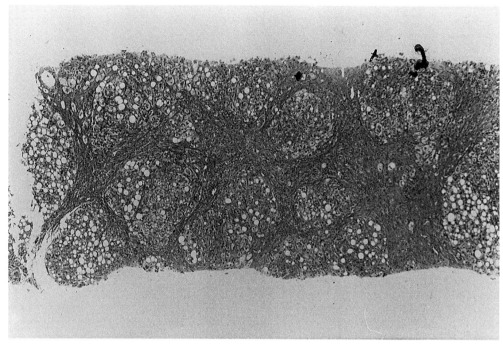

Clinical features
  Bleeding oesophageal varices
  Ascites
  Jaundice
  Other complications of cirrhosis

Fig. 14.6. Liver biopsy showing alcohol cirrhosis. The liver parenchyma is extensively disrupted by fibrous bands leading to micronodules. Fatty infiltration is present within the hepatocytes. (Courtesy of Dr S. Hubscher.)

the use of drugs such as amiodarone or perhexiline. Pericellular fibrosis may be found following chemotherapy or vitamin A toxicosis.

Clinically, the patient may be well but is usually ill with jaundice, fever and right upper quadrant abdominal pain. The blood tests show a characteristic pattern with a high polymorphonuclear leucocytosis (up to 50×10^9/litre) and a high serum bilirubin (which may exceed 900 micromol/litre) but a near normal alkaline phosphatase and transaminases.

Cirrhosis

Cirrhosis (Fig. 14.6) is characteristically micronodular in nature and is defined as transformation of the normal architecture with hepatocyte necrosis, regeneration nodules surrounded by fibrous septa. There are often features of fatty liver or alcoholic hepatitis. The cirrhosis is usually micronodular. There may be overload of iron, so that differentiation from haemachromatosis may be difficult. Hepatic iron index may help resolve the diagnosis.

Table 14.7. *Drug treatments for alcoholic liver diseases*

Drug	Effectiveness	Lesions particularly responsive
Nutritional support	+	Alcoholic hepatitis
Corticosteroids	+ +	Alcoholic hepatitis
Propylthiouracil	+ +	Cirrhosis
	+	Alcoholic hepatitis
Insulin + glucagon	±	Alcoholic hepatitis
Antifibrotics: D-penicillamine,	±	Cirrhosis
colchicine	±	Cirrhosis
Hepatoprotective agents + cyanidanol	±	Alcoholic hepatitis \ cirrhosis

Clinically, the patient may present with any of the complications of cirrhosis, such as bleeding oesophageal varices, ascites or jaundice.

Treatment

The mainstay of treatment of alcoholic liver disease is abstinence. This is associated with a marked improvement in prognosis and often with resolution of the abnormal liver function tests. A number of agents including propylthiouracil (to counteract the enhanced metabolism and hypoxia of cells), chlorpromazine and S-adenosyl methionine (to stabilise cell membranes), corticosteroids, anabolic steroids and anticytokine treatment (to reduce the immune effects) have all been tried (Table 14.7). Of these, propylthiouracil may be helpful in chronic liver disease and high-dose corticosteroids may be useful in reducing the short-term (30-day) mortality in those with severe alcoholic hepatitis.

Membrane-stabilising drugs and antioxidants, such as cyanidanol-3, and polyunsaturates, such as phosphatidylcholine, may also have some therapeutic benefit.

In the absence of specific therapy, the mainstay of therapy is abstinence (with counselling and support as necessary), nutritional support and replacement of vitamin and other nutritional deficiencies.

Liver replacement is a valuable treatment appropriate for only a limited few who have terminal liver disease that has progressed despite abstinence.

Summary

Alcohol remains a toxin that is enjoyed by many and yet it makes a significant contribution to national morbidity and mortality. Alcohol damage can affect every organ and system within the body. The hepatotoxicity of ethanol results primarily from metabolism within the liver and, to a lesser extent, within other organs by ADH, with the generation of acetaldehyde and reduced hepatic NADH. Acetaldehyde can also be produced by the microsomal ethanol oxidising system (MEOS) leading to the formation of free oxygen radicals which may lead to further damage. Although within the population there is a good correlation between the amount of alcohol drunk and the probability of developing liver disease, there are great individual variations. Some of these variations may be caused by additive effects of other hepatotoxins such as hepatitis B or C viral disease but factors such as sex and genetic make-up may also be important. The involvement of the immune system remains uncertain: patients with alcoholic liver damage have a variety of both cellular and humoral abnormalities of the immune system but the extent to which these are involved in the pathogenesis of liver disease rather than occurring as a consequence of liver disease is unclear.

Treatment of alcoholic liver disease is primarily that of abstinence. Drug therapy for alcoholic hepatitis has been tried including corticosteroids, colchicine and thiouracil, but none has been shown to reverse the liver damage.

FURTHER READING

Day, C. & Bassendine, M. (1992). Genetic predisposition to alcoholic liver disease. *Gut*, 33, 1444–1447.

Lieber, C.S. (1994). Alcohol and the liver. *Gastroenterology*, 106, 1085–1105.

Lumeng, L. & Crabb, D. (1994). Genetic aspects and risk factors in alcoholism and alcoholic liver disease. *Gastroenterology*, 107, 572–578.

Various authors (1993). *Seminars in Liver Diseases*, 13, No. 2.

Various authors (1994). *British Medical Bulletin*, 50, No. 1.

15

Diet and disease

G. NEALE

- Epidemiologically, diet is an important determinant of growth and development and of common disease processes.

- Some genetic disorders may be controlled by diet.

- Worldwide, protein–energy malnutrition is the most common cause of premature death. It is also a significant problem in chronically sick people at home and severely ill patients in hospital.

- Obesity is an increasing cause of disability in affluent countries. Understanding the pathogenesis of this condition is important in its management.

- Deficiencies of non-calorie nutrients, especially iron, folate and vitamin D, are common causes of disease worldwide. In addition, in developing countries, vitamin A deficiency, pellagra and beri-beri are still important problems.

Availability of food is a key aspect of the human environment. In a literal sense, the body is a product of dietary intake and genetic control. Nutritionists have provided many data on dietary intake and its effects on body composition and function, but we still know little about genetic control.

Research in clinical nutrition began at the beginning of the twentieth century when Voit in Germany and Atwater in the USA explored energy metabolism and the protein needs of the body. Some 20 years later the physician–scientists, Eijkman of Utrecht and Hopkins of Cambridge formulated the general concept that animals require more than protein, carbohydrate, fat, minerals and water. They had discovered vitamins. Between the two World Wars, the study of biochemistry concerned the identification of essential nutrients and the steps of intermediary metabolism. This task was essentially complete by the end of the Second World War. By then, it was becoming clear that it was necessary to do more than just define dietary requirements: the range of normality is too wide; dietary needs of individuals differ; their abilities to adapt to varying levels of nutrient intake are considerable; and the requirements for one nutrient may be influenced markedly by other dietary factors.

Immediately after the Second World War, clinicians interested in nutrition concentrated on the problems of protein–calorie malnutrition in the developing countries. The differences between hypoproteinaemic and normoproteinaemic malnutrition were

Table 15.1. *Nutritional disorders*

	Overnutrition	Undernutrition
Energy	Obesity	Wasting
Protein–calorie balance		Protein–calorie malnutrition
Essential fatty acids		Dermatitis, hair loss
Minerals		
Sodium	?Hypertension in salt sensitive	Weakness, lethargy
Potassium		
Calcium		?Osteoporosis
Magnesium		Tetany (often associated with hypocalcaemia, hypokalaemia)
Trace elements		
Iron	Haemochromatosis	Hypochromic anaemia
Iodine		Goitre, thyroid insufficiency
Zinc		Peristomal and acral dermatitis
Copper	Wilson's disease	Anaemia, kinky hair syndrome
Chromium		Neuropathy
Selenium		Cardiomyopathy (Keshan's disease)
Molybdenum		Encephalopathy
Flouride	Fluorosis	Increased incidence of dental caries
Vitamins		
A	Hypervitaminosis A (liver damage)	Night blindness, xerophthalmia
B_1		Peripheral neuropathy, cardiac failure, Wernicke–Korsakoff syndrome
B_2		Seborrhoea, glossitis
B_3		Pellagra
B_6	Neuropathy	Sideroblastic anaemia
B_{12}		Megaloblastic anaemia neuropathy
Folic acid		Megaloblastic anaemia
C	Renal stones	Scurvy
D	Hypercalcaemia	Rickets/osteomalacia
E		Spinocerebellar disorders, Haemolytic anaemia
K		Coagulation defect

defined and the body needs for energy and protein agreed. By now the complete range of primary nutritional disorders had been defined (Table 15.1). Slightly later, diet was identified as an important factor in the epidemiology of chronic degenerative diseases in wealthy industrialised countries. The concepts of 'the medical disorders of affluent societies', 'the saccharine disease' and 'nutrition, lipids and coronary artery disease'

Table 15.2. *Disorders believed to be related to diet*

Disorder	Nutrient
Ischaemic heart disease	Fat
Colonic disorders	
Constipation	Fibre
Polyps and cancer	Fat/protein/fibre
Diverticular disease	Fibre
(irritable bowel)	?Fibre
Metabolic diseases	
Obesity	Excess calories from refined food
Diabetes mellitus	
Vascular disease	
Hypertension	Salt (Na:K ratio)
Varicose veins	Fibre (?)
Deep venous thrombosis	Fibre (?)
Haemorrhoids	Fibre (?)
Stone disease	
Gall stones	
Renal stones	Affluent diet (?)
Tooth decay	
Dental caries	Sticky foods (refined sugar)
Inflammatory disorders	
Appendicitis	Fibre (?)
Inflammatory bowel disease	No clear evidence
Allergic disorders	Some foods implicated, e.g. dairy produce, wheat, shellfish

depend largely on the findings of epidemiologists. Accelerated atheroma, gastrointestinal cancer, the pathology of the biliary tract and a host of other disorders (Table 15.2) may indeed be related to dietary intake, but the mechanisms are not well understood and diet does not act in isolation.

Since the mid-1980s, there has been a new twist in the story relating nutrition to the health of the nation. There is reasonable epidemiological evidence that pre- and early post-natal nutrition has an important effect on cardiovascular disease and pancreatic islet cell function in adult life. To understand this, we must analyse nutrition at a molecular level. A start has been made. For example, the role of retinoids in lipid-linked carbohydrate transport and as components of visual purple have been clearly defined. In addition, epidemiological studies suggest that vitamin A may have a role in the aetiology of cancer. At a molecular level, retinoids appear to have an effect on the expression of proteins in epithelial cells. They are capable of activating and suppressing the transcription of genes and may act as nuclear mediators of cell differentiation.

In this book, we are trying to provide a knowledge of basic mechanisms to enable clinical students to build on a framework of understanding. Whatever his special interest, the clinician should know how pathological processes may be modulated by nutrition; should be able to recognise the signs of disease that may be nutritionally determined; must understand and be able to apply the results of laboratory investigations; should know how to help patients with nutritional problems; and should be prepared to interpret the epidemiological evidence that diet is a determinant of the overall health of the population.

This chapter attempts to give an understanding of a range of questions: how diet may modulate health; why a high protein diet is rarely useful in treating patients with hypoproteinaemia; why circulating iron is not a good marker of the iron status of the body; how a young woman with anorexia nervosa in the Western world differs nutritionally from a starved girl in a developing country; and why it is not enough to exhort an obese subject to eat less. To achieve these aims we will have to draw on knowledge from several of the basic sciences to provide a firm foundation for the understanding of the influence of nutrition on human health and disease.

Availability of food

Humans are able to adapt to a wide range of dietary intake (Table 15.3). Their food supply is dominated by cereals, which provide 85% of calorie requirements, but for optimal health this must be supplemented by at least some food with a higher protein content (Table 15.4, 15.5). Meat, fish and dairy produce are plentiful in temperate regions but supplies are limited in most tropical and subtropical countries, mainly because livestock farming is difficult but also because protein foods keep poorly in warm conditions. People in these areas are largely dependent on legumes to supplement the protein in their cereals, although milk and milk products are important sources of protein in some areas. In contrast, in cold temperate and Arctic regions, fish and sea mammals are important sources of food.

Food availability per capita in healthy adults ranges from less than 40 to well over 100 g protein per day and from 1500 to more than 3000 kcal (8400–12 500KJ) per day (Fig. 15.1). Within poor countries, there are large variations in the availability of food. The poor, particularly women and children, are most likely to suffer the ill effects of underconsumption. In the developing world, 25% of the total population is estimated to be seriously undernourished, with the greatest concentration of malnutrition occurring in Central Africa. The needs for energy and protein for the development and maintenance of healthy adult humans are not clearly defined. There is a complex interaction of genetic factors and environment. Suppose, for example, we take two boys (A and B) of different genotypes brought up by affluent well-educated parents in the Western world. A ends up 5 cm taller and 7 kg heavier than B and lives longer because B develops coronary artery disease at an early age. Transplant the same two genotypes to a peasant environment in Central Africa and one would find that they would grow fitfully in the face of recurrent famine, chronic infection, hard physical work and tropical heat. Both are likely to end up smaller, but A may no longer be bigger than B nor may A have an expectation of a longer life. For it is possible that B may have been programmed by genetic or developmental processes for growth under marginal circumstances.

Table 15.3. *Global variations in sources of energy and protein*

Region	Daily energy intake (g)	Protein intake		Quantitative daily intake	
		Vegetable (g)	Animal (g)	Energy (kcal)	Protein (g)
Western world	CHO (80 g sucrose lactose): 200–300 Fat: 100	Variable	Mainly meat/dairy produce	2750+	100+
Mediterranean	CHO (especially pasta): 250 Fat (especially vegetable oil): 75 Alcohol	Mixed		2200+	70
India	CHO (rice/wheat): 200–300	Pulse/beans: 25	Dairy produce: 10	1500	50
China	CHO (rice/wheat): 500	Mixed vegetables: 20	Animal protein: 7	2500	70
Central America	CHO (maize): 500	Beans: 20	Variable	2400	70
East Africa (Mozambique)	CHO (cassava/maize): 250	Pulses: 20	Variable	1300	30–40
Alaska (Eskimos)	CHO (imported cereals/sugar): 100–200 Fat: 50–100 High protein intake may be used for energy	Little	Fish, sea mammals: ~200 per day	1500+	50–500

Note:
CHO, carbohydrate.

Table 15.4. *Staple foods of humans*

	Nutrient content (% dry weight)			
	Protein	Carbohydrate	Fat	NSP
Cereals				
Wheat	16	72	2.5	10
Oats	12	72	8	8
Brown rice	7	89	3	2
Maize	8	81	3	7
Roots				
Potatoes	10	82	0.5	7
Yams	4.5	90	1.5	4.5
Cassava (tapioca)	0.5	98	0.1	0.5
Fruit				
Plantain (green banana-like food)	2.5	94	0.5	3

Note:
NSP, non-starch polysaccharides (a better term than 'fibre').

Table 15.5. *Main sources of vegetable protein*

	Nutrient content (% dry weight)			
	Protein	Carbohydrate	Fat	NSP
Legumes				
Butter beans	25	52	2	20
Peas	28	45	6	20
Lentils	29	57	2	13
Groundnuts (peanuts)	28	51	14	7
Soya beans	43	20	22	14

Note:
NSP, non-starch polysaccharides.
Leafy vegetables are an important source of beta-carotene, vitamin C and folic acid and also supply significant amounts of riboflavin, iron and calcium. Fruits are a major source of vitamin C.

Body composition

The main structural components of the body are shown in Fig. 15.2. These structural components are in a state of continuous metabolic flux. Adequate nutrition is necessary to maintain metabolic pathways and structural integrity. Body composition adapts during periods of dietary inadequacy, but this process may break down as a result of physical stress such as trauma and sepsis. Under such circumstances, nutritional support is often important in optimising the chances of recovery.

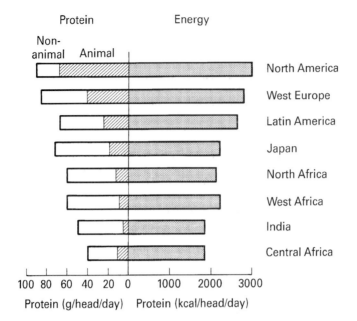

Fig. 15.1. Food availability per head of population (at a global level. (1 kcal ≈4.2 kJ.) (Data drawn from Lapedes, D. N. (ed.) (1977) *Encyclopedia of Food, Agriculture and Nutrition*. New York: McGraw-Hill.)

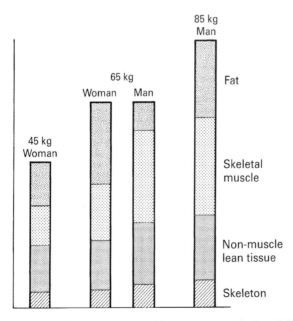

Fig. 15.2. The composition of humans. Note the big difference in fat and muscle in men and women of equivalent weights.

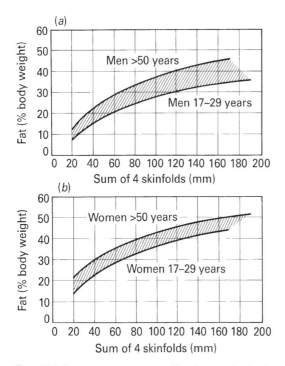

Fig. 15.3. Fat as a proportion of body weight for (*a*) men and (*b*) women. The percentage of body fat can be reasonably well estimated from the measurement of skin-fold thicknesses in four sites (posterior (triceps) and anterior (biceps) upper non-dominant arm midway between acromial and olecranon processes; subscapular in the line of dermatome; and suprailiac 1 cm above the left superior iliac crest in the mid-axillary line in a horizontal plane). (The graphs have been constructed from data published by Durnin and Womersley (1974)).

Water. In the average adult body 60% of the mass comprises water. A man weighing 65 kg contains 15 litres of extracellular water and 25 litres of intracellular water. The extracellular fluid integrates with fibrous proteins and mineral structures to provide the body supporting tissue.

Protein. About 17% of an average adult (10–12 kg) comprises protein. Half of this protein is found in muscle; 25% in the skin, skeletal and connective tissue; and the rest as intra- and extracellular proteins acting as enzymes, as transport vehicles and as mediators in the immune system.

Fat. About 15% of the average young adult, by weight, is fat, but the range varies over 5–50% (Fig. 15.3). About 1 kg fat is essential for body function (primarily as cell membranes); the rest represents an energy store.

Carbohydrate. The average adult carries only about 1 kg of carbohydrate. Of this, 100 g is as glycogen in the liver, 300 g as glycogen in muscles and much of the rest in nucleic acids as ribose phosphate. There is only a small amount of glucose readily available to satisfy immediate energy needs.

Energy sources in the body.   Glucose, fatty acids and amino acids are sources of fuel, acting through the intermediate ATP. Glycogen stores are small and muscle glycogen is not a source of glucose. Therefore, after only a few hours of fasting, the body starts to breakdown protein and fat. Carbohydrate and fat provide 4 kcal/g but both glycogen and structural protein are associated with two or three times their own weight as tissue fluid. Therefore, in tissue terms, neither are efficient sources of energy (1–2 kcal/g tissue weight). In contrast, fat provides 9 kcal/g and carries little in the way of extracellular supporting tissue. During prolonged starvation, there is a preferential use of fat and relative conservation of protein. These adaptive mechanisms break down under stress associated with infection, trauma (including surgery) and immobility (Table 15.13, below). It is important to remember that the body has no protein stores. Energy is released during protein catabolism but there is no non-structural source of nitrogen.

Body minerals.   Body minerals may be conveniently considered in three groups. The major minerals are present in molar quantities and include calcium, magnesium, phosphate, sodium, potassium and chloride. The minor minerals are in millimolar quantities and include iron and zinc. Trace elements such as copper, chromium, cobalt, selenium and iodine are present in micromolar quantities but are essential for life.

Variation in body composition

Body size adapts to allow the most efficient use of available nutritional resources. Such adaptation may be genetic (evolutionary change in several, perhaps many, genes) or phenotypic, resulting from the plasticity of growth of the individual in response to environmental influences. Body composition is not a simple concept – a big man may be very tall, very fat or very muscular; he may be long-legged or rotund; he may be active or sedentary. It is likely that selection will operate in different ways to produce these end results. Moreover, there will be different selective pressures on males and females because of sex differences in size and shape. In addition, the processes of development may themselves be subject to selection. For example, it may be advantageous to have periods of rapid and slow growth.

Birth weight

There is good evidence of strong genetic control of developmental processes in the fetus, with switch mechanisms producing specific substances at specific times. But the effect on birth weight is small. Correlations between the birth weights of siblings and half-siblings show that the fetal genotype is responsible for only 10% of the variance; most of the differences arise from the maternal environment (65%) and from the mother's genetic make-up (25%). Thus, processes of gene selection have little influence on normal fetal development.

Adult size

Normal height is accepted as an example of a multifactorial character responding to both genetic and environmental influences, the genetic component being polygenic. The individual genes involved may be synergistic (giving large phenotypic differences) or antagonistic (giving small phenotypic differences). As each gene has only a slight effect, it cannot be heavily selected for or against (unless there is some linkage of genes in the same system).

In polygenic inheritance, similar phenotypes develop from different genotypes and, therefore, genetic diversity and the potential for change is concealed by the phenotypic variation. The genes may act through endocrine systems (especially growth hormone), effects on carbohydrate and protein metabolism and the rate of timing of growth processes.The environmental component modifies the genetic potential by nutrition, the presence or absence of disease and physical factors. Family studies show a major genetic contribution to the variability of height, with correlations of 0.5–0.8 between first-degree relatives (0.95 for monozygotic twins). Therefore, inherited factors strongly influence adult size, which in itself is not a critical factor for a healthy life.

Variations in growth

Genetic control operates through growth, as seen by positive correlations in first-degree relatives for growth patterns for height, rates of skeletal maturation, onset of adolescence, dental development and neural development. Genes controlling the rate of growth are partly independent of those controlling final size. For some factors, single locus polymorphisms operate, as seen in the sequence of onset of ossification of the small bones of the wrist. The biometric evidence indicates the importance of the genetic component of variations in growth and development but leaves much room for nutritional modification of the phenotypic response. Body mechanisms respond readily to the available food supply, as will be demonstrated in the section on under- and overnutrition.

The potential effects of fetal nutrition

Nutrition during fetal and early infant life is important in determining the risk of disease, although we still know little about the processes involved. Many familiar conditions such as ischaemic heart disease, gall stones, colonic diverticulosis, cancer of the breast and so on have been termed 'Western diseases' because of their geographic distribution and their high prevalence in industrial society. It is often argued that the prevalence of these conditions is the result of the ready availability of cheap, highly palatable foods rich in fat and refined sugar and that their incidence would be reduced by the ingestion of diets high in complex carbohydrate and low in animal fat (Table 15.2). In fact, the issues are much more complex.

In the nineteenth century, industrialisation in temperate areas led to overcrowding, bad hygiene and changes in dietary intake. As living conditions improved, the prevalence of serious infectious disease such as diphtheria, tuberculosis and the streptococcal diseases declined, although other conditions associated with poor living standards, such as chronic bronchitis, cancer of the stomach and stroke, persisted. In contrast, increasing affluence is associated with an increase in the incidence of gall stones, renal stones and cancers of the breast, ovary and prostate. These reasonably simple patterns of change cannot be applied to certain other common disorders, such as ischaemic heart disease, appendicitis and duodenal ulceration. In the early years of the twentieth century, they were diseases of the well-to-do; now they are more common amongst the less well-off segment of the population. Why might this be so?

Circulating cholesterol, the level of which is influenced by dietary fat interacting with genetic predisposition, is a risk factor for ischaemic heart disease. In addition, it has been shown that the geographical distribution of ischaemic heart disease correlates with that for high infant mortality in the 1920s. The evidence is largely epidemiological but appears to be consistent over several studies from different populations. This additional factor has led to the concept of sensitive periods of development in infancy and fetal life. An early stimulus or insult operating at a critical period of development may result in 'programming', i.e. long-term changes in the structure and functioning of the body. In England and Wales, epidemiological analysis suggests that poor maternal physique and nutrition, and poor fetal infant growth, are associated with an increased risk of cardio-vascular diseases in adult life. Follow-up studies have shown strong relationships between perinatal growth and some major risk factors for cardiovascular disease: high blood pressure, high values for circulating cholesterol and fibrinogen, and non-insulin-dependent diabetes mellitus.

These observations have led to the fascinating hypothesis that if the fetus or infant is programmed for nutritional deficiency then it may respond adversely in a world of nutritional abundance. It is suggested that fetal malnutrition as a result of maternal malnutrition, maternal disease or placental abnormality leads to a reduced pancreatic beta cell mass and function which persists throughout life. Affected subjects may be less able to cope with abundant nutrition. The demand for insulin may outstrip supply. If such individuals become obese, they may develop insulin resistance and dyslipidaemia. There is also evidence that low-grade essential hypertension originates in early life. A rank order for blood pressure established in infancy persists throughout life (a process called 'tracking'). It is suggested that an accelerated growth rate of healthy babies of low birth weight during the first 6 months of life may be accompanied by an accelerated increase in blood pressure which persists into adult life. The concept of programming receives some support from experimental studies. Feeding low-protein diets to pregnant rats appears to reduce the vascularity of the islets of Langerhans in the embryos. As a result, they have less beta cells and show impaired glucose tolerance. These observations provide an interesting alternative to the concept of a 'thrifty genotype' in which the high incidence of diabetes mellitus in recently affluent societies is ascribed to diabetogenic genes which confer a survival advantage under conditions of nutritional deprivation.

Nutritional requirements

Previous considerations show that there are no absolute criteria for human requirements of nutrients. Estimates may be made from determining:

Table 15.6. *Nutritional requirements for energy and protein*

Age (years)	Estimated average requirements for energy (kcal/day)		Reference nutrient intake for protein (g/day)	
	Male	Female[a]	Male	Female[b]
under 1	545–920	515–865	12.5–14.9	
1–6	1230–1715	1165–1545	14.5–19.7	
7–14	1970–2220	1740–1845	28.3–42.1	28.3–41.2
15–18	2755	2110	55.2	45.0
19–60	2550	1940	55.5	45.0
60–74	2380	1900	53.3	46.5
75+	2100	1810	53.3	46.5

Notes:
[a] In the last trimester of pregnancy +200 kcal/day; in lactation +450–570 kcal/day.
[b] Throughout pregnancy +6 g/day; in lactation +8–11 g/day.

1. Biological markers of nutritional adequacy
2. Intakes required to maintain nutritional balance
3. Intakes needed to maintain concentrations of nutrients in the circulation or in the tissues
4. Diets associated with the absence of deficiency diseases
5. Intakes needed to correct nutritional deficiencies.

From such data, the Department of Health Committee on Medical Aspects of Food Policy have tried to establish ranges of intakes for individual nutrients, which they termed Dietary Reference Values (DRVs). For example, they have calculated Estimated Average Requirements (EAR) for many nutrients and by assuming that the requirements of individuals are normally distributed in the population, they have defined a Reference Nutrient Intake (RNI), which is two standard deviations (2 S.D.) above the mean and a Lower Reference Nutrient Intake (LRNI) 2 S.D. below the mean. LRNI values are regarded as inadequate for most individuals.

Protein

Protein requirements are based on consultations by the Food and Agriculture Organization of the UN and the World Health Organization (FAO/WHO) using growth, maintenance of well-being and nitrogen balance studies as appropriate criteria (Table 15.6). The DRVs assume a dietary protein pattern of sufficient variety to provide adequate amounts of indispensable amino acids. In the UK, average intakes (84 g for men, 64 g for women) far exceed the RNI and there is some concern that an excessive intake of protein may be associated with health risks such as an increase in age-related conditions including osteoporosis and a decline in renal function.

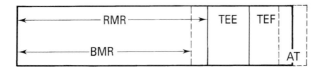

Fig. 15.4. Schematic representation of energy expenditure over 24 hours in a sedentery person. BMR, basal metabolic rate; TMR, resting metabolic rate, TEE, thermal effect of exercise; TEF, thermal effect of food; AT, adaptive thermogenesis (non-shivering thermogenesis, doubtful in humans).

Energy

It is not possible to determine DRV for energy nor for the amount of fat and carbohydrate of which it is comprised. The Department of Health provides proposals for average intakes that are consistent with good health given the present socio-cultural environment. This applies particularly to the intake of starches, sugars, fats and fatty acids. Total average energy intakes for individuals are shown in Table 15.6. Such data are of limited value because the range of normality is large.

Energy expenditure is necessary to cover basic or resting metabolism, which is the energy required to maintain metabolic processes in the post-absorptive state, activity of skeletal muscle and thermogenic responses induced by eating (diet-induced thermogenesis) and other physiological responses (such as the response of heat, cold and anxiety). Diet-induced thermogenesis in individuals is not predictable but makes up only 5–10% of total energy expenditure. Similarly, other physiological causes of thermogenesis make only a small contribution to total energy expenditure (Fig. 15.4). In the early 1980s, it was thought that brown fat allowed the body to generate heat and great excitement was generated by the discovery of a defect in brown fat metabolism in the obese rat. However, brown fat is not a significant control mechanism for energy expenditure in humans.

Physical exercise requires much less energy than commonly supposed. A 70 kg man may use 100 kcal in jogging for half an hour (equivalent to an average slice of bread without the butter) or 2000 kcal in running the marathon. Energy intake is, of course, the other side of the equation. Feeding may be initiated by hunger but is also markedly influenced by appetite and satiety. In affluent societies, people seldom eat primarily because they are hungry. Feeding is initiated by custom and habit, and it is usually terminated before the point of satiation.

Fat

The DRV for fat is complicated because apparent intake has been associated with many important diseases including atheroma, gall stones, cancer and obesity. The following considerations influence present thinking.

1. Polyunsaturated fatty acids (PUFA) include the essential fatty acids (EFA) (linoleic, linolenic and arachidonic acids) (Table 15.7) which are important for maintaining the structure and function of cellular and subcellular membranes.

Table 15.7. *The composition of dietary fat (%)*

	Saturated fatty acids	Monounsaturated fatty acids	PUFA (linoleic $C_{18:2}$)	Other PUFA
Butter, cream	61	30	2	1
Beef, pork	45	50	7	1
Fish oil	23	27	7	43
Soya oil	14	24	53	7
Olive oil	14	73	11	1
Sunflower seed oil	12	33	58	–

Notes:

Saturated fatty acids are primarily palmitic ($C_{16:0}$) and stearic ($C_{18:0}$) although butter cream contains considerable amounts of shorter chain fatty acids.

Monounsaturated fatty acids comprise palmitoleic ($C_{16:1}$, *n*-7)and Oleic ($C_{18:1}$, *n*-9).

Polyunsaturated fatty acids (PUFA), of which linoleic is the most important, have two or more double bonds. Fish oils have a high proportion of long chain polyunsaturated acids (C_{20}, C_{22}).

Essentially fatty acids (EFA) are linoleic ($C_{18:2}$, *n*-6) and alpha-linoleic ($C_{18:3}$,*n*-3). Other longer chain fatty acids that are physiologically important include arachidonic acid ($C_{20:4}$, *n*-6) eicosapentanenoic acid ($C_{20:5}$, *n*-3) and docosahexanenoic ($C_{22:6}$, *n*-3). They can be made in the tissues from linoleic and alpha-linolenic acids, but in EFA deficiency, intake from the diet may be critical.

They participate in the transport, breakdown and excretion of cholesterol. They are precursors for prostaglandins, thromboxane and leukotrienes. Moreover, there may be a specific requirement for EFAs in the rapid development of the infant brain. This has important implications for the composition of artificial infant feeds particularly for the premature baby.

2. The amount and type of fat in the diet is the main determinant of circulating cholesterol carried as LDL. Saturated fatty acids (chiefly palmitic) elevate circulating cholesterol. PUFA (chiefly linoleic acid) reduce circulating cholesterol but, gram for gram, their opposite effect is only half that of the saturated acids. Monounsaturated acids (e.g. oleic acid) have a smaller cholesterol-lowering effect.

3. HDL is protective because it plays a part in mobilising cholesterol from tissues. Dietary fat plays little part in controlling values of HDL, which are higher in women, are increased by ingesting alcohol and are lower in the obese.

4. Very long chain PUFA inhibit thrombosis.

5. PUFA are susceptible to lipid peroxidation by free radicals. It is claimed that lipid peroxidation may be pathogenic in the development of cancer and atherosclerosis and in promoting ageing. A balance between free radical activity and antioxidant status is important for the maintenance of cellular integrity. Antioxidants (such as beta-carotene, vitamin C and vitamin E) are important contributors to that balance, but there is no evidence that a high dietary intake of PUFA is harmful.

6. The double bonds of PUFAs allow geometric (*cis–trans*) isomerism. Unsaturated

Saturated FA (mainly palmitic and stearic acids)	*Cis*-monounsaturated FA (mainly oleic acids)	*Cis*-PUFA (mainly linoleic)	*trans*-FA

Fig. 15.5. DRVs for the proportion of fat in the diet (total fat intake to satisfy one-third of energy requirements). Not more than one-third of this fat should be in the form of saturated fatty acids.

fatty acids from all vegetable and most animal sources are in the *cis* configuration, so that the molecules are folded as is necessary in structural lipids. The production of margarines and other spreads includes processes that encourage the formation of *trans* fatty acids. These molecules are straight, so they cannot function as essential fatty acids although they are oxidised and used as fuels. The biological effects of *trans* fatty acids remain uncertain and extensive studies have failed to confirm suggested relationships between the intake of *trans* PUFA and atherosclerosis or cancer. Nevertheless, it is recommended that the average intake of *trans* fatty acids should not increase above the present average of 5 g per day. As a result of all these considerations, it is suggested that fat (fatty acids plus glycerol) should average 33% of dietary energy in the proportions shown in Fig. 15.5.

Carbohydrate

Carbohydrate remains the main source of energy in the diet, of which 80% should be in the form of complex polysaccharides (e.g. starches) and only 20% as simple sugars (sucrose causes dental caries; rapidly absorbed sugars stress the homeostatic mechanisms for circulating glucose and may predispose to obesity). It is also necessary to consider the role of indigestible plant polysaccharides in the diet. The term non-starch polysaccharides (NSP) has replaced the imprecise 'dietary fibre'. It should be noted that a small proportion of starch in the diet also resists digestion ('resistant starch') and will, therefore, behave as a NSP. NSP-rich foods (cereals, fruit and vegetables) (Tables 15.4 and 15.5) are generally less energy dense, more bulky and more capable of inducing satiety than NSP-free foods. In population studies, diets based on such foods have been related to a low prevalence of diverticular disease of the colon, appendicitis, cancer of the large intestine, haemorrhoids and constipation. Unfortunately, the studies on which these correlations are based are far from conclusive. At best, it seems possible that there may be a predisposition to such conditions by the consumption of a diet low in starch, low in NSP and high in fat. The available evidence suggests that diets rich in NSP are associated with some delay in the digestion and absorption of nutrients and some reduction in useable energy, even though NSPs contribute to energy intake as a result of fermentation in the colon, with the subsequent absorption and metabolism of volatile fatty acids. NSPs increase stool weight, which may not only lessen the prevalence of constipation but also reduce bowel pathology (stool weights of less than 100 g per day are associated with an increased risk of bowel disease). Therefore, DRVs have been provided for NSPs. An average of 18 g per day is suggested, which is 40% more than the present average intake.

Minerals

Calcium

The bones and teeth contain 99% of body calcium. The small quantity in tissues and body fluids is vital for inter- and intracellular metabolic functions and signal transmission. There are powerful homeostatic mechanisms maintaining circulating ionised calcium. Therefore, with respect to dietary intake, the main concern is the effect on skeletal structures. From the start of adult life, there is an age-related bone loss of approximately 0.3% peak bone mass per year. In females, this is accelerated in the first 5 years after the menopause. Osteoporosis may be ameliorated by ensuring a high peak bone mass or by decreasing the bone loss of the ageing process. Dietary calcium is only one and probably not the main modulating factor. Exercise, body build, vitamin D status and other dietary factors are of equal or greater importance. Body balance can be achieved over a wide range of calcium intake (250–1000 mg per day; 6.25–20 mmol per day) DRVs are of limited help with a RNI of 700 mg (17.5 mmol) per day.

Magnesium

The skeleton contains 60% of the body magnesium. Magnesium is physiologically important in maintaining electrical potential in nerve and muscle membranes, as a co-factor for enzymes requiring ATP and in nucleic acid metabolism. A low level of magnesium has been postulated as a risk factor in ischaemic heart disease, particularly with respect to ventricular dysrhythmias. In most cases, however, hypomagnesaemia appears to be related to other factors such as the use of diuretics and the intake of alcohol rather than to nutritional inadequacy. The RNI is 300 mg (12.3 mmol) per day, which is close to the average intake of the adult population.

Phosphorus

Although, 80% of phosphorus is in the skeleton, there is a vital intracellular component for the energy requirement of metabolic processes. An intake of 400 mg (12.9 mmol) per day is sufficient to maintain levels of circulating phosphate, and the average intake is well in excess of this (approximately 40 mmol per day of which about 10% is added in food processing). It is recommended that the intake of phosphorus should parallel that of calcium (mmole for mmole). Clinically it is important to monitor circulating phosphate in sick patients, particularly when they are receiving large amounts of glucose intravenously.

Sodium

Sodium is well distributed throughout the body. In the average adult, there are approximately 500 mmol in intracellular fluid, 1500 mmol in extracellular fluid and 2000 mmol in bone. Regulation of the extracellular sodium is closely related to the control of extracellular fluid volume. This control is normally very tight but is less good in infants and in the elderly. Humans can maintain sodium balance on a wide range of intake (5–500 mmol per day). Higher intakes may lead to an average increase in blood pressure by up to 5 mmHg, but the responses are very variable. It seems that up to 10% of the population may be particularly salt sensitive. In the assessment of hypertension in populations, it is difficult to disentangle the effect of the dietary intake of sodium from that of potassium and of other contributory factors such as smoking, alcohol and obesity. In the UK, average daily intakes for sodium are 180–200 mmol for men and 120–140 mmol for women. This is considerably more than the RNI of 70 mmol per day.

Potassium

Almost all potassium, 98%, is found in the intracellular compartment. Mechanisms of homeostasis are poorly understood and appear to be less effective than those of sodium. Deficiency of potassium alters the electrophysiology of cell membranes, leading to muscle weakness, dysrhythmias and cardiac arrest. Adequate quantities of potassium are needed for satisfactory sodium homeostasis. In the UK, the adult intake of potassium is 40–150 mmol per day. Higher intakes of potassium appear to reduce blood pressure and, therefore, it seems desirable that individuals reach the RNI of 90 mmol per day.

There is now good evidence that dietary electrolyte intake exerts a control on blood pressure and may also affect the risk of stroke and coronary heart disease by mechanisms independent of blood pressure. Epidemiologically, it is likely that a decrease in sodium intake (which is largely in the form of food additives) and an increase in potassium intake (as vegetables (including potatoes), fruit (especially bananas) and juices) would be beneficial.

Chloride

Chloride is the major extracellular and intracellular counter-anion to sodium and potassium. At present, there is insufficient evidence to show that it acts as an independent factor in disease processes. DRVs parallel those for sodium.

Vitamins

The vitamins are organic substances that the body requires in small amounts for the control of metabolic pathways. The body either cannot make these substances or fails to do so in sufficient quantity. The Cambridge scientist Gowland Hopkins described these as accessory food factors, a far more correct term than 'vital amine' which was coined by

Casimir Funk, a German scientist who made a major contribution to the understanding of vitamin B_1 (thiamin). With the successive discovery of vitamins in the first third of the twentieth century, they were labelled by letter. Now that their chemical structures are known they should be called by their specific names. Clearly few of the vitamins are amines. They are a heterogenous group of substances and have a wide range of physiological functions. Tradition dies hard, however, and there are practical reasons for maintaining a mixed nomenclature. Many of the vitamins consist of groups of closely related compounds (e.g. carotenoids, retinol and retinaldehyde, which make up vitamin A), so it is convenient to use an inclusive term. It is also useful to use the term vitamin B complex because the substances involved are found in the same foods even though chemically they are very different. The DRVs for vitamins are reasonably clearly defined and details can be found in reference books. Overt evidence of vitamin deficiency is uncommon in the Western world apart from folate and cholecalciferol (vitamin D) (Table 15.1).

Vitamin A

Vitamin A deficiency is common in some developing countries especially among young children. Night-blindness is the earliest sign of deficiency but xerophthalmia (dryness of the cornea and conjunctiva) is the major problem as it may cause permanent damage and blindness. Pre-formed vitamin A (as retinyl esters) occurs naturally only in animal food stuffs (liver, fish oils and dairy products are the richest sources). In the UK, up to one-third of vitamin A is derived from beta-carotene (in vegetables, especially carrots and tomatoes). Surveys show that mean intakes are well above RNI and post-mortem analyses of liver indicate that almost all the population has substantial reserves. Excess vitamin A damages liver and bone and causes headaches and vomiting. In pregnancy, retinol is teratogenic.

Vitamin B

Vitamin B group substances are widely distributed in the diet, especially in cereals, dairy produce and meat. Breakfast cereals are fortified.

Thiamin (B_1) is needed in intermediary metabolism, especially of carbohydrate and alcohol. Stores are limited to one month and so beri-beri is common in countries where there is dietary thiamin deficiency and a high intake of carbohydrate. 'Dry' beri-beri (a polyneuropathy) presents with paraesthesiae, cramps and impaired sensation; 'Wet' beri-beri causes dyspnoea and oedema secondary to biventricular cardiac failure. The Wernicke–Korsakoff syndrome is characteristic of thiamin deficiency associated with alcoholism and presents with ophthalmoplegia, nystagmus, ataxia and mental confusion.

Riboflavin (B_2) plays an essential role in the action of flavin-dependent enzymes, and deficiency leads to a reduced consumption of oxygen. Experimentally, riboflavin deficiency leads to glossitis and seborrhoeic dermatitis, but it is rarely identified in clinical practice because other features of vitamin B (complex) deficiency predominate. Subclinical deficiency may occur in the elderly and in the very sick.

Niacin (B_3) includes nicotinic acid and nicotinamide (substances that can also be synthesised from the essential amino acid *l*-tryptophan). This vitamin is vital for the generation of the nicotinamide nucleotide pro-enzymes NAD and NADP, which play a key part in intermediate metabolism. Deficiency results in pellagra, with pigmentation of exposed and pressured areas, diarrhoea and dementia.

Pyridoxine (B_6) is a co-factor catalysing the reaction of amino acids and is available in most foods. Some is synthesised by intestinal bacteria. Deficiency is rare but excess may lead to a peripheral sensory neuropathy. This has been recognised in women taking 50 mg or more a day for several months as treatment for pre-menstrual tension.

Cobalamins (B_{12}) are present in the body primarily in adenosyl-, methyl- and hydroxy-forms. They are involved in the recycling of folate co-enzymes and in the synthesis of methionine and tetrahydrofolate. The last is a precursor of folate compounds essential for the synthesis of thymidylate and ultimately for the production of DNA. Deficiency of vitamin B_{12} leads to a slowing in the replication of nucleic acid, with enlargement of precursor cells in the bone marrow (megaloblastosis). It also causes a disturbance of volatile fatty acid metabolism (especially that of propanyl-CoA), which leads to abnormal fatty acid synthesis for myelin. Therefore, severe vitamin B_{12} deficiency may lead to peripheral neuropathy and subacute combined degeneration of the spinal cord, as well as megaloblastic anaemia. The requirements for vitamin B_{12} are very small (RNI 1.5 µg per day). It is, however, found only in animal products (although it can also be produced by certain algae and bacteria). Thus, vegans are at risk of vitamin B_{12} deficiency. Turnover of the vitamin is extremely slow and the liver contains enough stores to cover requirements for several years.

Folic acid is the parent molecule of a large number of derivatives collectively known as folates. They are involved in single carbon-transfer reactions, especially in the synthesis of purines, pyrimidines, glycine and methionine. Deficiency causes a megaloblastic anaemia indistinguishable from that of vitamin B_{12} deficiency. Foods rich in folate include liver and green-leafy vegetables. A diet which is adequate in vitamin B and C is adequate in folic acid. The RNI for adults is 200 µg per day.

Vitamin C

Ascorbic acid (vitamin C) prevents scurvy, aids wound healing and reacts with free radicals containing oxygen. However, in the presence of some metal ions, it may also show pro-oxidant activity. Vitamin C is a labile nutrient easily destroyed by oxygen, increased pH, heat and light. The richest sources are citrus and soft fruits, peppers and the growing points of vegetables. Many studies have been undertaken to try to show that vitamin C has beneficial effects for normal humans at intakes and tissue levels well above those needed to prevent scurvy. It may improve cholesterol turnover, physical working capacity and immune function, and it has been claimed that it reduces the incidence of the common cold. But the evidence regarding these beneficial effects remains controversial and, therefore, the RNI remains based on turnover studies, biochemical indices of vitamin C status and the amount of vitamin C needed to prevent scurvy. The RNI is 40 mg per day. Possible risks of a very high intake of vitamin C (e.g. more than 1 g per day) include diarrhoea, increased production of oxalate (and hence renal stones) and systemic conditioning, whereby the sudden cessation of a high intake may precipitate scurvy through an enhanced turnover of the vitamin.

Vitamin D

Vitamin D is necessary for the absorption of calcium, the calcification of newly formed osteoid and assisting in the control of calcium homeostasis. It circulates primarily as 25-hydroxycholecalciferol, which is converted to the active substance 1,25-dihydroxy-cholecalciferol in the kidney. The precursor cholecalciferol is formed by ultraviolet irradiation of 7-dehydrocholesterol in the skin. Production is controlled by feedback mechanisms and thus vitamin D behaves like a hormone. In temperate regions, the appropriate ultraviolet radiation is available only during the spring and summer and so, for normal individuals, circulating 25-hydroxycholecalciferol shows a marked seasonal variation. Vitamin D status depends on factors influencing exposure of skin to sunlight (e.g. age, occupation, mobility, cultural behaviour) and the availability of calcium (a lowered availability enhances the catabolism of vitamin D). The normal range of plasma 25-hydroxycholecalciferol varies from 15–35 ng/ml in summer to 4–10 ng/ml in winter.

   Vitamin D is also acquired from the diet but only from fatty fish and in smaller amounts from eggs and fortified foods (margarine, some yoghurts and breakfast cereals). The intake of such foods is very variable and there are no DRVs for children over the age of three years or for normal adults. It is recommended that infants, pregnant and lactating women and the elderly should receive 10 μg per day. For this reason, mothers in the UK are sometimes advised to give their infants vitamin drops (A, C and D) in the first three years of life. Deficiency of cholecalciferol causes rickets in the young and osteomalacia and myopathy in the elderly.

DISEASE RESULTING FROM DIETARY IMBALANCE

The discussion above outlines the components of a healthy normal diet and the role these components play in maintaining a normally functioning metabolism. The disease states that follow arise from abnormal levels of these components. In genetic disorders, disease results from the inability to tolerate either a normal diet or some constituent of a normal diet. This often results in the accumulation of a metabolite that would be harmless at normal levels. Much more commonly, disease is caused by unhealthy diets, such as:

- protein–calorie malnutrition caused by undernutrition
- obesity caused by excess intake (overnutrition)
- iron deficiency, an example of a common disorder involving a non-calorie nutrient.

Table 15.8. *Genetic disorders resulting in a requirement for a modified diet*

Disorder	Incidence/prevalence
Uncommon inherited disorders managed primarily by diet	
Amino acid disorders	
Phenylketonuria	1:10 000 births
Maple syrup urine disease	1:100 000 births
Homocystinuria	1:200 000 births
Tyrosinaemia	1:1000 births in a localised area of French Canada; very rare elsewhere
Carbohydrate disorders	
Fructose intolerance	1:20 000 births
Galactosaemia	1:60 000 births
Sucrase–isomaltase deficiency	1:1 000 000 births
Lactase deficiency	Common normal variant
Common genetically predisposed disorders in which diet is important	
Hypercholesterolaemia	25% adults >250 mg/100 ml (6.5 mmol/l)
	5% adults >300 mg/100 ml (7.7 mmol/l)
	0.2–0.5% population are heterozygotes for monogenic familial disease
Obesity[a]	4% adults grade 2
	In the UK 0.05% adults grade 3
Coeliac disease	1:2000 to 1:10 000 births in Caucasians
Cystic fibrosis	1:2500 births in Caucasians

[a] Obesity is graded using Quetelet's index (weight (kg) divided by height ^{2} (m^2)). Grade 2 has an index value of 30–40; grade 3 an index value of >40.

Genetic disorders

Some single gene disorders cause clearly defined errors of metabolism (Table 15.8) as a result of which either a normal diet (e.g. as in phenylketonuria) or specific nutritional components (e.g. milk in adult lactose intolerance) cause disease.

Phenylketonuria

This exemplar condition affects approximately 1 per 10 000 live births in the Western world (much rarer in Africans and American Indians). Untreated, it leads to microcephaly, severe mental deficiency, hypertonicity, convulsions and hyperactivity with purposeless movements. The skin and hair are usually fair and the eyes blue because the accumulation of phenylalanine inhibits tyrosinase (Fig. 15.6). Phenylketonuria is interesting in that it was the first genetic disorder to be treated on a population basis by dietary control. Affected infants fed diets low in phenylalanine will develop satisfactorily as a group although the distribution of general intelligence will be shifted adversely by at least 1 S.D. As a result, at adolescence a quarter of those affected are more than 2 S.D. below the estimated population mean. It is known that the development of intelli-

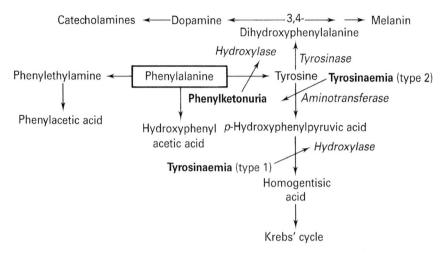

Fig. 15.6. Phenylalanine metabolism. The genetic error results in the absence of a particular enzyme; this causes a blockage in the metabolic pathway and an accumulation of the substrate.

gence is closely related to the degree of control of blood phenylalanine up to the age of eight years. Recently, magnetic resonance imaging has revealed progressive changes in intracerebral myelin in young adults on a normal diet. These changes have been correlated with decreased neuropsychological performance and, thus, long-continued dietary restriction is recommended in order to keep blood phenylalanine below 700 μmol/l. Unfortunately, even this level of control is insufficient to provide full protection to the fetus of a pregnant woman with phenylketonuria, in whom the risk of delivering a neurologically damaged infant is 90%.

Adult lactose intolerance

Other genetic disorders, for example the disaccharidase deficiencies, only cause disease when specific dietary components are ingested. Adult lactose intolerance is a good example.

Lactose is readily absorbed from the small intestine of normal infants. Milk sugar is hydrolysed by the appropriate enzyme, which is a constituent part of the brush border of the small intestinal mucosal cell. Glucose and galactose are released and actively transported into the circulation. In most mammals, intestinal lactase activity decreases markedly after weaning; in adults, little milk sugar can be absorbed. In humans there is much variation: the majority of Europeans can absorb lactose throughout adult life; few Chinese or south-east Asians are able to do so. In Africa, there are tribal differences. In Hamitic people, who keep cattle, lactase activity persists into adult life. The opposite is true of Bantus who drink little milk. It is suggested that persistent lactase activity provides a selective advantage among people who have access to animal milk. In areas where milk is not available or where milk is traditionally fermented and changed into yoghurt or cheese, the majority of the population are unable to metabolise lactose in

Table 15.9. *Causes of short stature*

Causes	Comments/Examples
Genetic	Normal physiological variation; small stock
Endocrine	Low growth hormone, hypothyroidism, Cushing's syndrome
Skeletal	Dysplastic conditions (e.g. achondroplasia)
Disease inhibiting growth and development	Congenital systemic disorders (cardiac, renal, neurological) Chronic infection (bronchiectasis, pyelonephritis) Inflammatory disorders (rheumatoid diseases, colitis) Metabolic disorders (e.g. diabetes mellitus) Malignant disease (e.g. Wilm's tumour) Malabsorption (e.g. coeliac disease, pancreatic disease)
Inadequate food supply throughout childhood and adolescence	Worldwide this is the most common cause of short stature

adult life. In such people, the gene for lactase is switched off after weaning. Providing a lactose-rich diet does not alter the situation and, therefore, there is no evidence to support the alternative hypothesis of direct environmental control of enzyme activity ('enzyme induction'),

Disease related to the intake of major nutrients

Now we must turn to the clinical problems caused by adverse nutrition: undernutrition and obesity.

Protein–calorie undernutrition

Undernutrition occurs when food intake is inadequate for needs. It occurs as a result of famine, reduced food intake for psychological reasons, disorders causing anorexia and/or malabsorption especially those affecting the gastrointestinal tract and severe pathology of any sort that enhances catabolism (e.g. infection, neoplastic conditions). Under all these circumstances, there is loss of body fat and wasting of skeletal muscle, with variable atrophy of the body viscera excluding the brain. In infants and children, growth and development are impeded (Table 15.9). The degree of wasting depends on the disease process, the adequacy of intake of specific nutrients and on hormonal responses. It is important to remember that, although body fat is a source of calories, the body has no store of unused protein.

The effects of starvation have been well characterised particularly in children. The FAO/WHO used a combination of one clinical sign (oedema) and two anthropomorphic indices (weight deficit for age and weight deficit for height) to provide an epidemiological classification for protein–energy malnutrition in children, based on the classical syndromes of *marasmus* and *kwashiorkor*. This classification has outlived its usefulness because it is too simple, it disregards pathogenesis and takes no account of the effects of non-nutritional pathology. Nevertheless, the terms marasmus and kwashiorkor are too well established to be replaced. Therefore, they must be set in context.

Marasmus

Clinicians interested in child growth and development have used the word marasmus for more than a century. It is derived from the Greek marasmus (meaning 'a dying away') and is usually applied to severe malnutrition in infants. Moderate or severe cases are instantly recognisable (Fig. 15.7). The condition may be precipitated or complicated by infection, which will alter the clinical picture. In particular, concentrations of circulating albumin are reasonably well maintained in uncomplicated marasmus but fall rapidly if the child gets an infection.

In developing countries, the health of many infants with nutritional marasmus is compromised by infection of the gut, especially by helminths, giardia, cryptosporidia and bacterial overgrowth of the small intestine, and by other pathology, e.g. that caused by malaria. As a result, the response to feeding a good diet is unpredictable. A good appetite and a lively infant are good signs. Anorexia and irritability often indicate a slow uncertain recovery, especially if there is persistent diarrhoea as well as malnutrition.

Stunting

In children, persistent suboptimal food intake leads to failure to thrive (Table 15.9, Fig. 15.8). Superficially, the child may appear normal but age-related weight and height are markedly reduced. Sexual maturation is retarded. The syndrome can be reproduced experimentally and is sometimes seen in other countries in children with malabsorption (especially coeliac disease) and those with a poor appetite secondary to pathology (such as chronic infection, chronic renal failure and cyanotic congenital heart disease). Stunting also occurs as a result of recurrent episodes of marasmus.

During the intervening periods of nutritional repletion, catch-up growth may fail to reach the curve for normal growth and development (Fig. 15.9).

Kwashiorkor

In 1933, the term kwashiorkor was introduced into medical literature. It comes from the language of the Ga tribe who live around Accra and it means 'the sickness of the older child when the next baby is born'. It is characterised by hypoproteinaemic oedema, a moon face and epidermal damage (thin, patchily ulcerated skin, sparse depigmented hair and thin nails) (Fig. 15.10, Table 15.10). Severely affected children are extremely irritable and, if left untreated, die within a few days. At post-mortem, the most characteristic finding is an extremely fatty liver. Yet, if the condition is uncomplicated and recognised early enough, it responds rapidly to a well-balanced diet (classically an adequate supply of good milk). Experimentally, a similar disorder can be produced in baboons by feeding a diet high in carbohydrate and low in first-class protein (with a deficiency of essential amino acids). Typical kwashiorkor is seen only in countries where the

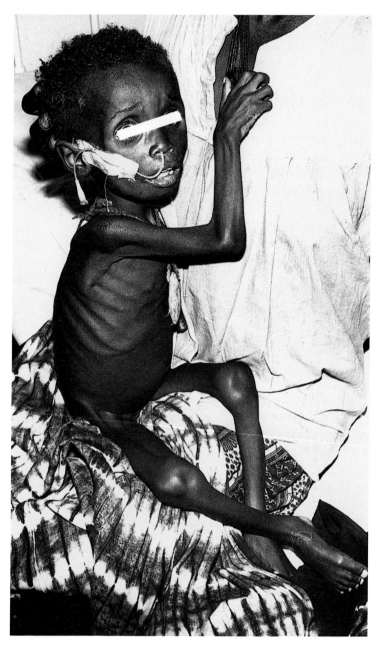

Fig. 15.7. Near absence of subcutaneous fat and severe muscle wasting in a child with marasmus. (Photograph by kind permission of R. G. Whitehead, MRC Dunn Nutrition Laboratory, Cambridge, UK.)

staple food is poor in protein and high in carbohydrate. Such foods include cassava, yams, plantain and poor-quality maize (Table 15.4). Weanlings fed solely on a pap made from the staple food are most likely to develop kwashiorkor. The carbohydrate intake tends to be sufficient to maintain body weight and the resulting high concentrations of

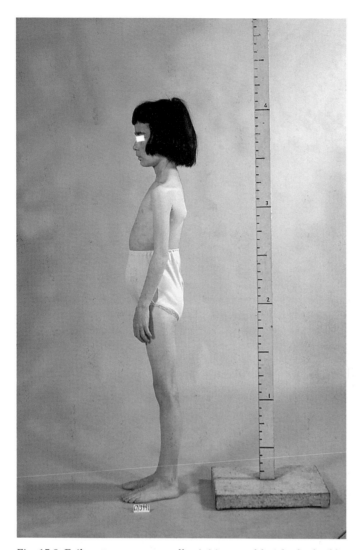

Fig. 15.8. Failure to grow normally. A 16-year-old girl who had been treated for four years for an eating disorder. She was referred for investigation and management of anaemia. Her haemoglobin was 9.5 g/100 ml and the blood film showed dimorphic red cells secondary to deficiencies of iron and folic acid. Note the stunting and delayed puberty. The correct diagnosis was coeliac disease. On a gluten-free diet she gained 8 inches in height in one year and developed secondary sex characteristics.

circulating insulin limit the breakdown of muscle. Therefore, there is a deficiency of circulating essential amino acids, which impairs the synthesis of body proteins. The liver and organs containing cells with a high rate of turnover (skin, gastrointestinal tract, marrow) are particularly affected. The condition is rarely seen in the Western world but has been described in infants taking unusual diets (e.g. rusks and Lucozade) and occasionally in adults with complex disorders of absorption. Unfortunately, the literature on malnutrition is often confusing because classifications are largely dependent on

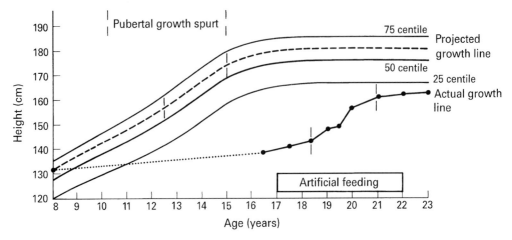

Fig. 15.9. Catch-up growth. The growth chart of a young man with Crohn's disease. The inflammatory condition of the bowel began in his ninth year. He was given various anti-inflammatory agents including corticosteroids. The symptoms were held in check but his pattern of growth was accepted as part of the disease process. Over eight years he gained only 8 cm in height. The normal pre-pubertal growth rate is 5 cm per annum.

At age 17, he showed only early signs of puberty (stage 2). He had marked ileocolonic Crohn's pathology and was treated with a regimen of 'bowel rest' – for a few months he was fed a standard 2000 kcal parenteral diet by a central venous catheter and he was subsequently weaned onto an oral elemental diet. He had a normal but seriously delayed pubertal growth spurt. Sexual development was also delayed but normal. The graph shows that he did not make up the additional 10 cm he should have grown in the first four years of his illensss. (Child Growth Foundation, 1995.)

anthropometric indices and the presence or absence of oedema (see next section). There would be less confusion if the term kwashiorkor was limited to individuals with classical signs of the condition, biochemical evidence of deficient essential amino acids, no other pathology and a prompt therapeutic response to feeding a high-quality diet (e.g. milk).

Oedematous malnutrition

Oedema is a common finding in malnourished people. Sometimes it occurs with normal or near-normal values for circulating albumin and is often seen when a severely malnourished person is re-fed ('war oedema', 're-feeding oedema'). The mechanism is far from clear but impaired integrity of the microvasculature secondary to an unbalanced generation of free radicals has been suggested. In addition, the activity of the cellular sodium pump is decreased, leading to an increase in total body sodium.

Hypoalbuminaemia

Most circulating proteins are produced in the parenchymal cells of the liver and they can be easily measured. As a result, serum protein concentrations have been used in the

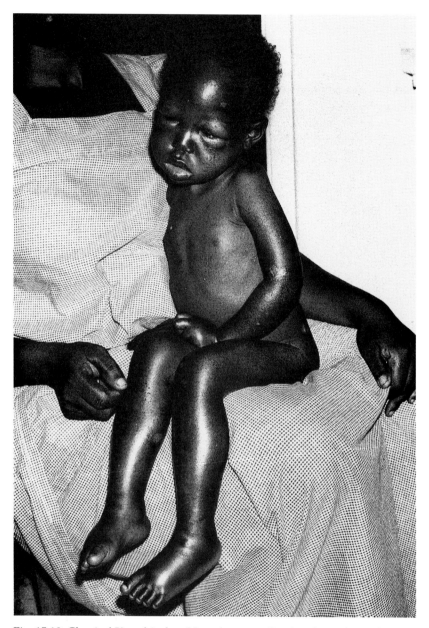

Fig. 15.10. Classical Kwashiorkor. Note the generalised oedema, moon face, patchy loss of skin, thin hair and general air of misery. The child is not wasted; compare it with the child with marasmus (Fig. 15.7). (Photograph by kind permission of R. G. Whitehead, MRC Dunn Nutrition Laboratory, Cambridge, UK.)

assessment of nutritional status. But the concentration of circulating albumin reflects not only synthetic rate but also the distribution of albumin in body pools, tissue catabolism of protein and loss of protein from the body (Fig. 15.11). It is important not to equate hypoproteinaemia with protein malnutrition. There are many causes (see Table 15.11).

Table 15.10. *Difference between marasmus and kwashiorkor in infancy*

	Marasmus[a]	Kwashiorkor[b]
Geographical prevalence	Areas of starvation	Primarily areas where staple food is of poor protein quality (cassava, plaintain, maize)
Upbringing	Often early weaning followed by diarrhoea–malnutrition syndrome	Weaning after the next child is born; thereafter fed pap (staple food soaked in water)
Appearance	Cachetic (Fig. 15.7)	Often bloated (Fig. 15.10)
Body fat	Very little	May be maintained, but there is often generalised oedema as well
Muscle protein	Very wasted	Often maintained
Skin	Intact (apart from frequent sores)	Depigmented, peeling
Hair	Normal	Depigmented, fine
Circulating albumin	Low normal	Subnormal
Liver	Not palpable	Enlarged and fatty

[a] Marasmus (cachexia) is seen at all ages.
[b] Classical kwashiorkor is rare outside infancy.

The total mass of albumin in an adult is about 300 g, of which more than half is extravascular. Passage of albumin from the intravascular space (transcapillary escape) occurs continuously at a rate of about 5% per hour. Extravascular albumin is returned to the circulation by the lymphatic system. In severe disease, there is usually an increased proportion of albumin in the extravascular pool, which contrasts with the effect of starvation, which is associated with a preferential preservation of the intravenous albumin mass. The concentration of plasma albumin is well maintained in obese patients losing weight and in patients with anorexia nervosa. Albumin has a half life of 12–20 days but this is considerably shortened in the presence of inflammatory disorders. As a result, the concentration of albumin is readily affected by any serious disease process and only rarely is this nutritionally determined.

Acute starvation reduces the concentration of some proteins with a short half life (e.g. transferrin (half life 5 days), pre-albumin (half life 2 days) and retinol-binding protein (half life 10 hours)) but values are often near-normal in individuals with well-established malnutrition. In assessing the significance of circulating proteins, it is necessary to consider possible confounding factors (Table 15.11) as well as the physiological pathways described in Fig. 15.11. In particular, inflammation enhances the synthesis of certain proteins by the liver, including C-reactive protein, which combines with phospholipid from damaged membranes to become an activator of the complement pathway; α_1-antitrypsin, which is a part of the control mechanism of inflammation; haptoglobin, which binds haemoglobin released by local haemolysis; fibrinogen, the precursor of fibrin; and caeruloplasmin and ferritin, which play an important part in copper and iron meta-

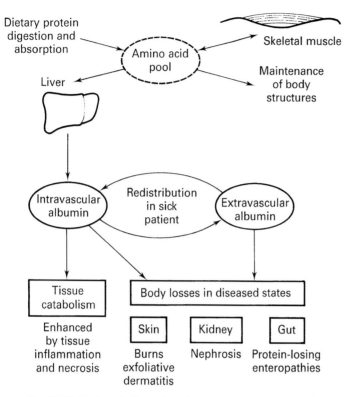

Fig. 15.11. Factors influencing the concentration of circulating albumin.

bolism, respectively. In contrast, the synthesis of albumin, pre-albumin, retinol-binding protein and transferrin fall with inflammation and so are sometimes termed negative acute-phase reactants.

The syndromes caused by deficiencies of macronutrients are outlined in Table 15.12. The nutritional problem can be defined by reference to the general principles outlined above. The integrated figure (Fig. 15.12) shows kwashiorkor-type malnutrition secondary to gastrectomy for severe haemorrhagic gastritis in a patient with severe exocrine pancreatic insufficiency.

The undernourished patient in hospital

Since the Second World War, it has been recognised that patients who have lost more than 10% of their body weight recover less well from surgical procedures than those who have not lost weight. But this may reflect the severity of the pathological process or the effect of co-existing disorders rather than malnutrition (Table 15.13). Although it is difficult to prove statistically that nutritional supplementation affects prognosis, in individual patients, it is important to recognise nutritional deficiencies in order to provide optimal care. The very thin are prone to hypothermia; muscle wasting, which leads to weakness and inanition; oedematous tissues, which heal poorly; and deficiencies of

Table 15.11. *Factors affecting the concentration of circulating proteins*

Protein	Increased concentrations	Decreased concentrations
All proteins	Dehydration	Overhydration, nephrotic syndrome, protein-losing enteropathy
Albumin		Injury/inflammation, cirrhosis
Pre-albumin		Acute starvation, injury/inflammation, liver disease
Transferin	Iron deficiency, in pregnancy (oestrogens)	As for pre-albumin
Retinol-binding protein	Renal insufficiency (corticosteroids)	As for pre-albumin, vitamin A deficiency, zinc deficiency
Acute-phase proteins Haptoglobins	Injury/inflammation	Haemolysis, ineffective erythropoiesis
Alpha-1 antitrypsin	Injury/inflammation (but variable)	
Orosomucoid	Injury/inflammation, renal insufficiency	
Ferritin	Injury/inflammation, iron overload	Iron deficiency

Table 15.12. *Deficiency of macronutrients*

Clinical disorders
Kwashiorkor
Marasmus
Stunting
Delayed maturation
Wasting

Aetiology
Famine in the Third World
Disadvantaged groups throughout the world
  The poor
  The elderly
  Alcoholics
  Chronically ill (e.g. post-gastrointestinal surgery, AIDS)
Undernutrition in illness
  Anorexia nervosa
  Intestinal failure
  Renal failure
  Chronic cardio-respiratory disease (cardiac cachexia)
  Severe injury: high resting energy expenditure, negative nitrogen balance (see Table 15.13)
  Cancer cachexia: anorexia, metabolic changes induced by the tumour

(a) 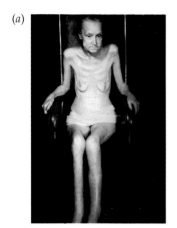 (b) 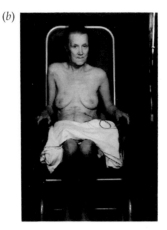 (c)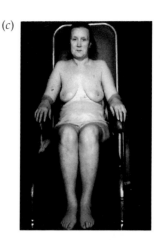

Symptoms
Anorexia
Diarrhoea
Miserable
Hair loss
Ankle swelling

Signs
Weight 44.5 kg, SFT (skin fold thickness) 23 mm
(falling to 38.9 kg with
resolution of oedema)
Apathy
Balding
Thin skin
Ankle oedema

Investigations
Haemoglobin 10.2 g/100 ml; mean cell value 85 Fe; mean cell haemoglobin content
30.2 pg (normocytic normochromic anaemia)
Urea 1.0 mmol/l; electrolytes normal
Total protein 52 g/l; albumin 18 g/l; low circulating essential amino acids
Faecal fat 920 mmol/day (equivalent to 50 g fat – at least 90% of intake)
Pancreo-lauryl test strongly positive for pancreatic insufficiency

Fig. 15.12. Kwashiorkor-type malnutrition secondary to severely impaired absorption of protein (and fat) because of a lack of gastic and pancreatic enzymes. Carbohydrate was moderately well absorbed through the action of enzymes in the intestinal mucosa. The malabsorption resulted from a partial gastrectomy because of severe haemorrhagic gastritis in the presence of severe exocrine pancreatic insufficiency. The 41-year-old patient subsequently developed severe diarrhoea and weight loss. (a) Severely malnourished; (b) gastrostomy feeding; (c) recovered patient.

Table 15.13. *Metabolic and nutritional effects of starvation and stress*

	Starvation		Stress	
	Early	Late	Early	Late
Energy expenditure	0	−	++	++
Preferred substrate	Glucose	Fat	Fat/amino acids	Fat/amino acids
Synthesis of protein	−	−	+	−
Lipogenesis	0	−	−−	+
Lipolysis	−	++	+++	+++
Rate of weight loss	++	+	++	+++
Fat stores	0	−−[a]	−	−−−
Muscle mass	0	−−[a]	−	−−−
Liver mass	−	−−	0	+
Heart mass	0	−−	0	+
Spleen size	−	−−−	++	++

Notes:
+, increase, −, decrease; 0, no change; ±, variable.
[a] Physical activity and the nature of the available food will affect the response. In starvation, fat disappears and muscle wastes, especially if the person is inactive. In anorexia nervosa, fat disappears but muscles are often well maintained (person is often hyperactive and protein intake is normal).

specific nutrients, which may impair organ function. By using the format in Table 15.14, one can determine the nutritional status of a patient and determine how best to provide nutritional support.

Overnutrition: obesity

So far we have examined the problems of undernutrition. In the prenatal period, undernutrition has implications for genetic expression and the possible long-term effects on growth, development and predisposition to disease in adult life. In the child, the problems are those of adaptation and effects on growth and development. In the adult, we are concerned with pathophysiology and the ability to withstand disease processes. Nutritional problems are also associated with a *plentiful* supply of processed food which may lead to the problem of overnutrition. Historical evidence would suggest that hunter–gatherer humans were well adapted to a feast/famine existence. The development of agriculture smoothed out variations in the availability of food, especially when humans developed effective means for its preservation and storage. It is only in the twentieth century, in the developed world, that food has become highly palatable, cheap and universally available to all sections of the population. As a result, people are bigger than their forebears. In addition, the epidemiology of disease has changed dramatically. Many life-threatening disorders of middle age are believed to be related to diet (Table 15.2). Until the mechanisms of these disorders are more clearly understood, we will not be able to separate the effects of programming in fetal life, life-time food intake and other

Table 15.14. *Assessing the nutritional status of the hospitalised patient*

1. History
    Anorexia
    Vomiting
    Diarrhoea
    Weakness
    Reduced activity
    Dietary intake: including food fads, alcohol

2. Appearance and examination
    Hydration
    Subcutaneous fat (SFT)
    Degree of muscle wasting
    Oedema
    Skinfolds
    Blood pressure (standing and lying)

3. Screening tests
    FBC: assessment of blood film
    Assessment iron, B_{12}, folate status if indicated by blood count and appearance of blood film
    Urea and electrolytes
    Liver function tests and proteins, including acute-phase reactants
    Calcium, magnesium and zinc (values corrected for albumin concentration)

4. Assess dietary intake

5. Correct specific nutritional deficiencies

6. Make an informed decision regarding feeding in hospital

7. Decide whether or not to supplement oral intake (or provide parenteral nutrition)

environmental influences on individual genotypes. As an examplar condition, we will take the disorder most clearly related to dietary imbalance – obesity – which will be discussed in some detail because of its clinical importance in the affluent world (Table 15.15).

The problem of obesity is usually regarded as primarily one of behaviour, but now there is increasing interest in other possibilities. The nature of programming in fetal life has already been considered and the possibility of identifying genetic causes for obesity has been boosted by the identification of an *ob* gene on chromosome 6 of the obese mouse. Sequence data suggest that this gene encodes a secreted protein (named leptin from the Greek *leptos* meaning thin). In *ob/ob* mice, the *ob* gene is mutated and no leptin is produced. When given leptin, *ob/ob* mice eat less and lose weight. In the human genome there is an *ob* homologue 84% identical with the mouse *ob* gene. Although, *ob* is a highly preserved biologically important gene, the *ob/ob* mouse model appears not to apply to humans. Obese humans have *elevated* levels of circulating leptin with *ob* mRNA elevated in adipocytes. As a result, it is suggested that obese humans have a decreased sensitivity to leptin (see Fig. 15.15 below).

Table 15.15. *Complications of obesity*

Area affected	Diseases
Metabolic	Diabetes mellitus
	Hyperlipidaemia
	Gout
	Gall bladder disease
	Decreased fertility
Cardiovascular	Hypertension
	Cardiac disease
	Cerebrovascular accidents
Respiratory	Sleep apnoea
Cancer	Breast, uterus, colon, prostate
Pregnancy risks	Toxaemia, glucose tolerance
Surgery risks	Pneumonia, wound infection, venous thrombosis
Lifespan	Early mortality

Basic mechanisms

Stores of body energy are regulated remarkably tightly in the majority of people. A small consistent change in the daily intake of calories will alter weight in an obvious way. For example, a positive balance of 100 kcal per day (one slice of bread, about 5% of dietary intake) might result in a weight gain of 4–5 kg over one year (Table 15.16). Yet, annual changes of weight of this degree are unusual. Progressive obesity occurs with a number of inherited disorders (e.g. Laurence Moon Biedl syndrome, Prader–Willi syndrome) and occasionally after damage to the hypothalamus. But these are rare conditions that probably do not shed light on the problem of common obesity.

Some nutritionists suggest that stores of body energy are actively regulated with a set point mechanism in the central nervous system. The simplest model requires efferent humoral and neural signals that monitor stored energy and recent food intake. These signals are received in the hypothalamus and result in efferent activators which modulate intake of food (satiety) and energy expenditure (Fig. 15.13). The system may maintain energy stores at a relatively constant level, although there are systematic changes with age. Evidence in favour of the set point hypothesis is derived from studies of energy expenditure after manipulations of body weight, genetic studies in humans and studies of obesity syndromes in experimental animals (especially those in which lesions have been produced in the hypothalamus).

Obese subjects who lose considerable weight reduce lean body mass and expend less energy. Usually they are persistently hungry and intolerant of cold. Women develop amenorrhoea. Conversely, experimental overfeeding of both obese and never-obese subjects results in a higher metabolic rate and a decrease in appetite. Therefore, there is a tendency for individuals to return to their pre-perturbation set point. The set point is not

Table 15.16. *Change in body weight: necessary data for simple calculations*

Calorific value

Carbohydrate	4 kcal/g
Protein	4 kcal/g
Fat	9 kcal/g

Assessment of body composition

The proportion of body weight that is fat
  Measured most accurately by underwater weighing
  Estimate clinically by the sum of skinfold thickness (Fig. 15..3)
The proportion of body weight that is lean body mass (LBM)
   Measured most accurately by estimation of ^{40}K (cellular content) or by estimating total body water (^{3}H dilution) (LBM is 75% water, 25% protein)
   Estimate clinically by subtracting fat mass from total body mass

Calorific exchange with change in body weight

Weight is gained as fat and LBM in a ratio of 3–4:1
Weight is lost as fat and LBM in a ratio of 2–3:1

Calculated energy required for a gain of weight of 1 kg (assuming stores of glycogen replete)

  0.8 kg fat+0.2 kg LBM
=0.8 kg fat+0.05 kg protein+0.15 kg water
=7200 kcal+200 kcal+0 kcal
=7400 kcal

Actual energy needed for a weight gain of 1 kg is, in fact, greater than predicted by this simple equation because

Energy is needed for metabolic conversion
Larger meals have a thermogenic effect
Intrinsic control mechanisms such as thermogenesis in brown fat (not proven in humans)
  may burn off some excess calories

absolute but its existence is supported by the high rate at which obese individuals return to their pre-dieting weight.

Behaviourists would offer an alternative explanation. Slim people condition themselves. They are sensitive to simple cues such as tightness of clothes, appearance in front of a mirror and breathlessness on exercise. This leads to a conscious or subconscious limit on food intake operating on a day-to-day basis.

Genetic studies

Genes are important in determining body weight. The prevalence of obesity among children of slim parents is less than 10%; with one obese parent the figure rises to 30% and with both parents obese it exceeds 60%. These correlations may, of course, reflect similarities of environment, but in studies of adopted children there are strong correlations between the weight class of adoptees and the body mass index of natural parents but not adoptive parents. In studies from Scandinavia, the body composition of identical twins reared apart was more concordant than that of fraternal twins reared together. Although

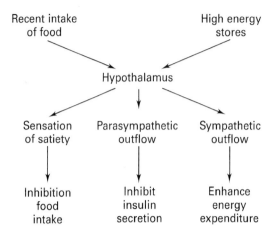

Fig. 15.13. Model for the regulation of stores of body energy by the hypothalamus.

the data are somewhat limited, it is estimated that 80% of the risk of obesity is heritable. The genetic transmission of a 'set point' would explain observations regarding heritability and the apparent resistance of adult body composition to long-term manipulation. Opponents of this hypothesis would stress that the nature of the genetic factors which may control body composition are unknown and seek to discuss genetic influences on behaviour.

The effect of diet

The normal adult contains, on average, about 140 000 kcal energy stored as fat. By comparison, the quantity of carbohydrate is minute – equivalent to only 800 kcal (glycogen of liver, muscle and kidney and circulating glucose). An individual eating 2000 kcal per day, of which 40% is carbohydrate, will take in an amount of carbohydrate equivalent to the total body stores; the calorific value of the fat intake will be less than 1% of body stores. Studies in animals suggest that day-to-day changes in the balance of body carbohydrate affects its intake in a reciprocal manner; in contrast, there is little obvious day-to-day relationship for the intake of fat.

A high-carbohydrate diet is less likely to produce obesity than a high-fat diet. Body storage of glycogen is limited and the conversion of carbohydrate to fat is energetically expensive. For nutrient balance, the net oxidation of each nutrient should equal the average composition of the macronutrients in the diet. On ingestion of a high-fat diet, there should be greater oxidation of fat; however, there seems to be considerable inter-individual variation in this respect, which may be genetically determined.

The standard laboratory rat will become obese when allowed free access to abundant highly palatable food (especially that containing sucrose and fat) rather than rat chow (an unappetising nutritionally balanced pelleted diet based on cereals). This contrasts with genetically obese animals, which produce fat preferentially, irrespective of diet.

Food in abundance may lead to obesity by distorting afferent feedback signals. The sight, smell, texture and taste of food act as sensory cues to initiate, maintain or abort

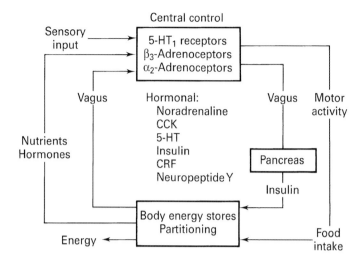

Modulating factors
  Food: quantity, digestibility, density
  Energy: exercise, vasodilatation, BMR
  Afferent signals: palatability, gastric distension, GI peptides
  Central control: adrenergic, serotoninergic, agonists, CCK, opioid antagonists
  Efferent mechanisms: jaw-wiring

Fig. 15.14. Model for nutrient balance, CCK, cholecystokinin; CRF, corticotrophin-releasing factor.

periods of eating. The ability of animals to avoid foods that have previously made them sick, a phenomenon known as bait shyness, is an example of afferent sensory signals integrated with a central learning system.

Figure 15.14 shows a model by which diet may modulate satiety.

Gastrointestinal signals may be initiated by one of three mechanisms: distension of the gastrointestinal tract (especially the stomach), the release of hormones and the effect of absorbed nutrients. Gastric and intestinal distension provide negative feedback by the vagus. Of the hormones, cholecystokinin (CCK) has received the most attention. CCK-A receptors in the antrum mediate pyloric constriction and, therefore, enhance gastric distension. CCK-B receptors in the brain allow direct action on the central controls of appetite. In hungry rats, intraperitoneal injections of CCK decrease food intake and in monkeys they inhibit foraging for food.

Nutrient signals may also act on the liver or brain to initiate satiety. In experimental animals, glucose, fatty acids and lactate have all been shown to provide signals that may modulate food intake. Observations that genetically obese animals become obese independent of diet suggest that there are effective mechanisms for the control of nutrient partitioning. Both sympathetic and parasympathetic systems may be involved. Experimental lesions of the hypothalamus causing obesity are associated with enhanced vagal activity and increased secretion of insulin. In contrast, the obese state is characterised by reduced sympathetic activity. The thermogenic response to food is activated by

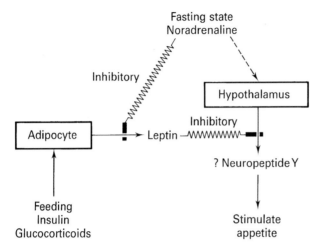

Fig. 15.15. Proposed role of leptin in relation to hypothalamic function. (From Rohner-Jeanrenaud, F. & Jeanrenaud, B. (1996). Obesity, leptin and the brain. *New England Journal of Medicine*, 34, 324–351.)

efferent sympathetic signals that activate β_3-adrenoceptors. Treating pigs and cattle with drugs that act on β-adrenoceptors increases the ratio of storage of protein to storage of fat.

Hormonal mechanisms are also important in the partitioning of nutrients. Increased levels of insulin are characteristic of obesity. This may be merely a reflection of high levels of nutrient intake but insulin is essential for the storage of nutrients as fat. Corticosteroids play a part. The adrenal insufficiency of Addison's disease is associated with leanness, whereas Cushing's syndrome is associated with obesity. Finally, growth hormone is also involved. In obese subjects, concentrations of growth hormone are high and its release in response to stimuli is blunted. Yet growth hormone stimulates metabolic rate and increases the secretion of protein at the expense of fat.

It is clear that the pathogenesis of obesity is complex, with metabolic, environmental and behavioural factors. Nevertheless, a candidate gene for obesity has now been identified and it is exciting to consider the implications of a circulating protein, synthesised and secreted by adipose tissue, which could signal satiety by interacting with specific factors in the brain. A suggested mechanism is described in Fig. 15.15. Normal body fat mass may be maintained by a central–peripheral loop system involving the brain, food ingestion and adipose tissue mass. Dysregulation of this system may be important in the severely obese. Our understanding of the genetics of human obesity changes by the month. In addition to the *ob* gene, there are at least 10 other candidate genes that show a statistical association with BMI or body fat.

Social and psychopathological aspects of obesity

Obesity is related to age, gender and social class. More females than males become obese; obesity increases with age and is more common in social classes IV and V. Psychological studies show that obesity correlates with low levels of anxiety in both males and females and low levels of depression in males. Furthermore, smoking tobacco correlates with being thin and being anxious as does excessive alcohol consumption in women. Therefore, there seem to be significant relationships between mood, certain addictive behaviours and obesity, which may be different for men and women.

Massive obesity leads to a life characterised by general inertia and sexual inactivity. This may become a protective and defensive strategy that serves to perpetuate the obesity, although women usually continue to show dysmorphophobia (a marked or even pathological fear of fatness). Psychoanalytical interpretations of obesity may also be important. Compliant overeating leading to early obesity may be the result of an excessively nurturing mother who has failed to come to terms with life and whose love is conditional on the child eating.

Knowledge of these aspects of obesity is essential in trying to understand the principles of treatment and its possible effects. Assessment of attitudes of the obese person can be determined by:

- factors contributing to weight gain (e.g. post-pregnancy, lifestyle)
- results of previous efforts to lose weight
- rate of weight loss patient believes possible (often unrealistic)
- expectations of effects of weight loss (often unrealistic)
- social class and educational achievements (important in understanding situation)
- drive and determination
- psychosocial history (stability is a desirable feature)
- drug habits (including alcohol and tobacco).

The effects of obesity and the potential benefits that may accrue from weight loss are summarised in Table 15.17. People who lose weight most effectively may make dramatic adjustments to their lives. They become more generally active, more assertive and regain sexual interest. This may have remarkable effects on their social relationships.

Disease related to the intake of non-calorie nutrients

Unlike fat, carbohydrate and protein, the body has homeostatic mechanisms for minerals, trace elements and vitamins. Body stores and the control of absorption and excretion protect against deficiency and excess but these mechanisms are by no means perfect. For example, deficiency syndromes of some nutrients are common because of poor intake and obligatory losses from the body (Table 15.1). Worldwide, this is particularly true for iron (causing anaemia), iodine (causing goitre), vitamin A (causing xerophthalmia) and vitamin B (causing pellagra and beri-beri). Diseases caused by excess intake of non-calorie nutrients are uncommon. They may occur with gene-related disorders (e.g. iron and haemochromatosis) and with excess intake of pharmaceuticals (e.g.hypervitaminosis D) (Table 15.1).

The assessment of nutritional status for minerals, trace elements and vitamins is not simply a matter of measuring the concentration of the nutrient in plasma. The well-informed clinician must be aware of nutrient intake, mechanisms of absorption and

Table 15.17. *Effects of obesity and the potential benefit of weight loss*

Findings in the obese	Results of weight loss
Metabolic changes	
Reduced glucose tolerance	Markedly improves
Increased plasma triglycerides, cholesterol uric acid	Improves
Increased prevalence of pathology	
Diabetes mellitus	Better control
Hypertension, vascular disease	Some improvement
Gall bladder disease	No effect
Fatty liver	May resolve
Osteoarthritis	Symptomatic improvement
Gout	Symptomatic improvement
Herniae	Symptomatic improvement
Varicose veins	Symptomatic improvement
Intertriginous dermatitis	Symptomatic improvement
Exercise tolerance	Considerable improvement
Sleep apnoea syndrome	Improves
Social disability	Often lessens

excretion, how the nutrient is carried in the circulation and stored in the body, the nature of obligatory losses and the functional effects of the deficiency (and much less commonly excess). These factors are illustrated by using iron deficiency as an exemplar condition.

Iron deficiency

Worldwide, iron deficiency is the most common nutritional deficiency disorder. Iron is the mineral for haemoglobin and myoglobin. It is vital for the transfer of oxygen. Moreover, the iron in cytochromes plays an essential role in electron transfer ($Fe^{2+} \rightarrow Fe^{3+} + e$), which is key to the oxidation of many substrates in pathways of intermediary metabolism.

Intake

An average diet provides about 10–20 mg iron per day of which 10–20% may be absorbed (Table 15.18). Iron in haem is in the ferrous state and is absorbed well (up to 40%). In contrast, vegetable iron is primarily ferric in non-haem complexes with proteins, phytates, oxalates and phosphates. Absorption is relatively poor but improved in the presence of animal foods, which allow the formation of soluble complexes, and in the presence of vitamin C, which reduces Fe^{3+} to Fe^{2+}. Gastric acid also facilitates the absorption of non-haem iron by reducing Fe^{3+} to Fe^{2+}, which helps to explain the high prevalence of iron deficiency in association with achlorhydria, for example after gastric

Table 15.18. *Sources of iron in the British diet*

Food	Average amount of of iron ingested per day[a] (mg)	Percentage of food-iron absorbed
Cereals	6	5–10
Meat	3.5	20–40
Vegetables	2.0	1–5
Eggs	0.5	10–20
Beverages	0.5	5–10
Other	1.5	5–10

Note:
[a] Average daily intake for men is 14 mg and for women is 12.5 mg. Supplementary iron is of considerable importance for women (provides 15% of intake)
Source: Data abstracted from *The dietary and nutritional survey of British adults.* OPCS, 1990.

resection. Conversely, prolonged iron deficiency will lead to gastric mucosal atrophy, which may be reversed on treatment with iron.

In a healthy person eating a normal diet, iron is best absorbed from the haem of meat (20% absorption), less well from cereals (5–10%) and least well from green vegetables (1–5%) (absorption from spinach is only about 1% despite the opinion of Popeye!). Therefore, intakes are low in diets based on refined cereals, sugars and fats. Milk is a poor source and in the first few months of life, infants rely on stores of iron laid down in the liver before birth. Percentage absorption is increased in iron deficiency and when the marrow is hyperplastic, as in haemolysis. Some simple arithmetic shows how difficult it is to balance the obligatory losses of iron from the body (Fig. 15.16).

Mechanisms of iron absorption

Iron in haem crosses into the intestinal mucosal cell unchanged and is then liberated by enzymatic breakdown. Non-haem iron is picked up by specific receptors (probably glycoproteins) and transferred into the cell where it links to a protein from which it is passed to transferrin, the carrier protein in plasma. Absorption occurs primarily from the duodenum and upper jejunum and is increased up to twofold by enhanced haematopoiesis (e.g. after a bleed), by diminished iron stores and by pregnancy. The nature of the signals influencing absorption are unknown.

Transport

Iron is carried in the plasma bound to transferrin. Each molecule of transferrin can carry two molecules of iron, giving a total binding capacity of 3–5 mg iron per litre (54–90 μmol/litre). Total iron-binding capacity increases in pregnancy and with iron deficiency. It is reduced by protein malnutrition and the acute-phase reaction. Normally the iron-

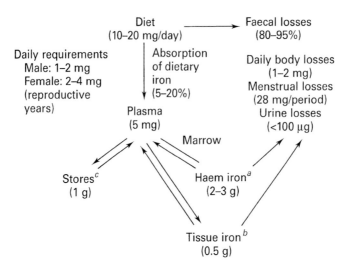

Fig. 15.16. Body stores of iron: absorption and excretion. [a] As haemoglobin; [b] as myoglobin, haem enzymes, non-haem enzymes; [c] in the liver, spleen and marrow as ferritin and haemosiderin.

binding capacity is 33% saturated, giving a serum iron of around 20 μmol/l. In an iron-deficient otherwise healthy person, the iron-binding capacity falls to less than 16%.

Stores

Iron is stored in cells as ferritin (a soluble complex of Fe^{3+} surrounded by protein) and insoluble complexes of haemosiderin. The total body store of 1 g is mostly as ferritin. As stores increase, haemosiderin accumulates, especially in the liver and spleen. It may be detected by adding ferrocyanide to sections of tissue, which stain Prussian blue.

Plasma ferritin is a good index of body iron stores, although it is also increased by the acute-phase reaction. Healthy men have plasma ferritin levels of around 150 μmol/litre, those with reduced iron stores around 50 μmol/litre and those with frank iron deficiency values of less than 5 μmol/litre.

Controlling factors

As ionic iron is toxic, virtually none is found in the circulation. Both Fe^{2+} and Fe^{3+} readily complex with proteins, the kidneys excrete virtually no iron and the only way in which the body can control iron status is by shedding the intestinal epithelium. Iron is also lost whenever there is bleeding. Female menstrual losses are approximately equal to the loss of iron by desquamation. In consequence, during their reproductive life, women have to absorb twice as much iron as men.

Correcting iron deficiency

It is difficult to correct iron deficiency by dietary means. In addition to correcting the red cell mass, a positive balance of about 1 g is needed to replenish stores. It is usual to give the patient an iron salt by mouth (e.g. ferrous sulphate) in a dose sufficient to provide 100–200 mg elemental iron per day. As only 10–20% of the iron salt is absorbed, it is necessary to continue treatment for several months. Nevertheless, this is usually preferable to blood transfusion (which provides 250 mg iron in 500 ml) or intramuscular injections of iron-sorbitol-citrate (Jectofer), which contain 25 mg iron per ml.

Summary

Diet is an important determinant of growth, development and disease. It interacts with the genetic profile of the individual and may influence programming, which appears to occur during fetal development.

The human body can adapt to a wide range of nutritional input. The interactions are complex but the general principles are reasonably well understood. Disease may arise not only from a deficiency and an excess of nutrients but also from imbalances such as the effect of sodium and potassium on blood pressure.

Deficiency of macronutrients gives rise to a variety of syndromes depending on the balance between the intake of protein and energy and the effect of associated conditions such as trauma, infection and neoplasia. Excess intake of macronutrients causes obesity, which is shown to have a complex aetiology. The discovery of obesity genes (or 'genes linked to obesity') provides an opportunity for the better understanding of satiety, which now appears to be a key factor in the pathogenesis of a condition which is becoming a major problem in the Western world.

Iron deficiency is used as an examplar condition for the understanding of the role of non-calorie nutrients in the pathogenesis of disease. The importance of individual nutrients in body physiology and biochemistry, the dietary sources and the mechanisms of absorption from the gut, the carriage of the nutrient in the circulation, its storage in tissue and the mode of loss from the body all need to be considered in the assessment and treatment of deficiency states.

FURTHER READING

General
Garrow, J.S. & James, W.P.T. (ed.) (1993). *Human Nutrition and Dietetics*, 9th ed. Edinburgh: Churchill Livingstone.
Truswell, A.S. (1992). *ABC of Nutrition*. London: British Medical Journal.
Eastwood, M., Edwards, C., Parry, D. (1992). *Human Nutrition: A Continuing Debate*. London: Chapman and Hall.
Neale, G. (1988). *Student Reviews: Clinical Nutrition*. London: Heinemann Medical Books.
Pennington, C.R. (1988). *Therapeutic Nutrition: A Practical Guide*. London: Chapman and Hall.

Specific topics

Payne-James, J., Grimble, G. & Silk, D. (ed.) (1995). *Artificial Nutritional Support in Clinical Practice.* London: Edward Arnold.

Kirby, D.F. & Dudrick, S.J. (ed.) (1994). *Practical Handbook of Nutrition in Clinical Practice.* Boca Raton, FL: CRC Press.

Schils, M.E., Olson, J.A. & Skike, M. (ed.) (1994). *Modern Nutrition in Health and Disease*, 8th ed. Philadelphia: Lea and Febiger.

Barker, D.J.P. (ed.) (1992). *Foetal and Infant Origins of Adult Disease.* London: British Medical Journal.

Department of Health and Social Security (1991). Dietary reference values for food energy and nutrients for the UK (Committee on Medical Aspects of Food Policy). *Reports on Health and Social Subjects No 41.* London: HMSO.

Bouchard, C. and Perusse, L. (1996). Current status of the human obesity gene map. *Obesity Research*, 4, 81–90.

16

Trauma

R. A. LITTLE

- Trauma is the most common cause of death in people less than 45 years of age and is responsible for major morbidity in the elderly.

- Death from hypotension and hypoxia can be prevented by application of the basic principles of resuscitation (ABC: airway, breathing, circulation).

- The neuroendocrine and autonomic nervous systems, cytokines and prostaglandins, and eicosanoids are the principle mediators of early physiological and tissue responses to injury.

- Later responses to injury include increased metabolic rate and fever, which are caused by cytokines such as IL-1, IL-6 and TNF, possibly in association with prostaglandins.

- Proteolysis, hyperglycaemia (with insulin resistance) and oxidation of fat have important implications for nutritional support following trauma. Large doses of corticosteroid post-trauma are without benefit and may even be deleterious in certain groups of patient; however other, more rational, therapies are being developed.

Trauma has been described as the last major plague of the young. It is responsible for more deaths in those aged less than 45 years than heart disease and malignancies combined. In the USA, injuries kill six times as many children as cancer, the second leading cause of death in children. Indeed the problem is such that life expectancy of those aged 15–24 years has fallen over the last few decades.

In Western Europe and the USA, the most common cause of injury is road traffic accidents, with annual death rates as high as 20–25 per 100 000 population being recorded, resulting in some 300 000 deaths per year from such accidents. The toll in the USA is greatly enhanced by the contribution from penetrating injuries resulting from bullets and knives. Every two years, more Americans are killed in their homes by firearms than were killed in all 11 years of the Vietnam war, and the most common cause of death in 15–24-year-old black American males is firearm homicide. Fortunately, this epidemic has not yet reached Western Europe. Although attracting the most publicity, deaths are only part of the problem caused by accidents; for every death there are as many as 100 seriously injured patients who require admission to hospital, often for very long periods. Recovery and rehabilitation may not be complete and a number of accident survivors suffer permanent disability; this is particularly the case after head injuries, which account for up to one-half of all trauma deaths.

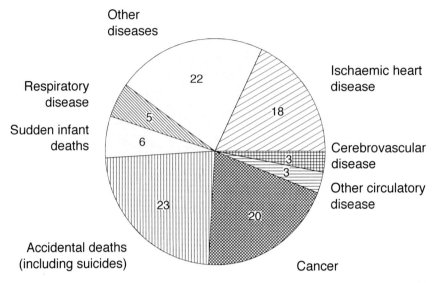

Fig. 16.1. Distribution of years of life lost, up to age 65 years (males), by cause of death (England and Wales, 1988). (Modified from *The Health of the Nation* (1991). London: HMSO.)

Most attention has been focused on the problem of injury in the young and its cost to society, expressed in terms of 'loss of productive life' (Fig. 16.1). However, the population is ageing, and although cancer and cardiovascular disease are the main causes of death in the geriatric population, trauma is still a problem. Improvements in many aspects of health care mean that the elderly are more active but, unfortunately, they live in environments that expose them to many dangers. For example, falls in the home are a major cause of injury in the elderly, and common injuries, such as a fractured neck or femur, cause an excess mortality of 35% at one year after the accident. A number of survivors fail to regain their independence even after long periods of hospitalisation, thereby putting increased strains on the provision of health care.

There are, therefore, compelling reasons to reduce the toll exacted by accidents and it is to be expected that increased knowledge of the epidemiology of trauma and the biological responses to it will improve treatment.

Trauma deaths

Death after trauma has a trimodal distribution (Fig. 16.2). The first peak of immediate deaths represents those who have sustained injuries that might be considered incompatible with life. This remains true for most injuries (e.g. decapitation, transection of the torso) but a few, involving, for example, major injuries to the heart, may respond to prompt intervention. However, the main hope for reductions in this group is prevention, including improvements in design and education, targeted at parents, for example, and enforcement of legislation relating to the wearing of seat belts, speed limits (Fig. 16.3) and drink-driving.

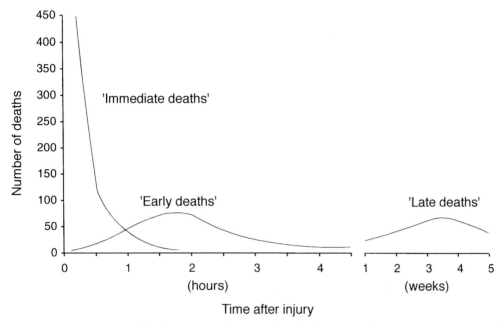

Fig. 16.2. Trimodal distribution of trauma deaths. (From Trunkey, D. D. (1983). *Scientific American*, 249, 28–35.)

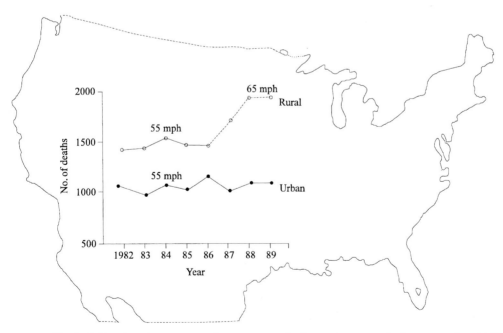

Fig. 16.3. Deaths of occupants of passenger vehicles on interstate highways in the 40 US states that increased the speed limit in rural areas from 55 mph (88 km/hour) to 65 mph (104 km/hour) at some time during April 1987 to July 1988. (From Editorial (1990). *British Medical Journal*, 301, 256.)

Table 16.1. *Effect of hypotension and/or hypoxia on outcome from severe head injury*

	Poor outcome (%)
Neither	34
Hypoxia	59
Hypotension	75
Hypoxia and hypotension	100

Source: From Gentleman, D. & Jennett, B. (1981). *Lancet*, ii, 853–854.

The second peak comprises those deaths that occur during the first few hours after injury. Many can be attributed to uncontrolled blood loss and/or inadequate pulmonary function, which frequently reflect failure to implement the basic principles of resuscitation. It has been clearly demonstrated, in a number of independent studies, that many of the deaths occurring in this second peak are preventable (i.e. the injuries sustained are not in themselves incompatible with life). For example, one study revealed that approximately 65% of non-head and 33% of head-injury deaths were preventable and an important factor in many of these was a failure to recognise the presence and/or magnitude of blood loss. It has also been clearly demonstrated that airway obstruction is not always recognised, even after admission to hospital. The compounding influences of hypotension and hypoxia on mortality have been most clearly demonstrated after head injuries (Table 16.1). The recognition that failure of treatment was so common led to the introduction, first in the USA and more recently in the UK, of Advanced Trauma Life Support (ATLS) courses. These courses present initial resuscitation and treatment in a didactic manner and are required learning for all those involved in the care of the acutely injured patient. The incorporation of such teaching within a co-ordinated system of trauma care that rigorously applies the basic principles of resuscitation (*airway*, *breathing* and *circulation*) and brings together relevant expertise can undoubtedly improve the early treatment of the injured patient and reduce the second peak of early deaths.

The third peak of late or delayed deaths is spread over a period extending for weeks or even months after injury. The elderly and those admitted to intensive care units with progressive multiple organ failure and underlying sepsis feature in this group. It seems that in many such patients the local inflammatory response initiated at the time of injury is not localised at the site of direct tissue damage but expands to involve all the body (the systemic inflammatory response syndrome: SIRS). The mechanism of the progression of inflammation from a protective local response to a destructive systemic response is unclear, but it does seem that failure to treat adequately the patient during the first few hours following injury may sow the seeds for the later phase of organ failure. Risk factors associated with the development of such multiple organ failure include prolonged hypovolaemic shock, head injury, peritoneal contamination following penetrating abdominal wounds and pre-existing malnutrition.

When considering these late deaths, it is, perhaps, worth considering that many of them occur in patients who without treatment (including resuscitation, surgery, mechanical and pharmacological organ support) would have died shortly after injury; therefore, a pattern of SIRS is being allowed to develop against which the host has no effective inherited defence mechanisms.

Biological responses

At first sight, the pathophysiological and metabolic changes associated with the general or systemic response to trauma appear to be an unrelated medley with no apparent association with outcome. Perhaps this is why these responses have provoked little serious attention despite the fact that the speciality of surgery arose from the treatment of physical injuries. The general body response to trauma is indeed very complex but progress towards its understanding has been revolutionised by the recognition that the events following injury can be related to the time interval from it and also to its severity. Sir David Cuthbertson in 1942 separated the early changes after injury from the late and these he called 'ebb' and 'flow'. These terms were chosen to describe what he saw as an early depression of vitality followed by a period of hypermetabolism. The concept of the early ebb phase was strengthened by animal studies that showed a reduction in metabolic rate and body temperature acutely after injury. It has been believed quite erroneously that these responses are secondary to a failure of oxygen transport; on the contrary, they are a result of a central inhibition of thermoregulation. As the term ebb phase is not synonymous with untreated shock, it has been used for many years to encompass the complex series of changes in homoeostatic reflex activity, fuel mobilisation, etc. initiated by injury. Another characteristic feature of the early response to injury is the pattern of changes in plasma protein concentration, known as the acute phase response or, more correctly, the acute phase protein response. The acute phase response has now become associated with all aspects of the systemic response to injury even if they persist for many weeks after major injury and/or when sepsis intervenes.

The ebb phase

Neuroendocrine changes

The ebb phase is the early stage after injury during which oxygen transport remains adequate and it may, therefore, be transient or it may persist for 24 hours or more. It includes the pattern of physiological and metabolic changes associated with the preparation for fight or flight (the defence or alerting reaction) on which are superimposed the responses to fluid loss from the circulation and/or tissue damage associated with injury.

It can be considered as a neuroendocrine response to these afferent excitatory and inhibitory inputs impinging on the endocrine neurones of the hypothalamus. The resultant changes in the release of hypothalamic hormones into the pituitary portal system influence the secretion of hormones from the anterior pituitary.

The hypothalamic–pituitary–adrenal axis is perhaps the most thoroughly investigated example of such a response to injury. Nociceptive stimuli increase (via a complex series of neuronal interactions involving 5-HT, GABA and the opioids) the release of corticotrophin-releasing factor (CRF) by the parvocellular nuclei of the posterior hypothalamus. The central injection of CRF mimics in experimental animals many of the features of the response to trauma. After injury, it is secreted into the capillary plexus of the hypophysial portal system and is then carried to the adenohypophysis where it stimulates adrenocorticotrophic hormone (ACTH) secretion. CRF is the main stimulus for ACTH production, but vasopressin released concomitantly from the neurohypophysis following activation of magnocellular nuclei (supraoptic) of the hypothalamus is also involved. ACTH stimulates the secretion of cortisol from the adrenal cortex, although the relationship between plasma ACTH and cortisol concentrations acutely after injury is complex. Plasma cortisol concentrations, both free and bound, are higher after injuries of moderate severity than after minor trauma, but more severe injuries are associated with lower concentrations (Fig. 16.4a). This cannot be attributed to low ACTH levels; after severe injury, plasma ACTH concentrations are raised to around the concentration needed for maximal stimulation of the adrenal cortex. However, reduced perfusion of the adrenal cortex may be important.

Of the other anterior pituitary hormones, growth hormone, the endorphins and prolactin are also released acutely after injury, and once again the relationships with severity are complex. Therefore, although rises in plasma prolactin concentration have been found acutely after injury in humans, animal studies have shown increased levels after minor stress but reductions in secretion after more serious injuries. The plasma concentrations of thyroid-stimulating hormone (TSH) appear to be normal acutely after injury. Although triiodothyronine (T_3) may start to fall at this time, changes in the control of thyroid hormone concentrations are a feature of the flow phase. The release of vasopressin from the posterior pituitary is increased in the ebb phase and its plasma concentration is directly related to the severity of injury.

The other major component of the neuroendocrine response to injury is a consequence of increased activity of the sympathetic nervous system. As mentioned above, many of the afferent inputs associated with the appreciation of danger, fluid loss from the circulation and tissue damage are integrated within the hypothalamus, which in turn modifies the activity of the pre-ganglionic sympathetic neurones in the intermediolateral columns of the spinal cord. Increased activity of the sympathetic nervous system leads to the release of noradrenaline from post-ganglionic nerve fibres and adrenaline from adrenal medullary cells, which are analogous to post-ganglionic neurones. Acutely after injury, there are rapid increases in the plasma concentrations of adrenaline, noradrenaline and dopamine, which are directly related to the severity of injury (Fig. 16.4b, c). The increases are sufficient to influence the secretion of other hormones and, as will be discussed below, for the mobilisation of energy substrates. Plasma insulin concentrations are often low acutely after severe injuries (Fig. 16.4d) despite a marked hyperglycaemia. This is a result of suppression of insulin secretion by adrenaline acting on pancreatic α-adrenoceptors. In contrast, the secretion of glucagon is stimulated by raised catecholamine concentrations, this time by a β-adrenoceptor mechanism. As expected, plasma glucagon levels are raised after injury.

(a)

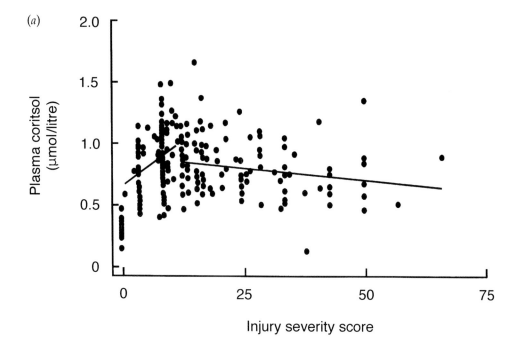

(b)

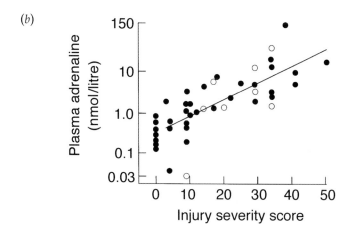

Fig. 16.4. Hormonal changes with severity of injury. Examples were taken within the first 2–3 hours after injury. (a) Plasma cortisol; (b) adrenaline; (c) noradrenaline; and (d) insulin. (From (a) Barton, R. N., Stoner, H. B. & Watson, S. M. (1987). *Journal of Trauma*, 27, 384–394; (b, c) Frayn, K. N., Little, R. A., Maycock, P. F. & Stoner, H. B. (1985). *Circulatory Shock*, 16, 229–240; (d) Frayn, K. N., Maycock, P. F., Little, R. A., Yates, D. W. & Stoner, H. B. (1987). *Archives of Emergency Medicine*, 4, 91–99.)

(c)

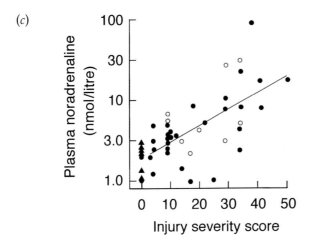

(d)

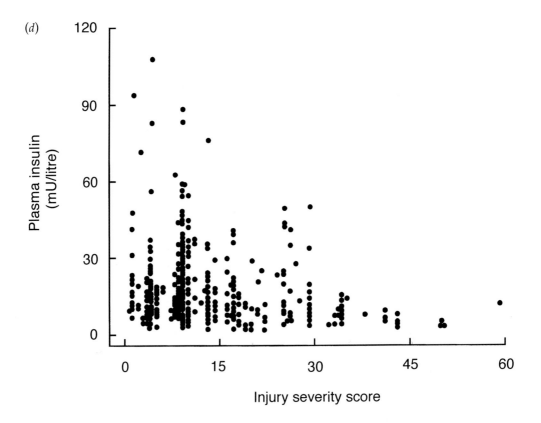

Fig. 16.4. (*cont.*)

Cytokines

Cytokines are a diverse group of regulatory proteins including:

- fibroblast growth factor
- epidermal growth factor (EGF)
- platelet-derived growth factor (PDGF)
- transforming growth factor (TGF-α, TGF-β)
- insulin-like growth factor (IGF-I, IGF-II)
- erythopoietin
- granulocyte colony-stimulating factor (G-CSF)
- macrophage colony-stimulating factor (M-CSF)
- interferons (α-IFN, β-IFN, γ-IFN)
- interleukins (IL-1 to IL-15)
- tumour necrosis factor (TNF-α, TNF-β)

Cytokines were originally isolated from immune cells but are now known to be released from many cell types both peripherally and within the central nervous system. They exert pleiotropic actions, including immune activation as well as several of the metabolic, behavioural and endocrine aspects of the response to injury. Of the growing number of identified cytokines, IL-1, IL-6, TNF-α are thought to play an important role in activation of the metabolic responses to injury.

Numerous studies have measured circulating concentrations of these cytokines in response to disease in experimental animals, human volunteers and patients, although the number of studies following uncomplicated injury is small. As with most other data derived from patients, the measured plasma concentrations of cytokines are variable. This may be the result of differences in the time samples were taken and the types of patient included in the study. In addition, although increased plasma concentrations of IL-1, IL-6 and TNF-α have been discovered after injury, many other studies have been unable to detect increases in circulating concentrations of these cytokines, particularly of IL-1. This variability is probably related to problems associated with the assay of cytokines, particularly in earlier studies, the sporadic release of cytokines and the presence of endogenous inhibitors, soluble receptors and biologically inactive (but immunoreactive) precursors or breakdown products. Increases in plasma concentrations of cytokines are not, however, prerequisites for their involvement and will not determine causal relationships. Indeed, more recent studies indicate that the local actions of cytokines, peripherally or within the brain, may be responsible for many of the metabolic responses to injury either directly or indirectly via the release of secondary mediators.

IL-1 is the cytokine most frequently studied in trauma. It was the first endogenous pyrogen to be isolated and is now known to exist in two forms, α and β. It can be produced from most cell types, including those within the central nervous system. Although increases in plasma IL-1 concentration have been observed following injury, this is usually after lethal or near-lethal stimuli and no correlations are observed between plasma IL-1 concentration and several aspects of the acute phase response. Nevertheless,

IL-1 is thought to play a pivotal role in metabolic responses to injury, probably by local actions within the target organ or at the brain.

TNF or cachectin was originally described for its ability to necrose haemorrhagic tumours and suppress lipogenesis; it was first described as an endogenous pyrogen in 1986. Although increased plasma concentrations have been observed following injury, raised circulating concentrations of TNF-α are more often associated with severe infection or sepsis, and plasma TNF-α levels often correlate with mortality in these situations. In the experimental situation, increases in plasma TNF-α occur transiently and often before the onset of acute phase responses, perhaps suggesting that raised plasma levels of TNF-α may act as a trigger for subsequent metabolic events.

IL-6 production is induced by peripheral administration of both IL-1 and TNF-α and even more potently by central IL-1 administration. Unlike IL-1 and TNF-α, plasma concentrations of IL-6 are often raised dramatically by injury. In addition, plasma IL-6 concentrations correlate with several aspects of the acute phase response, including fever, tachycardia and acute phase protein synthesis, in both experimental animals and patients (Fig. 16.5). On the basis of these observations IL-6 is the best candidate for the 'circulating mediator' of the acute phase response. IL-1 and TNF-α may be released locally following tissue injury; they may then stimulate the systemic release of IL-6, which will initiate a number of metabolic events.

Many of the actions of IL-1, IL-6 and TNF-α are mediated by the eicosanoids and, in particular, the prostaglandins. These cytokines cause prostaglandin release *in vitro* and administration of cyclo-oxygenase inhibitors prevents many of the actions of these cytokines both peripherally and within the brain. The prostaglandins and other eicosanoid derivatives (thromboxanes and leukotrienes) are produced from the liberation of membrane-bound arachidonic acid and, therefore, eicosanoid synthesis takes place in most cell types. As well as mediating the responses of the cytokines, eicosanoids can also regulate cytokine production. For example, prostaglandins inhibit IL-1 and TNF-α production, whereas leukotrienes augment production of these cytokines *in vitro*.

There has recently been much interest in the interaction between the endocrine and cytokine systems. Of particular interest in the area of metabolic responses to injury is the effect of cytokines on the release and action of the catabolic hormones (the catecholamines, cortisol and glucagon), although perhaps most interest has focused on cytokines and the hypothalamic–pituitary–adrenal axis. IL-1, IL-6 and TNF-α all activate the hypothalamic–pituitary–adrenal axis and thus stimulate glucocorticoid release by actions at the hypothalamic and pituitary level. Interestingly, administration of exogenous glucocorticoids inhibits cytokine production and action, thus completing a neuroendocrine–immune loop that regulates host responses to disease.

These cytokines also stimulate the release of the catabolic hormones and insulin. Exogenous administration of IL-1 or TNF-α causes release of insulin, glucagon and corticosterone in experimental animals and humans that is similar to that observed following injury. These two cytokines are able to act synergistically, as co-administration at doses that are ineffective individually stimulates insulin and glucagon release. IL-1 induced hyperinsulinaemia is much more potent when IL-1 is injected directly into the brain.

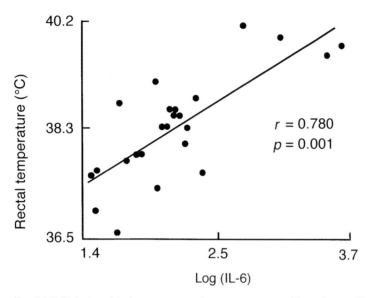

Fig. 16.5. Relationship between rectal temperature and log plasma IL-6 concentration in children during the first 24 hours following burning injury. (From Childs, C., Ratcliffe, R. J., Holt, I. *et al.* (1990). In *Physiological and Pathophysiological Effects of Cytokines.* ed. C. A. Dinerello *et al.*, pp. 295–300. New York: Liss.)

Mobilisation and utilisation of energy substrates

The increased activity of the sympathetic nervous system acutely after injury leads to mobilisation of energy substrates by stimulating glycogenolysis (Fig. 16.6) and lipolysis. The main stimulus for the breakdown of glycogen in both skeletal muscle and liver is adrenaline, although glucagon and vasopressin may also have a role in the liver. This glycogenolysis leads to hyperglycaemia either directly through liberation of glucose from the liver or indirectly, via the Cori cycle, from lactate released from skeletal muscle. It should always be remembered that raised plasma lactate concentrations can reflect this increase in skeletal muscle glycogenolysis as well as reflecting tissue hypoxia. The hyperglycaemia, which is directly related to the severity of injury, is potentiated after severe injuries by the reduction of glucose utilisation in skeletal muscle following the inhibition of insulin secretion by raised adrenaline levels and by the development of intracellular insulin resistance. The mechanism of this early insulin resistance is still unclear, although both glucocorticoids and cytokines may be involved.

The changes in carbohydrate metabolism in the ebb phase can be interpreted as defensive. In addition to providing a fuel for fight or flight, the hyperglycaemia may also play a role in the compensation of post-traumatic fluid loss, through the mobilisation of water associated with glycogen and through its osmotic effects. The decrease in glucose clearance associated with insulin resistance can also be considered protective in that it prevents the wasteful use of the mobilised glucose, which is an essential fuel for the brain and the wound, at a time when a supply of nutrients may be limited.

Plasma concentrations of non-esterified fatty acids (NEFA) and glycerol are also

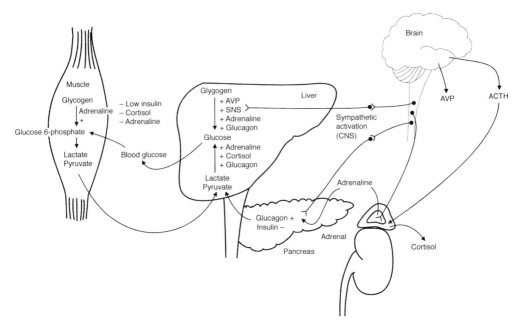

Fig. 16.6. Mobilisation of glycogen stores acutely after injury. AVP, vasopressin; SNS, sympathetic nervous system. (From Frayn, K. N. (1987). *Biochemical Society Transactions*, 15, 1030–1032.)

raised after injury, reflecting the mobilisation of triacyglycerol stores in adipose tissue. The relationship with severity is, however, complex; for example, plasma NEFA concentrations are lower after severe injuries than after moderate injuries. This may be related to metabolic (e.g. stimulation or re-esterification within adipose tissue by the raised lactate levels associated with severe injuries) or circulatory (e.g. poor perfusion of fat depots) factors.

The patterns of fuel mobilisation do not seem to be modified by the site of injury, but the age and sex of the patient may influence the changes seen. For example, for a given severity of injury, there is a suggestion that the plasma concentration of lipid metabolites (NEFA, glycerol and ketone bodies) is higher in elderly patients (see below). At the other extreme of life, children show an exaggerated hyperglycaemia, with plasma concentrations commonly exceeding 10 mmol/litre acutely after head injury and burns.

Protein metabolism

Although the major changes in protein metabolism following injury are associated with the flow phase (see below), the acute phase plasma protein response is initiated during the ebb phase. A number of plasma proteins increase in concentration (e.g. C-reactive protein and fibrinogen), although there is always a lag of approximately 6 hours before changes are seen. The cytokine IL-6 released from activated macrophages and other sites after injury may be responsible for inducing the hepatic synthesis of such acute phase proteins. After surgery, it has been shown that the rise in IL-6 precedes that of C-reactive

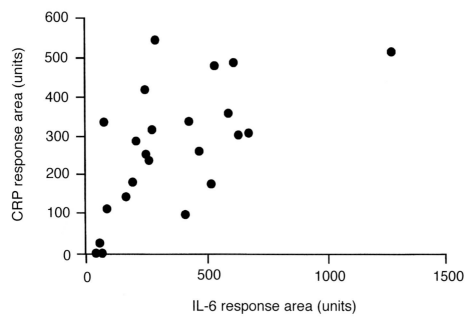

Fig. 16.7. Relationship between the responses of plasma IL-6 and C-reactive protein (CRP) to elective surgery in humans. (From Cruickshank, A. M. *et al.* (1990). *Clinical Science*, 79, 161–165.)

protein and a weak but significant positive correlation has been demonstrated between their serum levels (Fig. 16.7). Such a delay or lag is not seen for the proteins that show an acute-phase decrease in concentration after injury. The rapid fall in, for example, albumin concentration cannot be attributed to a reduction in its rate of synthesis but results from changes in its distribution between intra- and extravascular compartments secondary to an increase in microvascular permeability.

Heat production and thermoregulation

The concept of the ebb phase as a period of reduced energy metabolism arises from experimental studies which showed that after injury oxygen consumption and body temperature were reduced at ambient temperatures below the thermoneutral range. This impairment of heat production could not be reversed by reinfusion of blood or by the administration of 100% inspired oxygen, which are effective after simple haemorrhage. Therefore, although the fall in heat production after haemorrhage can be ascribed to a failure of oxygen delivery, this is not the case after tissue injury. In such cases, nociceptive afferent impulses triggered at the site of injury activate noradrenergic neurones in the hind-brain from where axons ascend in the ventral noradrenergic bundle to liberate noradrenaline in the region of the dorsomedial nucleus of the hypothalamus. The result is an inhibition of both thermoregulatory heat production and heat loss mechanisms. Thus lower temperatures have to be applied to the skin or the hypothalamus to induce shivering in skeletal muscle and higher temperatures have to be applied to the

Table 16.2. *Effects of injury (limb ischaemia) on the thresholds for the onset of heat production (shivering) and heat loss from the tail in the rat*

	Heat production threshold (°C)		Heat loss threshold (°C)
	Ta[a]	Thypo[b]	Thypo[b]
Control	20.0	34.8–36.4	39.8
During limb ischaemia	14.0	31	40.5
After limb ischaemia	11.3	No response	No response

Notes:
[a] Ambient temperature.
[b] Hypothalamic temperature when ambient temperature is 20°C.
Source: From Stoner, H. B. (1981). *Advances in Physiological Science*, 26, 25–33.

hypothalamus to initiate an increase in heat loss (Table 16.2). The inhibition of thermo-regulatory heat production by injury in the rat, which involves both skeletal muscle and brown adipose tissue, can eventually be overcome by lowering the ambient temperature sufficiently or by the injection of exogenous noradrenaline. This supports the suggestion that the reduction in heat production in the ebb phase of the response to injury in experimental animals is the result of a change in central control rather than an impairment of peripheral effector mechanisms.

The evidence for a similar pattern of change after injury in humans is not so good. Body temperature is reduced acutely after injury and the reduction is directly related to its severity (Fig. 16.8). It is, however, difficult to conclude that these changes are central in origin because plasma lactate concentrations are elevated after the most serious injuries and an impairment of oxygen transport cannot be excluded. There is some evidence for a change in thermoregulatory control at this time; patients do not shiver despite having body temperatures below the normal threshold for its onset and also the appreciation of thermal comfort is modified. Measurements of metabolic rate at this time after injury have not provided convincing evidence for a controlled reduction in metabolic rate, for example, as measured by indirect calorimetry.

Oxygen consumption calculated by a modification of the Fick equation is often higher than predicted in severely injured patients both before and after resuscitation. A possible limitation of this approach, especially after treatment, is that any manoeuvre that increases cardiac output might also be expected to increase the value for oxygen consumption, because this is calculated by a method that includes cardiac output. The consensus is that there is no evidence for a reduction in body temperature and metabolic rate acutely after injury in humans that cannot be attributed to a failure of oxygen transport or necrobiosis. However, this may not be too surprising if it is remembered that many of the measurements have been made at ambient temperatures close to or within the thermoneutral range, which may of course be extended after injury.

It is also important to realise that the continuous thermoregulatory variable in humans is heat loss, and not heat production as in the rat. Therefore, although changes

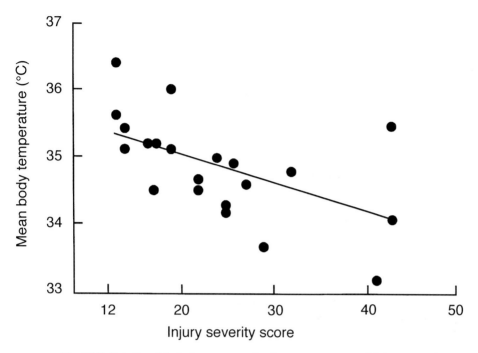

Fig. 16.8. Relationship between mean body temperature and injury severity score acutely after injury in humans. (From Little, R. A. & Stoner, H. B. (1981). *British Journal of Surgery*, 68, 221–224.)

in heat production (oxygen consumption) have been studied in the rat, clinical studies would, perhaps, be better focused on the mechanisms of heat loss at this time. Indeed, a detailed study of heat balance has shown an inhibition of heat loss and an upward resetting of thermoregulation to achieve an increase in heat content within the first 12 hours after a burning injury in children.

Cardiovascular response to haemorrhage and tissue injury

Haemorrhage

Haemorrhage induces a progressive increase in heart rate and peripheral vascular resistance as a result of activation of the baroreceptor reflex (Fig. 16.9). With blood losses of up to 10–15% of blood volume, this mechanism will maintain mean arterial blood pressure and oxygen delivery to flow-dependent organs such as the brain and heart at the expense of other vascular beds, for example those in the gut and skeletal muscle. This redistribution of cardiac output, mediated by a differential activation of efferent sympathetic vasoconstrictor activity, is certainly protective in the short term, but it is possible that the reduction in splanchnic flow may be of greater significance than thought previously. The integrity of the mucosa, especially at the tips of the villi, is susceptible to relatively small reductions in flow. This may be related to the increase in the translocation

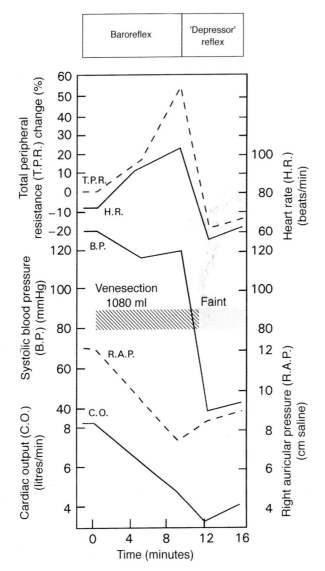

Fig. 16.9. Cardiovascular response to progressive simple haemorrhage. (From Barcroft, H. *et al.* (1944). *Lancet*, i, 489–491.)

of endotoxin and microorganisms from the gut lumen, which have been associated with hypovolaemia following injury and haemorrhage (see below).

    As the severity of haemorrhage increases and exceeds 20% of the blood volume, there is a dramatic change in the pattern of cardiovascular response. Heart rate and arterial blood pressure both fall dramatically (Fig. 16.9). The bradycardia does not result from failure of the heart but is reflex and mediated by the vagus following stimulation of cardiac vagal C-fibre afferents by distortions of the ventricular wall. The effects on blood pressure of this sudden reflex fall in heart rate will be exacerbated by the vasodilatation in skeletal muscle that also occurs following stimulation of cardiac vagal C-fibre afferents.

Since the efferent limb mediating the cardio-inhibitory component of the depressor reflex is carried in the vagus nerve, it is not surprising that the bradycardia associated with severe haemorrhage can be prevented by treatment with atropine. However, the administration of atropine alone under these circumstances is not to be recommended (unless there is very severe bradycardia or asystole), since it has been suggested that the depressor reflex may serve to protect the heart by reducing cardiac work at a time when coronary blood flow is compromised. Indeed, there have been clinical reports that the administration of atropine under these circumstances may be deleterious. The logical treatment is to restore blood volume and hence reduce the activation of the reflex, whereupon the bradycardia should correct itself.

A third reflex of importance in the cardiovascular response to haemorrhage is the arterial chemoreceptor reflex. The arterial chemoreceptors are found in the carotid and aortic bodies, close to the carotid sinus and aortic arch, respectively. They respond to changes in oxygen tension: a fall in oxygen tension increasing chemoreceptor afferent activity. In addition, increases in carbon dioxide tension and falls in arterial blood pH increase the sensitivity of the arterial chemoreceptors to hypoxia. Stimulation of arterial chemoreceptors produces an increase in respiration, while the primary cardiovascular effects are a vagally mediated bradycardia and a vasoconstriction in, for example, skeletal muscle, which is caused by increased sympathetic vasoconstrictor tone. This pattern of response is subsequently modified by the increased respiratory activity, which tends to inhibit both the vagal activity to the heart and the sympathetic vasoconstrictor activity.

Following a severe haemorrhage, the arterial chemoreceptors are activated as a result of a reduction in blood flow through the carotid and aortic bodies secondary to the fall in arterial blood pressure, and to sympathetic vasoconstriction in the bodies themselves, mediated by the local release of both noradrenaline and its co-transmitter neuropeptide Y. Therefore, during the hypotensive phase of a severe haemorrhage, stimulation of the arterial chemoreceptors may prevent arterial blood pressure falling even further and may be responsible for the increase in respiration noted following severe haemorrhage. Since an increase in respiratory activity has been shown to reduce the reflex bradycardia produced by stimulation of cardiac C-fibre afferents, it is possible that the enhanced respiratory activity seen following a severe haemorrhage may attenuate the bradycardia that occurs under these circumstances. This interaction between the respiratory and cardiovascular responses to chemoreceptor stimulation may also have implications for the treatment of injured patients. For example, procedures such as intubation, which inhibit respiratory activity, can unmask a dangerous bradycardia. The role of the chemoreceptors in helping to maintain blood pressure will, of course, be increased in the injured patient with thoracic injuries, which may impair pulmonary function.

Tissue injury

Simple haemorrhage is relatively uncommon and is usually accompanied by different amounts of tissue damage. Before considering how the presence of concomitant tissue injury modifies the cardiovascular response to haemorrhage, it is important to consider the cardiovascular changes elicited by tissue injury and their mediation. Tissue injury or ischaemia cause an increase in arterial blood pressure and a tachycardia, rather than the bradycardia that would be expected were the baroreceptor reflex functioning normally. This is a pattern of response similar to the defence reaction or preparation for fight or flight. This pattern of response is possible because there is a concomitant reduction in the sensitivity and a rightward resetting (i.e. towards a higher arterial blood pressure) of the baroreflex following 'injury'. The reduction in baroreceptor reflex sensitivity in humans is evident within 3 hours of injury of moderate severity (e.g. fracture of a long bone) and is persistent such that only partial recovery has occurred at 14 days after 'injury'. This impairment of the baroreceptor reflex is accompanied by a persistent tachycardia that is not related to hypovolaemia, and by a reduction in the variation in heart rate induced by respiration.

The afferent pathway for the response to injury runs in nociceptive fibres originating in the damaged tissues, ascends in the spinal cord and projects to a number of areas in the brain. The area of particular interest with regard to the response to injury is the periaqueductal grey region of the mid-brain, which is part of the brain's endogenous opioid system. Electrolytic lesions of this area prevent the reduction in baroreflex sensitivity normally seen following injury. Also the effects of injury on the baroreflex can be mimicked by the intracerebroventricular injection of metencephalin and prevented or reversed by naloxone (see below). This is just one example of the very complex central interaction between cardiovascular and nociceptive afferents associated with trauma and the descending pathways mediating antinociception and autonomic efferent activity.

Haemorrhage and tissue injury

When tissue injury is combined with haemorrhage, the cardiovascular responses to blood loss are markedly modified. Thus, the tachycardia elicited by small blood losses is reduced while the bradycardia associated with larger losses is prevented (Fig. 16.10).

This inhibition of the vagal bradycardia is central, since a long-lasting inhibition of cardiac pre-ganglionic motoneurones in the nucleus ambiguus has been demonstrated following electrical stimulation of nociceptive afferent fibres. Somatic afferent stimulation (e.g. of the sciatic nerve) is also able to block the vagal bradycardia evoked by stimulation of either the nucleus tractus solitarius or cardiac C-fibre afferents. This attenuation of the changes in heart rate normally associated with blood loss seems to offer some degree of protection against the hypotensive effects of a severe haemorrhage. However, this protection may be more apparent than real. Recent studies have demonstrated that superimposition of somatic afferent nerve activity (to simulate 'injury'), or a real injury, upon haemorrhage produces greater falls in cardiac index and systemic oxygen delivery than those produced by an equivalent 'simple' haemorrhage. Furthermore, animals subjected to haemorrhage and concomitant electrical stimulation of the sciatic nerve (to stimulate 'injury') had a lower survival rate compared with animals subjected to haemorrhage alone. It is possible that the better maintenance of

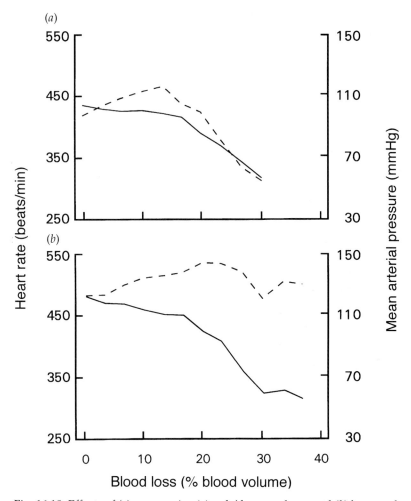

Fig. 16.10. Effects of (*a*) progressive 'simple' haemorrhage and (*b*) haemorrhage in the presence of limb ischaemia on heart rate (−−−) and mean arterial blood pressure (—) in the conscious rat. (From Kirkman, E. & Little R. A. (1994), In *Blood Loss and Shock*, ed. N. Secher *et al.*, pp. 61–75. London: Arnold.

blood pressure is achieved at the expense of intense peripheral vasoconstriction, leading to ischaemic organ damage that will exacerbate the severity of injury. It is tempting to speculate that the splanchnic circulation may be selectively vulnerable to such ischaemic damage, leading to the release of blood-borne factors that may impair cardiovascular function. Intestinal permeability may also be increased, leading to enhanced translocation of bacteria and endotoxin.

These studies of the changes in cardiovascular control after injury may help explain the limited value of heart rate as an index of blood loss, noted in casualties during the First and Second World Wars. Blood pressure is also a poor indicator of blood loss, falling only when homeostasis is overwhelmed. It has been proposed that the ratio of heart rate to blood pressure (the *Shock Index*) may be a more reliable guide (Fig. 16.11). The Shock

(*a*)

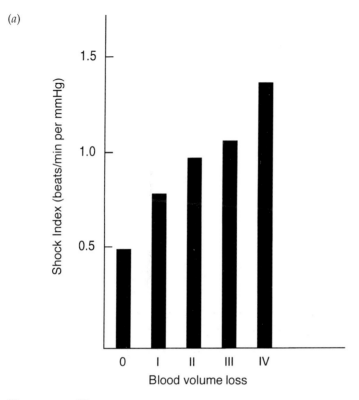

(*b*)

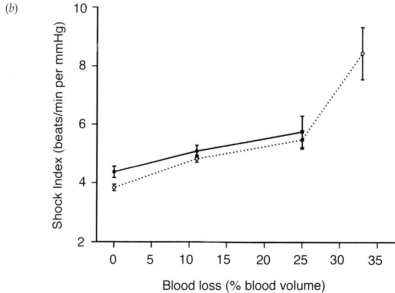

Fig. 16.11. (*a*) The relationship between the Shock Index and the magnitude of blood volume loss (grouped in increasing magnitude from O to IV) in humans. (*b*) Changes in the shock index with progressive 'simple' haemorrhage (●) and haemorrhage in the presence of limb ischaemia (○) in the conscious rat (compare with Fig. 16.10). ((*a*) From Allgöwer, M. & Burri, C. (1967). *Deutsche Medizinische Wochenschrift*, 43, 1–10.)

Table 16.3. *Resuscitation fluids*

Saline (0.9%)
Hypertonic saline (3, 5 & 7.5%)
Ringer's lactate
Gum acacia
Albumin
Plasma protein fraction
Dextran 40, 70
Hypertonic/hyperosmotic solution (7.5% NaCl/6% Dextran 70)
Hydroxyethylstarch
Pentastarch
Gelatin
Blood
Stroma-free haemoglobin
Fluosol

Index increases progressively with increasing blood loss and does not seem to be influenced by the presence of nociceptive afferent stimulation. Also abnormal Shock Index values have been noted in injured patients assessed as physiologically 'normal' by the Revised Trauma Score.

Fluid resuscitation

The goal of fluid resuscitation after injury is to replenish the intravascular volume and thereby maintain cardiac output and, more importantly, tissue oxygen delivery (the product of cardiac output and arterial oxygen content). The distribution of the cardiac output to those tissues with the lowest tolerance of oxygen-lack will, as already described, be helped by the non-uniform increase in sympathetic vasoconstrictor fibre activity elicited by hypovolaemia. The transfusion of asanguineous fluids will restore cardiac output but will, by lowering the haematocrit, reduce arterial oxygen content and hence tissue oxygen delivery. Fortunately, tissues can compensate for a reduction in delivery by increasing the extraction of oxygen from the blood delivered to them. Normally only 25% of the delivered oxygen is extracted, leaving a considerable margin for safety; however, some organs, such as the liver and heart, have a much higher oxygen extraction and are, therefore, very susceptible to a reduction in the tissue oxygen delivery.

   A range of resuscitation solutions (Table 16.3) has been suggested and a considerable debate has persisted over the relative merits of crystalloid versus colloid. The consensus seems to be that after trauma in young patients large volumes of lactated Ringer's solution can be given and this is very effective in restoring, for example, blood pressure. However, it is important to consider what 'end-point' should be used during resuscitation. Blood pressure, heart rate and central venous pressure are easy to measure but unfortunately they are poor indicators of blood volume and tissue oxygen delivery. If delivery is measured, it has been shown that colloids and, not surprisingly, blood are the more effective agents. Therefore, a given volume of colloid restores intravascular volume more efficiently than the same volume of lactated Ringer's solution.

A concern about the use of large volumes of crystalloid has been the risk of precipitating tissue oedema (especially in the lungs). Fortunately, these fears have proved unfounded in the young, previously healthy trauma patients, but care is needed in the treatment of the elderly or those with reduced physiological reserve as a result of pre-existing disease. In an attempt to minimise any adverse effects of giving large amounts of crystalloid solutions, hypertonic (7.5% NaCl) and hypertonic/hyperosomotic (7.5% NaCl/6% Dextran 70) solutions given in small volumes have been introduced. These have been shown to be effective in restoring whole body haemodynamics and microvascular perfusion. However, it must be remembered that such solutions replete the intravascular space at the expense of the extravascular and intracellular volumes.

In most cases of severe trauma, blood has to be given at some time because there is clearly a limit to the amount of haemodilution that can be offset by increases in oxygen extraction. The short shelf-life of blood and problems with incompatibility and, more recently, viral contamination have led to the development of a number of oxygen-carrying blood substitutes. These include preparations of haemoglobin and a range of perfluorochemicals. Whilst the haemoglobin solutions retain the characteristics of the oxyhaemoglobin dissociation curve of whole blood, the perfluorochemicals require a high 'inspired' oxygen concentration to dissolve enough oxygen to enhance tissue oxygen delivery.

Pharmacological modulation of the cardiovascular responses to haemorrhage and injury

The endogenous opioids

There is evidence suggesting that the endogenous opioid system may be involved in the response to severe hypovolaemia. Most of the evidence suggests a role for the opioid system in the sympatho-inhibitory response. However, there is also some, albeit weaker, evidence suggesting a role in the bradycardic response. Therefore, the opioid antagonist naloxone, when given intravenously, was shown to attenuate the reduction in sympathetic efferent activity and the associated hypotension (and possibly the bradycardia) that accompanies severe hypovolaemia. Naloxone is thought to exert its effect, in this case, via an antagonist action at δ-opiate receptors within the medulla. It should be stressed here that although the administration of naloxone, or of a more specific δ-opioid receptor antagonist, blocked the sympatho-inhibition, the effects of δ-receptor antagonism on the bradycardia were less clear. This may be because of the relatively small bradycardic response to severe hypovolaemia even in the absence of δ-receptor antagonism in these studies, which were conducted on rabbits. Since δ-opioid receptor antagonism appears to block *both* the vagal and the sympathetic component of the response to severe hypovolaemia, it is likely that the endogenous opioids are important early in the reflex pathway, before the two limbs diverge. One likely area for this effect is the nucleus tractus solitarius, which contains a dense population of δ-opioid receptors.

In addition to the δ-opioid receptors, the μ- and the κ-opioid receptors also appear to be capable of modifying the response to severe hypovolaemia. Thus, μ- and κ-receptor *agonists* can prevent the reflex sympatho-inhibition (and possibly the bradycardia) seen during severe hypovolaemia. However, it is unlikely that the μ-opioid receptor participates in the normal 'physiological' response to severe haemorrhage, although the use of μ-receptor agonists, e.g. the anaesthetics fentanyl and alfentanyl, may provide a pharmacological means of inhibiting the depressor effect of a severe haemorrhage.

Since 'injury' is also known to activate the endogenous opioid system, and cell bodies that synthesise and release encephalins are found in the periaqueductal grey, an area known to be involved in the cardiovascular response to 'injury' (see above), it is not surprising to learn that naloxone can modify the response to 'injury'. It has been demonstrated in experimental studies that the administration of naloxone, either centrally or intravenously, can prevent or reverse the reduction in baroreflex sensitivity produced by 'injury'. Conversely, some of the effects of 'injury' on the baroreflex can be mimicked by the central administration of a long-lasting analogue of metencephalin.

5-Hydroxytryptamine

There have been suggestions that 5-HT may also be involved in the central nervous pathways mediating the response to severe haemorrhage. For example, a cardiovascular response that includes the 'cardiac reflex' elicited by activation of cardiac-vagal C-fibre afferents can be blocked by methiothepin (a 5-HT_{1A} receptor antagonist) given centrally. Furthermore, blockade of the 5-HT system, either with *p*-chlorophenylalanine (PCPA, which blocks the synthesis of 5-HT), or with the 5-HT receptor antagonist methysergide has been reported to prevent or reverse both the sympatho-inhibitory and the bradycardic response to severe blood loss, while leaving baroreflex control intact. Although the 5-HT blocking agents were given intravenously in the latter study, their sites of action are likely to be central, since any effect of 5-HT on the ventricular receptors is mediated via 5-HT_3 receptors where methysergide has little activity.

However, the effects of 5-HT blockade on the response to severe blood loss are equivocal, since other studies have failed to show that PCPA blocks the depressor response to severe haemorrhage. They have also suggested that the action of agents such as methysergide is not blockade of 5-HT receptors but rather is agonistic at 5-HT_{1A} receptors. Also the 5-HT_{1A} receptor antagonist methiothepin fails to attenuate the reflex bradycardia that accompanies severe haemorrhage, unlike its effects on the 'cardiac reflex', suggesting that the two responses may be mediated via different central nervous pathways.

General anaesthetic agents

General anaesthetic agents merit consideration for at least two reasons; first, they are often given to trauma victims and, second, they may have differential effects on the reflexes involved in the responses to haemorrhage and injury and hence may alter the clinical signs in such patients. A number of agents, for example the barbiturates, attenu-

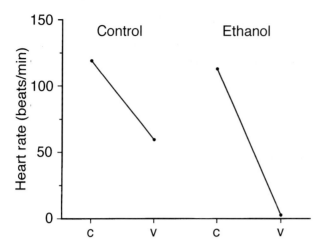

Fig. 16.12. Heart rate recorded before (C) and during stimulation of the cardiac C-fibre afferents with veratridine (V; 1.43 μg/kg) injected into the left atrium in an artificially ventilated dog anaesthetised with α-chloralose. The response was repeated before (control) and during an intravenous infusion of ethanol sufficient to produce blood levels of 138.9 mg% ethanol in the same dog. Note that although this is an unusually large potentiation of the response to cardiac C-fibre stimulation, it demonstrates the degree of potentiation that can be seen in some individuals.

ate the baroreceptor reflex, whereas other agents (e.g. propofol) attenuate the response to stimulation of the cardiac C-fibre afferents while leaving the baroreceptor reflex intact. Thus, a patient suffering a simple haemorrhage and anaesthetised with propofol may show the initial tachycardic response (see above) but not the later bradycardia as the haemorrhage progresses. Similarly, the barbiturates attenuate the cardiovascular response to injury while others, such as propofol, leave the response largely intact.

Ethanol

Ethanol is a drug taken socially, often preceding events such as an automobile accident that lead to trauma. The effects of ethanol on the cardiovascular response to haemorrhage and 'injury' are, therefore, of interest. Recent studies have shown that moderately raised blood levels of ethanol (100–200 mg%) can exacerbate the 'injury'-induced reduction in baroreflex sensitivity. Also, similar plasma ethanol concentrations can markedly increase the bradycardia elicited by stimulation of the cardiac C-fibres afferents (Fig. 16.12). This potentiation may be very marked and might underlie the association between acute alcoholic intoxication and the hypotension without a tachycardia reported following relatively minor trauma. Furthermore, it is possible that in susceptible individuals, ethanol may precipitate a cardiac arrest following a severe haemorrhage.

The ethanol-induced augmentation of the baroreflex-inhibitory effects of injury may reflect the ability of ethanol to potentiate the central effects of endogenous GABA, which is thought to be involved in the inhibition of the baroreflex induced by injury.

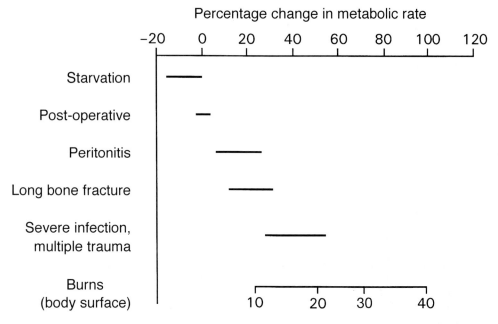

Fig. 16.13. Changes in metabolic rate during starvation and illness. The bars indicate ranges. (From Arnold, J. & Little, R. A. (1991)). *Current Anaesthesia and Critical Care*, 2, 139–148.)

The flow phase

Metabolic rate and thermoregulation

The characteristic features of the flow phase are increases in metabolic rate, body temperature and urinary nitrogen excretion plus reductions in body weight and, most importantly, lean body mass. The increase in metabolic rate has been claimed to be directly related to the severity of injury, with the largest increases occurring after burns exceeding 40–50% of body surface area (Fig. 16.13). This relationship is not always very obvious because the hypermetabolic response to injury is often superimposed on a background of reduced food intake and loss of muscle mass, both of which reduce metabolic rate. The situation can be further complicated by treatment, for example after head injury the use of neuromuscular blockade and steroids: the latter exacerbating the catabolic loss of lean body mass.

Metabolic rate may also be limited by the supply of oxygen to the tissue. It has been suggested that in the severely injured patients oxygen delivery should be increased to supranormal levels by the use of intravenous fluids, inotropic agents and artificial ventilation, with high inspired oxygen concentrations to ensure that oxygen consumption is not limited by its supply. Therapy directed towards increasing cardiac output, tissue oxygen delivery and arterial oxygen content to values that were associated with survival in retrospective studies have been shown to improve outcome in prospective clinical trials. However, the best results are achieved in patients who have enough physiological reserve to achieve such therapeutic goals with fluid loads and ventilation alone. If agents such as dopamine or dobutamine are used, it is important to realise that they, of themselves, increase oxygen consumption even in normal subjects. When oxygen delivery is inadequate and oxygen consumption cannot be maintained by increased oxygen extraction, then a vicious cycle of anaerobic metabolism, depletion of energy stores and increasing tissue damage will occur: the 'necrobiotic' or irreversible phase of the response to injury.

If it is accepted that metabolic rate is increased in the flow phase, it is important to understand its pathogenesis. Burns in which there are large increases in evaporative water loss have been the area studied most comprehensively. The energy costs of the latent heat of evaporation has to be met by an increase in metabolic rate; although the water loss can be reduced by the use of impermeable dressings, there is no agreement on the effect this has on metabolic rate. There is also little agreement on the effects of off-setting the increase in evaporative heat loss by reducing dry heat losses by increasing ambient temperature. In some hands, this abolishes the hypermetabolism while others have been able to demonstrate only a small reduction. Indeed it has been suggested that the dissociation between the evaporative water loss and hypermetabolism and the persistence of an elevated metabolic rate at a raised environmental temperature are evidence for an upward resetting in hypothalamic thermoregulatory control (see below).

Sympathetic nervous system

This upward resetting of thermoregulation after thermal injury leads to an increase in sympathetic nervous activity, and it is the increase in catecholamine release that mediates the increase in energy production. There is a positive relation between urinary catecholamine excretion and metabolic rate, which can be reduced by combined adrenergic blockade. However, although plasma catecholamine concentrations remain increased during the flow phase response to burns and to severe head injury, they have returned to normal after severe musculoskeletal injuries. Normal plasma catecholamine concentrations do not necessarily reflect normal activity of the sympathetic nervous system. In severe sepsis, increases in adrenaline release are balanced by increases in its uptake such that plasma adrenaline concentrations do not rise.

One way in which increased sympathetic activity may stimulate metabolic rate is by the enhanced exchange between NEFAs and triacylglycerol, both within adipose tissues and via plasma NEFAs, which can be blocked by propranolol. In addition, there is a concomitant increase in exchange between glucose and glycolytic products; it has been calculated that at least 15% of the flow-phase increase in metabolic rate can be accounted for by this substrate cycling.

The wound

The wound, which can be considered as an extra organ, also contributes to the glucose cycling. Lactate, produced by aerobic glycolysis in the wound, is transported to the liver where it is converted to glucose (via the Cori cycle), which is then returned to fuel the wound. The wound will also contribute to the increase in metabolic rate in a number of other ways. It has a hyperaemic circulation, which is not under neural control, and will require an increase in cardiac output, incurring extra energy expenditure by the heart. The inflammatory cells localised in the wound are themselves metabolically very active and will release a number of cytokines that have been implicated in the generation of fever via a prostaglandin-mediated upward resetting of the hypothalamic set-point.

Cytokines

The hypermetabolism that persists in injured patients for several weeks following the accident is often accompanied by a rise in body temperature: first described as 'traumatic fever'. By definition, fever represents a regulated rise in the hypothalamic set-point around which body temperature is normally maintained. It can be distinguished from hyperthermia, an uncontrolled rise in body temperature resulting from impaired heat dissipation or overwhelming environmental or metabolic heat. Apart from burn injury where the rise in body temperature is defended over a range of ambient temperatures, the thermoregulatory responses to other injuries have not been clearly defined. Investigation of the mechanisms involved in the hypermetabolic responses to disease has concentrated on experimental models of fever, whether they are induced following 'infectious' (endotoxin) or inflammatory (turpentine) stimuli. Following uncomplicated injury, it seems likely that similar mechanisms may be involved in the raised body temperature and metabolic rate, particularly since the cytokines IL-1, IL-6 and TNF-α are all endogenous pyrogens and are thought to be important in other metabolic aspects of the host response to injury.

IL-1 is the most potent endogenous pyrogen. Although raised plasma concentrations of IL-1 are rarely observed during fever and hypermetabolism, the use of neutralising antibodies and antagonists to IL-1 action have enabled the precise role of IL-1 during fever and hypermetabolism to be investigated. One of the most useful tools for these studies has been the discovery of the naturally occurring IL-1 receptor antagonist (IL-1RA). IL-1RA is co-secreted with IL-1 and is observed in the circulation following a number of inflammatory stimuli. In rodents, IL-1RA binds preferentially but not specifically to the type I IL-1 receptor, although in humans it has equal affinity for both the type I and type II receptor subtypes. Therefore, administration of IL-1RA, at least to rodents, can help to distinguish between the IL-1 receptor subtypes, as well as determine the role of endogenous IL-1 in fever and hypermetabolism. Peripheral but not central administration of IL-1RA inhibits the sustained febrile and hypermetabolic responses to turpentine injection in the rat. Since no detectable increases in plasma IL-1 concentrations are observed following turpentine injection, IL-1 is presumably released at the site of injury and via a secondary mediator induces fever and hypermetabolism. IL-1RA also inhibits endotoxin-induced fever but, as with turpentine-induced fever, it is only effective when administered peripherally.

Raised plasma concentrations of TNF-α are observed during experimentally induced fever and hypermetabolism; however, this response is transient and precedes the metabolic response (Fig. 16.14). Following intramuscular turpentine injection, no increase in

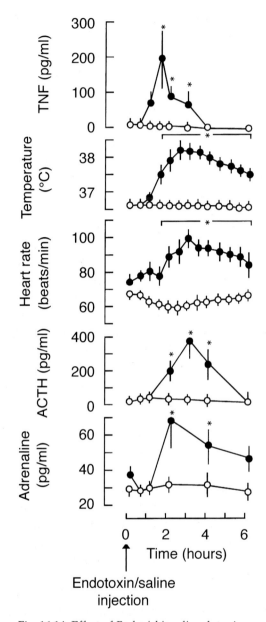

Fig. 16.14. Effect of *Escherichia coli* endotoxin on plasma TNF, ACTH and adrenaline concentrations and heart rate and body temperature in humans: ●, endotoxin; ○, saline; *$p < 0.05$. (From Mitchie, H. R. *et al.* (1988). *New England Journal of Medicine.* 318, 1481–1486.)

circulating TNF-α is observed; however peripheral injection of a neutralising TNF-α antiserum reduces the fever and hypermetabolism associated with turpentine injection. This indicates that local production of this cytokine presumably at the site of tissue injury (as with IL-1) causes fever and hypermetabolism, at least in this model of localised tissue injury.

Plasma concentrations of IL-6 are often correlated with the magnitude of a fever; it has been suggested that IL-6 is the putative circulating endogenous pyrogen. Following turpentine injection, the source of IL-6 is the inflamed limb (site of turpentine injection), and as inhibition of IL-1 and TNF-α action can markedly suppress the rise in plasma IL-6 concentration, it would appear that IL-6 does act as the circulating pyrogen for locally released IL-1 and TNF-α in this model.

How IL-6 or any circulating cytokine enters the brain to increase the set-point for body temperature and stimulate thermogenesis is unclear, as these peptides are probably too large (17–26 kDa) to diffuse passively across the blood–brain barrier. A carrier system for IL-1 has been identified; however, the amount of IL-1 that can enter the brain from the periphery via this mechanism is less than 1%. As circulating concentrations of IL-1 during disease are usually low, it is unlikely that enough IL-1 could pass into the brain to elicit centrally mediated responses. An alternative explanation is that cytokines act on, or near, the circumventricular organs, particularly the OVLT (organum vasculosum laminae terminalis), which lack a blood–brain barrier, and induce the release of brain-derived cytokines or secondary mediators such as the prostaglandins.

During fever, the cerebrospinal fluid concentrations of prostaglandins, particularly PGE_2 increases. As prostaglandins, but not other eicosanoid products such as the thromboxanes and leukotrienes, are able to act directly on thermosensitive neurones within the hypothalamus, they have been proposed as the final common mediators of fever, particularly as they mediate the pyrogenic and thermogenic actions of IL-1, IL-6 and TNF-α both peripherally and centrally within the brain. Administration of cyclo-oxygenase inhibitors attenuates febrile responses following injury in the rat and burn injury and endotoxin administration in humans. Interestingly, topical application of a cyclo-oxygenase inhibitor to the wound also reduces the hypermetabolic responses to burn injury in animals, suggesting that locally released prostaglandins are responsible for burn-induced hypermetabolism.

Although the cytokines and prostaglandins are the most likely mediators of the febrile and hypermetabolic responses to injury, release of the catabolic hormones may also stimulate these responses. The simultaneous infusion of the catabolic hormones cortisol, glucagon and adrenaline into healthy volunteers increases resting energy expenditure but does not cause a rise in body temperature. Infusion of the hormones individually increases resting energy expenditure; however, the magnitude of these responses are less than that observed during the combined infusion. The infusion rates of hormones used in these studies were chosen to mimic the plasma concentrations usually observed in injured patients. However, although the plasma hormone concentrations achieved did reflect those found acutely after injury, they were higher than those observed during the later hypermetabolic response to injury (see below) (Table 16.4). The modest increases in energy expenditure observed in these studies suggest that the catabolic hormones are not the principal mediators of the hypermetabolic responses to injury. Instead, it is far more likely that a combination of endocrine- and cytokine-mediated responses are responsible.

Table 16.4. *Plasma concentrations of counter-regulatory hormones in the flow phase of injury response in humans*

	Adrenaline (nmol/1)	Cortisol (nmol/l)	Glucagon (mg/l)
Sepsis	0.8±0.3	674±88	154±20
Trauma	0.29±0.04	420±30	170±20
Triple hormone infusion[a]	2.4±1.8	1050±400	480±160
Normal levels	0.3	300	130

Notes:
Results expressed as mean±S.D.
[a] The infusion rate was chosen to mimic the plasma concentrations usually observed in injured patients.
Source: Data for triple hormone from Bessey, P. Q. *et al.* (1984), *Annals of Surgery*, 200, 264–280.

Protein and amino acid metabolism

The increased urinary output of nitrogen and the muscle wasting observed after injury have led to the suggestion that an increased rate of amino acid oxidation was largely responsible for the hypermetabolism of the flow phase. It now seems that the contribution of protein oxidation is not as great as previously assumed, representing no more than 20% of whole body expenditure in the severely catabolic patient. An exception may be after head injuries where, even in the absence of steroid treatment, the contribution of protein oxidation is as high as 30%.

Whole body protein turnover is increased after injury, with the balance between synthesis and breakdown being modified by the severity of injury and the influence of nutritional intake on synthesis. Thus, increasing severity of injury causes increasing rates of both synthesis and breakdown, whilst accompanying undernutrition reduces synthesis. However, after the most severe injuries, the increase in breakdown predominates and cannot be countered by even the most aggressive nutritional support.

The most obvious site of the net increase in protein breakdown is skeletal muscle, although it is likely that, just as in starvation, muscle in the diaphragm, the wall of the gut and the heart is also affected. The breakdown of myofibrillar protein is reflected by the increase in urinary excretion of 3-methylhistidine, which is directly related to the amount of damaged muscle. However, the use of 3-methylhistidine as a specific marker of skeletal muscle breakdown is complicated by its liberation from other organs such as the gut. The increases in urinary creatine after injury is, however, directly related to the degree of injury as indicated by the injury severity score (Fig. 16.15), although much of the creatine comes from muscle distant from the site of injury, emphasising the general nature of the catabolic flow phase.

The increase in proteolysis provides amino acids as precursors for hepatic gluconeogenesis. Although the plasma levels of a number of amino acids, such as alanine, fall at this time, their hepatic extraction is increased because of increases in hepatic blood flow. The increase in hepatic gluconeogenesis, at a time when plasma

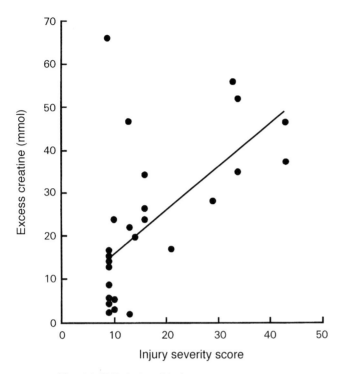

Fig. 16.15. Relationship between excess creatine output in the urine and the injury severity score. (From Threlfall, C. J. *et al.* (1984). *Journal of Trauma* 24, 516–523.)

concentrations of glucose and insulin are increased, is one of the facets of insulin resistance discussed in more detail below. One amino acid of particular interest is glutamine, the intracellular concentration of which falls after injury from its normally high levels. The glutamine released from muscle is an important fuel for the lymphocytes and macrophages activated by injury. Also, it has recently been implicated in the maintenance of the gut mucosa, the integrity of which may be compromised after injury.

Carbohydrate metabolism

Hyperglycaemia and inappropriately high plasma insulin concentrations are features of the flow phase although an exception to this pattern may be seen after very severe injuries, such as burns, where the prolonged rise in plasma catecholamine concentrations maintains adrenergic suppression of insulin secretion. There is also an exaggerated pancreatic insulin response to glucose, which may be related to the increased plasma concentration of arginine, an insulin secretagogue. The concomitant elevations of plasma glucose and plasma insulin concentration are the hall-marks of insulin resistance, which involves both liver and muscle. Also hepatic glucose production is not inhibited as expected by hyperglycaemia and hyperinsulinaemia during the flow phase.

There is an increase in glucose turnover at this time, although because of the prevailing insulin resistance, the peripheral utilisation of glucose is less than expected from

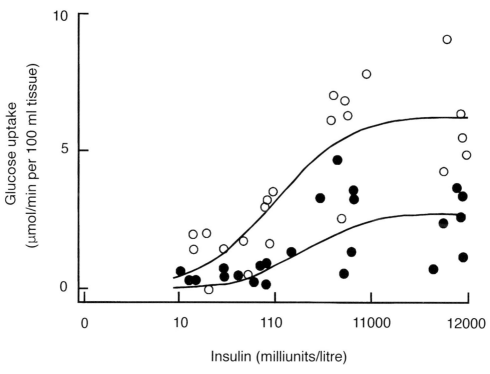

Fig. 16.16. Effect of insulin on forearm glucose uptake in injured patients (●) and control subjects (○). (From Henderson, A. A. *et al.* (1991). *Clinical Science*, 80, 25–32.)

the raised glucose and insulin concentrations (Fig. 16.16). This impairment of glucose disposal has been demonstrated using glucose/insulin clamp techniques after thermal and non-thermal injuries and also in septic surgical patients. As expected, part of the insulin resistance is found in uninjured skeletal muscle. The relationship between glucose uptake and plasma insulin concentration shows a marked reduction in the maximum response and in the sensitivity to insulin, suggesting changes in both receptor binding of insulin and intracellular pathways.

An important role has been suggested for the counter-regulatory or catabolic hormones (e.g. glucagon, adrenaline, cortisol and growth hormone) in the pathogenesis of insulin resistance. The plasma concentrations of all these hormones are elevated at sometime during the response to injury. Infusions of glucagon, adrenaline and cortisol over a 3 day period mimic some of the features of the flow phase: peripheral insulin resistance and increases in metabolic rate (see above) and urinary nitrogen excretion. However, as mentioned above, the plasma concentrations of these hormones needed to elicit this pattern of response are closer to those found in the acute ebb phase rather than in the flow phase. In the latter, the endogenous levels of these hormones are falling, except after the most severe injuries, to or close to normal. The suggestion is that other humoral factors may have a role, and once again the cytokines are likely candidates. They are able to reproduce by central and peripheral mechanisms many of the acute- and flow-phase responses to injury, such as acute-phase protein synthesis, central resetting of metabolic activity (see above), muscle protein catabolism and changes in glucose homeostasis. It is perhaps an oversimplification to assume that any single cytokine is predominant; they may have an important role by acting collectively in a co-ordinated way, both locally and systemically.

Once glucose has been taken up during the flow phase, it seems that in those receiving low-dose glucose infusions or those receiving enteral carbohydrate its rate of oxidation is increased. However in clamp studies when large amounts of glucose or insulin are given to either injured or septic patients, there is evidence that glucose oxidation is impaired. Indeed, in such patients fat oxidation, which should be suppressed, persists (see below).

Fat metabolism

As the flow phase progresses, plasma NEFA concentrations fall as the sympathetic drive to lipolysis wanes, although after major injuries such as severe burns they may remain high. Fatty acid oxidation is, however, greater than expected from the plasma NEFA concentration. Turnover, which is normally directly proportional to concentration is also disproportionately increased, although there is no clear relationship between NEFA turnover and oxidation. The turnover of endogenous and of infused triacylglycerol is also enhanced in the hypermetabolic state. Injury causes similar changes in the relationship between the turnover and the plasma concentration of glycerol. Thus, in patients with burns, glycerol turnover is increased in relation to its concentration and also to the turnover of NEFAs, implying increased re-esterification within adipose tissue.

In the fasted uninjured subject, fat oxidation is suppressed by insulin released after the intravenous administration of large amounts of glucose. However in hypermetabolic patients, this suppression is incomplete and fat oxidation continues. The reason for this continuing preferential oxidation of fat is not known, but it is an important factor to be considered when planning the nutritional support of the injured/septic patient.

Modification of the responses to injury

The factors modifying the responses to injury can be considered as constitutional (e.g. age and nutritional status) or external (e.g. ambient temperature and drugs).

Age

The acute metabolic and hormonal responses to injury are certainly not reduced in the elderly compared with the young. Instead, there is evidence that for a given severity of injury the plasma concentrations of glucose and lipid metabolites (NEFAs, triacylglycerol and ketone bodies) are higher in elderly patients. This may, however, be explained in part by the preponderance in this age group of females, who exhibit greater lipolysis than men after surgical trauma. These results must be interpreted in the light of the finding of increased 'resting' concentrations of NEFAs and glycerol in the elderly.

In other words, a similar response to injury may be superimposed on a different background.

When considering the flow-phase metabolic response, the contributions of fat oxidation and of NEFA/triacylglycerol cycling to total energy expenditure are less in the elderly than in younger injured patients. Ageing causes changes in carbohydrate metabolism, but little is known of the interaction with the response to injury. An impairment of peripheral glucose uptake is associated with ageing that does not seem to be caused by the loss of muscle mass. Immobility and an impairment of insulin secretion may play a part, but the major factor seems to be a reduction in peripheral tissue sensitivity to insulin. A study of elderly patients following accidental injury has suggested that insulin resistance may last for longer in the aged than in the younger patients. This may be a result of the persistent elevation of plasma cortisol concentrations, which is a feature of the response to injury in the elderly. The mechanism of this is unclear, although it may involve changes in cortisol clearance and in the central control of cortisol secretion. In addition to its effects on carbohydrate metabolism, the persistently elevated plasma cortisol levels may increase skeletal muscle catabolism.

Ageing is associated with a reduction in resting metabolic rate that has been attributed to a loss of lean body mass. This reduction in skeletal muscle mass may be responsible for the reduced capacity for shivering thermogenesis on cold exposure in the elderly, an impairment that is exacerbated by pre-existing protein malnutrition. The elderly also have a reduced ability to discriminate differences in environmental temperature, to select thermal comfort and to control heat loss. Aged animals have been shown to have reduced febrile and thermogenic responses to endotoxin. Therefore, it seems likely that the effects of the inhibition of thermoregulation elicited acutely by injury could be exaggerated in the elderly, who have a pre-existing impairment of thermoregulation. The ability to mount a prolonged increase in metabolic rate may also be impaired in the elderly, although the magnitude of the hypermetabolic responses on the first 2–3 days after severe injury are similar in elderly and young patients. As discussed above, an increase in metabolic rate is dependent on increases in cardiac output and tissue oxygen delivery. However, the myocardium of the elderly becomes infiltrated with collagen and they are less able to maintain an increase in cardiac output. Also pulmonary function may be limited in the elderly by a reduction in compliance of the rib cage, loss of muscle from the diaphragm and an impairment of pulmonary gas exchange. Therefore, it is possible that a failure to achieve the goals of increases in cardiac output and tissue oxygen delivery needed to fuel the hypermetabolic flow phase may be one of the reasons why the elderly are more vulnerable to the effects of injury.

The age-related reduction in muscle mass also means that the elderly are less able to accommodate the additional loss of muscle mass associated with injury. For example, a loss of 10–15% muscle mass is well tolerated by a young person who on standing uses only 50% of the maximal voluntary contraction generated by, for example, the quadriceps muscles. In contrast, the elderly may normally require nearly 100% of that maximal voluntary contraction to stand and are, therefore, unable to compensate for any further reduction in muscle function.

Environmental temperature

The recognition of the complex interaction between the level of energy expenditure and environmental temperature during the response to injury has stimulated a number of studies of the effects of raising ambient temperature on that response. Nursing the burned patient with exposed wounds at a high ambient temperature may improve energy balance, although the situation may be different if the burns are covered with occlusive dressings. Increasing environmental temperature reduces urinary nitrogen excretion following injury (e.g. fractured femur or scald) in the rat. Complementary clinical studies have also demonstrated a reduction in urinary nitrogen loss and improvement in nitrogen balance. Although exposure to a high ambient temperature may seem advantageous, enthusiasm should be tempered by the observation that, although blood pressure, acid–base status and core temperature were better maintained in animals placed in a thermoneutral environment immediately after injury, survival was markedly reduced.

Drugs

As discussed above, afferent nociceptive impulses are important initiators of the response to injury. It would, therefore, seem logical that a reduction in this afferent input should reduce and/or modify this response. Indeed, either the injection of local anaesthetics at the site of injury or the production of discrete lesions in the spinal cord abolish the effects of hind-limb ischaemia on cardiovascular and thermoregulatory reflex control in the rat. Regional opiate analgesia attenuates the early metabolic and endocrine responses to surgery, but it is not as effective as regional anaesthesia. The efficacy of regional anaesthesia is determined by the site and severity of surgery; for example, patients subjected to major upper abdominal surgery are more resistant to suppression of the acute stress response than those undergoing hysterectomy. Maintenance of epidural anaesthesia for 24 hours following hysterectomy reduced accumulative nitrogen loss over the next 5 days compared with women operated on under general anaesthesia, although it did not decrease nitrogen excretion after major surgery.

As an increase in sympathoadrenal activity is important in the mediation of many of the responses to injury, it is not surprising that adrenoceptor-blocking agents are able to modify these responses. For example, β-adrenoceptor blockade reduces the increases in both plasma glucose and NEFA concentration after injury. Phentolamine-induced α-adrenoceptor blockade also reduces the hyperglycaemia, but this may be a result of antagonism of adrenergic inhibition of pancreatic insulin secretion, a suggestion supported by the finding of plasma insulin concentrations commensurate with the prevailing hyperglycaemia in acutely injured patients pre-treated with chlorpromazine. Also, as already discussed, combined α- and β-adrenoceptor blockade reduces the hypermetabolism and β-adrenoceptor blockade abolishes the increased activity in the triglyceride–fatty acid cycle associated with burning injury.

Although it is well established that a reduction in the adrenocortical response to injury/sepsis is deleterious both in experimental animals and in humans, there is no

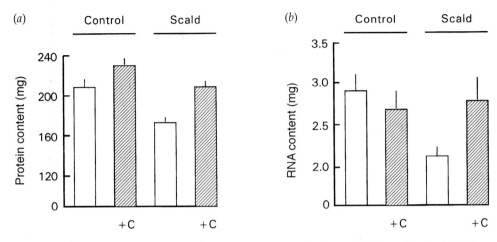

Fig. 16.17. Effect of the α_2-adrenoceptor agonist clenbuterol (12 mg/kg diet), (+C) on gastrocnemius protein (*a*) and RNA (*b*) content in paired control and scalded (+3 days) rats. (From Martineau, L. *et al.* (1993). *Burns*, 19, 26–34.)

evidence that treatment with exogenous steroids is of any benefit, even after head injuries. It is possible that treatment with corticosteroids may, by increasing insulin resistance and the urinary excretion of nitrogen, exacerbate the loss of muscle mass. Indeed a large, well-controlled study has shown that treatment with corticosteroids, even in massive doses, is without benefit and may even be deleterious in certain groups of patients.

It has been known for some time that β-adrenoceptor agonists increase muscle mass in farm animals, and recently a similar effect has been reported in humans. If such agents are also effective after injury and sepsis, and recent evidence suggests that they are (e.g. Fig. 16.17), then they may offer a novel means for the treatment of the skeletal muscle catabolism associated with injury. Anabolic steroids (e.g. stanozol) have also been demonstrated to improve nitrogen balance after surgery for colorectal cancer, although there is a complex interaction with nutritional intake. Growth hormone and insulin-like growth factor have been shown to improve nitrogen balance and protein synthesis in patients with severe burns and after surgery. It has recently been suggested that short-term use of growth hormone may be of most value in the treatment of the aged patient in whom post-traumatic muscle wasting adversely affects morbidity and mortality.

It has to be emphasised that such therapies are not a substitute for but rather an adjunct to nutrition. However, in the absence of such pharmacological agents, the negative nitrogen balance associated with severe injury cannot be prevented even when positive energy balance is achieved. At the moment, it seems that feeding should be started enterally as soon after injury as possible. In some cases, for example after major abdominal injuries, the parenteral route has to be used, but the adverse effects this has on gut function and integrity should not be forgotten. It is the consensus that the severely injured or septic patient requires some 35–40 kcal/kg daily based on a mixture of carbohydrate and fat together with approximately 14 g nitrogen per day. Considerable interest has been expressed in the theoretical advantages of enriching feeding regimens with, for example, branched-chain amino acids, but unfortunately results from clinical studies have been disappointing. Supplementation with the dipeptide alanyl-glutamine increases protein synthesis, reduces negative nitrogen balance and provides a fuel for inflammatory cells and the gut mucosa.

Recently, a number of novel therapies have been introduced for the treatment of sepsis and septic shock, which may be relevant to trauma. First, there are core-directed anti-endotoxin antibodies, which are effective in animal models of endotoxin shock (especially when given as a pre-treatment) but have not yet been shown to be of clinical benefit. It is likely that endotoxin is released early in the response to sepsis and trauma (e.g. from the gut) and has triggered the inflammatory response before the antibody is given. Treatment aimed at endotoxin will, of course, only be effective against Gram-negative infections and have no impact on Gram-positive infections. A more useful approach might be directed against the inflammatory response. A distinction should be made between attenuating the protective local inflammatory reaction and reducing the systemic response. The latter occurs when the ability of endogenous IL-1 receptor antagonists, soluble receptors for TNF and anti-inflammatory cytokines to limit the inflammatory response is overwhelmed. Unfortunately, both IL-1 receptor antagonists and anti-TNF therapies have not improved survival in prospective randomised controlled clinical trials. Indeed, one of the trials using p75-sTNF receptors resulted in a dose-related increase in mortality! One cytokine that might be introduced as a therapy for shock is IL-10, or cytokine synthesis inhibitory factor. This is produced by T_H2 cells and inhibits the production of IL-1, IL-6 and TNF by stimulated human monocytes. Prominent among other possible treatments are (i) a competitive antagonist against bradykinin, which is generated during tissue injury and increases microvascular permeability, activates neutrophils and increases macrophage cytokine production; (ii) inhibitors of nitric oxide synthase (based on the hypothesis that enhanced nitric oxide formation contributes to the hypotension and hyporeactivity to vasoconstrictor agents seen in shock); (iii) selective digestive decontamination (SDD) to reduce the occurrence of primary endogenous infections by both community- and hospital-derived pathogenic microorganisms; and (iv) platelet-activating factor antagonists. Unfortunately, it seems that basic scientific knowledge of the complex medley of responses to injury is still insufficient to develop successful therapeutic interventions.

Summary

From this review of selected aspects of the response to injury, it is suggested that a successful strategy for reducing the toll exacted by injury would be based on the following.

1. Prevention, education and legislation.
2. Rapid transfer to a hospital committed to the treatment of trauma.
3. Resuscitation based on ATLS guidelines to ensure adequacy of cardiac output and tissue oxygen delivery whilst recognising that supranormal values are needed.

4. Pharmacological intervention to reduce nociceptive input to the central nervous system and modulate inflammatory and immune responses (perhaps including anti-endotoxin therapy).

5. Early reduction in the size of a wound (e.g. reduction of fractures, debridement of dead tissues).

6. Initiate antibiotic therapy to reduce primary endogenous infections.

7. Start feeding (using the enteral route if at all possible) with pharmacological support (e.g. growth hormone/factors) and novel substrates (e.g. alanyl-glutamine).

8. Recognition of special problems in groups such as the elderly.

9. Improve rehabilitation.

10. Increase research into the biological responses to trauma.

FURTHER READING

Barton, R.N. (ed.) (1985). Trauma and its metabolic problems. *British Medical Bulletin*, 41.

Barton, R.N. (1987). The neuroendocrinology of physical injury. *Ballière's Clinical Endocrinology and Metabolism*, 1, 355–374.

Barton, R.N., Frayn, K.N. & Little, R.A (1990). Trauma, burns and surgery. In *The Metabolic and Molecular Basis of Acquired Disease*, vol. 1, (ed.) R.D. Cohen, B. Lewis, K.G.M.M. Alberti, & A.M. Denman, pp. 684–717. Baillière Tindall.

Frayn, K.N. (1986). Hormonal control of metabolism in trauma and sepsis. *Clinical Endocrinology*, 14, 577–599.

Horan, M.H. *et al.* (1992). Injury responses in old age. In *Oxford Textbook of Geriatric Medicine*, (ed.) J.G. Evans, & T.F.C. Williams, pp. 88-93. Oxford: Oxford University Press.

Kinney, J.M. & Tucker, H.N. (ed.) (1994). *Organ Metabolism and Nutrition: Ideas for Future Critical Care*. New York: Raven Press.

Kirk, R.M., Mansfield, A. & Cochrane, J. (ed.) (1993). *Clinical Surgery in General: RCS Course Manual*. Edinburgh: Churchill Livingstone.

Schlag, G. & Redl, H. (1993). *Pathophysiology of Shock, Sepsis and Organ Failure*. Berlin: Springer Verlag.

Secher, N., Pawelczyk, J. & Ludbrook, J. (ed.) (1994). *Blood Loss and Shock*. London: Edward Arnold.

INDEX

abl oncogene 34, 37
acanthosis nigricans 230
acetaldehyde
  as hapten 399
  complement activation 402
  metabolism of 395
  toxicity of 400–1
acetaldehyde dehydrogenase (ALDH) 392, 395
  isozymes of 397–8
acetoacetate 206
acetyl coenzyme A 206–7
acetylator status 385
acquired immunodeficiency syndrome (AIDS)
    186–7, 384
acromegaly 34
activating transcription factors (ATFs) 31
activation domains 17
activator protein-1 (AP-1) 17, 30, 31, 32
acute myelogenous leukaemia 90
acute myocardial infarction 255
  atherosclerotic plaque rupture and 251–2
  see also heart failure
Addison's disease 450
adenomas 339–41, 342
  adenomatous polyposis coli 329, 343
  familial adenomatous polyposis (FAP) 341–7
adenovirus 155
  as vector 91
adenylate cyclase 27, 30, 273
  constitutive activation 33, 54
adhesion molecules 100, 141–4, 145
  adhesins 170
  asthma and 157–8
  leucocyte adhesion molecule (LAM-1) 197
  role in alcoholic liver disease 402–3
  selectins 141–2, 144, 158, 197, 402
  see also intercellular adhesion molecules; vascular
    cell adhesion molecule-1
adrenaline
  in diabetic ketoacidosis 222
  in heart failure 273
  trauma response 462, 463, 467, 488
adrenocorticotrophic hormone (ACTH) 462

adult respiratory distress syndrome (ARDS) 190,
    193
advanced glycosylation end-products (AGE) 241
adverse drug reactions, *see* drug toxicity
aflatoxin 163
age
  as risk factor for Alzheimer's disease 295
  drug toxicity and 380
  trauma response and 489–90
AIDS (acquired immunodeficiency syndrome)
    186–7
alanine aminotransferase (ALT) 405
albumin 438–41
alcohol dehydrogenase (ADH) 392–4
  isoenzymes of 396–7
alcohol toxicity 389–411
  alcohol metabolism 392–5
  clinical aspects 403–10
    history 403–4
    investigations 404–6
    liver lesions 406–10
    treatment 410
  epidemiology 390
  extrahepatic manifestations 391
  fibrosis and 403
  genetic factors in ethanol metabolism 396–8
  immunological factors 402–3
  metabolic toxicity 399–402
    acetaldehyde 400–1
    acetaldehyde adducts 402
    ethanol 399–400
    ethanol as enzyme inducer 401–2
  mortality 390, 391
  treatment 410
  see also liver
aldehyde dehydrogenase 395
aldose reductase 241–2
alleles 14, 64
  frequency of 68
allergens 134–5
  see also haptens
allergy 129–35
  adhesion molecules and 141–4